6

SIXTH EDITION

Ignatavicius • Workman

Medical-Surgical Nursing

Patient-Centered Collaborative Care

Chris Winkelman, RN, PhD, CCRN, ACNP
Assistant Professor
Frances Payne Bolton School of Nursing
Case Western Reserve University;
Clinical Nurse
Trauma/Critical Care Float Pool
MetroHealth Medical Center
Cleveland, Ohio

M. Linda Workman, PhD, RN, FAAN
Senior Volunteer Faculty
College of Nursing
University of Cincinnati
Cincinnati, Ohio;
Formerly Gertrude Perkins Oliva Professor
    of Oncology
Frances Payne Bolton School of Nursing
Case Western Reserve University
Cleveland, Ohio

Kathy A. Hausman, PhD, RN
Chair of Nursing and Allied Health
Baltimore City Community College
Baltimore, Maryland

SAUNDERS

ELSEVIER

SAUNDERS
ELSEVIER

11830 Westline Industrial Drive
St. Louis, Missouri 63146

ISBN: 978-1-4160-5189-3

Notice

Knowledge and best practice in this field are constantly changing. As new research and experience broaden our knowledge, changes in practice, treatment and drug therapy may become necessary or appropriate. Readers are advised to check the most current information provided (i) on procedures featured or (ii) by the manufacturer of each product to be administered, to verify the recommended dose or formula, the method and duration of administration, and contraindications. It is the responsibility of the practitioner, relying on their own experience and knowledge of the patient, to make diagnoses, to determine dosages and the best treatment for each individual patient, and to take all appropriate safety precautions. To the fullest extent of the law, neither the Publisher nor the Authors assumes any liability for any injury and/or damage to persons or property arising out of or related to any use of the material contained in this book.

The Publisher

Previous editions copyrighted 2006, 2002

Senior Editor: Lee Henderson
Developmental Editor: Julie Eisen
Publishing Services Manager: Deborah Vogel
Project Manager: Brandilyn Tidwell
Designer: Margaret Reid

Working together to grow
libraries in developing countries
www.elsevier.com | www.bookaid.org | www.sabre.org

ELSEVIER | BOOK AID International | Sabre Foundation

Printed in Canada

Last digit is the print number: 9 8 7 6 5 4 3 2 1

This new edition of the *Clinical Companion* for *Medical-Surgical Nursing: Patient-Centered Collaborative Care* is a succinct reference to conditions and interventions seen in the acute care setting. We've added new content, revised each section, and updated each page. Look for these clinical pearls throughout the text: Critical Rescue 🔲 gives cues to engage in an activity or intervention that promotes optimal outcomes; Clinical Landmine 🖐 signals actions to avoid or indications for additional surveillance and intervention; and National Patient Safety Guideline ▽ indicates application of information from The Joint Commission to promote safe, effective care (*www.jointcommission.org*). Considerations for older adults, people of specific ethnicities, and women have been retained and updated to reflect current research and practice.

Part 1, renamed Concepts of Medical-Surgical Nursing, covers common clinical conditions, providing an overview of the physiology, pathophysiology, and collaborative management using the nursing process to integrate assessment, diagnostic testing, interventions, and evaluation of patient responses. New content on cancer, infection, inflammation, and immunity summarize key concepts for bedside clinicians.

Part 2 also has new content reflecting current trends in admission diagnoses. This section continues to feature a brief, prioritized snapshot of the diseases and disorders. Designed to be a reference for nurses in a variety of settings delivering acute care to adults, the *Clinical Companion* stands alone. But for the reader who desires more information, we recommend Ignatavicius and Workman's *Medical-Surgical Nursing: Patient-Centered Collaborative Care*, 6th edition.

There are now 11 appendixes designed as quick capsules of concentrated knowledge. The appendixes include four common situations (head-to-toe assessment, normal lab values, discharge planning, and sources for additional information) and five less typical situations (electrocardiogram interpretation, care for a patient with chest tubes and mechanical ventilation, environmental and bioterrorism emergencies, and vocabulary for Spanish-speaking patients) that need quick responses. Medical-surgical nursing is both the most and least specialized practice in the acute care setting; we tried to balance general and specialty knowledge in a book that can be carried with you in a variety of medical-surgical settings.

Let us know if we left out important information you need to practice at the bedside; we are already making plans for the 7th edition.

ACKNOWLEDGMENTS

We want to acknowledge the insight and skillful assistance of Lee Henderson, Julie Eisen, and Brandi Tidwell from Elsevier—their insight, persistence, and good humor have made this edition clean, crisp, and user-friendly.

—CW and MLW

I've been mentored by awesome clinicians, dedicated educators, and insightful researchers—nurses all. Thanks especially to my co-author, Linda Workman. I am always grateful for my family: Craig, Alli, Sam, and Leah.

—CW

I would like to acknowledge students everywhere whose enthusiasm keeps me going.

—MLW

CONTENTS

APPENDIXES

PART ONE

CONCEPTS OF MEDICAL-SURGICAL NURSING

CANCER PATHOPHYSIOLOGY

OVERVIEW

- *Neoplasia* is any new or continued cell growth not needed for normal development or replacement of dead and damaged tissues. This new growth may be benign or cancerous.
- *Benign tumor cells* are normal cells growing in the wrong place or at the wrong time. They are not needed for normal growth and development. Although benign tumors do not invade other tissues, depending on their location, they can damage normal tissue and may need to be removed.
- *Cancer cells*, also called *malignant cells*, are abnormal, serve no useful function, and are harmful to normal body tissues. Without treatment, cancer leads to death.
- Cancer can develop in any tissue or organ but tends to occur more commonly in tissues that continue to grow by cell division (mitosis) throughout the life span.
- All cancers start from normal cells that undergo changes at the gene level. These changes result in a loss of control over cell growth.
- *Carcinogenesis* and *oncogenesis* are additional names for cancer development.
- *Malignant transformation* is the process of changing a normal cell into a cancer cell.
- *Carcinogens* are substances that can damage normal cell DNA and activate genes that allow a normal cell to become a cancer cell. Carcinogens may be chemicals, physical agents, or viruses.
- Biologic features of cancer cells and malignant tumors are:
  1. Poorly controlled or continuous cell division
  2. No response to normal cellular signals for programmed cell death (i.e., apoptosis)
  3. An anaplastic appearance, the loss of the specific appearance of their parent cells, and becoming small and round
  4. A large nuclear-cytoplasmic ratio
  5. Loss of specific functions
  6. Loose adherence to each other
  7. Ability to migrate throughout the body

8. Invasion and destruction of normal tissues
9. Abnormal chromosomes (aneuploidy)

- A *primary tumor* is the original tumor, identified by the normal tissue from which it arose.
- When primary tumors are located in vital organs, such as the brain or lungs, they can grow excessively and lethally damage the vital organ or crowd out healthy organ tissue and interfere with that organ's ability to perform its vital function.
- A *metastatic tumor* is one that has spread from the original site, usually through the blood, into other tissues and organs, where it can establish metastatic or secondary tumors that grow and cause more damage and dysfunction.
  1. When a metastatic tumor is in another organ, it is still a cancer from the original altered tissue.
  2. For example, when breast cancer spreads to the lung and the bone, it is breast cancer in the lung and bone, not lung cancer and not bone cancer.

CARCINOGENESIS/ONCOGENESIS

- The process of carcinogenesis or oncogenesis occurs through the steps of initiation, promotion, progression, and metastasis.
  1. *Initiation* is damage to genes controlling cell division, resulting in the activation and overexpression of oncogenes, beginning the change of a normal cell into a cancer cell. After initiation, a cell can become a cancer cell if the cellular changes that occurred during initiation continue and cell division is not impaired. *If growth conditions are right, widespread metastatic disease can develop from just one cancer cell.*
  2. *Promotion* is the enhancement of growth of an initiated cell. Many normal hormones and body proteins, such as insulin and estrogen, can act as promoters and make initiated cells divide more frequently.
  3. *Progression* is the continued change of a cancer, making it more malignant over time. Particular changes include the development of a separate blood supply and changes that provide the cancer cells with advantages that allow them to live and divide no matter how the conditions around them change. These changes allow cancer cells to become more malignant and have fewer normal cell features.
  4. *Metastasis* is the spread of a tumor into nearby or remote tissue areas by invasion.
- Cancers are classified by the type of tissue from which they arise. For example, glandular cancers are carcinomas, and connective tissue cancers are sarcomas.

- About 100 different types of cancer arise from various tissues or organs.
- Solid tumors develop from specific tissues (e.g., breast cancer, lung cancer). Hematologic cancers (e.g., leukemias, lymphomas) arise from blood cell–forming tissues and lymphatic tissues.
- Systems of cancer grading and staging are used to standardize cancer diagnosis, prognosis, and treatment.
- *Grading* of a tumor classifies cellular aspects of the cancer and ranks cancers for degree of malignancy on the basis of cancer cell appearance, growth rates, and aggressiveness compared with the normal tissues from which they arose. *Low-grade* cancers have fewer malignant features; *high-grade* cancers have more malignant features.
- Tumor *ploidy* classifies tumor chromosomes as normal or abnormal. When cancer cell chromosomes are abnormal, they are called *aneuploid*. The degree of aneuploidy usually increases with the degree of malignancy.
- *Staging* classifies clinical aspects of the cancer. It determines the exact location of the cancer and its degree of metastasis at diagnosis, and it influences selection of therapy.
  1. *Clinical staging* assesses the patient's clinical manifestations and evaluates clinical signs for tumor size and possible spread.
  2. *Surgical staging* assesses the tumor size, number, sites, and spread by inspection at surgery.
  3. *Pathologic staging* is the most definitive type, determining the tumor size, number, sites, and spread by pathologic examination of tissues obtained at surgery.

CANCER ETIOLOGY AND GENETIC RISK

- Carcinogenesis takes years and depends on several tumor and patient factors.
- Three interacting factors influence cancer development: exposure to carcinogens, genetic predisposition, and immune function.
- *Oncogene activation* with overexpression is the main mechanism of carcinogenesis regardless of the specific cause.
- When a normal cell is exposed to any carcinogen (initiator), the normal cell's suppressor genes (which control cell growth and prevent oncogene overexpression) can be damaged or mutated. As a result, the oncogenes are overexpressed and can cause the cells to change from normal cells to cancer cells.
- Both external and personal factors can activate oncogenes and lead to cancer development.

- External factors causing cancer include:
  1. Exposure to chemical carcinogens, such as many known chemicals, tobacco, drugs, and other products used in everyday life
  2. Exposure to physical carcinogens, such as radiation and chronic irritation
  3. Exposure to carcinogenic viruses, such as certain strains of the human papillomavirus (HPV)
  4. Possible dietary factors, such as low fiber intake, high intake of red meat, and high animal fat intake. Preservatives, contaminants, preparation methods, and additives (e.g., dyes, flavorings, sweeteners) also may have cancer-promoting effects.
- Personal factors in cancer development include:
  1. Immune function, with decreased immune function increasing cancer risk
  2. Advancing age, the single most important risk factor for cancer
  3. Genetic predisposition, resulting from the inheritance of specific gene mutations

Genetic Considerations

- Genetic risk for cancer occurs in a small percent of the population; however, people who have a genetic predisposition are at very high risk for cancer development, and these predispositions can be passed from generation to generation.
- The development of cancer depends on more than just the presence of oncogenes. The oncogene must be overexpressed for cancer to occur. In some people, the sequence of a specific oncogene is different (has been mutated), which may allow it to be activated more easily. In other people, the oncogene is normal, but the gene controlling oncogene activity, the *suppressor gene*, is mutated and allows overexpression of one or more oncogenes, leading to a huge increase in cancer risk.
- Patterns of genetic risk for cancer have been identified, including inherited predisposition for specific cancers, inherited conditions associated with cancer, familial clustering, and chromosomal aberrations.

Cultural Awareness

- The incidence of cancer varies among races. African Americans have a higher incidence of cancer than white Americans do, and the death rate is higher for African Americans.
- Cancer sites and cancer-related mortality also vary along racial lines. One explanation for this difference is that more African

Americans have less access to health care. They are more often diagnosed with later stage cancer that is more difficult to cure or control. However, this disparity in health care access does not explain all differences.

DISEASE-RELATED CONSEQUENCES OF CANCER

- Reduced immunity and blood-producing functions
  1. Occur most often in patients with leukemia and lymphoma but can occur with any cancer that invades the bone marrow
  2. Increase patient risk for infection, anemia, and bleeding
  3. Cause patient weakness and fatigue
- Altered GI structure and function
  1. Obstruction or compression of structures anywhere along the GI tract
  2. Reduced ability to absorb nutrients and eliminate wastes
  3. Increased metabolic rate and increased need for protein, carbohydrates, and fat
  4. Metastasis to liver, leading to malnutrition and death
  5. Change in taste sensation
  6. Anorexia
  7. Cachexia (extreme body wasting and malnutrition) from an imbalance between food intake and energy use
- Motor and sensory deficits
  1. Bone pain and fractures
  2. Hypercalcemia
  3. Reduced mobility
  4. Compression of nerves leading to sensory changes
  5. Brain metastasis with loss of motor function, sensory function, and cognition
  6. Pain
- Decreased respiratory function
  1. Airway obstruction
  2. If lung tissue is involved, decreased lung capacity
  3. Pulmonary edema and dyspnea
  4. Thickened alveolar membrane leading to reduced gas exchange
  5. Development of pulmonary effusion and pneumothorax
  6. Hypoxia and poor tissue oxygenation
- Death

CANCER TREATMENT ISSUES

- The purpose of cancer treatment is to prolong survival time or improve quality of life.

- Therapies for cancer include surgery, radiation therapy, chemotherapy, hormonal manipulation, photodynamic therapy, immunotherapy, gene therapy, and targeted therapy.
- Various therapies may be used separately or, more commonly, in combination to kill cancer cells.
- The types and amount of therapy used depend on the specific type of cancer, whether the cancer has spread, and the health of the patient.

CANCER SURGERY

OVERVIEW

- Surgery for cancer involves the removal of diseased tissue and may be used for prophylaxis, diagnosis, cure, control, palliation, determination of therapy effectiveness, and reconstruction.
  1. *Prophylactic surgery* is the removal of at-risk tissue to prevent cancer development and is performed when a patient has an existing *premalignant* condition or a known family history that strongly predisposes the person to the development of a specific cancer.
  2. *Diagnostic surgery* (biopsy) is the removal of all or part of a suspected lesion for examination and testing. It provides proof of the presence of cancer.
  3. *Curative surgery* is focused on removal of *all* cancer tissue and alone can result in a cure rate of 27% to 30% when all visible and microscopic tumor is removed or destroyed.
  4. Cancer control, or *cytoreductive surgery*, is the removal of part of the tumor and leaving a known amount of gross tumor. It is also known as *debulking surgery*, and it does not alone result in a cure.
  5. *Palliative surgery* is focused on improving the quality of life during the survival time and is not focused on cure.
  6. *Second-look surgery* is used for a re-diagnosis after treatment. The results of this surgery are used to determine whether a specific therapy should be continued or discontinued.
  7. *Reconstructive or rehabilitative surgery* increases function or enhances appearance, or both.

PATIENT-CENTERED COLLABORATIVE CARE

- Care usually involves the loss of a specific body part or its function. The amount of function lost and how much the loss affects patients depend on the location and extent of the surgery.
- Some cancer surgery results in major scarring or disfigurement.
- The physical nursing care needs of the patient having surgery for cancer are similar to those related to surgery for other reasons.

- Two additional priority care needs are psychosocial support and assisting the patient to achieve or maintain maximum function.
  1. Assess the patient's and family's ability to cope with the uncertainty of cancer and its treatment and with the changes in body image and role.
  2. Coordinate with the health care team to provide support for the patient and family.
  3. Encourage the patient and family to express their feelings and concerns.
  4. Encourage the patient to look at the surgical site, touch it, and participate in any dressing changes or incisional care required.
  5. Provide information about support groups such as those sponsored by the American Cancer Society or specialty cancer organizations.
  6. Discuss with the patient the idea of having a person who has coped with the same issues come for a visit.
  7. Teach the patient about the importance of performing and progressing the intensity of any prescribed exercises to regain as much function as possible and prevent complications.
  8. Coordinate with the physical therapist, occupational therapist, and family members to plan strategies individualized to each patient to regain or maintain optimal function.

RADIATION THERAPY

OVERVIEW

- The purpose of radiation therapy for cancer is to destroy cancer cells with minimal exposure of the normal cells to the damaging actions of radiation.
- Because the effects of radiation are seen only in the tissues in the path of the radiation beam, this type of therapy is a *local* treatment.
- Radiation doses used vary according to the size, location, and radiation sensitivity of the tumor and surrounding normal tissues.
- Radiation therapy is classified in two categories:
  1. *Teletherapy*: The radiation source is external to the patient and remote from the tumor site. It is also called *external beam radiation. Because the source is external, the patient is not radioactive and is not a hazard to others.* This type of therapy usually is given as a series of divided doses.
  2. *Brachytherapy*: The radiation source comes into direct, continuous contact with the tumor tissues for a specific period of time. It is delivered in a solid, sealed form or unsealed within

body fluids. *With all types of brachytherapy, the patient emits radiation for a period of time and is a hazard to others.*

- Side effects of radiation therapy are limited to the tissues exposed to the radiation and vary according to the site. Skin changes and hair loss are local but are likely to be permanent. Other common side effects include altered taste sensations and severe fatigue.
- Radiation damage to normal tissues during cancer therapy can start the inflammatory responses that cause tissue fibrosis and scarring. These effects may not be apparent for many years after radiation treatment.

PATIENT-CENTERED COLLABORATIVE CARE

- For teletherapy, teach patients to:
    1. Wash the irradiated area gently each day with water or with a mild soap and water.
    2. Use the hand rather than a washcloth to be gentler.
    3. Rinse soap thoroughly from the skin.
    4. Not remove any ink or dye markings that indicate exactly where the beam of radiation is to be focused.
    5. Dry the irradiated area with patting motions rather than rubbing motions; use a clean, soft towel or cloth.
    6. Use no powders, ointments, lotions, or creams on the skin at the radiation site unless they are prescribed by the *radiologist* or the radiation therapy advanced practice nurse.
    7. Wear soft clothing over the skin at the radiation site.
    8. Avoid wearing belts, buckles, straps, or any type of clothing that binds or rubs the skin at the radiation site.
    9. Avoid exposure of the irradiated area to the sun.
        a. Protect this area by wearing clothing over it but *not* by applying sunscreening agents.
        b. Avoid going outdoors between 10:00 AM and 4:00 PM to avoid the more intense sunrays.
        c. Use awnings, umbrellas, and other forms of shade when outdoors during the times when the sunrays are most intense.
    10. Avoid heat exposure.
- For patients receiving brachytherapy:
    1. Assign the patient to a private room with a private bath.
    2. Place a "Caution: Radioactive Material" sign on the door of the patient's room.
    3. If portable lead shields are used, place them between the patient and the door.
    4. Keep the door to the patient's room closed as much as possible.

5. Wear a dosimeter film badge at all times while caring for patients with radioactive implants. Each badge should be used only by one individual.
6. Wear a lead apron while providing care. Always keep the front of the apron facing the source of radiation (do not turn your back toward the patient).
7. Pregnant nurses should not care for these patients; do not allow pregnant women or children younger than 16 years to visit.
8. Limit each visitor to one-half hour per day. Be sure visitors are at least 6 feet from the source.
9. Never touch the radioactive source with bare hands. In the rare instance that it is dislodged, use a long-handled forceps to retrieve it. Deposit the radioactive source in the lead container kept in the patient's room.
10. Save all dressings and bed linens until after the radioactive source is removed.

CHEMOTHERAPY

OVERVIEW

- Chemotherapy is the treatment of cancer with chemical agents. It is used to cure and to increase survival time because it has some selectivity for killing cancer cells over normal cells.
- The tumors most sensitive to chemotherapy are those that have rapid growth.
- Its effects are systemic, providing the opportunity to kill metastatic cancer cells that may have escaped local treatment.
- Drugs used for chemotherapy usually are given systemically and exert their cell-damaging (cytotoxic) effects against healthy cells and cancer cells.
- The normal cells most affected by chemotherapy are those that divide rapidly, including skin, hair, intestinal tissues, spermatocytes, and blood-forming cells.
- Chemotherapy drugs are classified by the specific types of action they exert in the cancer cell and include antimetabolites, antitumor antibiotics, antimitotic agents, alkylating agents, topoisomerase inhibitors, and miscellaneous agents.
- Successful cancer chemotherapy most often involves giving more than one anticancer drug in a timed manner, known as *combination chemotherapy.*
- Drugs are selected based on known tumor sensitivity to the drugs and the degree of side effects expected.
- Dosages for most chemotherapy drugs are calculated according to the type of cancer and the patient's size, usually based on

milligrams per square meter of total body surface area or on weight in kilograms.

- Although most chemotherapy drugs are given IV, they may also be given by the oral, intra-arterial, isolated limb perfusion, intracavitary, and intrathecal routes.

- Administration of IV chemotherapy is usually performed by a registered nurse who has completed an approved chemotherapy course.

- Extravasation or infiltration is a serious complication of IV chemotherapy administration that can lead to:
  1. Pain
  2. Infection
  3. Tissue loss

- The most important nursing intervention for extravasation is prevention by close monitoring of the access site during chemotherapy administration.

- Immediate treatment of extravasation depends on the specific drug. Coordinate with the oncologist and pharmacist to determine the type of compress and specific antidote needed for the extravasated drug.

- Perform and document the following activities for an extravasation event:
  1. Date and time when extravasation was suspected or identified
  2. Date and time when the infusion was started
  3. Time when the infusion was stopped
  4. The exact contents of the infusion fluid and the volume of fluid infused
  5. The estimated amount of fluid extravasated
  6. Diagram the exact insertion site, and indicate whether this is a venous access device, implanted port, or a tunneled catheter.
  7. The method of administration (e.g., pump, controller; rate of infusion)
  8. The needle type and size
  9. Indicate on the diagram the location and number of venipuncture attempts.
  10. Record the time between the extravasation and the last fully documented blood return.
  11. Identify all agents administered in the previous 24 hours through this site (list agent administered, dosage and volume, and order of administration).
  12. Take and record the patient's vital signs.
  13. Ask and record the patient's subjective sensations and symptoms.
  14. Record all observations of the site, including size, color, and texture.

15. Take a photograph of the site.
16. Document the administration of neutralizing or antidote agents.
17. Document the application of compresses and their temperature.
18. Document other nursing interventions.
19. Record the patient's responses to nursing interventions.
20. Document notification of the prescribing physician (including the time).
21. Document the written and oral instructions given to the patient about follow-up care.
22. Document any consultation request.
23. Sign the documentation.

- Nurses and other health care workers who prepare or give these drugs or who handle the excreta from patients within 48 hours of receiving IV chemotherapy must use extreme caution and wear personal protective equipment (PPE), including eye protection, masks, double gloves, and gown.
- Side effects of chemotherapy often include bone marrow suppression (e.g., neutropenia, anemia, thrombocytopenia), nausea and vomiting, mucositis, alopecia, changes in cognitive function, and peripheral neuropathy.

PATIENT-CENTERED COLLABORATIVE CARE

- For patients with neutropenia:
  1. Administer biological response modifiers as prescribed.
  2. Assess the skin and mucous membranes, lung sounds, mouth, and venous access device insertion sites every 8 hours.
  3. Urge the patient to report any indicator of infection, such as a change in skin and mucous membranes (e.g., pimple, sore, rash, open area), presence of a cough, burning on urination, pain around the venous access site, or new drainage from any location.
  4. Use good handwashing before contact with the patient.
  5. Use aseptic technique when performing any invasive procedure.
  6. Ensure that mouth care and washing of the axillary and peri-anal regions is performed at least every 12 hours.
  7. Monitor for manifestations of infection.

> ⬛ **Critical Rescue** ◆ The patient with neutropenia often does not develop a high fever or have purulent drainage, even when a severe infection is present. Any elevation of temperature in a patient with neutropenia is significant and is considered a sign of infection, and it should be reported to the health care provider immediately.

8. Initiate standard protocols regarding obtaining cultures, tests, and administering antibiotics for suspected infection in neutropenic patients according to institution policy.
9. Teach patients and family members precautions to reduce the risk for infection.

- For patients with anemia:
    1. Administer biological response modifiers as prescribed.
    2. Assess for tachycardia and increased respiratory rate.
    3. Encourage the patient to rest.
    4. In collaboration with other members of the health care team, postpone or cancel activities that do not have a direct impact on the health of the patient.

- For patients with thrombocytopenia, provide a safe hospital environment by:
    1. Handling the patient gently
    2. Using and teaching unlicensed assistive personnel (UAP) to use a lift sheet when moving and positioning the patient in bed
    3. Avoiding IM injections and venipunctures
    4. Applying firm pressure to needle stick sites for 10 minutes
    5. Testing all urine and stool for the presence of occult blood
    6. Observing IV sites every 4 hours for bleeding
    7. Avoiding rectal temperatures, even on unconscious patients
    8. Administering prescribed suppositories carefully with liberal lubrication
    9. Instructing the patient and UAP to use an electric shaver rather than a razor
    10. When providing mouth care or supervising others in providing mouth care, instruct about:
        a. Using a soft-bristled toothbrush or tooth sponges
        b. Not using floss
        c. Checking to ensure that dentures fit and do not rub

- For patients with chemotherapy-induced nausea and vomiting (CIN):
    1. Administer prescribed antiemetics on a scheduled, rather than PRN, basis.
    2. Ensure that premedication with antiemetics occurs before each session of IV chemotherapy.
    3. Assess patients for dehydration and electrolyte imbalances.
    4. Teach patients to continue the therapy as prescribed, even when the nausea and vomiting appear controlled.

Considerations for Older Adults

- Sometimes, older patients have received lower doses of chemotherapy drugs because it was thought the older person would not be able to tolerate the side effects of nausea and vomiting.

- The older adult can become dehydrated more quickly if CIN is not adequately controlled. Teach older adult patients to be proactive with taking their prescribed antiemetics and to contact their health care provider if the CIN does not resolve within 12 hours or becomes worse.
- For patients with mucositis:
  1. Examine the patient's mouth, including the roof, under the tongue, and between the teeth and cheek, every 4 hours.
  2. Document the location, size, and character of fissures, blisters, sores, or drainage.
  3. Brush the teeth and tongue with a soft-bristled brush or sponges every 8 hours.
  4. Rinse the mouth with a solution of one-half peroxide and one-half normal saline every 12 hours. (Rinsing with lukewarm water can be done as often as the patient desires.)
  5. Avoid the use of alcohol or glycerin-based mouthwashes.
  6. Encourage the patient to drink 3 or more liters of water per day, if another health problem does not require limiting fluid intake.
  7. Administer antimicrobial and topical analgesic drugs as prescribed.
  8. Assist the patient in using *artificial saliva* as needed, if prescribed.
  9. Urge the patient to avoid using tobacco or drinking alcoholic beverages.
  10. Assist the patient in menu choices to avoid spicy, salty, acidic, dry, rough, or hard food.
  11. Suggest that dentures be worn only during meals.
  12. Offer complete mouth care before and after every meal.
- For patients with alopecia:
  1. Reassure patients that hair loss is temporary and that hair regrowth usually begins about 1 month after completion of chemotherapy.
  2. Inform the patient that the new hair may differ from the original hair in color, texture, and thickness.
  3. Teach the patient to protect the scalp from injury by avoiding direct sunlight on the scalp by using hats or other head coverings.
  4. Teach the patient to wear some head covering underneath helmets, headphones, headsets, and other items that rub the head.
  5. Assist patients in selecting a type of head covering (e.g., wigs, scarves, turbans, caps, hats) that suits their income and lifestyle.

- For patients with changes in cognitive function:
    1. Support the patient who reports this side effect. Listen to the patient's concerns and tell him or her that other patients have also reported such problems.
    2. Warn patients against participating in other behaviors that could alter cognitive functioning, such as excessive alcohol intake, recreational drug use, and taking part in activities that increase the risk for head injury.
- For patients with peripheral neuropathy, teach patients to prevent injury by:
    1. Not walking around in bare feet or stocking feet
    2. Always wearing shoes with a protective sole
    3. Making sure shoes are long enough and wide enough to prevent creating sores or blisters (avoid pointed-toe shoes and high heels)
    4. Providing a long break-in period for new shoes; not wearing new shoes for longer than 2 hours at a time
    5. Inspecting feet daily (with a mirror) for open areas or redness
    6. Avoiding extremes of temperature; wearing warm clothing in the winter, especially over hands, feet, and ears
    7. Testing water temperature with a thermometer when washing dishes or bathing and using warm water rather than hot water (less than 110° F)
    8. Setting hot water heater temperature at or below 110° F
    9. Using potholders when cooking
    10. Using gloves when washing dishes or gardening
    11. Not eating foods that are "steaming hot"
    12. Getting up from a lying or sitting position slowly
    13. Looking at the feet and the floor or ground when walking to assess how the ground, floor, or step changes
    14. Not using area rugs, especially those that slide easily
    15. Using handrails when going up or down steps

HORMONAL MANIPULATION

- Hormonal manipulation can help control some types of cancer by decreasing the amount of hormones reaching hormone-sensitive tumors.
- Some drugs are hormone antagonists that compete with natural hormones at the tumor's receptor sites, preventing a needed hormone from binding to the receptor.
- Hormone inhibitors suppress the production of specific hormones in the normal hormone-producing organs.
- Androgens and the antiestrogen receptor drugs cause masculinizing effects in women, with increased chest and facial hair,

interruption of the menstrual period, and shrinkage of breast tissue.

- Other effects for men and women receiving androgens include acne, fluid retention, hypercalcemia, deep vein thrombosis, and liver dysfunction (with prolonged therapy).
- Feminine manifestations often appear in men who take estrogens, progestins, or antiandrogen receptor drugs, including thinning facial hair, smoother skin, and gynecomastia. Testicular and penile atrophy also occurs to some degree.

PHOTODYNAMIC THERAPY

OVERVIEW

- Photodynamic therapy (PDT) is the selective destruction of cancer cells through a chemical reaction triggered by different types of laser light.
- It is most commonly used for non-melanoma skin cancers, ocular tumors, GI tumors, and lung cancers located in the airways.
- An agent that sensitizes cells to light is injected IV along with a dye. These drugs enter all cells but leave normal cells more rapidly than cancer cells. Usually, within 48 to 72 hours, most of the drug has collected in high concentrations in cancer cells. At this time, a laser light is focused on the tumor. The light activates a chemical reaction within those cells retaining the sensitizing drug that induces irreversible cell damage.

PATIENT-CENTERED COLLABORATIVE CARE

- The patient has general sensitivity to light for up to 12 weeks after the photosensitizing drug is injected.
- The most intense period of light sensitivity is after injection and before the laser treatment. During this time, the patient is at high risk for sunburn and eye pain.
- Before photosensitizing therapy, teach the patient to:
  1. Bring protective clothing (e.g., shirts with long sleeves and high collars, long pants or skirt, gloves, socks, wide-brimmed hat) and UV-protective sunglasses when he or she comes to be injected with the photosensitizing agent.
  2. If possible, have someone else drive the patient home so that he or she can be covered with a sheet or light blanket.
  3. Plan to avoid leaving home during daylight hours for anywhere from 1 to 3 months.
  4. Cover all windows with light-blocking shades or heavy drapes or curtains.
  5. Replace high-wattage light bulbs with lower-wattage ones, and use as few as possible.

- After photosensitizing therapy, teach the patient to:
  1. Continue to wear all protective clothing, avoid sunlight in any form, and high wattage indoor lights.
  2. Drink plenty of water to prevent becoming dehydrated.
  3. Do not take any newly prescribed or over-the-counter (OTC) drugs without contacting the physician who performed the PDT. Some drugs make the light sensitivity even worse; others interact with the photosensitizing drug.
  4. When starting re-exposure to sunlight and other bright lights, do so slowly. Start out exposing only about 1 inch of skin to sunlight at a time. Start out with 10 minutes, and increase the time by about 5 minutes each day.
  5. Remember that sunscreen cannot prevent severe sunburn during this time.
  6. If pain or blistering occurs, notify the PDT health care team.
  7. Continue to wear dark glasses, even indoors, until eye pain no longer occurs when in a normally lighted environment.
  8. After 3 months, see an ophthalmologist to check for retinal damage.

IMMUNOTHERAPY: BIOLOGICAL RESPONSE MODIFIERS

OVERVIEW

- Biological response modifiers (BRMs) modify the patient's biologic responses to tumor cells, and those in use for cancer therapy are *cytokines*, which are small protein hormones made by WBCs.
- Cytokines made by macrophages, neutrophils, eosinophils, and monocytes are *monokines*; cytokines produced by lymphocytes (especially the T-lymphocytes) are *lymphokines*.
- Cytokines for cancer therapy generally enhance the immune system and can:
  1. Stimulate the immune system to recognize cancer cells and take actions to eliminate or destroy them.
  2. Serve a supporting role by stimulating faster recovery of bone marrow function after treatment-induced suppression.
- Two common types of BRMs used as cancer therapy are:
  1. *Interleukins* (ILs), which help different immune system cells recognize and destroy abnormal body cells. In particular, IL-1, -2, and -6 appear to "charge up" the immune system and enhance attacks on cancer cells by macrophages, natural killer (NK) cells, and tumor-infiltrating lymphocytes.

2. *Interferons* (IFNs), which can:
   a. Slow tumor cell division.
   b. Stimulate the growth and activation of NK cells.
   c. Help cancer cells resume a more normal appearance and function.
   d. Inhibit the expression of oncogenes.

PATIENT-CENTERED COLLABORATIVE CARE

- Side effects of interleukins include manifestations of inflammatory reactions:
  1. Widespread edema
  2. Chills, fever
  3. Rigors (severe shaking with chills)
  4. Flu-like general malaise
  5. Skin reactions
  6. Peripheral neuropathy (later, with high doses)
- Management includes:
  1. Giving meperidine (Demerol) for rigors
  2. Giving acetaminophen for fever
  3. Advising patients to apply moisturizers (perfume free) to the skin and to use mild soap to clean the skin
  4. Teaching patients to protect involved skin areas from the sun with clothing or the use of sunscreen agents, to avoid swimming, and to refrain from using topical steroid creams on affected areas

TARGETED THERAPY

- Targeted therapies take advantage of one or more differences in cancer cell growth or metabolism that are not present or only slightly present in normal cells.
- Agents used as targeted therapies often are antibodies that work to disrupt cancer cell division by:
  1. Targeting and blocking growth factor receptors, especially the epithelial growth factor receptors (EGFRs) or the vascular endothelial growth factor receptors (VEGFRs). When a cancer cell's growth depends on having the growth factors bind to their specific receptors, blocking the receptor slows or eliminates the cancer cell's growth.
  2. Blocking signal transduction pathways in cancer cells so that the signals for turning on cell division genes do not get through to the cancer cell's nucleus
- Targeted therapies work only on cancer cells that overexpress the actual target substance. Each person's cancer cells are evaluated to determine whether the cells have enough of a target to be affected by targeted therapy.

- Allergic reactions are an issue in patients receiving monoclonal antibodies because most were developed in animals and may express some animal proteins.
- For therapies that bind to the EGFR and VEGFR receptors, normal cells in the skin, GI tract, and mucous membranes also express these receptors and may develop open sores, rashes, and acne-type lesions.

ONCOLOGIC EMERGENCIES

- Oncologic emergencies are acute conditions associated with cancer and its treatment that often require immediate intervention to avoid life-threatening situations. These conditions include sepsis and disseminated intravascular coagulation (DIC), syndrome of inappropriate antidiuretic hormone (SIADH), spinal cord compression, hypercalcemia, and tumor lysis syndrome (TLS).
- Sepsis and DIC
  1. Microorganisms enter the bloodstream and grow unchecked because the patient often has low WBC counts and impaired immune function. This problem can lead to septic shock and death.
  2. DIC is a clotting problem triggered by sepsis, by the release of clotting factors from cancer cells, or by blood transfusions. Extensive, abnormal clotting occurs throughout the small blood vessels, using up the existing clotting factors and platelets. This process is then followed by extensive bleeding that can range from minimal to fatal hemorrhage.
  3. Management focuses on prevention, early detection, and prompt aggressive treatment.
  4. For prevention:
     a. Identify those patients at greatest risk for sepsis and DIC.
     b. Practice strict adherence to aseptic technique during invasive procedures and during contact with nonintact skin and mucous membranes in immunocompromised patients.
     c. Teach patients and family members the early manifestations of infection and sepsis and when to seek medical assistance.
  5. For treatment:
     a. IV antibiotic therapy
     b. Cryoprecipitated clotting factors therapy
     c. Possible administration of synthetic activated protein C (drotrecogin alpha [Xigris])

- SIADH
  1. Certain cancers secrete or stimulate the secretion of antidiuretic hormone (ADH) when it is not needed by the body for fluid and electrolyte balance. The result is retention of pure water and dilution of electrolytes. In addition to lung and other cancers, SIADH can be caused by morphine sulfate and cyclophosphamide.
  2. Assess for:
     a. Weight gain
     b. Decreased urine output
     c. Weakness and fatigue
     d. Muscle cramps
     e. Low serum sodium levels of 115 to 120 mEq/L (normal range is 135 to 145 MEq/L)
     f. Seizures, coma, and death (when sodium levels are lower than 110 mEq/L)
  3. Management includes:
     a. Fluid restriction
     b. Increased sodium intake
     c. Drug therapy, most often with demeclocycline
     d. Immediate cancer therapy to cause tumor regression
  4. Monitor for indications of fluid overload and pulmonary edema:
     a. Increased pulse quality
     b. Increasing neck vein distention
     c. Presence of crackles in lungs
     d. Increasing peripheral edema
- Spinal cord compression (SCC)
  1. SCC and damage occur when a tumor directly enters the spinal cord or when the vertebrae collapse from tumor degradation of the bone. It most commonly occurs with lung, prostate, breast, and colon cancers.
  2. Manifestations include:
     a. Back pain
     b. Numbness or tingling
     c. Reduced motor and sensory function
     d. Paralysis (which may be permanent)

> 🔲 **Critical Rescue** ◆ Early recognition and treatment of spinal cord compression are key to a good outcome. Assess any cancer patient with new-onset back pain, muscle weakness or a sensation of "heaviness" in the arms or legs, numbness or tingling in the hands or feet, loss of ability to distinguish hot and cold, or an unsteady gait, and report these findings to the oncologist immediately.

  3. Teach patients and families the manifestations of early SCC and instruct them to seek help as soon as problems are apparent.
  4. Management is often palliative and may include:
      a. High-dose corticosteroids to reduce swelling around the spinal cord
      b. High-dose radiation to the site
      c. Intense chemotherapy to reduce tumor size
      d. Surgery to remove the tumor from the area (less common)
      e. External back or neck braces to reduce pressure on the spinal cord or spinal nerves
- Hypercalcemia
  1. Hypercalcemia (increased serum calcium level) occurs most often in patients with bone metastasis. Tumors can also secrete parathyroid hormone, causing bone to release calcium. Decreased mobility and dehydration worsen hypercalcemia.
  2. Early manifestations of hypercalcemia include:
      a. Fatigue
      b. Loss of appetite
      c. Nausea and vomiting
      d. Constipation
      e. Polyuria (increased urine output)
  3. Later manifestations include:
      a. Severe muscle weakness
      b. Loss of deep tendon reflexes
      c. Paralytic ileus
      d. Dehydration
      e. Electrocardiographic (ECG) abnormalities
  4. Management includes:
      a. Oral hydration
      b. Parenteral hydration with normal saline
      c. Drug therapy to reduce calcium levels *temporarily*:
          (1) Oral glucocorticoids
          (2) Calcitonin
          (3) Bisphosphonates
          (4) Diphosphonate
          (5) Mithramycin
      d. Dialysis (if renal impairment is present)
- Superior vena cava (SVC) syndrome
  1. SVC syndrome occurs when the SVC is compressed or obstructed by tumor growth or by the formation of clots in the vessel. It is most common in patients with lymphomas, lung cancer, and cancers of the breast, esophagus, colon, and testes.
  2. Manifestations result from blockage of blood flow from the head, neck, and upper trunk. Early manifestations include:
      a. Facial edema, especially around the eyes, on arising
      b. Tightness of the shirt or blouse collar (Stokes' sign)

3. Later manifestations include:
   a. Edema in the arms and hands
   b. Dyspnea
   c. Erythema of the upper body
   d. Epistaxis (nosebleeds)
4. Late manifestations include:
   a. Hemorrhage
   b. Cyanosis
   c. Mental status changes
   d. Decreased cardiac output and hypotension
5. Management includes:
   a. High-dose radiation therapy to the mediastinal area
   b. Stenting of the vena cava
   c. Surgery (rarely)
- Tumor lysis syndrome (TLS)
  1. TLS occurs when large numbers of tumor cells are destroyed rapidly and their intracellular contents, including potassium and purines (DNA components), are released into the bloodstream faster than the body can eliminate them. The purines are converted to uric acid. Untreated TLS can cause renal failure and death by hyperkalemia and cardiac arrest.
  2. TLS is most often seen in patients receiving radiation or chemotherapy for cancers that are very sensitive to these therapies, including leukemia, lymphoma, small cell lung cancer, and multiple myeloma.
  3. Prevention through hydration is the best management for TLS.
     a. Instruct at-risk patients to drink at least 3000 mL (5000 mL is more desirable) of fluid the day before, the day of, and for 3 days after treatment.
     b. Stress the importance of following the antiemetic regimen so that oral hydration can be accomplished.
     c. Instruct patients to contact the cancer clinic immediately if nausea and vomiting prevent adequate fluid intake so that IV fluids can be started.
     d. Management of actual TLS includes:
        (1) Aggressive fluid resuscitation
        (2) Osmotic diuretics
        (3) Drug therapy to increase the excretion of purines
            i. Allopurinol (Aloprim, Zyloprim)
            ii. Rasburicase (Elitek)
        (4) Drug therapy to reduce serum potassium levels
            i. Sodium polystyrene sulfonate
            ii. IV infusions of glucose and insulin
        (5) Dialysis (for severe hyperkalemia and hyperuricemia)

END-OF-LIFE CARE

OVERVIEW

- *Death* is the cessation of integrated tissue and organ function, manifested by cessation of heartbeat, absence of spontaneous respirations, or irreversible brain dysfunction.
- Although dying is part of the normal life cycle, it is often feared as a time of pain and suffering.
- A *good death* is one that is free from avoidable distress and suffering for patients, families, and caregivers; in agreement with patients' and families' wishes; and consistent with clinical practice standards.
- A *bad death* is one that is associated with pain, not having one's wishes followed at the end of one's life, isolation, abandonment, and constant agonizing about losses.
- The Patient Self-Determination Act of 1990 requires that all patients admitted to any health care agency be asked if they have written advance directives, including a durable power of attorney (DPOA) for health care and a living will.
- As death nears, patients may manifest fear, anxiety, and physical symptoms of distress that require management and control.
- The desired outcomes for a patient near the end of life are:
  1. Identification of patient needs
  2. Control of symptoms of distress
  3. Promotion of meaningful interactions between the patient and family
  4. Facilitation of a peaceful death
- Hospice care philosophy uses an interdisciplinary approach to assess and address the holistic needs of patients and families to facilitate quality of life and a peaceful death. This approach neither hastens nor postpones death, but it provides relief of symptoms experienced by the dying patient.

PATIENT-CENTERED COLLABORATIVE CARE

Assessment

- Obtain patient information to identify the risks for symptoms of distress at the end of life.
  1. Diagnosis
  2. Past medical history
  3. Recent state of health
- Assess any symptom of distress in terms of intensity, frequency, duration, quality, exacerbating (worsening) and relieving factors, and effect on the patient's comfort when awake or asleep.

- A consistent method for rating the intensity of symptoms should be used to facilitate ongoing assessments and evaluate treatment response.
- Assess and document the intensity of the symptom before and after an intervention.
- Assess the patient for:
  1. Physical manifestations of approaching death
     a. Pain
     b. Coolness and mottling of extremities
     c. Increased sleeping
     d. Decreased fluid and food intake
     e. Incontinence
     f. Dyspnea
     g. Congestion and gurgling
     h. Breathing pattern change
     i. Disorientation
     j. Restlessness
  2. Emotional manifestations of approaching death
     a. Withdrawal
     b. Vision-like experiences
     c. Agitation
     d. Letting go
     e. Saying goodbye

> **Clinical Landmine** ◆ Do not deny or argue with what the dying person claims about talking to people you cannot see or hear and seeing objects and places not visible to you.

  3. Family's perception of patient's symptoms
  4. Vital signs
  5. Psychosocial issues that may have an influence on the dying experience, control of symptoms, and family bereavement
     a. Values and religious beliefs of patient and family
     b. Cultural considerations
     c. Fear, anxiety
     d. Knowledge deficits regarding the process of dying
  6. Signs that death has occurred
     a. Breathing stops
     b. No heartbeat
     c. Pupils become fixed and dilated
     d. Body color becomes pale and waxen
     e. Body temperature drops
     f. Muscles and sphincters relax
     g. Urine and stool may be released
     h. Eyes may remain open and there is no blinking

    j. Jaw may fall open

    k. Trickling of fluids internally may be heard

🌐 Cultural Awareness

- Death-related beliefs and practices vary by ethnicity, religion, and race.
    1. African American
        a. Primarily Protestant or Muslim but there is diversity among different communities
        b. Belief in an afterlife and judgment
        c. Funerals tend to be highly involved ceremonies with defined rituals; family, friends, and acquaintances of the deceased make an effort to attend.
    2. Asian
        a. Encompasses several countries and religions (e.g., Chinese, Filipino, Japanese, Laotian, Cambodian, Korean, Vietnamese)
        b. There is a traditional strong family and extended family with male dominance.
        c. Herbal medicine plays an important role.
        d. Direct eye contact is considered impolite.
        e. For Southeast Asians, discussing dying brings bad luck, and hospitals and treatments are alien. Some Southeast Asians, especially if uneducated, are likely to avoid visiting terminally ill family members for fear of contracting the disease.
        f. The number or character "4" is avoided because it symbolizes death.
        g. Funeral and burial customs vary greatly, depending on culture, religion, and generation involved.
    3. Latino or Hispanic
        a. Many subcultures within this population with diverse cultural variations exist (e.g., Mexico, Central America, the Caribbean, South America).
        b. Catholicism is the predominant religion, but many people depend on folk healers for treatment of ailments.
        c. Death is viewed as a direct result of life; one naturally follows the other.
        d. There is an acceptance of death based on religious and cultural beliefs.
        e. Family and family life are important, especially regarding deaths and funerals.
        f. Expression of grief is open, especially among women.
    4. Native Americans or American Indians
        a. More than 350 distinct tribes in the United States exist, with variations in cultural practices.

   b. The focus of identity is on the tribe or council, rather than on ancestry; each tribe has its own belief system.
   c. Most tribes have the belief that spirits are attached to living things.
   d. Indian healers (Shamans) are common.
   e. Family is usually a large extended unit, often including as many as a hundred or more.
   f. Family may not want the patient to die at home, but to allow a family member to die alone is also not appropriate.
   g. Material possessions often are dispersed before or after death to friends and family members.
   h. Bereavement follow-up may not be appropriate because some tribes have a taboo against speaking of the dead.
5. Judaism
   a. This religion encompasses Orthodox, Conservative, and Reformed Jews.
   b. There is a strong belief in the sacredness of life and one, indivisible God.
   c. Funerals have two common themes: honor the dead and comfort the mourners.
   d. The body must not be left unattended until burial, which should take place as soon as possible, preferably within 24 hours.
   e. Autopsies and cremation are opposed.
   f. The deceased is often dressed in a white shroud and buried in a plain pine box.
   g. A 7-day mourning period, called Shiva, follows the person's death for the immediate next of kin.
   h. Due to acculturation to American society, there may be variations in funeral and mourning traditions.

Interventions
- Weakness management: Patients commonly experience weakness and fatigue as death nears, which may impair the ability to swallow.
  1. After the patient is unable to swallow, oral intake should stop.
  2. Warn families of the risk for aspiration and reassure them that anorexia is normal at this stage.
  3. Reinforce that the cessation of food and liquids and dehydration is a natural process and that giving fluids can actually *increase* discomfort.
  4. Apply emollient to the lips, and moisten the mouth and lips with applicators to help prevent or relieve dryness.
  5. In collaboration with a pharmacist experienced in palliative care, identify alternative routes and or alternative drugs to maintain control of symptoms.

6. Choose the least invasive route, such as oral, buccal mucosa, transdermal, or rectal.

> 🏴 **Clinical Landmine** ◆ Avoid the subcutaneous or IV routes for drug delivery because these methods are invasive and painful, and they can cause infection.

- Pain management: Pain is the symptom that dying patients fear the most.
  1. Patients who have had their pain controlled with long-acting opioids should continue their scheduled doses of opioids to prevent pain recurrence.
  2. Depending on the brand of long-acting opioid, oral capsules may be given rectally (same dose and same capsule) when swallowing is impaired.
  3. Increases in pain require immediate-relief analgesics (e.g., morphine sulfate, immediate-release).
  4. Morphine sulfate elixir can be given sublingually, rectally (even to comatose patients), or through the buccal mucosa.
  5. Nonpharmacologic pain management strategies can be incorporated with pharmacologic therapy and include:
     a. Massage
     b. Music therapy
     c. Therapeutic touch
     d. Aromatherapy
- Dyspnea management: Dyspnea is a subjective experience in which the patient has an uncomfortable feeling of breathlessness, which is often described as terrifying. It can manifest itself as air hunger, copious secretions, cough, chest pain, or fatigue.
  1. Treatment is based on physical assessment and the underlying condition. *Pharmacologic interventions should begin early in the course of dyspnea near death.* Nonpharmacologic interventions can be used in conjunction with, but not in place of, drug therapy.
  2. Opioids such as morphine elixir are the standard treatment for dyspnea near death.
  3. Patients who have not been receiving opioids are given starting doses of 5 to 6 mg orally. Those who have taken morphine or other opioids for pain may need much higher doses of morphine (up to 50% more than their usual dose) for relief of dyspnea.
  4. Bronchodilators may be used for bronchospasms and corticosteroids may be used for inflammatory responses that reduce airway lumens.

5. Diuretics may be given for pulmonary fluid overload due to heart failure.
6. Antibiotics may be indicated for dyspnea from a respiratory infection.
7. Anticholinergics, such as transdermal or subcutaneous scopolamine, reduce the production of secretions.
8. Administer oxygen if other methods to reduce dyspnea are not effective; monitor responses, and continue this therapy if dyspnea is relieved.
9. Use nonpharmacologic interventions to relieve dyspnea, including:
   a. Increasing the circulation of cool air (e.g., with an air conditioner and fan)
   b. Applying wet cloths on the patient's face
   c. Positioning the patient (head of bed elevation) to facilitate chest expansion
   d. Providing frequent rest periods to conserve energy
   e. Encouraging imagery and deep breathing

- Nausea and vomiting management: Nausea and vomiting occur in almost one half of terminally ill patients during the last week of life.
  1. When constipation is the cause of nausea and vomiting, administer a biphosphate enema, or a mineral oil enema followed by disimpaction.
  2. Administer prescribed antiemetic drugs.
  3. Remove sources of odors and keep the room temperature at a level that the patient desires.
  4. For some patients, aromatherapy has been found to be helpful in relieving nausea.

- Restlessness and agitation management: Agitation at the end of life is common and may be caused by pain, urinary retention, constipation, or another reversible cause.
  1. If constipation is ruled out as the cause and if analgesia and catheterization do not relieve the restlessness, sedatives should be administered.
  2. Benzodiazepines such as lorazepam (Ativan) elixir or a tablet (1 to 2 mg) dissolved in 0.5 mL of water can be placed against the buccal mucosa.
  3. To prevent agitation from occurring, Ativan should be given every 3 to 4 hours around the clock.
  4. Music therapy and aromatherapy may produce relaxation by quieting the mind and removing a patient's inner restlessness.

- Seizure management: Seizures may occur with brain tumors, advanced AIDS, and pre-existing seizure disorders.

1. If patients have been taking antiepileptic drugs (AEDs), give drugs around-the-clock to maintain a high seizure threshold.
2. Drug therapy may include benzodiazepines (e.g., diazepam [Valium], lorazepam [Ativan]) or barbiturates given by the oral or rectal routes.

- Management of the refractory symptoms of distress: A few patients experience symptoms of distress that are refractory, or resistant to treatment, near the end of life.
  1. High doses of analgesia that cause sedation may be needed to control distressing symptoms.
  2. Use established protocols for drug doses with the intention of alleviating suffering, not hastening death.

> 🔲 **Critical Rescue** ◆ The ethical responsibility of the nurse in caring for patients near death is to follow guidelines for drug use to manage symptoms and to facilitate prompt and effective symptom management.

- Psychosocial management: The personal experience of dying or of losing a loved one through death can be extremely difficult. Sudden, unexpected deaths of younger people tend to be more traumatic for families than deaths after longer terminal illnesses; however, grief, bereavement, and mourning are usually experienced regardless of the circumstances of death.
  1. Perform an assessment to identify the patient's spiritual needs and to facilitate open expression of his or her beliefs and needs.
  2. Incorporate the patient's specific beliefs and customs regarding death when planning and providing care.
  3. Allow patients and their families to verbalize their fears and concerns.
  4. Offer physical and emotional support by *being with* the patient and family. *Being with* implies that you are physically and psychologically with the grieving patient, empathizing to provide emotional support.
  5. Avoid trite assurances such as, "Things will be fine. Don't cry" or "Don't be upset."
  6. Be realistic, keeping patients and families involved in health care decisions and emphasizing that the patient will remain as comfortable as possible until death.
  7. Encourage the patient and family to participate in reminiscence and life review.
  8. Foster hope by listening and caring, but remain realistic.
  9. Avoid explanations of the loss.

10. Teach about the physical signs of death (described earlier) using common terms.
11. Ensure that the patient is receiving palliative care, with an emphasis on symptom management.
12. Provide referrals to bereavement specialists.

> **Clinical Landmine** ◆ Do not try to explain the loss in philosophic or religious terms. Statements such as "Everything happens for the best" or "God sends us only as much as we can bear" are not helpful when the bereaved person has yet to express feelings of anguish or anger.

- Provide for the care of the patient after death.
  1. Ensure that the nurse or physician has completed and signed the death certificate.
  2. Ask the family or significant others if they wish to help wash the patient.
  3. If no autopsy is planned, remove or cut all tubes and lines according to health care agency policy.
  4. Close the patient's eyes.
  5. Insert dentures if the patient wore them.
  6. Straighten the patient, and lower the bed to a flat position.
  7. Place a pillow under the patient's head.
  8. Wash the patient as needed; comb and arrange the patient's hair.
  9. Place pads under the patient's hips and around the perineum to absorb feces and urine.
  10. Clean the patient's room or unit.
  11. Allow the family or significant others to see the patient in private and to perform any religious or cultural customs they wish.
  12. Notify the hospital chaplain or appropriate community religious leader if requested by the family or significant others.
  13. Prepare the patient for transfer to a morgue or funeral home. Wrap the patient in a shroud, and attach identification tags per agency policy (if the patient is to be transferred to the morgue).

INFECTION

OVERVIEW

- An infection is the invasion of a body tissue by microorganisms that allows replication of the microorganism and results in tissue damage.

- A pathogen is any microorganism, also called an agent, capable of producing disease.
- Virulence is the degree to which a pathogen can invade the body and cause disease after infection.
- Normal flora are microorganisms that live in or on the human host without causing disease. Some microbes are beneficial, but when these flora move to another body area, they can be pathogenic.
- Colonization is the process of having pathogenic organisms living and growing in or on a body area without causing disease or damage.
- Toxins are protein molecules released by bacteria to affect host cells at a distant site.
  1. Exotoxins are released by the bacteria into the host's body.
  2. Endotoxins remain within the bacterial cell walls and are released when the bacterium is attacked.
- Microorganisms are parasites that live at the host's expense.
- Infectious diseases can be communicable (transmitted from person to person, such as influenza) or not communicable (e.g., peritonitis).
- Transmission of infection requires these factors:
  1. Reservoir (or source) of infectious agents
     a. Animate reservoirs include people, animals, and insects
     b. Inanimate reservoirs include soil, water, other environmental sources, or medical equipment
  2. Susceptible host with a portal of entry
  3. Mode of transmission
  4. Portal of exit (exit of the microbe from the host often occurs through the portal of entry but can exit by other routes)
- Prevention of infection transmission involves disrupting the three factors or breaking the chain of infection at any point.
- Host factors that increase the susceptibility to infection are:
  1. Congenital or acquired immune deficiencies
  2. Alteration of normal flora by antibiotic therapy
  3. Advancing age
  4. Hormonal changes (e.g., pregnancy, diabetes, corticosteroid therapy, adrenal insufficiency)
  5. Defective phagocytosis
  6. Breaks in skin or mucous membranes
  7. Interference with flow of urine, tears, or saliva
  8. Impaired cough reflex or ciliary action
  9. Malnutrition or dehydration
  10. Smoking, alcohol consumption, inhalation of toxic chemicals
  11. Invasive therapy, chemotherapy, radiation therapy, steroid therapy, surgery

- Common modes of infection transmission are:
  1. Contact transmission (most common)
     a. Direct (person-to-person) contact, in which the source and host have physical contact and microorganisms are transferred directly (e.g., common cold)
     b. Indirect contact, in which the transfer of microorganisms occurs from a source to a host by passive transfer from a contaminated object (e.g., staphylococcal organisms)
  2. Droplet transmission from contact with infected secretions or droplets (e.g., influenza)
  3. Airborne transmission from small airborne particles containing pathogens that leave the infected source, are suspended in the air, and enter a susceptible host (e.g., *Mycobacterium tuberculosis,* the varicella zoster virus)
  4. Vector transmission, in which insects carry pathogens between two or more hosts, such as the deer tick that causes Lyme disease
- Human physiologic defenses against infection include:
  1. Intact skin and mucous membranes
  2. Normal flora
  3. Secretions and natural movements of the respiratory, GI, and genitourinary tracts
  4. Inflammation and phagocytosis (natural immunity)
  5. Antibody-mediated immunity (AMI) and cell-mediated immunity (CMI)
- A hospital-acquired infection (HAI) is an infection acquired while the patient was in an inpatient setting. It occurs while the patient is receiving health care. Old terms for this include *nosocomial* and *iatrogenic.*
- HAIs can be prevented or controlled in at least five major ways:
  1. Hand hygiene
     a. Handwashing (wetting, soaping, lathering, applying friction under running water for at least 15 seconds, rinsing, and adequate drying)
     b. Alcohol-based hand rubs (ABHRs)
  2. Use of personal protective equipment (PPE), also called *barriers*
  3. Adequate staffing
  4. Disinfection or sterilization
  5. Patient placement and transport

> Clinical Landmine ◆ Do not use an ABHR before inserting eye drops, ointments, or contact lenses. Alcohol can irritate the patient's eyes, causing burning and redness.

- Centers for Disease Control and Prevention (CDC) Transmission-Based Guidelines include:
  1. *Standard Precautions* assume that all body excretions, secretions, and moist membranes and tissues, excluding perspiration, are potentially infectious, and the precautions should be used in the care of all patients.
     a. Respiratory Hygiene/Cough Etiquette (RH/CE) for respiratory illnesses
        (1) Patient, staff, and visitor education
        (2) Posted signs
        (3) Hand hygiene
        (4) Covering the nose and mouth with a tissue and prompt tissue disposal or using surgical masks
        (5) Separation from the person with respiratory infection by more than 3 ft (1 m)
     b. Safe injection practices, using a sterile, single-use disposable needle and syringe for each injection; prevention of contamination of injection equipment and drug; and use of retractable needles
  2. Transmission-Based Precautions
     a. *Airborne Precautions* for patients known or suspected to have infections transmitted by the airborne transmission route (e.g., tuberculosis, measles [rubeola], and chickenpox [varicella])
        (1) Negative airflow rooms
        (2) Enclosed booths with high-efficiency particulate air (HEPA) filtration or ultraviolet light
     b. *Droplet Precautions* for patients known or suspected to have infections transmitted by the droplet transmission route (e.g., influenza, mumps, pertussis, meningitis)
     c. *Contact Precautions* for patients known or suspected to have infections transmitted by direct contact or contact with items in the environment (e.g., significant multidrug-resistant organism [MDRO] infection or colonization, pediculosis, scabies, respiratory syncytial virus [RSV], and *Clostridium difficile*)

> **Critical Rescue** ◆ The CDC recommends that private rooms always be used for patients on Airborne Precautions and those in a Protective Environment.

- A number of microorganisms have become resistant to certain antibiotics, and once useful drugs no longer control these infectious agents (multidrug-resistant organisms [MDROs]).
  1. Methicillin-resistant *Staphylococcus aureus* (MRSA)

2. Community-associated MRSA (CA-MRSA)
3. Vancomycin-resistant *Enterococcus* (VRE)
4. Vancomycin-intermediate *S. aureus* (VISA)
5. Vancomycin-resistant *S. aureus* (VRSA)

> 🔲 **Critical Rescue** ◆ Help prevent development of drug resistance by teaching patients to complete their prescribed antibiotic therapy and not stop the drug when they are feeling better.

- Complications from infection are relapse, cellulitis, pneumonia, abscess formation, sepsis, septic shock, disseminated intravascular coagulation (DIC), multi-system organ failure, and death.

PATIENT-CENTERED COLLABORATIVE CARE
Assessment
- Obtain patient information about:
  1. Age
  2. History of tobacco or alcohol use
  3. Current illness or disease (e.g., diabetes)
  4. Past and current drug use (e.g., prescribed, OTC, recreational, injection)
  5. Nutritional status
  6. Previous vaccinations or immunizations
  7. Exposed to infectious agents
  8. Contact with animals, including pets
  9. Insect bites
  10. Travel history
  11. Sexual history
  12. Transfusion history
  13. Previous infection history
  14. Onset order of symptoms
- Assess for and document:
  1. Skin manifestations
     a. Redness
     b. Warmth
     c. Swelling
     d. Drainage or pus
     e. Pain
  2. Generalized manifestations
     a. Fever (usually a temperature above 101° F [38° C] or 99° F [37° C] for older adults)
     b. Chills
     c. Malaise and fatigue
     d. Lymphadenopathy

    e. Joint pain
    f. Muscle aches
    g. Photophobia
3. GI tract manifestations
    a. Nausea and vomiting
    b. Diarrhea
4. Genitourinary manifestations
    a. Dysuria
    b. Frequency
    c. Urgency
    d. Hematuria
    e. Purulent drainage
    f. Pelvic or flank pain
5. Respiratory tract manifestations
    a. Cough
    b. Congestion
    c. Rhinorrhea
    d. Sore throat
    e. Chest pain
6. Psychosocial dysfunction
    a. Anxiety and frustration
    b. Lack of knowledge
    c. Social isolation
7. Abnormal laboratory findings
    a. Positive culture
    b. Positive serologic results
    c. High or low WBC count
    d. Elevated erythrocyte sedimentation rate (ESR)
8. Abnormal imaging findings
    a. Chest x-ray, sinus or joint films, GI studies
    b. CT
    c. MRI
    d. Ultrasonography
9. Biopsy

Planning and Implementation

❖ **NDx:** Hyperthermia

*   Interventions to reduce fever include:
    1. Antimicrobials
    2. Antipyretics
    3. External cooling

> 🛡️ **Clinical Landmine** ◆ Avoid making the patient shiver during any form of external cooling. Shivering may indicate that the patient is being cooled too quickly.

    4. Fluid administration

- Effective anti-infective therapy requires:
  1. Agent appropriate for the known organism
  2. Sufficient dosage
  3. Proper rate of administration
  4. Sufficient duration
- Nursing interventions include:
  1. Obtaining an allergy history before giving antibiotics
  2. Monitoring the patient for side effects of antibiotics, such as nausea, vomiting, or rash
  3. Applying a hypothermia blanket and monitoring for shivering
  4. Sponging the patient with tepid water
  5. Monitoring for manifestations of dehydration
     a. Thirst
     b. Decreased skin turgor
     c. Dry skin and mucous membranes
  6. Encouraging fluid intake
  7. Measuring intake and output
  8. Monitoring vital signs and oxygen saturation
  9. Monitoring skin color and temperature
  10. Assessing level of consciousness and for seizure activity
  11. Monitoring laboratory values
  12. Providing or assisting with oral hygiene

❖**NDx:** Social Isolation

- Teach the patient and family about the mode of transmission of infection and mechanisms that prevent spread to others.
- Assess coping mechanisms that the patient has used in the past.
- Collaborate with the chaplain or social worker to help reduce the patient's stress, anxiety, or depression.
- Encourage staff to maintain contact with the patient.
- Encourage family members and friends to visit and to use appropriate infection control measures.
- Assist the family in providing contact by telephone or e-mail.
- Encourage the use of television, Internet, and iPods or other MP3 players.

Community-Based Care

- Urge immunization against respiratory infections for adults older than 50 years, anyone with a chronic illness, and anyone who lives with an older adult or a person with a chronic illness.
- Remove indwelling urinary catheters as soon as possible to prevent urinary tract infections.
- Emphasize the importance of a clean home environment, especially for the patient who continues to be immunocompromised or who is uniquely susceptible to superinfection.
- Demonstrate proper handwashing with the patient and family and obtain a repeat demonstration.

- Teach the patient and family about:
  1. What is causing the illness
  2. Whether the infection can be spread to others
  3. Modes of transmission
  4. Specific precautions for transmission prevention, including:
     a. Whether any special household cleaning is necessary and, if so, what those special steps include
     b. How to dispose of any used needles and syringes safely and legally
     c. Cleaning clothing soiled with blood or other body fluids by washing them with bleach or disinfectant (e.g., Lysol)
     d. Cleaning measures to be based on actual available equipment and facilities
  5. The importance of adhering to the prescribed antibiotic therapy regimen, including:
     a. Timing of doses
     b. Number of days
     c. Any specific drug administration instructions (e.g., before meals, with meals, and without other agents) and the possible side effects
     d. Allergic manifestations and the need to notify a health care provider if an adverse reaction occurs
     e. What to do if a drug dose is missed (e.g., doubling the dosage, waiting until the next dose time)
  6. Managing IV drug therapy
- Refer to home health care agencies as needed.

INFLAMMATION AND IMMUNITY

OVERVIEW

- Immunity is composed of many cell functions that protect people against the effects of injury or microscopic invasion.
- The purpose of inflammation and immunity is to meet the human need for protection by neutralizing, eliminating, or destroying organisms that invade the internal environment.
- To meet protection needs without harming the body, immune system cells use protective actions only against non-self proteins and cells by distinguishing between the body's own healthy self cells and other, non-self proteins and cells. This process is called *self-tolerance.*
- The immune system cells are the only body cells capable of determining self from non-self.
- Self-tolerance is possible because of the different kinds of proteins present on cell membranes. Each person's cells have a unique protein sequence on the surface that serves as a *universal*

product code or a *cellular fingerprint* for that person; the proteins are known as human leukocyte antigens (HLAs) and constitute the tissue type of the person. These proteins are recognized as *foreign*, or non-self, by the immune system of another person.

- The HLA is key for recognition and self-tolerance. At any encounter with an invader, the immune system cells compare the surface protein HLAs to determine whether the encountered cell is self or non-self. If the encountered cell's HLA does not perfectly match the HLA of the immune system cell, the encountered cell is non-self, or foreign. The immune system cell then takes action to neutralize, destroy, or eliminate this foreign invader.
- Immune function is most efficient when people are in their 20s and 30s and slowly declines with increasing age. Disease and drugs can reduce immune function.
- Whenever inflammation and immunity are reduced, the risk for infection and cancer dramatically increases.

ORGANIZATION OF THE IMMUNE SYSTEM

- The immune system is not located in any one organ or body area, but most immune system cells come from the bone marrow. Some cells mature in the bone marrow; others leave the bone marrow and mature in different body sites.
- When mature, many immune system cells are released into the blood, where they circulate to most body areas and have specific effects.
- The WBCs, also known as *leukocytes*, are the inflammatory and immune system cells. Each type has specific functions.
- The leukocytes provide protection through many defensive actions, including:
  1. Recognition of self versus non-self
  2. Destruction of foreign invaders, cellular debris, and unhealthy or abnormal self cells
  3. Production of antibodies directed against invaders
  4. Complement activation
  5. Production of cytokines that stimulate increased formation of leukocytes in bone marrow and increase specific leukocyte activity
- The three processes needed for human protection through immunity are:
  1. Inflammation
  2. Antibody-mediated immunity (AMI)
  3. Cell-mediated immunity (CMI)

- Each process uses different defensive actions, and each influences or requires assistance from the other two processes. Full immunity (*immunocompetence*) requires the function and interaction of all three processes.

INFLAMMATION

- Inflammation, also called *natural immunity*, provides immediate protection against the effects of tissue injury and invading foreign proteins.
- The purpose of inflammation is to start blood vessel and tissue reactions to rid the body of harmful microorganisms and other invaders.
- Inflammation differs from immunity in two important ways:
  1. Inflammatory protection is immediate but short term against injury or invading organisms. It does not provide true immunity on repeated exposure to the same organisms.
  2. Inflammation is a *nonspecific* body defense to invasion or injury and can be started by almost any event, regardless of where it occurs or what causes it.
- The classic manifestations of inflammation are:
  1. Warmth
  2. Redness
  3. Swelling
  4. Pain
  5. Decreased function
- How widespread the symptoms of inflammation are depends on the intensity, severity, and duration of exposure to the initiating injury or invasion.
- Inflammation occurs in response to tissue injury and to invasion by organisms. Infection is usually accompanied by inflammation; however, inflammation can occur without infection.
  1. Examples of inflammation without infection include sprain injuries to joints, myocardial infarction, sterile surgical incisions, blister formation, and thrombophlebitis.
  2. Examples of inflammation caused by noninfectious invasion by foreign proteins include allergic rhinitis, contact dermatitis, and other allergic reactions.
  3. Examples of inflammation caused by infection include otitis media, appendicitis, peritonitis, and viral hepatitis.

CELL TYPES INVOLVED IN INFLAMMATION

- Four types of WBCs (leukocytes) are involved in inflammation:
  1. Neutrophils
  2. Macrophages

3. Eosinophils
4. Basophils

- Neutrophils and macrophages use phagocytosis to destroy and eliminate foreign invaders. Basophils and eosinophils release chemicals that act on blood vessels to cause tissue-level responses.

PHAGOCYTOSIS

- Phagocytosis is the engulfing and destruction of invaders. This action also rids the body of debris after tissue injury. Neutrophils and macrophages are most efficient at phagocytosis.
- Phagocytosis involves seven steps:
  1. *Exposure and invasion:* For phagocytosis to start, leukocytes must first be exposed to organisms, foreign proteins, or debris from damaged tissues.
  2. *Attraction:* To ensure the WBC comes into direct contact with the target (antigen, invader, or foreign protein), damaged tissues and blood vessels secrete chemotaxins (chemical attractants) that can combine with the surface of invading foreign proteins to improve attraction.
  3. *Adherence:* This process allows the phagocytic cell to bind to the surface of the target.
  4. *Recognition:* This process occurs when the phagocytic cell sticks to the surface of the target cell and recognizes it as non-self. This action ensures that phagocytosis occurs only against non-self or unhealthy self cells.
  5. *Cellular ingestion:* Phagocytosis (engulfment) into the phagocyte is needed because the destruction of the target cell occurs inside the phagocytic cell.
  6. *Phagosome formation:* This occurs when the phagocyte's granules are inside the vacuole and fuse to the invader.
  7. *Degradation:* The phagosome enzymes digest the engulfed target, which is the final step.

SEQUENCE OF INFLAMMATORY RESPONSES

- Inflammatory responses occur in a predictable sequence of three stages. The sequence is the same regardless of the triggering event and the timing may overlap.
  1. *Stage I* is the vascular part of the inflammatory response. Injured tissues and the leukocytes in this area secrete histamine, serotonin, and kinins that constrict the small veins and dilate the arterioles in the area of injury. These blood vessel changes cause redness and warmth of the tissues. This increased blood flow increases delivery of nutrients to injured tissues, causing redness, swelling, and pain. The duration of

these responses depends on the severity of the initiating event, but they usually subside within 24 to 72 hours.

  a. The macrophage is the major cell involved in stage I of inflammation.

  b. Cytokines, such as colony-stimulating factors (CSFs), are secreted to trigger the bone marrow to increase the rate of WBC production from 14 days to a matter of hours.

2. *Stage II* is the cellular exudate part of the response in which neutrophilia (increased number of circulating neutrophils) occurs. Exudate in the form of pus occurs, containing dead WBCs, necrotic tissue, and fluids that escape from damaged cells.

  a. The most active cell in this stage is the neutrophil, which can increase in count up to five times within 12 hours after the onset of inflammation as a result of cytokine stimulation.

  b. Neutrophils attack and destroy organisms and remove dead tissue through phagocytosis.

  c. The arachidonic acid (AA) cascade starts to increase the inflammatory response by converting fatty acids in plasma membranes into AA. Enzymes (including cyclooxygenase) then convert AA into many chemicals that are further processed into the substances that continue the inflammatory response in the tissues. Some of these substances include histamine, leukotrienes, prostaglandins, serotonin, and kinins.

3. *Stage III* features tissue repair and replacement. Although this stage is completed last, it begins at the time of injury and is critical to the final function of the inflamed area.

  a. Some of the WBCs involved in inflammation start the replacement of lost tissues or repair of damaged tissues by inducing the remaining healthy cells to divide.

  b. In tissues that are unable to divide, WBCs trigger new blood vessel growth (angiogenesis) and scar tissue formation. Because scar tissue does not behave like normal tissue, loss of function occurs wherever damaged tissues are replaced with scar tissue.

CONSEQUENCES OF INFLAMMATION

- When inflammation occurs in response to invasion by infectious microorganisms, its actions can eliminate or destroy the invaders and prevent the person from becoming ill.

- Inflammation alone cannot provide immunity but its actions are needed to trigger both antibody-mediated immunity (AMI) and cell-mediated immunity (CMI).

- When inflammatory responses are prolonged or occur at inappropriate times or in inappropriate places, they can cause tissue damage with extensive fibrosis, scarring, and loss of healthy tissue function.
- Long-lasting immune actions develop through antibody-mediated immunity (AMI) and cell-mediated immunity (CMI).

IMMUNITY

ANTIBODY-MEDIATED IMMUNITY

- Antibody-mediated immunity (AMI), also known as *humoral immunity*, involves antigen-antibody interactions to neutralize, eliminate, or destroy foreign proteins. Antibodies are produced by B-lymphocytes (B-cells).
- B-cells become sensitized to a specific foreign protein (antigen) and produce antibodies directed specifically against that protein. The expressed antibody (rather than the B cell) causes one of several actions to neutralize, eliminate, or destroy that antigen.
- B-cells start as lymphocytes in the bone marrow, the primary lymphoid tissue, and migrate into many secondary lymphoid tissues, where maturation is completed. The secondary lymphoid tissues for B-cell maturation are the spleen, parts of lymph nodes, tonsils, and the mucosa of the intestinal tract.
- The body learns to make enough of any specific antibody to provide long-lasting immunity and protection against specific organisms or toxins.
- Seven steps are needed to produce a specific antibody directed against a specific antigen whenever the person is exposed to that antigen:
  1. *Exposure or invasion* is needed because antibody actions occur inside the body or on a few body surfaces. Without exposure, an antibody cannot be made.
  2. *Antigen recognition* is the recognition of the invader by an unsensitized B-cell. This process involves macrophages and helper/inducer T-cells.
  3. *Lymphocyte sensitization* occurs when the B-cell recognizes the antigen as non-self and becomes *sensitized* to this antigen. A single naive B-cell can become sensitized only once.
  4. *Antibody production and release* occurs at a rate as high as 300 molecules of antibody per second by each sensitized B-lymphocyte. These antibody molecules are released and can bind to their specific antigen. *Circulating antibodies can be transferred from one person to another to provide the receiving person with immediate immunity of short duration.*

5. *Antibody-antigen binding* occurs when the tips of the Y-shaped antibody recognize the specific antigen and bind to it. The binding stimulates reactions to neutralize, eliminate, or destroy the antigen.

6. *Antibody-binding actions* include agglutination, lysis, complement fixation, precipitation, and inactivation or neutralization, all of which can neutralize, eliminate, or destroy the antigen.

7. *Sustained immunity (memory)* is critical in providing long-lasting immunity to a specific antigen. It results from memory B-cells made during the lymphocyte sensitization stage. These memory cells remain sensitized to the specific antigen to which they were originally exposed. On re-exposure to the same antigen, the memory cells rapidly respond, and each new cell can rapidly make large amounts of the antibody specific for the sensitizing antigen. This ability of the memory cells to respond on re-exposure to the same antigen that originally sensitized the B-cell allows a rapid and large immune (anamnestic) response to the antigen. Such large quantities of antibody are made that the invading organisms usually are removed completely, and the person does not become ill. Because of this process, most people do not become ill with chickenpox or other infectious diseases more than once, even though they are exposed many times to the causative organism. Without the action of memory, people would remain susceptible to specific diseases on subsequent exposure to the organisms, and no sustained immunity would be generated.

- All antibodies are immunoglobulins (Ig), also called gamma globulins because they are globular proteins that confer immunity.
- There are five antibody types:
  1. IgA is the secretory antibody found on body surfaces and secretions to prevent antigen entry.
  2. IgM is the antibody type a sensitized B-cell makes on first exposure to an antigen. Because it is large and is a complex, it has 10 binding sites to efficiently bind antigen even though it is produced in small amounts. This antibody ensures that an initial infectious illness, such as chickenpox, lasts only 5 to 10 days.
  3. IgG is the most common antibody found in the blood. On re-exposure to the same antigen, the already sensitized B-cell makes large amounts of the IgG type of antibody against that antigen. The enormous numbers produced make IgG antibodies efficient at clearing the antigen and protecting the person from again becoming ill with the disease.

4. IgE is the antibody type that is responsible for many allergic reactions.
5. IgD activates B-cells and modifies the activity of IgM.

ACQUIRING ANTIBODY-MEDIATED IMMUNITY

- Two broad categories of immunity are innate-native immunity and adaptive (acquired) immunity.
- *Innate-native immunity* (sometimes called *natural immunity*) is any natural protective feature, including inflammation and barriers (e.g., skin, mucosa). This type of immunity cannot be developed or transferred from one person to another and is not an adaptive response to exposure or invasion by foreign proteins.
- *Adaptive immunity* is the immunity that a person's body learns to make (or can receive) as an adaptive response to invasion by organisms or foreign proteins. AMI is an acquired immunity, is active or passive, and is acquired naturally or artificially.
  1. *Active immunity* occurs when antigens enter the body and the body responds by actively making specific antibodies against the antigen.
     a. Natural active immunity occurs when an antigen enters the body without human assistance and the body responds by actively making antibodies against that antigen (e.g., chickenpox virus). *This type of immunity is the most effective and the longest lasting.*
     b. Artificial active immunity is the protection developed by vaccination or immunization. Small amounts of specific antigens are placed as a vaccination into a person and the immune system responds by actively making antibodies against the antigen.
  2. *Passive immunity* occurs when antibodies against an antigen are in a person's body but were transferred to the person's body after being made in the body of another person or animal. It provides only immediate, short-term protection against a specific antigen.
     a. Natural passive immunity occurs when antibodies are passed from the mother to the fetus through the placenta or to the infant through colostrum and breast milk.
     b. Artificial passive immunity involves injecting a person with antibodies that were produced in another person or animal.
- AMI works with inflammation to protect against infection. However, AMI can provide the most effective, long-lasting immunity only when its actions are combined with those of cell-mediated immunity (CMI).

CELL-MEDIATED IMMUNITY

- CMI, or cellular immunity, involves many WBC actions and interactions. This type of immunity is provided by lymphocyte stem cells that mature in the secondary lymphoid tissues of the thymus and pericortical areas of lymph nodes. These cells are known as T-lymphocytes (T-cells).
- Certain CMI responses influence and regulate the activities of AMI and inflammation by producing and releasing cytokines. For total immunocompetence, CMI must function optimally.
- Cytokines are small protein hormones produced by the many WBCs. One cell produces a cytokine, which exerts its effects on other cells of the immune system and on other body cells.
  1. The cells responding to the cytokine may be located close to or remote from the cytokine-secreting cell.
  2. Cytokines act like *messengers* that tell specific cells how and when to respond.
  3. Cytokines include the interleukins, interferons, colony-stimulating factors, and tumor necrosis factor.
- Four T-lymphocyte subsets that are critically important for the development and continuation of CMI are:
  1. *Helper/inducer T-cells* (T4 cells, T_H cells, CD4$^+$ cells) that easily recognize self cells versus non-self cells. In response to the recognition of non-self (antigen), helper/inducer T-cells secrete cytokines that can enhance the activity of other WBCs.
  2. *Suppressor T-cells* (T8 cells, CD8$^+$ cells, T_S cells) regulate CMI by preventing hypersensitivity (continuous overreactions) when a person is exposed to non-self cells or proteins. These cells secrete cytokines that inhibitor immune system cell action and work in opposition to helper/inducer T-cells. Immune function is well balanced when T4$^+$ cells outnumber T8$^+$ cells by a 2:1 ratio.
  3. *Cytotoxic/cytolytic T-cells* are a subset of suppressor cells that destroys cells containing a processed antigen's major histocompatibility complex (MHC). This activity is most effective against self cells infected by parasites, such as viruses or protozoa.
  4. *Natural killer (NK) cells* (CD16 cells) have direct cytotoxic effects on some non-self cells that are independent of the interactions of other WBCs. NK cells conduct "seek and destroy" missions in the body to eliminate non-self cells. NK cells are most effective in destroying unhealthy or abnormal self cells such as cancer cells and virally infected body cells.
- CMI helps protect the body through the ability to differentiate self from non-self.

- The non-self cells most easily recognized by CMI are cancer cells and the self cells infected by organisms that live within host cells.
- CMI watches for and rids the body of self cells that might potentially harm the body.
- It is important in preventing the development of cancer and metastasis.

PAIN

OVERVIEW

- Pain is an unpleasant sensory and emotional experience associated with actual or potential tissue damage.
- It is whatever the experiencing person says it is and exists whenever he or she says it does.
- Self-report is always the most reliable indication of pain.
- The nurse's primary role in pain management is to advocate for the patient by *believing* reports of pain.
- The Joint Commission states that patients in all health care settings, including home care, have a right to effective pain management.
- There are two main types of pain:
  1. *Acute pain* results from acute injury, disease, or surgery. It is usually temporary, of sudden onset, and easily localized. Features include:
     a. Physiologic responses
        (1) Increased heart rate
        (2) Increased blood pressure
        (3) Increased respiratory rate
        (4) Dilated pupils
        (5) Sweating
     b. Common behavioral responses
        (1) Restlessness
        (2) Inability to concentrate
        (3) Apprehension
        (4) Overall distress
  2. *Chronic pain* or *persistent pain* is further divided into two subtypes:
     a. Chronic cancer pain is pain associated with cancer or another progressive disease, such as AIDS. Sources of cancer pain are:
        (1) Nerve compression
        (2) Invasion of tissue
        (3) Bone metastasis
        (4) Surgery
        (5) Toxicities from chemotherapy and radiation therapy

   b. Chronic non-cancer pain is the more common type and is associated with tissue injury that has healed or is not associated with cancer, such as arthritis or chronic back pain.

   c. Major features of chronic pain may include:

     (1) Serves no biologic purpose

     (2) Persists or recurs for indefinite periods, usually for more than 3 months

     (3) Onset is gradual, and the character and quality of the pain change over time.

     (4) Usually poorly localized (hard to pinpoint) and often difficult to describe

     (5) Physiologic adaptation occurs, and the symptoms often associated with acute pain, such as increased pulse, are *absent* with chronic pain.

     (6) Interferes with personal relationships and ADLs

     (7) May result in emotional and financial burdens

     (8) Depression is common.

> **Critical Rescue** ◆ Although many characteristics of chronic pain are similar in different patients, be aware that each situation is unique and requires a highly specialized plan of care.

- Other pain categories by processing:
  1. Nociceptive pain (normal processing of pain)
     a. Somatic pain (arising from the skin and musculoskeletal structures)
     b. Visceral pain (arising from organs)
  2. Neuropathic pain (abnormal processing of pain)
     a. Burning
     b. Shooting
     c. Stabbing
     d. Pins and needles feeling
- The attitudes of health care professionals toward pain influence the way they perceive and interact with patients in pain.
- Many patients are reluctant to report pain. When they do, they may underreport its severity.
- Some patients, especially older adults, are reluctant to take pain medications, especially opioid analgesics, because they fear becoming addicted to or used to the drug.
- Although pain is familiar to everyone, it is so complex that there is no single, universal treatment.

Considerations for Older Adults

Age can influence how pain is perceived, assessed, and treated. The incidence of pain in older adults is high, as is risk for undertreatment.

Women's Considerations

Certain painful conditions are more common in men or women. Most chronic pain sufferers are women. Women have more migraine headaches, tension headaches, rheumatoid arthritis and osteoarthritis, fibromyalgia, and multiple sclerosis. Men have more cluster headaches, back pain, gout, peripheral vascular disease, and postherpetic neuralgia.

- Definitions important to pain management:
  1. *Addiction* is a primary, chronic neurobiologic disease with one or more of the following: impaired control over drug use, compulsive use, continued use despite harm, and craving.
  2. *Pseudoaddiction* is a health care–induced syndrome created by the undertreatment of pain. Features include patient behaviors such as anger and escalating demands for more or different medications, and results in suspicion and avoidance by staff.
  3. *Tolerance* is a state of adaptation in which exposure to a drug induces changes that result in a decrease in one or more of the drug's effects over time.
  4. *Physical dependence* is adaptation manifested by a drug class–specific withdrawal syndrome that can be produced by abrupt cessation, rapid dose reduction, decreasing blood level of the drug, or administration of an antagonist. It occurs in *everyone* who takes opioids over a period of time.
  5. *Withdrawal* or *abstinence syndrome* results when a patient who is physically dependent on opioids abruptly ceases using them.
  6. *Placebo* is any medical treatment or nursing care that produces an effect in a patient because of its therapeutic intent and not because of its actual physical or chemical properties.

> Critical Rescue ◆ Carefully explain the difference between physical dependence and addiction when a patient starts on opioid therapy.

> Clinical Landmine ◆ Because of the deception involved and the need for informed consent, *never* administer a placebo to your patient.

PATIENT-CENTERED COLLABORATIVE CARE

Assessment

- Assess and record pain history information:
  1. Precipitating factors
  2. Aggravating factors
  3. Localization of pain
  4. Character and quality of pain
  5. Duration of pain
- Assess for these clinical manifestations in cognitively intact and verbal patients:
  1. Tachycardia (acute pain)
  2. Increased blood pressure (acute pain)
  3. Patient's statement of pain (acute and chronic pain)
  4. Splinting (acute and chronic pain)
  5. Functional status impairment (acute and chronic pain)
  6. Level and location of pain (acute and chronic)
     a. Localized pain (confined to the site of origin)
     b. Projected pain (pain along a specific nerve or nerves)
     c. Radiating pain (diffuse pain around the site of origin, not well localized)
     d. Referred pain (pain perceived in an area distant from the site of painful stimuli)
  7. Intensity and quality of pain
     a. Pain intensity scales
     b. Verbal descriptive scales
     c. Faces Pain Rating scale of smile to frown
- To assess pain in cognitively impaired or nonverbal patients:
  1. Use self-report (when possible).
  2. Search for potential causes of pain.
  3. Observe patient behaviors.
  4. Use surrogate reporting (e.g., family member).
  5. Attempt an analgesic trial.

Considerations for Older Adults

- Six common pain indicators among older adults are:
  1. Facial expression (e.g., grimacing, crying)
  2. Verbalizations or vocalizations (e.g., screaming)
  3. Body movements (e.g., restlessness)
  4. Changes in interpersonal interactions
  5. Changes in activity patterns or routines
  6. Mental status changes (e.g., confusion, increased confusion)

Interventions

Nonsurgical Management

- Drug therapy

1. The non-opioid analgesics are the first-line therapy for mild to moderate pain.
   a. Acetylsalicylic acid (aspirin)
   b. Acetaminophen (Tylenol)
2. NSAIDs
   a. Ketorolac (Toradol)
   b. Ibuprofen (Motrin)
   c. Naproxen (Naprosyn)
   d. Ketoprofen (Orudis)
   e. Celecoxib (Celebrex)
3. Opioid analgesics
   a. Hydromorphone (Dilaudid)
   b. Morphine (Roxanol, Avinza, Kadian)
   c. Fentanyl (Sublimaze)
   d. Codeine
   e. Hydrocodone
   f. Oxycodone
   g. Methadone (Dolophine)
   h. Tramadol (Ultram)
   i. Meperidine (Demerol)
   j. Oxymorphone (Opana, Numorphan)

> **Clinical Landmine** ◆ Meperidine use is considered to be outdated pain management. It should not be used for pain control.

- WHO Analgesic Ladder is used for drug therapy selection based on a 1-to-10 (10 being the worst pain) pain intensity scale.
  1. Level 1 pain (1 to 3 rating): Use non-opioids , such as acetaminophen or NSAIDs.
  2. Level 2 pain (4 to 6 rating): Use weak opioids alone or in combination with an adjuvant drug, such as Ultram or Vicodin.
  3. Level 3 pain (7 to 10 rating): Use strong opioids, such as morphine, hydromorphone (Dilaudid), or fentanyl (Duragesic patch or Fentanyl Oralets).
- Common routes of opioid drug delivery are:
  1. Oral
  2. Transdermal patch
  3. IV or subcutaneous
  4. Rectal
  5. Intrathecal
  6. Epidural

- Nursing care issues related to opioid therapy:
  1. Side effects can include constipation, nausea and vomiting, urinary retention, pruritus (itching), sedation, and respiratory depression.
  2. Whenever a patient is started on regular doses of opioids at home, teach him or her how to prevent constipation.
  3. Sedation occurs before opioid-induced respiratory depression, so nurse-monitored sedation levels are recommended by use of a sedation scale for opioid-naive (not currently on an opioid) patients or those receiving opioids IV or epidurally. The key to assessing sedation is determining how easily the patient is aroused.
  4. Monitor respiratory rate and depth, especially while sleeping.

> ▣ **Critical Rescue ◆** Stop the opioid if the patient is difficult to arouse.

> ▣ **Critical Rescue ◆** Respiratory depression is managed with an opioid antagonist, naloxone (Narcan). It is a fast-acting drug given IV to reverse the opioid effect. It should be administered only when absolutely necessary because it removes all of the pain-relieving effects of the opioid and leads to withdrawal symptoms. The respiratory-depressant effect of the opioid is usually longer acting than naloxone. Continue to monitor the patient after giving the drug because respiratory depression can recur. If respiratory depression recurs, additional naloxon is given.

- Nursing care issues with patient-controlled analgesia (PCA):
  1. PCA allows the patient to control the dosage of opioid received, improving pain relief and increasing patient satisfaction.
  2. PCA is achieved through the use of a PCA infusion pump. The infusion pump delivers the desired amount of drug through an IV access for pain.
  3. Morphine, fentanyl, and hydromorphone are the most commonly used drugs for PCA.
  4. Drug security to avoid overdosing is achieved through a locked syringe pump system or locked drug reservoir system.
  5. When the patient presses the button or pendant (on ambulatory pumps), the appropriate bolus or demand dose is delivered.

> ▣ **Critical Rescue** ◆ All PCA pumps should have warning labels with large print that read "Patient Only to Push Button" to prevent other people or staff from administering the drug.

6. Teach patients how to use the PCA and to report side effects, such as dizziness, nausea and vomiting, and inability to void.
7. Monitor the patient's vital signs, particularly respirations, and check sedation level at least every 2 hours or per agency protocol.

- Nursing care issues for epidural analgesia are:
  1. Epidural analgesia is the instillation of a pain-blocking agent, usually an opioid analgesic alone or in combination with a local anesthetic, such as bupivacaine, into the epidural space.
  2. Epidural analgesia is most commonly used for the management of acute pain.
  3. Morphine (preservative free), hydromorphone (Dilaudid), and fentanyl (Sublimaze) are the most commonly used opioids for epidural administration.
  4. Pruritus (itching), nausea, and vomiting are common side effects of epidural opioids.
  5. A temporary, externalized epidural catheter is used for acute pain control. This device is not sutured to the skin and is easily dislodged. Be sure to tape the catheter in two places to anchor it properly.
  6. Complications that occur with epidural analgesia are directly related to catheter placement, catheter maintenance, and the type of analgesic.
  7. Infection is rare but can occur as a result of failure to maintain aseptic technique during catheter placement, through direct drug instillation, during infusion of solution and tubing changes, and from a failure to maintain aseptic conditions for indwelling catheters at the site of insertion or at the site of tube junctions.

> ▣ **Critical Rescue** ◆ To prevent infections, ensure that all catheter line connections are secure and that an occlusive, sterile dressing is maintained over the catheter site.

  8. There is a risk for respiratory depression resulting from high plasma or cerebrospinal fluid concentrations of the instilled drug. Monitor the patient's respirations and sedation level at frequent intervals during and after the administration of epidural opioids and immediately report any concerns to the health care provider.

9. Urinary retention is a common problem associated with epidural analgesia, which is more likely to occur in men than in woman.

10. Lower motor weakness is common when an epidural local anesthetic is used in combination with an opioid. Assist patients who get out of bed for the first time to determine the degree of leg weakness.

> **Clinical Landmine** ◆ Do not delegate this activity and assessment to unlicensed assistive personnel!

- Adjuvant analgesics may be used to relieve pain alone or in combination with other analgesics by potentiating or enhancing the effectiveness of the analgesic.
  1. Antiepileptic drugs (AEDs or anticonvulsants)
     a. Gabapentin (Neurontin)
     b. Pregabalin (Lyrica)
     c. Topiramate (Topamax)
  2. Tricyclic antidepressants
     a. Amitriptyline (Elavil)
     b. Nortriptyline (Pamelor)
     c. Imipramine (Tofranil)
  3. Other antidepressants
     a. Trazodone (Desyrel)
     b. Paroxetine (Paxil)
     c. Sertraline (Zoloft)
  4. Antianxiety drugs
     a. Alprazolam (Xanax)
     b. Lorazepam (Ativan)
     c. Oxazepam (Serax, Zapex)
     d. Clonazepam (Klonopin)
  5. Oral local anesthetics
  6. Local anesthesia infusion pumps
  7. Topical drugs
     a. Lidocaine patch (Lidoderm patch)
     b. Lidocaine and prilocaine (EMLA cream)
     c. Lidocaine (ELA-Max cream)
  8. Local, short-acting gels and creams for cryotherapy
     a. BioFreeze
     b. Ben Gay
- Nonpharmacologic interventions
  1. Physical measures
     a. Cutaneous (skin) stimulation strategies
        (1) Application of heat, cold, and pressure
        (2) Therapeutic touch

      (3) Massage
      (4) Vibration
   b. Physical and occupational therapy
      (1) Exercises
      (2) Heat, cold, or massage
      (3) Splinting of joints
   c. Transcutaneous electrical nerve stimulation (TENS)
  2. Cognitive-behavioral measures
   a. Distraction
   b. Imagery
   c. Relaxation
   d. Hypnosis
   e. Music therapy
   f. Aromatherapy
   g. Prayer and meditation
  3. Other complementary and alternative therapies
   a. Magnet therapy
   b. Acupuncture
   c. Herbal supplements
- Invasive techniques for chronic pain
  1. Nerve blocks
  2. Spinal cord stimulation

Surgical Management

- *Rhizotomy* is the destruction of specific sensory nerve roots at the point where they enter the spinal cord. In a *closed* rhizotomy, a percutaneous catheter is inserted into the area, and the sensory nerve roots are destroyed by chemicals, coagulation, or cryodestruction (extreme cold). A laminectomy is necessary for an *open* rhizotomy. During this surgery, the health care provider isolates and destroys the nerve roots.
- *Cordotomy* is severing of the pain pathways at the midline portion of the spinal cord to prevent nerve impulses from ascending to the spinothalamic tract. As with the other surgical procedures, patients may experience impaired bowel, bladder, or sexual function.
- After surgical intervention, assess the nature of the neurologic deficits, if any, and teach the patient how to adapt to them.
- If the patient has lost sensation in a body area, teach him or her how to protect that area from harm.
- Assess expectations in relation to the surgery and help the patient to express realistic expectations.

Community-Based Care

- Ensure that the patient, especially one who is on opioids, has enough pain medication to last at least until the first follow-up visit.

- Collaborate with the patient and family, case manager or discharge planner, and occupational therapist to determine whether modifications are necessary for maintaining a reasonably pain-free regimen after discharge.
- Make appropriate referrals for physical therapy, a clinical nurse specialist in pain management, a social worker, and hospice or palliative care.
- Well-defined home agency practices and professional support at home are required if patients leave the hospital with infusion therapy for pain management.
- Teach the patient and family about analgesic regimens, including any technical skills needed to administer or deliver the analgesic, the purpose and action of various drugs, their side effects or adverse reactions, and the importance of dosage intervals.
- If the patient is on a flexible analgesic schedule, teach the patient and family how to safely increase the drug within the prescribed dosing guidelines.
- Evaluate family support systems to assist the patient in adhering to and continuing the proposed medical treatment and nursing plans.
- Suggest ways for the patient to continue participation in household, social, sexual, and work-oriented activities after discharge.
- Help identify important activities and plan them around adequate rest schedules.
- Help the patient and family to identify coping strategies that have worked in the past.
- Plan a home care nurse referral for patients who will require assistance or supervision with their pain relief regimen at home.
- When severe chronic or intractable pain exists, direct the patient and family to appropriate resources, such as pain centers or providers who specialize in pain management.

PERIOPERATIVE CARE

PREOPERATIVE ISSUES

OVERVIEW

- The preoperative period begins when the patient is scheduled for surgery and ends at the time of transfer to the surgical suite.
- The primary roles of the nurse are educator, patient advocate, and promoter of health.

- *Inpatient* refers to a patient who is admitted to a hospital the day before or the day of surgery and requires hospitalization after surgery.
- *Outpatient* and *ambulatory* refer to a patient who goes to the surgical area the day of the surgery and returns home on the same day (i.e., same-day surgery [SDS]).
- The primary reasons for surgery are:
  1. Diagnostic
  2. Curative
  3. Restorative
  4. Palliative
  5. Cosmetic
- The urgency of surgery may be:
  1. Elective
  2. Urgent
  3. Emergency
- The risk of surgery may be:
  1. Minor
  2. Major
- The extent of surgery can be:
  1. Simple
  2. Radical
  3. Minimally invasive surgery (MIS)

Considerations for Older Adults

- The older adult may have a variety of physical changes and psychosocial issues that can have an impact on the planning of care and outcome of surgery.
- Physical changes may include:
  1. Greater incidence of chronic illness
  2. Greater incidence of malnutrition
  3. Decreased ability to withstand the stress of surgery and anesthesia
  4. Increased risk for cardiopulmonary complications after surgery
  5. Risk of a change in mental status when admitted (related to unfamiliar surroundings, change in routine, drugs given, and so forth)
  6. Increased risk of a fall and resultant injury
- Psychosocial issues may include:
  1. Increased incidence of impaired self-care abilities
  2. Inadequate support systems

PATIENT-CENTERED COLLABORATIVE CARE

Assessment

- Obtain patient information about:
  1. Age
  2. Use of tobacco, alcohol, or illicit substances, including marijuana
  3. Current drugs, especially:
     a. Antihypertensives
     b. Tricyclic antidepressants
     c. Anticoagulants
     d. NSAIDs
  4. Use of complementary or alternative practices, such as herbal therapies, folk remedies, or acupuncture
  5. Medical history, especially:
     a. Decreased immunity, infection
     b. Diabetes
     c. Pulmonary disease
     d. Cardiac disease or hemodynamic instability
     e. Multisystem disease
     f. Anemia or coagulation defect or disorder
     g. Dehydration
     h. Hypertension or hypotension
     i. Any chronic disease
  6. Prior surgical procedures, experience with anesthesia, pain control, and how these were tolerated
     a. Less-than-optimal emotional reaction
     b. Anesthesia reactions or complications
     c. Postoperative complications
  7. Autologous or directed blood donations

▼ National Patient Safety Goal

If the patient has made arrangements for an autologous blood transfusion, verify that the patient is wearing the identification band provided by the blood bank. This band or tag is used to match up with the identification on the blood bag to ensure the patient receives his or her own blood in a transfusion.

  8. Allergies, including sensitivity to latex products
  9. General health
     a. Malnutrition
     b. Obesity
     c. Poor coping skills
  10. Family history
     a. Malignant hyperthermia
     b. Cancer
     c. Bleeding disorder

11. Type of surgery planned
    a. Neck, oral, or facial procedures (airway complications)
    b. Chest or high abdominal procedures (pulmonary complications)
    c. Abdominal surgery (paralytic ileus, deep vein thrombosis [DVT])
12. Knowledge about and understanding of events during the perioperative period
13. Adequacy of the patient's support system
- Perform a complete physical assessment before surgery to obtain baseline data, and identify current health problems, potential complications related to anesthesia, and possible complications that may occur after surgery.

> 🗋 **Critical Rescue** ◆ Report and document any abnormal findings to the surgeon and the anesthesia provider immediately. Some abnormalities must be corrected before surgery.

1. Vital signs
2. Cardiovascular status
   a. Assess for hypertension.
   b. Auscultate heart sounds for rate, regularity, and abnormalities.
   c. Assess hands and feet for temperature, color, peripheral pulses, capillary refill, and edema.
   d. Ask about chest pain, shortness of breath, and dyspnea.
3. Respiratory status
   a. Obtain a smoking history (including exposure to second-hand smoke).
   b. Observe posture; respiratory rate, rhythm, and depth; overall respiratory effort; and lung expansion.
   c. Check for clubbing of the fingertips or cyanosis.
   d. Auscultate the lungs for crackles, wheezes, or rubs.
   e. Assess oxygen saturation.
4. Renal status—ask about or check:
   a. Frequency of urination
   b. Dysuria
   c. Nocturia
   d. Difficulty starting urine flow
   e. Oliguria
   f. Appearance and odor of the urine
   g. Usual fluid intake and degree of continence
5. Neurologic status—ask about or check:
   a. Level of consciousness and orientation
   b. Ability to follow commands

    c. Specific motor or sensory deficits

    d. Any hearing or vision problems

    e. Risk for falls (check ability to ambulate and the steadiness of gait)

  6. Musculoskeletal status—ask about or check:

    a. Arthritis

    b. Any limited joint motion

    c. Presence of joint replacements

    d. Skeletal deformities

    e. Shape and length of the neck and the shape of the chest cavity

  7. Nutritional status (malnutrition and obesity can increase surgical risk), assessing for these indicators of poor fluid or nutritional status:

    a. Brittle nails

    b. Muscle wasting

    c. Dry or flaky skin, decreased skin turgor

    d. Dull, sparse, or dry hair

    e. Orthostatic (postural) hypotension

    f. Decreased serum protein levels

    g. Abnormal serum electrolyte values

- Psychosocial issues can affect the patient's ability to learn, cope, and cooperate with operative procedures or postoperative interventions. Determine the level of:

  1. Anxiety and fear

  2. Coping skills

- Laboratory assessment, report any abnormalities in:

  1. Urinalysis

  2. Blood type and screen

  3. CBC or hemoglobin level and hematocrit

  4. Clotting studies (prothrombin time [PT], international normalized ratio [INR], activated partial thromboplastin time [aPTT], and platelet count)

  5. Electrolyte levels

    a. Hypokalemia

    b. Hyperkalemia

  6. Serum creatinine and blood urea nitrogen levels

  7. Possible pregnancy testing

  8. Other studies based on the patient's medical history

- Other assessment data may include:

  1. Chest x-ray

  2. Electrocardiogram

  3. Additional studies based on the patient's history

Planning and Implementation

❖NDx: Deficient Knowledge

- Explore the patient's level of knowledge and understanding, and then provide information about informed consent, dietary restrictions, specific preparation for surgery (bowel and skin preparations), exercises after surgery, and plans for pain management.

- *Informed consent* is obtained from the patient (or legal designee) by the surgeon before sedation is given and before surgery is performed.
- Clarify facts that have been presented by the surgeon and dispel myths that the patient or family may have about the surgical experience. Ensure that the consent form is signed by serving as a witness to the signature, not to the fact that the patient is informed.
- *Consent* implies that the patient has sufficient information to understand:
  1. The nature of and reason for surgery
  2. Who will perform the surgery and whether others will be present during the procedure
  3. All available options and the risks associated with each option
  4. The risks associated with the surgical procedure and its potential outcomes
  5. The risks associated with the use of anesthesia

> 🛟 **Critical Rescue** ◆ If you believe that the patient has not been adequately informed, contact the surgeon and request that he or she see the patient for further clarification.

- A competent adult has the right to refuse treatment for any reason, even when refusal might lead to death.

🚩 National Patient Safety Goal

For surgical procedures that are site specific, such as left, right, or bilateral, ask the competent patient to mark the site with a marker to ensure the correct site is used and the wrong site is avoided. At a minimum, the patient's identity, correct side and site, correct patient position, agreement on the proposed procedure, and availability of correct implants and equipment must be verified by all members of the surgical team.

- Routine preoperative care includes:
  1. Determining the existence and nature of the patient's advance directives
  2. Implementing dietary restrictions
     a. NPO means no eating, drinking (including water), or smoking.
     b. Recommendations are 6 or more hours for easily digested solid food and 2 hours for clear liquids.

    c. Failure to adhere to NPO status can result in cancellation of surgery or increase the risk for aspiration during or after surgery.

3. Administering regularly scheduled drugs
   a. Most drugs are discontinued before surgery or given IV.
   b. Others, especially for cardiac disease, respiratory disease, seizures, and hypertension, are usually allowed before surgery with a sip of water.

4. Ensuring intestinal preparation
   a. Before bowel or intestinal surgery, using "enemas until clear," GoLYTELY (in the prescribed strength), or antibiotics to ensure bacterial reduction
   b. Bowel evacuation before major abdominal, pelvic, perineal, or perianal surgery, using simple enema or laxative, according to agency policy and surgeon preference

5. Performing skin preparation
   a. Showering with an antiseptic solution to remove oil or debris and reduce the number of organisms at the site
   b. Clipping hair with electrical clippers
   c. Shaving of the area (controversial) immediately before the start of the surgical procedure

6. Preparing the patient for tubes, drains, and vascular access
   a. Describe the purpose and placement of each device.
   b. Show the devices to the patient and family.
   c. Reassure the patient that these are temporary and that efforts will be made to reduce discomfort.
   d. Common devices include:
      (1) Foley catheter
      (2) NG tube
      (3) Drains (Penrose, Jackson-Pratt, Hemovac)
      (4) Vascular access

7. Teaching about procedures and exercises to prevent respiratory complications
   a. Deep, diaphragmatic breathing
   b. Expansion breathing
   c. Incentive spirometry
   d. Coughing and splinting
   e. Turning

8. Teaching about procedures and exercises to prevent cardiovascular complications
   a. Assessing for deep vein thrombosis (DVT)
   b. Swelling in one leg

    c. Presence of calf pain that worsens with ambulation

    d. Antiembolism stockings (TED or Jobst stockings) and elastic (Ace) wraps

    e. Pneumatic compression devices

    f. Leg exercises

    g. Early ambulation

    h. ROM exercises

❖**NDx:** Anxiety

- Assess the patient's knowledge about the surgical experience.
- Provide factual information.
  1. Allow ample time for questions.
  2. Respond to questions accurately.
  3. Ensure unanswered questions are addressed by the proper person.
- Incorporate support systems into the plan of care.
- Provide prescribed antianxiety drugs.
- Encourage communication.
- Promote rest and relaxation.
- Provide opportunity for distraction.
- Teach family members.
- Ensure family members remain in the information loop.
  1. Explain the routines expected before, during, and after surgery.
  2. Direct family to appropriate waiting area.

Final Preoperative Preparation

- Review the preoperative chart for:
  1. Completion of surgical informed consent form and any other special consent forms
     a. Patient's signature
     b. Date
     c. Witnesses' signatures
  2. Confirmation that the scheduled procedure is what is listed on the consent form

🛡️ **National Patient Safety Goal**

For surgical procedures that are site specific, such as left, right, or bilateral, ask the patient to mark the site with a marker to ensure the correct site is used and the wrong site is avoided.

  3. Documentation of allergies
  4. Accurate height and weight
  5. Documentation of the results of all laboratory, radiographic, and diagnostic tests are on the chart
  6. Presence of autologous blood donor or directed blood donations slips (if appropriate)

7. Documentation of current vital signs (within 1 to 2 hours of the scheduled surgery time)
8. Documentation of any significant physical or psychosocial observations
9. Communication of special needs, concerns, and instructions to the surgical team
   a. Advance directives
   b. No use of blood products
   c. Communication difficulties (visually impaired, hearing impaired, does not speak the main language of the institution)

- Patient preparation
   1. Appropriate clothing removal
   2. Application of prescribed antiembolism stockings or pneumatic compression devices
   3. Ensuring proper storage of valuables
   4. Ensuring proper patient identification
   5. Removing and safe-keeping of dentures, prosthetic devices, contact lenses, glasses, wigs, toupees, and hairpins and clips
   6. Taping rings securely or removing them (with the patient's permission)
   7. Following agency policy for removal of fingernail polish and artificial nails
   8. Ensuring the patient empties his or her bladder

- Prescribed preoperative drugs:
   1. Positively identifying the patient (using the arm band and asking the patient to state his or her name)
   2. Ensuring the operative permit is signed
   3. Administering the correct drugs in the correct dosages
   4. Raising the siderails
   5. Placing the call system within easy reach of the patient
   6. Reminding him or her not to try to get out of bed
   7. Placing the bed in a low position

- Patient transfer to the surgical suite

INTRAOPERATIVE ISSUES

OVERVIEW

- The intraoperative period begins when the patient enters the surgical suite and ends at the time of transfer to the postanesthesia recovery area, same-day surgery unit, or the intensive care unit.
- Basic surgical team members include:
   1. The *surgeon*, a physician who assumes responsibility for the surgical procedure and any surgical judgments about the patient

2. The *anesthesia provider*, who gives anesthetic drugs to induce and maintain anesthesia and delivers other drugs as needed to support the patient during surgery
    a. *Anesthesiologist*, a physician who specializes in giving anesthetic agents
    b. *Certified registered nurse anesthetist (CRNA)*, who is a registered nurse with additional education and credentials and who delivers anesthetic agents under the supervision of an anesthesiologist, surgeon, dentist, or podiatrist
3. *Perioperative nursing staff*, whose main concerns are the safety and advocacy for the patient during surgery
    a. *Holding area nurse* coordinates and manages the care of the patient in the presurgical holding area next to the main operating room (OR). This nurse assesses the patient's physical and emotional status, gives emotional support, answers questions, and provides additional education as needed.
    b. *Circulating nurse* is responsible for coordinating all activities within that particular OR. He or she sets up the OR and ensures that supplies, including blood products and diagnostic support, are available as needed. This nurse positions the patient, assists the anesthesia provider, inserts a Foley catheter if needed, and scrubs the surgical site before the patient is draped with sterile drapes. Other responsibilities include:
        (1) Monitoring traffic in the room
        (2) Assessing the amount of urine and blood loss
        (3) Reporting findings to the surgeon and anesthesia provider
        (4) Ensuring that sterile technique and a sterile field are maintained
        (5) Communicating information about the patient's status to family members
        (6) Documenting care, events, interventions, and findings
        (7) Completing documentation in the OR and nursing records about the presence of drains or catheters, the length of the surgery, and a count of all sponges, "sharps" (needles, blades), and instruments
    c. *Scrub nurse* sets up the sterile field, drapes the patient, and hands sterile supplies, sterile equipment, and instruments to the surgeon and the assistant. This person also maintains an accurate count of sponges, sharps, instruments, and amounts of irrigation fluid and drugs used.
    d. *Specialty nurse* may be in charge of a particular type of surgical specialty (e.g., orthopedic, cardiac, ophthalmologic)

and is responsible for nursing care specific to patients needing that type of surgery.

- Safe environment
  1. All members of the surgical team and other support personnel in the surgical suite are free of communicable diseases.
  2. Good personal hygiene and no jewelry
  3. Appropriate use of surgical attire (e.g., shirt and pants, cap or hood, shoe coverings)
  4. Use of protective attire (e.g., mask, eyewear, gloves, gown)
  5. Scrubbed team members also wear sterile fluid-resistant gown, sterile gloves, and eye protectors, or face shields.
- Types of anesthesia and complications
  1. *General anesthesia* is a reversible loss of consciousness induced by inhibiting neuronal impulses in several areas of the central nervous system (CNS). The patient is unconscious, unaware, and has loss of muscle tone and reflexes. Agents are administered by inhalation and IV injection.
     a. Complications include malignant hyperthermia (MH), an acute, life-threatening complication of certain drugs in which skeletal muscle exposed to specific agents increase calcium levels and metabolism leading to acidosis, cardiac dysrhythmias, and a high body temperature.
        (1) MH is a genetic disorder with an autosomal dominant pattern of inheritance and is most common in young, well-muscled men.
        (2) Drugs most associated with it are halothane, enflurane, isoflurane, desflurane, sevoflurane, and succinylcholine.
     b. Overdose of anesthesia can occur when the patient's metabolism and drug elimination are slower than expected, such as in an older patient or one who has liver or kidney problems.
     c. Unrecognized hypoventilation with failure to exchange gases adequately can lead to cardiac arrest, permanent brain damage, and death.
     d. Intubation complications from improper neck extension or anatomic differences in a patient can lead to broken or injured teeth and caps, swollen lip, or vocal cord trauma.
  2. *Local or regional anesthesia* can briefly disrupt sensory nerve impulse transmission from a specific body area or region. The patient remains conscious and able to follow instructions.
     a. Local anesthesia is delivered topically (applied to the skin or mucous membranes of the area to be anesthetized) and by local infiltration.

b. Regional anesthesia is a type of local anesthesia that blocks multiple peripheral nerves in a specific body region. Types of regional anesthesia include field block, nerve block, spinal, and epidural.

c. Complications are most associated with overdoses, inadvertent systemic drug delivery, or patient allergic reactions to the agent.

3. *Conscious sedation* is the IV delivery of sedative, hypnotic, and opioid drugs to reduce the level of consciousness but allow the patient to maintain a patent airway and to respond to verbal commands. It is used most often in the emergency department or in procedures rooms before short but uncomfortable procedures.

PATIENT-CENTERED COLLABORATIVE CARE

Assessment

- Correct identification of the patient is the responsibility of every member of the health care team (i.e., National Patient Safety Goals).
  1. Verify the patient's identity with *two types of identifiers* (name, birth date, medical record number, or social security number).
     a. Check the patient's identification bracelet.
     b. Ask the patient, "What is your name, and what is your birth date?"
  2. Validate that the surgical consent form has been signed and witnessed.
     a. Ask the patient, "What kind of operation are you having today?"
     b. Compare patient responses to the information on the operative permit and the operative schedule.
     c. When the procedure involves a specific site, validate the side on which a procedure is to be performed.
     d. Investigate *any* discrepancy and notify the surgeon.
- Validate that all aspects of the checklist are complete.
  1. Ask the patient about any allergies.
  2. Determine whether autologous blood was donated.
  3. Check the patient's attire to ensure adherence with facility policy.
  4. Remove dentures, dental prostheses (e.g., bridges, retainers), jewelry (including body piercing), eyeglasses, contact lenses, hearing aids, wigs, and other prostheses.
- Review the medical record for:
  1. Advance directives and do not resuscitate orders
  2. Previous reactions to anesthesia or blood transfusions
     a. Allergies to iodine products or shellfish
     b. Latex allergies

3. Laboratory and diagnostic test results
4. Medical history and physical examination findings

Planning and Implementation

❖**NDx:** Risk for Perioperative-Positioning Injury
- Ensure proper positioning.
  1. Padding the operating bed with foam or silicone gel pads, or both
  2. Properly placing the grounding pads
  3. Assisting the patient to a comfortable position
  4. Assessing the skin for bruising or injury, and applying extra padding as needed
  5. Modifying the patient's position according to the patient's safety and special needs
  6. Avoiding excessive joint abduction
  7. Securing the arms firmly on an arm board, positioned at shoulder level
  8. Supporting the wrist with padding and not overtightening wrist straps
  9. Placing safety straps above or below the nerve locations
  10. Maintaining minimal external rotation of the hips
  11. Supporting the lower extremities
  12. Not placing equipment on lower extremities
  13. Urging OR personnel to avoid leaning on the patient's lower extremities
  14. Maintaining the patient's extremities in good anatomic alignment by slightly flexing joints and supporting with pillows, trochanter rolls, or pads
- Observe for complications of special positioning, such as wrist-drop or footdrop, loss of sensation, changes in extremity temperature or circulation, and inflammation.

❖**NDx:** Risk for Infection
- Identify patients with preexisting health problems such as diabetes mellitus, immunodeficiency, obesity, and renal failure.
- Perform prescribed skin preparation.
- Protect the patient's exposure to cross contamination.
- Ensure the use of sterile surgical technique, protective drapes, skin closures, and dressings.

❖**NDx:** Potential for Hypoventilation
- Continuously monitor the patient according to official standards, including:
  1. Breathing
  2. Circulation
  3. Cardiac rhythm
  4. Blood pressure
  5. Heart rate
  6. Oxygen saturation

POSTOPERATIVE ISSUES

OVERVIEW

- The postoperative period starts at the completion of surgery and transfer of the patient to the postanesthesia care unit (PACU), SDS unit (ambulatory care unit), or the intensive care unit (ICU).
- The postoperative period continues after the patient's condition is stabilized and after the patient is discharged from the ambulatory surgery facility or hospital.
- On arrival to the PACU, the anesthesia provider and the circulating nurse give the PACU nurse a verbal "hand-off" report to communicate the patient's condition and care needs.

⧫ National Patient Safety Goal

A hand-off report requires effective communication between health care professionals and is at least a two-way verbal interaction between the professional giving the report and the nurse receiving it. The language used by the report giver is clear and cannot be interpreted in more than one way. The nurse receiving the report focuses on the report and is not distracted by the environment or other responsibilities. The receiving nurse takes the time to restate (report back) the information to verify what was said and to make certain the reporting professional and the receiving nurse have the same understanding. The receiving nurse takes the time to ask questions, and the reporting professional must respond to the questions until a common understanding is established.

- The handoff report should contain the following information:
  1. Type and extent of the surgical procedure
  2. Type of anesthesia and length of time the patient was under anesthesia
  3. Tolerance of anesthesia and the surgical procedure
  4. Allergies (especially to latex or drugs)
  5. Pathologic condition
  6. Oxygen saturation
  7. Status of vital signs
  8. Core body temperature
  9. Type and amount of IV fluids and drugs administered
  10. Estimated blood loss (EBL)
  11. Any intraoperative complications, such as a traumatic intubation
  12. Preoperative drugs and patient responses
  13. Primary language, any sensory impairments, any communication difficulties
  14. Anxiety level before receiving anesthesia

15. Special requests that were verbalized by the patient preoperatively
16. Preoperative and intraoperative respiratory function and dysfunction
17. Pertinent medical history, including substance abuse
18. Location and type of incisions, dressings, catheters, tubes, drains, or packing
19. Intake and output, including current IV fluid administration and estimated blood loss
20. Prosthetic devices
21. Joint or limb immobility while in the OR, especially in the older patient
22. Other intraoperative positioning that may be relevant in the postoperative phase
23. Intraoperative complications, how managed, patient responses
24. Any other important intraoperative occurrences

PATIENT-CENTERED COLLABORATIVE CARE

Assessment

- The initial assessment of the patient immediately after surgery includes respiration, oxygen saturation, level of consciousness, temperature, pulse, and blood pressure.
- Examine the surgical area for bleeding.
- Assess vital signs on admission and then at least every 15 minutes until the patient's condition is stable. Frequency of assessment is then based on agency policy and patient responses.
- Routine postoperative monitoring and assessment includes:
  1. Respiratory status by assessing:
     a. Patent airway and gas exchange by oxygen saturation and end-tidal carbon dioxide levels
     b. Presence of an artificial airway (endotracheal tube, a nasal trumpet, oral airway)
     c. Type of delivery device and the concentration or liter flow of the oxygen

> **Critical Rescue** ◆ If the SpO₂ drops below the level of 95% or the patient's baseline, notify the surgeon or anesthesia provider. If it drops by 10 percentage points and you are certain it is an accurate measure, call the Rapid Response Team.

     d. Rate, pattern, and depth of breathing
     e. Auscultate all lung fields for breath sounds.
     f. Check symmetry of breath sounds and chest movement.
     g. Listen for snoring and stridor.

   h. Check for skeletal muscle weakness by assessing.
     (1) Inability to maintain a head lift
     (2) Weak hand grasps
     (3) Abdominal breathing pattern.
2. Cardiovascular status by assessing:
   a. Heart rate, quality, and rhythm
   b. Blood pressure
   c. Compare findings for trends.

> 🔲 **Critical Rescue** ◆ Report blood pressure changes that are 25% higher or lower than values obtained before surgery (a 15- to 20-point difference, systolic or diastolic) to the anesthesia provider or the surgeon.

   d. Electrocardiography for dysrhythmias
   e. Comparing distal pulses, color, temperature, and capillary refill on extremities
   f. Checking feet and legs for manifestations of DVT (e.g., redness, pain, warmth, swelling)
   g. Applying prescribed compression devices or antiembolic stockings
3. Neurologic status by assessing:
   a. Level of consciousness or awareness
   b. Presence of lethargy, restlessness, or irritability
   c. Patient responses to stimuli (calling the name, touching the patient, and giving simple commands such as "Open your eyes" and "Take a deep breath")
   d. Degree of orientation to person, place, and time by asking the conscious patient to answer questions such as "What is your name?" (person), "Where are you?" (place), and "What day is it?" (time)
   e. Comparing the patient's baseline neurologic status (obtained before surgery) with the findings after surgery
4. Motor and sensory function status by:
   a. Asking the patient to move each extremity
   b. Assessing the strength of each limb and comparing the results on both sides
   c. Gradually elevating the patient's head and monitoring for hypotension
5. Assessing fluid, electrolyte, and acid-base balance by:
   a. Measuring intake and output (including IV fluid intake, vomitus, urine, wound drainage, nasogastric tube drainage)
   b. Checking hydration status (e.g., inspecting the color and moisture of mucous membranes; the turgor, texture, and

"tenting" of the skin; the amount of drainage on dressings; and the presence of axillary sweat)

   c. Comparing total output with total intake to identify a possible fluid imbalance

6. Renal or urinary status by:
   a. Measuring intake and output
   b. Assessing for urine retention by inspection, palpation, percussion of the lower abdomen for bladder distention, or use of a bladder scanner
   c. Performing prescribed intermittent catheterization
   d. Assessing urine for color, clarity, and amount
   e. Assessing voiding for frequency, amount per void, and any symptoms

> 🛟 **Critical Rescue** ◆ Report a urine output of less than 30 mL/hr (240 mL per 8-hour nursing shift) to the surgeon.

7. GI status by:
   a. Listening for bowel sounds in all four abdominal quadrants and at the umbilicus
   b. Assessing for nausea and vomiting
   c. Administering prescribed antiemetic drugs
   d. Assessing for manifestations of paralytic ileus (few or absent bowel sounds, a distended abdomen, abdominal discomfort, vomiting, and no passage of flatus or stool)
   e. Assessing and recording the color, consistency, and amount of the NG tube drainage
   f. Checking NG tube placement

> 🛠 **Clinical Landmine** ◆ After gastric surgery, do not move or irrigate the tube without an order from the surgeon.

8. Skin status by:
   a. Assessing the incision (if visible) for redness, increased warmth, swelling, tenderness or pain, and the type and amount of drainage
   b. Condition of the sutures or staples
   c. Presence of open areas

9. Dressings and drains for:
   a. Color, amount, consistency, and odor of drainage
   b. Leakage around or under the patient
   c. Patency of drains
   d. Any restriction of circulation or sensation

10. Pain

11. Psychosocial issues of anxiety, restlessness, fear

Planning and Implementation

❖**NDx:** Impaired Gas Exchange

- Interventions in the PACU may include:
  1. Monitoring for snoring or stridor that indicate obstruction
  2. Inserting an oral airway or a nasal airway (nasal trumpet) to keep the airway open
  3. Keeping the manual resuscitation bag and emergency equipment for intubation or tracheostomy nearby
  4. Positioning the patient in a side-lying position to prevent aspiration
  5. Suctioning the mouth, nose, and throat to keep the airway clear of mucus or vomitus as needed
  6. Keeping the patient's head flat to prevent hypotension and possible shock, unless this position is contraindicated by the condition or surgical procedure
  7. Applying prescribed oxygen by face tent, nasal cannula, or mask
  8. Raising the head of the bed (after the patient is fully reactive and stable)
  9. Assisting the patient to cough (with the incision splinted), deeply breathe, and use the incentive spirometer
  10. Performing mouth care after removing secretions
- Interventions for inpatients after PACU care may include:
  1. Encouraging the patient to continue coughing, deep breathing, and incentive spirometry exercises
  2. Assisting the patient out of bed and to ambulate as soon as possible
  3. Assisting the patient to turn at least every 2 hours (side to side)
  4. Offering prescribed pain medication 30 to 45 minutes before the patient gets out of bed

❖**NDx:** Impaired Skin Integrity

Nonsurgical Management

- Wound care includes reinforcing the dressing, changing the dressing, assessing the wound for healing and infection, and caring for drains, including emptying, measuring, and documenting drainage features.
  1. The initial dressing is often changed by the surgeon.
     a. Reinforce the dressing (add more dressing material to the existing dressing) if it becomes wet from drainage.
     b. Document the added material and the color, type, amount, and odor of drainage fluid and time of observation.
  2. Routine wound care and dressing changes include:
     a. Changing gauze dressings at least once during a nursing shift or daily

   b. Cleaning the area with sterile saline or some other solution as prescribed

   c. Assessing the skin in areas where tape has been used for redness, rash, or blisters

   d. Assessing the incision for integrity, condition, and healing stage

   e. Assessing the incision for wound infection:
     (1) Redness, heat, and swelling
     (2) Drainage of purulent or foul-smelling material

   f. Removing sutures or staples according to agency policy and surgeon request

   g. Removing or advancing drains according to agency policy and surgeon request

   h. Administering prescribed antibiotic therapy

Surgical Management

- Poorly healing wounds, infected wounds, or complicated wounds may require surgical intervention.
- Management of *dehiscence*, which is opening of all or part of a wound down to the visceral peritoneum
  1. Apply a sterile nonadherent (e.g., Telfa) or saline dressing to the wound and notify the surgeon.
  2. Instruct the patient to bend the knees and to avoid coughing.
  3. The surgeon may reclose the wound or leave it open to heal by second intention.
- Management of *evisceration*, which is a wound opening with protrusion of internal organs. *This condition is a surgical emergency.*
  1. Call for help! Instruct the person who responds to notify the surgeon or Rapid Response Team immediately and to bring any needed supplies into the patient's room.
  2. Stay with the patient.
  3. Cover the wound with a nonadherent dressing premoistened with warmed sterile normal saline.
  4. If premoistened dressings are not available, moisten sterile gauze or sterile towels in a sterile irrigation tray with sterile saline, and then cover the wound.
  5. If saline is not immediately available, cover the wound with gauze and then moisten with sterile saline using a sterile irrigation tray as soon as someone brings saline.
  6. Do not attempt to reinsert the protruding organ or viscera.
  7. While covering the wound, observe the patient's response and assess for manifestations of shock.
  8. Place the patient in a supine position with the hips and knees bent.

9. Raise the head of the bed 15 to 20 degrees.
10. Take vital signs and document them.
11. Provide support and reassurance to the patient.
12. Continue assessing the patient, including vital signs assessment, every 5 to 10 minutes until the surgeon arrives.
13. Keep dressings continuously moist by adding warmed sterile saline to the dressing as often as necessary. *Do not let the dressing become dry.*
14. When the surgeon arrives, report your finding and your interventions. Then follow the surgeon's directions.
15. Document the incident, the activity the patient was engaged in at the time of the incident, your actions, and your assessments.
16. The surgeon performs surgery in the OR with the patient under general, regional, or local anesthesia to close the wound. Stay or retention sutures of wire or nylon are usually used in addition to or instead of standard sutures or staples.

❖**NDx:** Acute Pain

- Opioids and non-opioids are routinely given in the early postoperative period.
- Drugs are given IV initially and then are administered orally.
- Around-the-clock scheduling is more effective than "on-demand" scheduling because more constant blood levels are achieved.
- PCA by IV infusion or internal pump (the catheter is sutured into or near the surgical area) may be used.
- Epidural analgesia can be given intermittently by the anesthesia provider or by continuous drip through an epidural catheter left in place after epidural anesthesia.
- See the "Pain" section on p. 45 for an in-depth presentation of pain assessment and pain control interventions.

❖**NDx:** Potential for Hypoxemia

- The highest incidence of hypoxemia after surgery occurs on the second postoperative day. Those at highest risk are older adults and patients with lung disease.
- The key to preventing hypoxemia is to follow the interventions for the nursing diagnosis of "Impaired Gas Exchange" (p. 71).
- Monitor the patient's oxygen saturation (Spo_2) with pulse oximetry.
- Apply prescribed oxygen as needed.
- Prevent hypothermia.
- Ensure that prescribed respiratory treatments are performed.
- Mechanical ventilation may be needed if other interventions are not successful in maintaining adequate oxygen saturation.

Community-Based Care

- Discharge planning, teaching, and referral begin before surgery and continue after surgery.
- Provide written discharge instructions for the patient to follow at home.
- Assess the need for assistance with wound care and ADLs.
- The teaching plan for the patient and family after surgery includes:
  1. Prevention of infection
  2. Care and assessment of the surgical wound
  3. Management of drains or catheters
  4. Nutrition therapy
  5. Pain management
  6. Drug therapy
  7. Progressive increase in activity
  8. Follow-up with the surgeon
- Ensure that appropriate referrals are made to a social worker, home care agency, skilled nursing care, Meals on Wheels, support groups, and homemaker services.

SUBSTANCE ABUSE

OVERVIEW

- Substance abuse is the excessive use of a chemical substance, such as drugs and alcohol, and the resulting physical and psychological dependence that interferes with life's activities.
- It is a documented nursing diagnosis when the patient:
  1. Loses control in use of the drug
  2. Ingests the drug even though the drug has caused adverse conditions in the body
  3. Demonstrates cognitive, behavioral, and physiologic disturbances with the abuse of drugs or inhalants
- *Dependence* is a condition that causes a habitual, compulsive, and uncontrollable urge to use a substance. Without the substance, the body experiences severe physiologic, psychological, and emotional disturbances.
- *Substance use* is taking chemicals for pleasure without dependence.
- *Substance misuse* occurs when people use chemicals for reasons other than their intended action.
- *Addiction* causes negative outcomes after abusers stop using the substances. It is a disease caused by changes in the brain that affect human behavior, and it is manifested by substance craving, seeking, and subsequent use.

- *Withdrawal syndrome* symptoms may result if the drug is eliminated suddenly, such as hallucinations, severe irritability, and hyperactivity.
- Many people abuse substances for stress relief.
- Family history of substance abuse increases a person's risk for this behavior.

🌐 Cultural Awareness

- An understanding of the patient's culture helps avoid making assumptions about substance abuse.
- Some behaviors that are interpreted within the Western culture as negative responses are considered normal, even reverent in some cultures, as in the case of avoiding eye contact.

🧬 Genetic Considerations

- Genetic factors appear to contribute to misuse, abuse, or dependence from illicit drug use, as evidenced by studies of twins showing genetic-associated susceptibility to drug abuse and dependence.
- Genes associated with illegal drug abuse are not the same as those associated with abuse of legal substances such as alcohol and nicotine.

〰️ Considerations for Older Adults

- Substance abuse should not be overlooked in the older adult population; the potential is high because of the number of different drugs taken by this age group.
- Common substances abused by older adults include alcohol, drugs, OTC drugs, and herbal preparations.
- Impaired memory may also result in overdosing of OTC or prescribed drugs.

TYPES OF DEPENDENCIES

ALCOHOL

- *Alcoholism (alcohol dependence)* is a disease in which the patient:
  1. Has a strong need (craving) or compulsion to consume alcohol
  2. Is unable to limit alcohol consumption once drinking has begun (loss of control)
  3. Experiences physical dependence
  4. Has a need to increase the amount of alcohol to get the desired effect (tolerance)
- *Alcohol dependence* is present when the person experiences alcohol withdrawal symptoms after habitual use is suddenly

stopped, resulting in nausea, sweating, shakiness, and disorientation.

- When drinking alcohol relieves the symptoms of withdrawal, the person has developed a true physical dependence on alcohol and is considered an *alcoholic.*
- *Alcohol abuse* exists when a person *does not* have a strong craving for alcohol, loss of control, or physical dependence but has problems resulting from alcohol use (e.g., failing to fulfill responsibilities at home, work, or school; drinking in unsafe situations; continuing to drink when problems have been caused or worsened by use of alcohol).
- *At-risk drinking* is five or more of these beverages for men or four or more for women:
  1. 12 ounces of beer
  2. 5 ounces of wine
  3. 1.5 ounces of 80 proof spirits

PATIENT-CENTERED COLLABORATIVE CARE

Assessment

- Tools to identify risk for alcohol problems
  1. CAGE
  2. T-ACE
- Blood alcohol levels (BALs)
  1. Breathalyzer, a BAL of 0.08 is the legal limit.
  2. Standard BALs
     a. 80 to 200 mg/dL (mild to moderate intoxication), with mood and behavior changes, impaired judgment, poor motor coordination, and hypotension (levels greater than 100 mg/dL)
     b. 250 to 400 mg/dL (marked intoxication), with staggering ataxia and emotional liability. May progress to confusion and stupor or coma
     c. Greater than 500 mg/dL (severe intoxication), possible death from respiratory depression
- Manifestations of alcohol withdrawal
  1. Mild (6 to 24 hours after the last drink)
     a. Restlessness, anxiety
     b. Low-grade fever, diaphoresis
     c. Tremors
     d. Headache
     e. Palpitations
     f. Mild hypertension
     g. GI discomfort
     h. Insomnia

2. More severe (24 to 72 hours after the last drink, in addition to mild symptoms)
   a. Delirium tremens (DTs)
   b. Hallucinations (visual or auditory)
   c. Disorientation
   d. Tachycardia and hypertension
   e. Low-grade fever and pronounced diaphoresis
   f. Agitation
   g. Vomiting

Interventions

- Priority during alcohol withdrawal is to protect the patient from self-harm and from harming others.
- Drug therapy
  1. Benzodiazepines to prevent seizures
     a. Chlordiazepoxide (Librium)
     b. Diazepam (Valium)
  2. Beta blockers to reduce cravings, decrease blood pressure
  3. Alpha-adrenergic blockers to decrease withdrawal symptoms
  4. IV fluids
  5. Vitamins (e.g., thiamine)
- Nursing interventions include:
  1. Creating a low-stimulation environment
  2. Monitoring vital signs during withdrawal
  3. Monitoring for DTs
  4. Administering prescribed anticonvulsants or sedatives, as appropriate
  5. Medicating to relieve physical discomfort, as needed
  6. Addressing hallucinations in a therapeutic manner
  7. Maintaining adequate nutrition and fluid intake
  8. Administering prescribed vitamin therapy
  9. Providing emotional support to patient and family
  10. Providing reality orientation

NICOTINE

- Nicotine is one of the most addictive substances in the United States and is the addictive component of tobacco.
- Tobacco use remains the leading cause of *preventable* death in the United States and nicotine continues to be a major contributing factor to the occurrence of cardiovascular disease.
- Several nicotine products are available: cigarettes, pipe tobacco, chewing tobacco, and "spit tobacco."
- Secondhand smoke contributes to the development of cardiovascular disease and lung cancer in nonsmokers.
- The addictive power of nicotine is similar to that of cocaine, and withdrawal symptoms occur when nicotine is discontinued.

PATIENT-CENTERED COLLABORATIVE CARE

- Motivate the patient to quit using nicotine through education.
- Exhibit sensitivity to the actual addiction present with tobacco use.
- Refer patients to community-based support groups and smoking cessation programs, many of which use behavioral models, hypnosis, acupressure, or other modalities tailored to the individual.
- Drug therapy
  1. Bupropion (Zyban, Wellbutrin) can help diminish nicotine craving.
  2. Nicotine patches, gums, or tablets
  3. Low-dose naltrexone (ReVia, Depade) along with a nicotine patch

STIMULANTS

- Stimulants are drugs that excite the cerebral cortex of the brain producing a variety of behavioral responses.
  1. Commonly used stimulants
     a. Amphetamines (street names include *black beauties, cross, hearts*)
     b. Methamphetamines (street names include *biker dope, chalk, speed, crank, crystal, glass, hillbilly crack, meth*)
     c. Cocaine
     d. Minor stimulants (caffeine, nicotine)
  2. Therapeutic effects of stimulants
     a. Improved sense of well-being
     b. Increased mental alertness
     c. Increased capacity to work
     d. Improved performance of motor skills
  3. Manifestations of overdose
     a. Respiratory distress
     b. Hypertension
     c. Ataxia
     d. Fever
     e. Myocardial infarction
     f. Convulsions
     g. Coma
     h. Stroke
     i. Death
  4. Emergency care for overdose
     a. Monitoring vital signs (especially heart rate, blood pressure, temperature)
     b. Maintaining a safe environment
     c. Providing respiratory support
     d. Applying cooling blanket

   e. Administering anticonvulsants
   f. Administering anti-psychotics
   g. Administering ammonium chloride (to acidify urine for excretion of amphetamines [bases])
5. Manifestations of stimulant withdrawal
   a. Fatigue
   b. Depression
   c. Agitation
   d. Apathy
   e. Anxiety
   f. Insomnia
   g. Disorientation
   h. Craving
6. Management of withdrawal focuses on drug therapy with:
   a. Antianxiety drugs
   b. Antidepressants
   c. Dopamine agonists (to reduce tremors)

> **■ Critical Rescue ◆** For the patient with an overdose of or withdrawal from cocaine, essential care includes observing for cardiac symptoms and assessing for depression and potential suicide gestures.

HALLUCINOGENS AND RELATED COMPOUNDS

- Hallucinogens are chemical substances that possess mind-altering or mental perception-altering properties.
- Lysergic acid (street names include *LSD, acid*)
  1. Manifestations
     a. Dilated pupils
     b. Tachycardia
     c. Palpitations
     d. Diaphoresis
     e. Tremors
     f. Poor coordination
     g. Elevated body temperature
     h. Increased pulse and respiration
     i. Psychological symptoms (paranoid ideas, anxiety, depression, sensory experiences, bizarre thoughts)
     j. Brain damage, psychosis, death
  2. Management involves one-to-one observation to keep the patient safe and to help the person sort reality as the effects subside and includes:
     a. Reducing environmental stimuli
     b. Administering prescribed antianxiety drugs (e.g., benzodiazepines, haloperidol)

- Phencyclidine (street names include *PCP, angel dust*)
  1. Manifestations
     a. Feelings of detachment
     b. Heart rate and blood pressure instability
     c. Eye flickering
     d. Flushing
     e. Increased perspiration
     f. Aggression
     g. Incoherence
     h. Seizures
     i. Progression to hallucinations, catatonia, coma, and death
  2. Management
     a. Calm environment
     b. Cardiac and respiratory support
  3. With long-term use, symptoms may persist for a year or cause permanent disabilities.
- Ketamine (street names include *businessman's LSD, Special K, K, Kat*)
  1. Manifestations of moderate doses
     a. Euphoria
     b. Loss of inhibition
     c. Confusion
     d. Ringing in the ears
     e. Quick burst of energy
     f. Drunken feeling
  2. Manifestations of overdose
     a. Tunnel vision
     b. Shortness of breath
     c. Loss of balance
     d. Numbness of the body
     e. Clinical depression
     f. No sense of time
     g. Seizures
     h. Coma
  3. Management
     a. Providing a calm and stimulus-free environment
     b. Respiratory support
- Methylenedioxymethamphetamine or MDMA (street names include *Adam, ecstasy, XTC, hug, beans, date rape drug*) is an altered amphetamine that produces hallucinogenic responses.
  1. Manifestations
     a. Development of trust in others
     b. Reduced inhibitions
     c. Increased confidence
     d. Euphoria

    f. Relaxation of voluntary muscles
    g. Heightened sexual experiences
    h. Amnesia
    i. Hyperthermia
    j. Psychological symptoms of depression, sleep disturbances, drug craving, severe anxiety, paranoia
    k. Long-term use leads to parkinsonism, brain damage, multiorgan failure, and death.
  2. Management
    a. Symptom-based support
    b. Safe environment
    c. Reduction or elimination of adverse drug effects

- Marijuana (street names include *weed, smoke, pot, grass, Mary Jane, herb*)
  1. Manifestations
     a. Euphoria
     b. Sexual arousal
     c. Relaxation
     d. Increased heart rate and hypertension
     e. Impaired short-term memory
     f. Paranoia, panic attacks
     g. Increased appetite
     h. Impaired coordination
  2. Withdrawal symptoms
     a. Insomnia
     b. Decreased appetite
     c. Nausea
     d. Irritability
     e. Anxiety
  3. Management
     a. Frequent vital sign assessment
     b. Symptom management
     c. Pain control

DEPRESSANTS

- Depressants are drugs that reduce the activity of the CNS. They include the commonly prescribed drug categories of benzodiazepines and barbiturates, as well as many illicit drugs.
- All benzodiazepines can produce the same effects; however, some are much more potent than others and produce the effects at low doses.
- Rohypnol (flunitrazepam) is a frequently abused benzodiazepine (street names include *rophies, ruffies, R2s, Mexican Valium, Rib, roach, Roches, Forget Me Pill, Forget Pill*).
  1. Manifestations

        a. Reduced anxiety
        b. Lowered inhibitions
        c. Lowered heart rate and blood pressure
        d. Lowered respirations
        e. Fatigue
        f. Poor concentration, confusion, impaired coordination, amnesia
        g. Impaired judgment
    2. Manifestations of overdose
        a. Respiratory depression
        b. Excessive sedation
        c. Cardiac arrest
        d. Death
    3. Management
        a. Respiratory support
        b. Close monitoring
        c. Symptomatic relief and comfort measures
        d. Drug therapy for acute overdose is flumazenil (Romazicon)
        e. Long-term therapy for abuse is detoxification with titrating doses

- Gamma hydroxybutyrate (street names include *GHB, liquid ecstasy*)
    1. Manifestations of low doses
        a. Reduced social inhibitions
        b. Increased libido
        c. Euphoria and anxiety
        d. Impaired judgment and loss of coordination
        e. Nausea
    2. Manifestations of higher doses and overdose
        a. Dizziness
        b. Respiratory depression
        c. Memory loss
        d. Muscle fatigue
        e. Coma and death
    3. Death is most common when the drug is combined with alcohol.

- Barbiturates are common drugs and include amobarbital (Amytal) and phenobarbital (Nembutal) (street names include *barbs, reds, red birds, phennies, tooies, yellows, yellow jackets*).
    1. Manifestations
        a. Sedation
        b. Drowsiness
        c. Decreased motor activity
    2. Manifestations of overdose
        a. Respiratory depression

    b. Pinpoint pupils
    c. Coma
  3. Manifestations of withdrawal
    a. Nausea, vomiting, abdominal cramping
    b. Seizures
    c. Variable behavioral responses
  4. Management for overdose or withdrawal
    a. Drug tapering (for overdose to prevent withdrawal)
    b. Frequent vital signs checks
    c. Frequent neurologic checks
    d. Emotional support
    e. Food, fluids
    f. Calm environment

OPIOIDS

- Opioids is a broad term encompassing all drugs that are made from the Asian poppy or produced as a synthetic drug which produces the same effects of the opium plant.
- Other terms for opioids are *narcotics* or *narcs*. Street names include *horse*, *junk*, *H*, and *smack*.
- Drugs included in this category are codeine, morphine, heroin, methadone, hydromorphone (Dilaudid), meperidine (Demerol), and oxycodone (OxyContin).
- They are used for pain relief and have potential for abuse or addition.
  1. Manifestations of opiate intoxication
    a. Constricted pupils
    b. Decreased blood pressure
    c. Decreased respirations
    d. Drowsiness
    e. Slurred speech
    f. Initial euphoria followed by dysphoria (depression)
    g. Cognitive impairments resulting in judgment and memory losses
  2. Manifestations of opiate overdose
    a. Dilated pupils
    b. Respiratory depression
    c. Coma
    d. Shock
    e. Convulsions
    f. Respiratory arrest
    g. Death
  3. Manifestations of opiate withdrawal
    a. Yawning
    b. Insomnia

    c. Irritability
    d. Rhinorrhea
    e. Diaphoresis
    f. Abdominal cramps
    g. Nausea and vomiting
    h. Muscle aches
    i. Chills, cold flashes with goose bumps (referred to as *cold turkey*)

4. Management of opiate overdose
    a. Drug therapy with anticonvulsants, opioid antagonists, and antianxiety agents
    b. Frequent vital sign and neurologic checks
    c. Supportive measures

INHALANT ABUSE

- Inhalants are breathable chemical vapors that produce psychoactive effects.
- Common or street names for these abused drugs include *glue*, *kick*, *bang*, *sniff*, *huffing*, *poppers*, *whippets*, and *Texas shoe-shine*.

1. Commonly abused inhalants
    a. Solvents such as paint thinners, gasoline, glues, paper correction fluid, felt-tip markers, and electronic contact cleaners
    b. Gases such as butane lighters, propane tanks, whipping cream aerosols, spray paints, hair or deodorant sprays, chloroform, ether, and nitrous oxide (laughing gas)
    c. Nitrites such as cyclohexyl nitrite, amyl nitrite, and butyl nitrite

2. Manifestations of inhalant use
    a. Slurred speech
    b. Drunken, dizzy, or dazed appearance
    c. Chemical smell on the person
    d. Paint stains on the face or body
    e. Red eyes
    f. Rhinorrhea

3. Management is supportive, based on manifestations.

STEROIDS

- Anabolic-androgenic steroids are synthetic substances that mimic the actions of testosterone and are sometimes abused by athletes to increase strength and performance.
- Their legal use is for people with hormonal difficulties such as delayed puberty or impotence.
- Street names include *roids*, *juice*, *hype*, and *pump*.

- Effects of steroid use
  1. In men
     a. Shrunken testicles
     b. Reduced sperm count
     c. Infertility
     d. Baldness
     e. Development of breasts
     f. Increased risk for cancer
  2. In women
     a. Growth of facial hair
     b. Male pattern baldness
     c. Changes or cessation of menses
     d. Enlargement of the clitoris
     e. Deepened voice
  3. General complications
     a. Negative emotional effects such as *roid rage*, with severe, aggressive behavior with the potential for violence
     b. Mood swings
     c. Hallucinations, paranoia, anxiety or panic attacks, depression, or thoughts of suicide
     d. High blood pressure and heart disease
     e. Liver damage
     f. Stroke and blood clots
     g. Urinary and bowel problems such as diarrhea
     h. Headaches, muscle cramps, aching joints
     i. Sleep problems
     j. Increased risk of ligament and tendon injuries
     k. Severe acne

PART TWO

DISEASES AND DISORDERS

ABSCESS, ANORECTAL

- Anorectal abscesses result from obstruction of the ducts of glands in the anorectal region by feces, foreign bodies, or trauma.
- Stasis of the obstructing contents results in infection that spreads into adjacent tissue.
- Rectal pain is the first clinical manifestation.
- Local swelling, erythema, and tenderness on palpation appear a few days after the onset of pain.
- The diagnosis is made by physical examination and history.
- Simple perianal and ischiorectal abscesses can be excised and drained with local anesthesia; more extensive abscesses require incision using regional or general anesthesia.
- Intervention includes:
  1. Giving systemic antibiotics only to patients who are immunocompromised, including patients who have diabetes, valvular disease or prostheses, or extensive cellulitis
  2. Assisting the patient to maintain comfort and optimal perineal hygiene by providing warm sitz baths, analgesics, bulk-forming agents, and stool softeners, as ordered
  3. Emphasizing the importance of ongoing perineal hygiene and the maintenance of a regular bowel pattern with a high-fiber diet

ABSCESS, BRAIN

OVERVIEW

- A brain abscess is an infection of the brain in which encapsulated pus forms in the extradural, subdural, or intracerebral area.
- The number of patients with a brain abscess resulting from immunosuppression, organ transplantation, and acquired immunodeficiency syndrome (AIDS) has rapidly increased over the past 2 decades.
- The causative organisms are most often bacteria, such as *Streptococcus* and *Staphylococcus*.
- Most brain abscesses occur in the frontal and temporal lobes.

87

PATIENT-CENTERED COLLABORATIVE CARE

- A brain abscess typically manifests with symptoms of a mass and of mildly increased intracranial pressure, including:
  1. Headache
  2. Fever
  3. Focal neurologic deficits
  4. Lethargy and confusion
  5. Visual field deficits
  6. Nystagmus and disconjugate gaze
  7. Generalized weakness, hemiparesis
  8. Ataxic gait
  9. Seizures
  10. Various degrees of aphasia with a frontal or temporal lobe abscess
  11. Elevated WBC count
- Drug therapy includes:
  1. Antibiotics, typically administered IV or intrathecally
  2. Metronidazole (Flagyl, Novonidazol) if an anaerobic organism is the causative agent
  3. Antiepileptic drugs, as ordered, to prevent or treat seizures
  4. Analgesics, as ordered, to treat the patient's headache
- Surgical drainage of an encapsulated abscess or an exploratory craniotomy may be performed.

ABSCESS, HEPATIC

- Hepatic (liver) abscesses occur when the liver is invaded by bacteria or protozoa.
- Liver tissue is destroyed, producing a necrotic cavity filled with infected agents, liquefied liver cells and tissue, and leukocytes.
- Liver abscess occurs infrequently and is associated with a high mortality rate.
- Pyrogenic abscesses are caused by bacteria such as *Escherichia coli*, *Klebsiella*, *Enterobacter*, *Salmonella*, *Staphylococcus*, and *Enterococcus*.
- Abscesses can result from acute cholangitis, liver trauma, peritonitis, or sepsis, or an abscess can extend to the liver after pneumonia or bacterial endocarditis.
- Amebic hepatic abscesses occur after amebic dysentery as a single abscess in the right upper quadrant of the liver.
- Assessment findings include:
  1. Right upper quadrant abdominal pain
  2. Tender, palpable liver
  3. Anorexia

4. Weight loss
5. Nausea and vomiting
6. Fever and chills
7. Shoulder pain
8. Dyspnea
9. Pleural pain if the diaphragm is involved
10. Jaundice

- Hepatic abscesses are usually diagnosed by contrast-enhanced CT or ultrasound.
- Abscesses may be drained under CT or ultrasound guidance. Drainage is sent for laboratory analysis so optimal antibiotic treatment can be selected.

ABSCESS, LUNG

- A lung abscess is a localized area of lung destruction caused by liquefaction necrosis, which is usually related to pyogenic bacteria.
- Common causes are pneumonia, aspiration of mouth or stomach contents, and obstruction as a result of a tumor or foreign body.
- Lung abscess also can be caused by any condition that alters the ability to swallow, such as alcoholic blackouts, seizure disorders, other neurologic deficits, and swallowing disorders.
- Assessment findings include:
  1. Recent history of any pulmonary infection (influenza or pneumonia)
  2. Fever
  3. Cough and foul-smelling sputum
  4. Decreased breath sounds on affected side, crackles
  5. Fatigue and unplanned weight loss
  6. Abnormal chest x-ray
- Nursing diagnoses and interventions are similar to those for pneumonia.
- Medical management includes percutaneous drainage of the abscess and antibiotic therapy.

ABSCESS, PANCREATIC

- A pancreatic abscess consists of infected, necrotic pancreatic tissue.
- Pancreatic abscess usually occurs after severe acute pancreatitis, exacerbations of chronic pancreatitis, and biliary tract surgery.

- The problem may occur as a single abscess or multiloculated abscesses resulting from extensive inflammatory necrosis of the pancreas readily invaded by infectious organisms such as *Escherichia coli*, *Klebsiella*, *Bacteroides*, *Staphylococcus*, and *Proteus*.
- Temperature spikes may be as high as 104° F (40° C).
- The mortality rate is 100% if the abscess is not surgically drained; multiple drainage procedures are often required.
- Insulin-secreting beta-cells may be destroyed with infection, leading to hyperglycemia.
- Antibiotic therapy alone does not resolve the abscess.
- Pleural effusions often accompany the abscess.

ABSCESS, PERITONSILLAR

- Peritonsillar abscess (PTA), or *quinsy*, is a complication of acute tonsillitis.
- The infection spreads from the tonsil to the surrounding tissue, forming an abscess.
- The most common cause is infection with group A beta-hemolytic streptococci.
- Signs of infection are pronounced on examination. Pus forms behind the tonsil and causes one-sided swelling with deviation of the uvula toward the unaffected side. The swelling causes drooling, severe throat pain radiating to the ear, a voice change, and difficulty swallowing.

> 🔲 **Critical Rescue** ◆ Check the patient for respiratory obstruction, which also may occur from swelling. If obstruction is present, notify the Rapid Response Team.

- Management includes:
  1. Percutaneous needle aspiration
  2. Antibiotics
  3. Analgesics
  4. Warm saline gargles or irrigations
  5. Ice collar
  6. Tonsillectomy after the abscess has healed

ABSCESS, RENAL

- A renal abscess is a collection of fluid and cells resulting from an inflammatory response to bacteria in the renal parenchyma, renal fascia, or flank.
- An abscess is suspected when fever and symptoms of kidney infection are unresponsive to antibiotic therapy.

- Symptoms include:
  1. Fever
  2. Flank pain
  3. General malaise
  4. Local edema
- Treatment includes:
  1. Broad-spectrum antibiotics
  2. Drainage by surgical incision or needle aspiration

ACIDOSIS, METABOLIC

OVERVIEW

- Acidosis is *not* a disease; it is a condition caused by a metabolic problem, a respiratory problem, or both.
- Metabolic acidosis is a problem in which the acid-base balance of the blood and other extracellular fluid (ECF) is upset by reduction of the number of bicarbonate ions that is out of proportion to the number of hydrogen ions (H^+).
- It is reflected by arterial blood gas (ABG) values of a pH below 7.35, low HCO_3^-, normal Po_2, and normal or low Pco_2.
- Metabolic acidosis often is accompanied by potassium excess (hyperkalemia).
- An *actual metabolic acidosis* occurs as a result of too much acid from overproduction of acids (and release of hydrogen ions) or underelimination of normally produced acids (retention of hydrogen ions). This type of acidosis is known as an *acid excess* acidosis.
- A *relative acidosis* occurs when the amount or strength of acids is normal, but the amount or strength of the bases (especially bicarbonate) decreases. This type of acidosis is known as a *base deficit* acidosis.
- Common causes of metabolic acidosis include:
  1. Conditions that overproduce hydrogen ions
     a. Diabetic ketoacidosis
     b. Fever
     c. Heavy exercise
     d. Hypoxia, anoxia, ischemia
     e. Starvation, carbohydrate-free diets
     f. Aspirin or other salicylate intoxication
     g. Ethanol, methanol, or ethylene glycol intoxication
  2. Conditions that undereliminate hydrogen ions (renal failure)
  3. Conditions that underproduce bicarbonate ions (liver failure, pancreatitis, or dehydration)
  4. Conditions that overeliminate bicarbonate (diarrhea)

PATIENT-CENTERED COLLABORATIVE CARE

Assessment

- Assessment findings include:
  1. Central nervous system (CNS) changes
     a. Depressed activity (lethargy, confusion, stupor, and coma)
  2. Neuromuscular changes
     a. Hyporeflexia
     b. Skeletal muscle weakness
     c. Flaccid paralysis
  3. Cardiovascular changes
     a. Delayed electrical conduction (bradycardia to heart block)
     b. Tall T waves
     c. Widened QRS complex
     d. Prolonged PR interval
     e. Hypotension
     f. Thready peripheral pulses
  4. Respiratory changes
     a. Increased respiratory rate
     b. Kussmaul respirations (greatly increased rate and depth of ventilation)
  5. Skin changes
     a. Warm, flushed
     b. Dry

Interventions

- Management focuses on:
  1. Correcting the underlying cause of the acid imbalance
  2. Administering IV fluids and maintaining IV access
  3. Monitoring arterial blood gas values and serum potassium levels
  4. Cardiac monitoring
  5. Monitoring intake and output

ACIDOSIS, RESPIRATORY

OVERVIEW

- Respiratory acidosis is a problem in which the acid-base balance of the blood and other extracellular fluid (ECF) is upset by an excess of hydrogen ions (H^+) that is out of proportion to the number of bicarbonate ions.
- It results when any area of respiratory function is impaired, reducing the exchange of oxygen (O_2) and carbon dioxide (CO_2), and leading to CO_2 retention.

- Because any increase in CO_2 levels causes the same increase in hydrogen ion levels, CO_2 retention leads to acidosis.
- Respiratory acidosis results from only one mechanism: retention of CO_2, causing increased production of free hydrogen ions. It is always an *acid excess* acidosis.
- It can be an acute condition or a chronic condition.
- Acute respiratory acidosis is reflected by arterial blood gas (ABG) values of a pH below 7.35, normal HCO_3^-, low Po_2, and high Pco_2. Usually, the serum potassium level is normal.
- Chronic respiratory acidosis is reflected by arterial blood gas (ABG) values of a pH below 7.35, high HCO_3^-, low Po_2, and high Pco_2. Usually, the serum potassium level is above normal.
- Common causes of respiratory acidosis include:
  1. Respiratory depression
     a. Anesthetics
     b. Drugs (especially opioids and benzodiazepines)
     c. Head trauma
     d. Electrolyte imbalance
     e. Cerebral edema
  2. Reduced alveolar-capillary diffusion
     a. Disease (emphysema, pneumonia, tuberculosis, fibrosis, cancer)
     b. Pulmonary edema
     c. Atelectasis
     d. Pulmonary emboli
     e. Chest trauma
  3. Airway obstruction
     a. Foreign object
     b. Disease (asthma, epiglottitis)
     c. Tight clothing
     d. Strangulation
     e. Regional lymph node enlargement
  4. Inadequate chest expansion
     a. Skeletal deformities (kyphosis, scoliosis), trauma (flail chest, broken ribs), spinal cord injury
     b. Hemothorax or pneumothorax
     c. Respiratory muscle weakness
     d. Obesity
     e. Abdominal or thoracic masses
     f. Ascites

Considerations for Older Adults

- The older adult is at higher risk for respiratory acidosis because of cardiac, respiratory, and renal problems.

- The older adult is more likely to be taking drugs that interfere with acid-base balance, such as aspirin, diuretics, laxatives, antihypertensives, and cardiac glycosides.

PATIENT-CENTERED COLLABORATIVE CARE

Assessment

- Assessment findings include:
  1. Central nervous system (CNS) changes
     a. Depressed activity (lethargy, confusion, stupor, and coma)
  2. Neuromuscular changes
     a. Hyporeflexia
     b. Skeletal muscle weakness
     c. Flaccid paralysis
  3. Cardiovascular changes
     a. Delayed electrical conduction (bradycardia to heart block)
     b. Tall T waves
     c. Widened QRS complex
     d. Prolonged PR interval
     e. Hypotension
     f. Thready peripheral pulses
  4. Respiratory changes
     a. Respirations rapid and shallow
     b. Diminished respiratory effort
  5. Skin changes
     a. Cool, pale to cyanotic
     b. Moist

Interventions

- Management focuses on:
  1. Ensuring adequate oxygenation:
     a. Assessing the airway and breathing effectiveness
     b. Administering nebulized oxygen cautiously, as prescribed
     c. Placing the patient in the high-Fowler or semi-Fowler position
  2. Administering appropriate drugs to improve ventilation and gas exchange
     a. Inhaled bronchodilator drugs, such as albuterol (Proventil, Ventolin), ipratropium (Atrovent, Apo-Ipravent ✦), theophylline (Elixophyllin, Theo Dur, Uniphyl, Theolair, many others)
     b. Inhaled or systemic anti-inflammatory drugs, such as fluticasone (Flovent), prednisone
     c. Mucolytic drugs, such as acetylcysteine (Mucomyst) or dornase alfa (Pulmozyme)

A

3. Monitoring respiratory status at least every 2 hours for response to therapy or worsening of breathing effectiveness
   a. Respiratory rate and depth
   b. Oxygen saturation or arterial blood gas (ABG) values
   c. Ease of ventilation and use of accessory muscles
   d. Breath sounds
   e. Color of nail beds and mucous membranes
   f. Level of consciousness and cognition
   g. Oxygen flow rate

> 🔲 **Critical Rescue** ◆ Notify the Rapid Response Team about any patient whose respiratory rate remains at less than 8 to 10 breaths/min with stimulation or whose oxygen saturation suddenly drops by 8 to 10 percentage points and does not improve within a few minutes.

> 🔲 **Clinical Landmine** ◆ Avoid excessive oxygen flow rates for patients with chronic respiratory acidosis who are not being mechanically ventilated. A decrease arterial oxygen level is this patient's only drive for breathing.

ACUTE RESPIRATORY DISTRESS SYNDROME

OVERVIEW

- Acute respiratory distress syndrome (ARDS) is acute respiratory failure with the following indicators:
  1. Hypoxemia that persists even when 100% oxygen is given
  2. Decreased pulmonary compliance
  3. Dyspnea
  4. Noncardiac-associated bilateral pulmonary edema
  5. Dense pulmonary infiltrates on x-ray (ground-glass appearance)
- ARDS often occurs after an acute lung injury (ALI) as a traumatic event in people who have no previous pulmonary disease.
- Common conditions or events that can lead to ARDS include sepsis, pulmonary embolism, shock, aspiration or inhalation injury, and multiple transfusions with whole blood, packed RBCs, platelets, and fresh-frozen plasma. All of these conditions can activate the inflammatory response.
- Nonpulmonary causes of ARDS include serious nervous system injury, such as head or spinal trauma, strokes, tumors, and

sudden increases in cerebrospinal fluid pressure. These conditions cause massive sympathetic discharge and systemic blood vessel constriction that move large volumes of blood into lung circulation.

- The inflammatory response injures the alveolar-capillary membrane, causing protein-containing fluid to leak into and between the alveoli.
- Surfactant production is reduced, making the alveoli unstable and at risk for collapse unless they are filled with fluid. These fluid-filled or collapsed alveoli cannot exchange gases.
- Edema forms around terminal airways, which are compressed, are closed, and can be destroyed. Lung volume and compliance are further reduced. Poorly inflated alveoli receive blood but cannot oxygenate it, increasing the shunt. Hypoxemia and ventilation-perfusion ($\dot{V}/\dot{Q}$) mismatch result.
- Patients have a rapidly deteriorating respiratory status that does not respond to increased oxygen therapy. The mortality rate is high even when intensive interventions are used.

▼ National Patient Safety Goal

Reduce the risk of health care–associated infections by good hand-washing and using appropriate precautions to reduce transmission of infection from one patient to another or from one body area to another on the same patient.

> 🕒 **Critical Rescue** ♦ A nursing priority in the prevention of ARDS is early recognition of patients at high risk for the syndrome. Two important areas for prevention are aspiration of gastric contents and prevention of sepsis. Closely assess and monitor those receiving tube feeding and those with problems that impair swallowing and gag reflexes. Follow meticulous infection control guidelines, including hand-washing, invasive catheter and wound care, and body substance precautions.

PATIENT-CENTERED COLLABORATIVE CARE
Assessment
- Assessment findings include:
  1. Decreasing oxygen saturation or Pao_2
  2. Increased respiratory rate
  3. Increased work of breathing (grunting respiration, cyanosis, pallor, and intercostal retractions or substernal retractions)
  4. Diaphoresis

5. Normal breath sounds on auscultation (because the edema of ARDS occurs first in the interstitial spaces and *not* in the airways)
6. Hypotension
7. Pallor and cyanosis
8. Tachycardia
9. Dysrhythmias
10. Mental status changes
11. Hazy or "whited-out" areas of lung fields on chest x-ray

Interventions

- Medical management includes drug therapy:
  1. Anti-inflammatories such as corticosteroids may be used to reduce the inflammatory response and prevent fibrosis.
  2. Other agents that may be used to modify the inflammatory responses and reduce oxidative stress include vitamins C and E, *N*-acetylcysteine, nitric oxide, and surfactant replacement.
  3. Antibiotics are given to manage identified infections.
  4. Conservative IV fluid volume replacement is preferred to prevent hypotension and inadequate perfusion.

> **Clinical Landmine** ◆ Avoid excessive IV fluid administration in these patients because it leads to fluid overload and more edema in the pulmonary and systemic circulation.

  5. Enteral nutrition (tube feeding) or parenteral nutrition is started as soon as possible to prevent malnutrition, loss of respiratory muscle function, and reduced immune response.
- The course of ARDS and its management are divided into four phases:
  1. Phase 1 includes early changes of dyspnea and tachypnea. Early interventions involve supporting the patient and providing oxygen.
  2. In phase 2, patchy infiltrates form from increasing pulmonary edema. Interventions include intubation and mechanical ventilation and prevention of complications. Usually, positive end-expiratory pressure (PEEP) or continuous positive airway pressure (CPAP) are used. Because one of the side effects of PEEP is tension pneumothorax, assess lung sounds hourly and suction as often as needed to maintain a patent airway. Patient positioning may include the prone position, continuously turning the patient to 40 degrees from side to side, or using a 90-degree lateral position. Sedation and paralysis may be needed for adequate ventilation and to reduce tissue oxygen needs.

3. Phase 3 occurs over days 2 to 10, and the patient has progressive hypoxemia that responds poorly to high levels of oxygen. Interventions focus on maintaining adequate oxygen transport, preventing complications, and supporting the failing lung until it has had time to heal.

4. In phase 4, pulmonary fibrosis with progression occurs after 10 days. This phase is irreversible and is often called *late* or *chronic* ARDS. Patients who develop and survive this stage will have some permanent lung damage. Interventions focus on preventing sepsis, pneumonia, and multiple organ dysfunction syndrome (MODS), and on weaning the patient from the ventilator.

ALKALOSIS, METABOLIC

OVERVIEW

- Alkalosis is *not* a disease; it is a condition caused by a metabolic problem, a respiratory problem, or both.
- Metabolic alkalosis is a problem in which the acid-base balance of the blood and other extracellular fluid (ECF) is upset by an excess of bicarbonate ions that are out of proportion to the number of hydrogen ions (H^+).
- It is reflected by arterial blood gas (ABG) values of a pH above 7.45, high HCO_3^-, normal Po_2, and normal or rising Pco_2.
- Often, metabolic alkalosis is accompanied by a low serum potassium level (hypokalemia).
- An *actual metabolic alkalosis* occurs when a base (usually bicarbonate) is overproduced or undereliminated. This type of alkalosis is known as a *base excess* alkalosis.
- A *relative alkalosis* occurs when the amount or strength, or both, of the acids decreases, making the blood more basic than acidic as a result of overelimination or underproduction of acids. This type of alkalosis is known as an *acid deficit* alkalosis.
- Common causes of metabolic alkalosis include:
  1. Increase of base (especially bicarbonate)
     a. Excessive use of antacids or bicarbonate
     b. Milk-alkali syndrome
     c. Multiple transfusions of blood products
     d. IV administration of bicarbonate
     e. Total parenteral nutrition
  2. Acid loss
     a. Prolonged vomiting
     b. Continuous nasogastric suctioning
     c. Use of thiazide diuretics
     d. Hypercortisolism
     e. Hyperaldosteronism

PATIENT-CENTERED COLLABORATIVE CARE

A

Assessment

- Assessment findings include:
  1. Central nervous system (CNS) changes
     a. Light-headedness
     b. Decreased ability to concentrate
     c. Anxiety, irritability
     d. Paresthesia
     e. Positive Chvostek's sign
     f. Positive Trousseau's sign
     g. Tetany, seizures
  2. Neuromuscular changes
     a. Skeletal muscle weakness
     b. Muscle cramping and twitching
     c. Hyperreflexia
  3. Cardiac changes
     a. Weak, rapid pulse
     b. Hypotension (if hypovolemia is also present)
     c. Increased myocardial sensitivity to digoxin
  4. Respiratory changes
     a. Decreased respiratory effort (a late manifestation of metabolic alkalosis, occurring as a result of weakness of respiratory skeletal muscles)
     b. Decreased oxygen saturation

Interventions

- Management focuses on:
  1. Drug therapy to resolve the causes of alkalosis (e.g., antiemetics for severe vomiting)
  2. Oral or IV fluid replacement to restore normal fluid, electrolyte, and acid-base balance
  3. Monitoring patient responses to therapy
     a. Respiratory effectiveness (rate, depth, oxygen saturation)
     b. Cardiac effectiveness (pulse, blood pressure)
     c. Intake and output
     d. Serum electrolytes and arterial blood gas (ABG) values
     e. Hand grasps and deep tendon reflexes

ALKALOSIS, RESPIRATORY

OVERVIEW

- Respiratory alkalosis is *not* a disease; it is a condition caused by a respiratory problem that usually involves an excessive rate or depth of ventilation, or both.
- Respiratory alkalosis is a problem in which the acid-base balance of the blood and other extracellular fluid (ECF) is upset by a

reduction of the number of hydrogen ions (H^+) in proportion to the number of bicarbonate ions.

- It is reflected by arterial blood gas (ABG) values of a pH above 7.45, normal HCO_3^-, normal Po_2, and low Pco_2.
- Often, it is accompanied by a low serum potassium level (hypokalemia).
- Respiratory alkalosis occurs because of an excess loss of acids in the form of carbon dioxide.
- The main cause of respiratory alkalosis is hyperventilation, which leads to excessive exhalation of carbon dioxide. Common conditions leading to hyperventilation include:
  1. Anxiety or fear
  2. Improper settings on mechanical ventilators (too high a ventilation rate or too great a tidal volume, or both)
  3. Direct stimulation of central respiratory centers
     a. Fever
     b. Hyperthyroidism
     c. Drugs (salicylates, catecholamines, progesterone)
     d. High altitudes or low atmospheric oxygen levels

PATIENT-CENTERED COLLABORATIVE CARE

Assessment
- Assessment findings include:
  1. Central nervous system (CNS) changes
     a. Light-headedness
     b. Decreased ability to concentrate
     c. Anxiety, irritability
     d. Paresthesia
     e. Positive Chvostek's sign
     f. Positive Trousseau's sign
     g. Tetany, seizures
  2. Neuromuscular changes
     a. Skeletal muscle weakness
     b. Muscle cramping and twitching
     c. Hyperreflexia
  3. Cardiac changes
     a. Weak, rapid pulse
     b. Hypotension (if hypovolemia is also present)
     c. Increased myocardial sensitivity to digoxin
  4. Respiratory changes
     a. Rapid, deep ventilation (cause of respiratory alkalosis)

Interventions
- Management focuses on:
  1. Ensuring ventilator settings are appropriate for patient size
  2. Rebreathing exhaled air to increase carbon dioxide levels

3. Attempting to calm the patient and work with him or her to control ventilation
4. Drug therapy to resolve the causes of alkalosis (e.g., antipyretics for fever, anxiolytics for acute anxiety)
5. Oral or IV fluid replacement (if hyperventilation leads to dehydration) to restore normal fluid and electrolyte
6. Monitoring patient responses to therapy
   a. Respiratory effectiveness (rate, depth, oxygen saturation)
   b. Cardiac effectiveness (pulse, blood pressure)
   c. Intake and output
   d. Serum electrolytes and arterial blood gas (ABG) values
   e. Hand grasps and deep tendon reflexes

ALLERGY, LATEX

- Latex allergy is a type I hypersensitivity reaction in which the specific allergen is a protein found in processed natural latex rubber products.
- Allergic reactions to latex vary from contact dermatitis to anaphylaxis.
- People at greatest risk for latex allergy are those with a high-level exposure to natural latex products, such as patients with spina bifida, people who routinely use latex condoms, and health care workers who use latex gloves.
- Ask all patients about their use of and known reactions to natural latex products and to specific foods (e.g., banana, kiwi, avocado, tomato, chestnut).

> 🔲 **Critical Rescue** ♦ It is essential to use latex-free products in the care of a patient with a known latex allergy.

- Teach latex sensitive patients to avoid products containing latex.
- When caring for a patient with a known latex allergy:
  1. Remove any latex-containing product from your person (e.g., erasers, tourniquets, blood tubes).
  2. Wear a cover gown before entering the room or touching the patient.
  3. Wash hands before entering the room or touching the patient.

AMPUTATION

OVERVIEW

- Amputation is the removal of a part of the body.

- The psychosocial aspects of the procedure are often more devastating than the physical impairments that result. The loss is complete and permanent and causes a change in body image and often in self-esteem.
- *Traumatic amputation* occurs when a body part is severed unexpectedly, most often resulting from accidents. Depending on the extent of damage, body parts that are severed may be reattached or reimplanted.

> 🔲 Critical Rescue ♦ For prehospital care with any traumatic amputation:
> - Call 911.
> - Assess the patient for airway or breathing problems.
> - Apply direct pressure to amputation site with layers of dry gauze or other cloth.
> - Elevate the extremity above the patient's heart to decrease the bleeding.

> 🔲 Critical Rescue ♦ For prehospital care for finger amputation:
> - Wrap the completely severed finger in a dry, sterile gauze or clean cloth.
> - Put the finger in a watertight, sealed plastic bag.
> - Place the bag in ice water—never directly on ice—at one part ice and three parts water.
> - Prevent contact between the finger and the water.
> - Keep semidetached parts of the digit in contact with the digit.
> - Be sure that the amputated part goes with the patient to the hospital.

- Surgical amputations are planned *elective* procedures performed for a variety of disorders and complications.
- Regardless of the reason for the surgical amputation, every effort is made to preserve maximum possible patient function.
- Loss of any or all of the small toes presents a minor disability.
- Loss of the great toe is significant because it affects balance, gait, and *push-off* ability during walking.
- Midfoot amputations (e.g., Lisfranc, Chopart, or Syme amputation) remove most of the foot but retain the intact ankle so that weight bearing can be accomplished without the use of prosthesis and with reduced pain.
- Other *lower extremity amputations* are below-the-knee amputation (BKA), above-the-knee amputation (AKA), hip disarticula-

tion, or removal of the hip joint, and hemipelvectomy (removal of half of the pelvis with the leg).

- The higher the level of amputation, the more energy is required for ambulation.
- *Upper extremity (UE) amputations* usually are more incapacitating than those of lower extremities. Early replacement with a prosthetic device is vital for the patient with UE amputation.

🌐 Cultural Awareness

The incidence of lower extremity amputations is greater in the black, Hispanic, and American Indian populations because the incidence of major diseases leading to amputation, such as diabetes and arteriosclerosis, is greater in this population. Limited access to health care for these minority groups may also play a major role in limb loss.

- Complications of elective or traumatic amputation include:
  1. Hemorrhage
  2. Infection
  3. Phantom limb pain
  4. Neuroma
  5. Flexion contractures

PATIENT-CENTERED COLLABORATIVE CARE

Assessment

- Assess:
  1. Neurovascular status of extremity to be amputated
     a. Examine skin color, temperature, sensation, capillary refill, and pulses.
     b. Compare findings with those of the unaffected extremity.
     c. Check and document the presence of discoloration, edema, ulcerations, hair distribution, and any necrosis.
  2. Psychosocial responses
     a. Preparation for a planned amputation
     b. Presence of bitterness, hostility, depression
     c. Expectations of how the loss of a body part may affect employment, social relationships, recreational activities
     d. Current self-concept and self-image
     e. Willingness and motivation to withstand prolonged rehabilitation after the amputation
     f. How he or she has dealt with previous life crises
  3. Family reaction to the surgery or trauma
  4. Patient and family coping abilities
  5. Patient's religious, spiritual, and cultural beliefs
  6. Diagnostic assessment may include:
     a. Segmental limb blood pressures

b. Ankle-brachial index (ABI)
c. Blood flow by Doppler ultrasonography or laser Doppler flowmetry or use of transcutaneous oxygen pressure ($TcPo_2$)

National Patient Safety Goal

With the patient, identify the limb or digit to be amputated preoperatively, and mark it with indelible ink. Follow time-out rules before amputation so that the correct patient and digit or limb is identified by at least two people.

Interventions

- Monitor for signs indicating that there is sufficient tissue perfusion but no hemorrhage:
  1. Skin flap at the end of the residual limb should be pink in a light-skinned person and not discolored.
  2. Area is warm, not hot.
  3. Assess the closest proximal pulse for strength and compare it with that in the other extremity.
- Pain management for residual limb pain (RLP) is like that for any patient in pain.
- Phantom limb pain (PLP) management
  1. Recognize that the pain is real, and manage it promptly and completely.

> **Clinical Landmine** ♦ It is not helpful to respond to the patient with PLP by telling him or her that the limb is no longer present and therefore cannot be causing pain.

  2. Handle the residual limb carefully to prevent stimulating PLP.
  3. Opioid analgesics are usually not the first choice for PLP but can be used.
  4. Common drugs for PLP are:
     a. IV infusions of calcitonin (Miacalcin, Calcimar)
     b. Beta-blocking agents such as propranolol (Inderal, Apo-Propranolol, Detensol) for constant, dull, burning pain
     c. Antiepileptic drugs, such as carbamazepine (Tegretol) and gabapentin (Neurontin), for knifelike or sharp, burning pain
     d. Antispasmodics such as baclofen (Lioresal) for muscle spasms or cramping
  5. Complementary and alternative therapies
     a. Transcutaneous electrical nerve stimulation (TENS)
     b. Ultrasound therapy

    c. Massage
    d. Exercises
    e. Biofeedback
    f. Distraction therapy
    g. Hypnosis
    h. Psychotherapy
    i. Acupuncture/acupressure

- Infection prevention
  1. Drug therapy with broad-spectrum prophylactic antibiotics may be used before, during, and after surgery.
  2. The initial pressure dressing and drains are usually removed by the surgeon 48 to 72 hours after surgery.
  3. Inspect the wound site for signs of inflammation (e.g., redness, swelling) and monitor the healing process.
  4. Record the characteristics of drainage, if present.
  5. Change the soft dressing every day until the sutures or staples are removed.
  6. Dressings usually include an elastic bandage wrapped firmly around the residual limb after application of sterile gauze dressing over the incision.

- Promotion of mobility
  1. Coordinate with the physical therapist to begin exercises as soon as possible after surgery.
  2. For patients with AKAs or BKAs, teach ROM exercises for prevention of flexion contractures, particularly of the hip and knee.
  3. Ensure that a trapeze and an overhead frame are used to aid in strengthening the upper extremities and allow the patient to move independently in bed.
  4. Provide a firm mattress for the patient with a lower extremity amputation.
  5. Assist the patient into a prone position every 3 to 4 hours for 20- to 30-minute periods if tolerated and not contraindicated.
  6. Instruct the patient to pull the residual limb close to the other leg and contract the gluteal muscles of the buttocks.
  7. For patients with BKAs, teach how to push the residual limb down toward the bed while supporting it on a pillow.
  8. Follow health care provider and agency policy for elevation of a lower-leg residual limb on a pillow while the patient is in a supine position.

- Preparation for prosthesis
  1. Coordinate with a certified prosthetist-orthotist (CPO) for appropriate postoperative planning.

2. Instruct the patient being fitted for a leg prosthesis to bring a sturdy pair of shoes to the fitting.
3. After surgery, apply the prescribed device, such as the Jobst air splint, or elastic bandages to shape and shrink the residual limb in preparation for the prosthesis. If elastic bandages are used, reapply the bandages in a figure-eight wrap every 4 to 6 hours or more often if they become loose.
   a. Decrease the tightness of the bandages while wrapping in a distal-to-proximal direction.
   b. After wrapping, anchor the bandages to the most proximal joint, such as above the knee for BKAs.
- Promotion of body image and lifestyle adaptation
  1. If possible, arrange for the patient to meet with a rehabilitated amputee who is about the same age as him or her.
  2. Assess the patient to determine what term for the remaining limb (e.g., "stump") seems less offensive.
  3. Assess the patient's verbal and nonverbal references to the affected area.
  4. Ask the patient to describe his or her feelings about changes in body image and self-esteem.
  5. Check whether the patient looks at the area during a dressing change.
  6. Document behavior that indicates acceptance or nonacceptance of the amputation.
  7. Teach the patient and family about available resources and support from organizations such as the Amputee Coalition of America (ACA) (*www.amputee-coalition.org*) and the National Amputation Foundation (NAF) (*www.nationalamputation.org*).
  8. Stress the patient's personal strengths.
  9. Collaborate with a social worker or vocational rehabilitation specialist to evaluate the skills of a patient who may need to change employment.
  10. Discuss sexuality issues with the patient and the patient's partner together as needed.
  11. If appropriate, refer the patient and family for professional assistance from a sex therapist, intimacy coach, or psychologist.
  12. Help the patient and family set realistic desired outcomes and take 1 day at a time.
  13. Teach the patient and family how to care for the limb and the prosthesis if it is available.
  14. Teach the patient or family to care for the limb after it has healed by cleaning it each day with the rest of the body during bathing with soap and water.

15. Teach the patient and family to inspect the limb every day for signs of inflammation or skin breakdown.

AMYOTROPHIC LATERAL SCLEROSIS

- Amyotrophic lateral sclerosis (ALS), also known as Lou Gehrig's disease, is a progressive degenerative disease involving the motor tract of the central nervous system.
- Changes in cognition, memory, or mood do not occur as a result of the pathology.
- The disease is characterized by atrophy of muscles used with talking, dysphagia, weakness of the hands and arms, nasal quality to speech, fasciculations of the face, and dysarthria.
- As the disease progresses, muscle atrophy and eventually flaccid quadriplegia develops. As respiratory muscles, including the diaphragm, fail, respiratory failure and increased risk for pneumonia occurs.
- There is no known cure.
- Treatment is symptomatic and directed toward the following: preventing complications of immobility, promoting comfort, providing ongoing support and counseling to the patient and family, and informing the patient about the need for advance directives such as a living will and durable power of attorney.
- The drug riluzole (Rilutek) is associated with increased survival time.

ANAPHYLAXIS

OVERVIEW

- Anaphylaxis is the most dramatic and life-threatening example of a type I hypersensitivity reaction.
- It occurs rapidly and systemically.
- Anaphylaxis affects many organs within seconds to minutes after allergen exposure; the episodes can vary in severity and can be fatal.

PATIENT-CENTERED COLLABORATIVE CARE

Assessment

- Assessment findings include:
  1. Subjective feelings of uneasiness, apprehension, weakness, and impending doom
  2. Generalized itching and urticaria (hives)
  3. Erythema
  4. Angioedema (diffuse swelling) of the eyes, lips, or tongue

5. Intensely itchy skin wheals or hives that merge to form large, red blotches
6. Bronchoconstriction, mucosal edema, and excess mucus production
7. Nasal congestion and rhinorrhea
8. Dyspnea, increasing respiratory distress, audible wheezing
9. Crackles, wheezing, drooling, and reduced breath sounds on auscultation
10. Laryngeal edema (hoarseness, and stridor)
11. Respiratory failure and hypoxemia
12. Hypotension
13. Rapid, weak, irregular pulse
14. Dysrhythmias
15. Diaphoresis
16. Increasing anxiety and confusion

> 🔲 Critical Rescue ◆ Immediately call the Rapid Response Team if anaphylaxis is suspected. If the patient is not treated immediately, he or she may lose consciousness. Dysrhythmias, shock, and cardiac arrest may occur within *minutes* as intravascular volume is lost and the heart becomes hypoxic.

Interventions
- Emergency respiratory management
  1. Immediately assess the respiratory status, airway, and oxygen saturation of patients who show any symptoms of an anaphylactic reaction.
  2. If the airway is compromised in any way, call the Rapid Response Team before proceeding in any other intervention.
  3. Ensure that intubation and tracheotomy equipment is ready.
  4. Apply oxygen using a high-flow, non-rebreather mask at 40% to 60%.
- Drug therapy
  1. Immediately discontinue the IV drugs of a patient having an anaphylactic reaction to that drug.

> 🔳 Clinical Landmine ◆ Do not remove the IV catheter, but change the IV tubing, and hang normal saline.

  2. If the patient does not have an IV access, start one immediately, and run normal saline.
  3. Be prepared to administer diphenhydramine (Benadryl) and epinephrine IV.

a. Diphenhydramine: 25 mg to 50 mg IV push (immediately)
b. Epinephrine, 1:1000 concentration: 0.3 to 0.5 mL IV push (immediately); repeat as needed every 10 to 15 minutes until the patient responds
c. Theophylline: 6 mg/kg IV over 20 to 30 minutes for severe bronchospasms
d. Once stabilized, inhaled beta-adrenergic agonist such as metaproterenol (Alupent) or albuterol (Proventil) by means of a high-flow nebulizer every 2 to 4 hours
e. Corticosteroids (IV) are added to emergency interventions but are not effective immediately.

4. Document all drugs administered (accurately and up to the minute).

- Supportive care
  1. Keep the head of the bed elevated about 10 degrees (if hypotension is present); if blood pressure is normal, elevate the head of the bed to 45 degrees or higher to improve ventilation.
  2. Raise the feet and legs to improve blood return to the heart.
  3. Monitor pulse oximetry to determine oxygenation adequacy.
  4. Use suction to remove excess mucous secretions.
  5. Continually assess the patient's respiratory rate and depth.
  6. Stay with the patient.
  7. Reassure the patient that the appropriate interventions are being instituted.
  8. Observe the patient for fluid overload from the rapid drug and IV fluid infusions.
  9. Before discharge, instruct the patient to obtain and wear a medical alert bracelet or ID about the specific allergy.

ANEMIA, APLASTIC

- Aplastic anemia is a deficiency of circulating RBCs because of failure of the bone marrow to produce these cells. It is caused by an injury to the immature precursor pluripotent stem cell for RBCs. It usually occurs with leukopenia (reduction in WBCs) and thrombocytopenia (reduction in platelets).
- *Pancytopenia* is a deficiency of all three blood cell types.
- Disease onset may be slow or rapid.
- The most common cause of acquired aplastic anemia is long-term exposure to toxic agents and drugs, ionizing radiation, or viral infection.

- Often, the cause of aplastic anemia is unknown.
- Assessment findings include:
  1. Weakness
  2. Pallor
  3. Petechiae or ecchymosis
  4. CBC shows severe macrocytic anemia, leukopenia, and thrombocytopenia.
  5. Bone marrow biopsy may show replacement of marrow-forming cells with fat.
- Management includes:
  1. Blood transfusions when the anemia causes disability or when platelet counts are so low that risk for hemorrhage is high
  2. Immunosuppressive therapy with drugs such as prednisone, antithymocyte globulin (ATG), cyclosporine (Sandimmune), or cyclophosphamide (Cytoxan, Procytox ✦)
  3. *Splenectomy* (removal of the spleen) may be needed when an enlarged spleen is destroying normal RBCs or suppressing their development.
  4. Hematopoietic stem cell transplantation (bone marrow transplantation) can replace defective stem cells and may cure the disorder. Cost, availability, and complications limit this treatment of aplastic anemia.

ANEMIA, FOLIC ACID DEFICIENCY

- Folic acid deficiency causes anemia because folic acid is essential for RBC formation.
- The most common cause of folic acid deficiency is poor nutrition, especially a diet lacking green leafy vegetables, liver, yeast, citrus fruits, dried beans, and nuts.
- Malabsorption, such as Crohn's disease and chronic alcohol abuse, also is a common cause.
- Drugs, such as anticonvulsants and oral contraceptives, cause folic acid deficiency by slowing or preventing the absorption of folic acid and its conversion to the active form.
- Clinical manifestations are similar to those of vitamin B_{12} deficiency, but without the accompanying nervous system manifestations. The absence of neurologic problems helps distinguish folic acid deficiency from vitamin B_{12} deficiency.
- The disease develops slowly, and symptoms may be attributed to other problems or diseases.
- Prevention of folic acid deficiency anemia is aimed at identifying high-risk patients, such as older, debilitated patients with alcoholism; patients at risk for malnutrition; and those with increased folic acid requirements.

- Management includes:
  1. Teaching the patient to eat a diet rich in foods containing folic acid and vitamin B$_{12}$ to prevent a deficiency
  2. Providing scheduled folic acid replacement therapy

ANEMIA, IRON DEFICIENCY

- Iron deficiency produces anemia because iron is an essential component needed to make fully functional RBCs.
- Depletion of iron stores occurs first, followed by a reduction in hemoglobin. As a result, the RBCs are small (microcytic).
- Iron deficiency anemia can result from blood loss, poor intestinal absorption, and dietary inadequacy.
- Management first involves identifying the cause of the iron deficiency.
- If bleeding is the cause, it is identified and treated.
- The patient is instructed to increase his or her oral intake of iron from common food sources, such as liver and other organ meats, red meat, kidney beans, whole wheat breads and cereals, green leafy vegetables, carrots, egg yolks, and raisins and other dried fruit.
- When iron deficiency is mild, oral iron preparations are prescribed.
- Teach the patient that iron preparations often change the color of stool to black and can promote constipation.
- When iron deficiency is more severe, iron preparations may be given parenterally.

ANEMIA, VITAMIN B$_{12}$ DEFICIENCY

- A deficiency of vitamin B$_{12}$ indirectly causes anemia by inhibiting folic acid transportation and limiting DNA synthesis in RBC precursor cells. As a result, the immature precursor cells increase in size. This is called megaloblastic (macrocytic) anemia.
- Anemia caused by failure to absorb vitamin B$_{12}$ is called *pernicious anemia*.
- Anemia as a result of vitamin B$_{12}$ deficiency may be mild or severe, usually develops slowly, and produces few symptoms.
- Assessment findings include:
  1. Pallor
  2. Jaundice
  3. Glossitis (smooth, red, "beefy" tongue)
  4. Fatigue
  5. Weight loss

6. Paresthesias in the feet and hands
7. Disturbances of balance and gait

- Management
  1. Teach the patient to eat foods high in vitamin B_{12}, such as animal proteins, eggs, and dairy products.
  2. Provide vitamin supplements.
  3. For pernicious anemia, administer vitamin B_{12} parenterally on a regular basis (usually monthly for life). After pernicious anemia has been found to respond to parenteral vitamin B_{12}, the patient may start cyanocobalamin (CaloMist), which delivers vitamin B_{12} by nasal spray to maintain vitamin levels.
  4. Encourage the patient to rest as needed.

AORTIC ANEURYSM

OVERVIEW

- An aneurysm is a permanent, localized dilation of an artery accompanied by weakening of the vessel wall.
- An aneurysm forms when the media, or the middle layer of the artery, is weakened, producing a stretching effect in the intima (the inner layer) and adventitia (the outer layer of the artery).
- The effect of blood pressure on the artery wall produces further weakness in the media and enlarges the aneurysm.
- The most common cause is atherosclerosis; atheromatous plaque weakens the intimal surface.
- Hypertension and cigarette smoking are contributing factors.
- The three types of aneurysms are:
  1. Saccular, an outpouching from a distinct portion of the artery wall
  2. Fusiform, the diffuse dilation involving the total circumference of the artery
  3. Dissecting, a cavity formed when blood separates the layers of the artery wall (more commonly referred to as aortic dissection)
- Abdominal aneurysms are located below the renal arteries and above the iliac bifurcation.
- Thoracic aneurysms develop between the origin of the left subclavian artery and the diaphragm.
- The thoracic aorta is the most common site for dissecting aneurysms.
- Femoral and popliteal aneurysms are relatively uncommon.
- Aneurysms can thrombose, embolize, or rupture (rupture is the most frequent and life-threatening complication).

PATIENT-CENTERED COLLABORATIVE CARE

Assessment

- Most patients with abdominal or thoracic aneurysm often are asymptomatic.
- Assess for clinical manifestations of abdominal aortic aneurysms:
    1. Prominent pulsation in the upper abdomen (Do not palpate.)
    2. Abdominal bruit
    3. Abdominal, flank, or back pain (Pain is usually steady with a gnawing quality, is unaffected by movement, and may last for hours or days.)
    4. Femoral bruits
- Assess for clinical manifestations of thoracic aneurysms:
    1. Hoarseness
    2. Shortness of breath
    3. Difficulty swallowing
    4. Visible mass above the suprasternal notch (occasional)
    5. Sudden and excruciating back or chest pain (if rupture occurs)
- Assess for abdominal or thoracic aortic dissection:
    1. Pain that is described as tearing, ripping, and stabbing
    2. Pain that is located in the anterior chest, back, neck, throat, jaw, or teeth
    3. Diaphoresis
    4. Nausea, vomiting
    5. Faintness, apprehension
    6. Decreased or absent peripheral pulses
    7. Severe and sudden pain, abdominal distention, and hypovolemic shock
- Assess also for:
    1. Presence of a mass on thoracic or abdominal x-ray or CT scan
    2. Results of ultrasonography

Planning and Implementation

Nonsurgical Management

- Antihypertensive drugs are prescribed to maintain normal blood pressure and to decrease stress on an aneurysm < 5-6 cm or when surgery is not feasible.
- Teach the patient the importance of keeping scheduled CT scan appointments to monitor size of the aneurysm for possible surgery.
- Review with the patient the clinical manifestations of aneurysms that need to be promptly reported and to avoid lifting or activity that increases abdominal pressure.

Surgical Management
- Surgical removal of the aneurysm is reserved for symptomatic lesions or aneurysm > 6 cm. The excised portion of the aorta is replaced with a graft. Ruptures always require emergency surgery.
- Provide preoperative care.
  1. Administer large volumes of IV fluids if the aneurysm has ruptured to maintain tissue perfusion and blood pressure.
  2. Assess all peripheral pulses to serve as a baseline for comparison after surgery; mark where the pulse is heard.
- Provide routine postoperative care.
  1. Care of the patient with an abdominal aneurysm repair is similar to that provided for patients undergoing other abdominal surgeries. The patient is admitted to the critical care unit and is often maintained on a mechanical ventilator overnight.
- In addition to routine postoperative care:
  1. Assess vital signs every hour.
  2. Assess circulation by checking pulses distal to the graft site with vital signs.
  3. Report signs of occlusion immediately to the physician, such as pulse changes, severe pain, cool to cold extremities below the graft, white or blue extremities or flanks, abdominal distention, and decreased urinary output.
- Abdominal aortic aneurysm repair requires assessment of renal function because the aorta is clamped during the repair, potentially compromising the blood flow to the kidneys.
- Additional postoperative care specific to abdominal aortic repair includes:
  1. Assessing hourly urinary output and urine color
  2. Monitoring daily blood urea nitrogen and creatinine levels
  3. Limiting elevation of the head of the bed to 45 degrees to avoid flexion of the graft
  4. Assessing the patient's respiratory rate and depth and breath sounds hourly
  5. Managing pain as for postoperative care by administering opioid analgesics for pain
  6. Avoiding nausea, vomiting, or other occasions of increased intra-abdominal pressure, typically using a nasogastric tube that empties the stomach for 3 or 4 days until bowel sounds return
  7. Monitoring for complications such as myocardial infarction, graft occlusion or rupture, hypovolemia or renal failure, respiratory distress, and paralytic ileus related to cardiovascular disease or hypotension

A

- Care of the patient undergoing thoracic aneurysm repair is similar to that for other thoracic surgeries. Additional postoperative care includes:
  1. Reporting signs of hemorrhage immediately; assessing for bleeding and separation at the graft site by monitoring chest tube drainage for excess drainage
  2. Monitoring for cardiac dysrhythmias, paraplegia, and respiratory distress
  3. Instructing the patient with thoracic aneurysm repair to report back pain, shortness of breath, difficulty swallowing, or hoarseness
- Endovascular stent grafts are becoming the treatment of choice. The stent graft is inserted through a skin incision into the femoral artery by means of a catheter-based system and advanced to a level above the aneurysm, away from the renal arteries. The graft is deployed into place with a series of hooks. Monitor the patient closely in the hospital and at home for the development of complications, such as bleeding, aneurysm rupture, peripheral embolization, and misdeployment of the stent graft. All of these complications require surgical intervention.

⛊ **National Patient Safety Goal**

Before any procedure, use a time-out process to conduct a final verification of the procedure, patient, and site using active communication techniques.

⚇ **Critical Rescue** ♦ Report signs of hemorrhage or graft occlusion to the physician immediately.

Community-Based Care
- Emphasize the importance of compliance with the schedule of CT scans to monitor the size of the aneurysm in patients who have not had surgery.
- Emphasize the importance of controlling blood pressure.
- Educate the patient and family.
  1. Teach the patient to restrict activities (if surgery was performed), including:
     a. Avoiding lifting heavy objects for 6 to 12 weeks postoperatively
     b. Using discretion in activities that involve pulling, pushing, or straining, such as vacuuming, changing bed linens, moving furniture, mopping or sweeping, raking leaves, mowing grass, and chopping wood

    c. Avoiding hobbies such as tennis, swimming, golf, and horseback riding

    d. Deferring driving a car for several weeks

2. Provide written and oral wound care instructions, if needed.

3. Provide pain management instruction.

- Refer to home health nursing and other community agencies as needed.

ANTHRAX, CUTANEOUS

- Cutaneous anthrax is an infection caused by the spores of the bacterium *Bacillus anthracis.*
- In the United States, the most common risk factor is contact with an infected animal. Those most at risk for cutaneous anthrax include farm workers, veterinarians, and tannery and wool workers. This organism has become a tool for terrorism. *When lesions that are consistent with cutaneous anthrax appear in people who have no exposure to infected animals, consider the possibility of bioterrorism.*
- The infection can be confined to the skin, or it may be systemic. At first, a raised vesicle appears on an exposed body area such as the head or arms. The lesion may itch and often resembles an insect bite. Within a few days, the center of the vesicle becomes hemorrhagic and sinks inward. An area of necrosis and ulceration begins and eschar forms. Usually, this process is painless.
- It is distinguished from insect bites or other skin lesions by the fact that it is painless and that eschar forms regardless of treatment. Patients may have only one lesion, or there may be multiple lesions, usually in the same body area.
- Diagnosis is made based on the appearance of the lesions, a culture that is positive for the organism, or the presence of anthrax antibodies in the patient's blood.
- Management involves oral antibiotics for 60 days for patients who have no edema, systemic symptoms, and the lesions are not located on the head or neck. The antibiotics of choice are ciprofloxacin (Cipro) or doxycycline (Doryx, Vibramycin). For patients who have a fever, have lesions on the head or neck, are pregnant, or have extensive edema, antibiotics are given IV and then followed by an oral course of 60 days.

ANTHRAX, INHALATION

OVERVIEW

- Inhalation anthrax is a bacterial infection caused by the grampositive, organism *Bacillus anthracis,* which lives as a spore in contaminated soil. Infection with this organism can occur through the skin, the intestinal tract, or the lungs.

- Inhalation anthrax is a rare natural occurrence in the United States, but it has a fatality rate of nearly 100% without treatment.
- *It is not spread by person-to-person contact. Because the inhalation form of the disease is rare, any occurrence is considered unnatural or an intentional act of bioterrorism.*
- This organism first forms a *spore*, an encapsulated organism that is inactive until engulfed by macrophages. The organisms then leave their capsules and replicate. The active bacteria produce several toxins that they release into the infected tissues and the blood. The organisms can enter the blood and spread rapidly, causing sepsis and meningitis.

PATIENT-CENTERED COLLABORATIVE CARE

Assessment

- Inhalation anthrax is a two-stage illness, and manifestations may not begin until as long as 8 weeks after exposure to the organism.
- The *prodromal stage* is the first stage and is difficult to distinguish from influenza or pneumonia. Manifestations are non-specific and include:
  1. Fever
  2. Fatigue
  3. Mild chest pain
  4. Dry, harsh cough

> 🆘 Critical Rescue ◆ A special feature of inhalation anthrax is that it is not accompanied by upper respiratory manifestations of rhinitis, headache, watery eyes, or sore throat. Notify the infection control department of your facility for any patient who fits this profile.

- The *fulminant stage* is the second stage and begins after the patient feels a little better. Manifestations include:
  1. A sudden onset of a feeling of breathlessness
  2. Rapid progression to severe respiratory distress, dyspnea, diaphoresis, stridor on inhalation and exhalation, and cyanosis
  3. High fever
  4. Mediastinitis and pleural effusions
  5. Septic shock
  6. Meningitis

7. Death often occurs within 24 to 36 hours after the onset of breathlessness, even if antibiotics are started in this stage.

Interventions

- Drug therapy for suspected or diagnosed inhalation anthrax includes:
  1. Prophylaxis drug therapy
     a. Ciprofloxacin (Cipro): 500 mg orally twice daily *or*
     b. Doxycycline (Vibramycin): 100 mg orally twice daily *or* (if the organism proves susceptible to penicillin)
     c. Amoxicillin (Amoxil, Trimox): 500 mg orally every 8 hours
     d. Prophylaxis must continue for 60 days (or longer if exposure was heavy).
  2. Treatment drug therapy
     a. Ciprofloxacin (Cipro IV): 400 mg IV every 12 hours *or*
     b. Doxycycline (Doxy 100): 100 mg IV every 12 hours
     c. Plus one or two of the following secondary agents (parenteral form; dosage based on patient's weight and age):
        (1) Rifampin (RIF)
        (2) Clindamycin (Cleocin)
        (3) Vancomycin (Vancocin, Vancoled)
     d. Treatment with IV drugs continues for at least 7 days. When the response is good and the patient improves, IV drugs are changed to oral agents, which are continued for at least 60 days.
- Teach patients with any type of lower respiratory infection to be especially vigilant for changes after they think they are getting well. They need to seek medical attention immediately on having a setback that starts with breathlessness.

APPENDICITIS

OVERVIEW

- Appendicitis is an acute inflammation of the vermiform appendix, the small finger-like pouch attached to the cecum of the colon.
- Inflammation of the appendix can occur when the lumen of the appendix is obstructed.
- Inflammation leads to infection as bacteria invade the wall of the appendix.
- Appendicitis is the most common cause of acute inflammation in the right lower abdominal quadrant.
- Appendicitis may occur at any age, but the peak incidence is between 20 and 30 years of age.

~~~~ **Considerations for Older Adults** A

- Appendicitis is not common in older adults, but when it occurs, perforation is a common complication.
- The diagnosis of appendicitis is difficult to establish for the older adult because symptoms of pain and tenderness are not as pronounced in older adults as they are in younger persons.

PATIENT-CENTERED COLLABORATIVE CARE
Assessment
- Assessment findings include:
    1. Abdominal pain originating in the epigastric or periumbilical area and shifting to the right lower quadrant (McBurney's point); pain may not be localized.
    2. Nausea and vomiting
    3. Anorexia after the initial diagnosis of pain
    4. Urge to defecate or pass flatus
    5. Muscle rigidity and rebound tenderness
    6. Normal or slightly elevated temperature
    7. Increased WBC count with possible increased segs (polys) (i.e., left shift)
- Abdominal pain that increases with cough or movement and is relieved by flexion of the right hip or knees suggests a perforated appendix with peritonitis.
Planning and Implementation
- Withhold oral fluids 2 to 4 hours preoperatively to surgical appendectomy (removal of the appendix).
- Keep the patient in a semi-Fowler position so that abdominal drainage, if any, can be contained in the lower abdomen.
- Appendectomy may be performed as a traditional procedure through a small incision or, if not ruptured, by means of laparoscopy.
- Routine postoperative care for a traditional appendectomy includes:
    1. Assessing the abdominal drains for excess drainage. Drains are placed only if an abscess is present.
    2. Maintaining the patient's nasogastric tube or other drainage devices if inserted intraoperatively for peritonitis
    3. Administering IV antibiotics
    4. Assisting the patient out of bed on the evening of surgery
    5. Typical postoperative pain management, including administering opioid analgesia
- Care after a laparoscopic procedure includes:
    1. Monitoring puncture sites
    2. Providing routine postoperative care, anticipating discharge within 24 hours of surgery

> ⚙ **Critical Rescue** ◆ A change in pain from localized to generalized abdominal pain may indicate the appendix has ruptured. Immediately inform the surgeon of this finding, along with vital signs.

ARTERIAL DISEASE, PERIPHERAL

OVERVIEW

- Peripheral arterial disease (PAD) is a condition in which partial or total arterial occlusion deprives the lower extremities of oxygen and nutrients.
- Tissue damage generally occurs below the arterial destruction, and the location of the occlusion determines the location of tissue damage.
- Obstructions are characterized as inflow or outflow according to the arteries involved and their relationship to the inguinal ligament.
- Patients with chronic PAD seek treatment for the characteristic leg pain known as intermittent claudication.
- The four stages of chronic PAD are:
  1. Stage I: Asymptomatic
     a. No claudication is present.
     b. Bruit or aneurysm may be present.
     c. Pedal pulses are decreased or absent.
  2. Stage II: Claudication
     a. Muscle pain, cramping, or burning is exacerbated by exercise and relieved by rest.
     b. Symptoms are reproducible with exercise.
  3. Stage III: Rest Pain
     a. Pain while resting commonly awakens the patient at night.
     b. Pain is described as a numb, burning, toothache-type of pain.
     c. Pain usually occurs in the distal portion of the extremity (toes, arch, forefoot, or heel) and only rarely the calf or ankle.
     d. Pain is relieved by placing the extremity in a dependent position.
  4. Stage IV: Necrosis or Gangrene
     a. Ulcers and blackened tissue occur on the toes, forefoot, and heel.
     b. A distinctive gangrenous odor is present.
- To detect cyanosis in a dark-skinned patient, assess the skin and nail beds for a dull, lifeless color.

- Acute peripheral vascular disease occurs when there is an acute obstruction by a thrombus or embolus, causing severe, acute pain below the level of the obstruction.
- Risk factors for acute disease include hypertension, hyperlipidemia, diabetes mellitus, cigarette smoking, obesity, and familial predisposition.

PATIENT-CENTERED COLLABORATIVE CARE

Assessment

- Assessment findings include:
  1. Leg pain with exercise or rest
  2. Discomfort in the lower back, buttocks, or thighs (inflow disease)
  3. Burning or cramping in the calves, ankles, feet, and toes (outflow disease)
  4. History of acute or chronic pain
  5. Ischemic changes of the extremity
     a. Loss of hair on the lower calf, ankle, and foot
     b. Dry, scaly skin
     c. Thickened toenails
     d. Color changes (elevation pallor or dependent rubor)
     e. Mottled and cool or cold extremity
  6. Presence or absence of pulses
  7. Ulcer formation
     a. Arterial ulcers develop on the toes, between the toes, or on the upper aspect of the foot; they are painful.
     b. Diabetic ulcers develop on the plantar surface of the foot, over metatarsal heads, on the heel, or on pressure areas; they may not be painful.
     c. Venous stasis ulcers occur at the ankles, with discoloration of the lower extremity at the ulcer; they cause minimal pain.
- Diagnostic assessment includes:
  1. Segmental systolic blood pressure measurement using a Doppler probe
  2. Exercise tolerance test
  3. Plethysmography

Planning and Implementation

Nonsurgical Management

- Teach the following methods of increasing arterial blood flow in chronic arterial disease:
  1. Exercise, which promotes collateral circulation
  2. Positioning to promote circulation and decrease swelling
     a. Legs should be elevated but not above the level of the heart.

    b. Teach patients to avoid crossing their legs and wearing restrictive clothing.

3. Providing warmth to the affected extremity
   a. Teach the patient to wear socks or insulated bedroom shoes and maintain a warm home environment.
   b. Caution the patient not to apply direct heat to the lower limbs, which may cause burns because of decreased sensitivity.
4. Decreasing exposure to cold and avoiding nicotine, caffeine, and emotional stress
5. Drug therapy, including antiplatelet therapy
6. Control of hypertension

- Endovascular procedures may be used to restore arterial circulation. Treat the patient with typical preoperative interventions. The procedural approach is one of the following:
  1. Percutaneous transluminal angioplasty (PTA) dilates arteries that are occluded or stenosed with a balloon catheter; a stent may be placed.
  2. Laser-assisted angioplasty may be used to open an occluded artery.
  3. Mechanical rotational abrasive atherectomy is used to improve blood flow to ischemic limbs for scraping plaque while minimizing danger to the vessel wall.
- After PTA, care of the patient includes:
  1. Observing the puncture site for bleeding
  2. Closely monitoring vital signs
  3. Checking the distal pulses of both limbs
  4. Encouraging the patient to maintain bedrest for 6 to 8 hours, as ordered, with the limb straight
  5. Administering anticoagulation therapy, which may continue for 3 to 6 months after the procedure
  6. Encouraging the patient to take aspirin on a permanent basis, as ordered

Surgical Management

- An emergency surgical embolectomy is performed on patients who experience an acute peripheral artery occlusion by an embolus.
- Acute arterial insufficiency often presents with the "6 P's" of ischemia:
  1. Pain
  2. Pallor
  3. Pulselessness
  4. Paresthesia
  5. Paralysis
  6. Poikilothermia (coolness)

- Arterial revascularization surgery is used to increase arterial blood flow in an affected limb and includes inflow procedures such as aortoiliac bypass, aortofemoral bypass, and axillofemoral bypass and outflow procedures, including femoropopliteal bypass and femorotibial bypass.
- Grafting materials for bypass surgeries include the autogenous saphenous vein and synthetic graft material such as polytetrafluoroethylene.
- Provide postoperative care.
  1. Monitor for the patency of the graft by checking for changes in the extremity.
     a. Color
     b. Temperature
     c. Pulse intensity
     d. Pain intensity (Typical pain is described as throbbing pain, which occurs from increased blood flow to the affected limb.)
  2. Mark the site of the distal pulses, located by palpation or auscultated with Doppler ultrasonography.
  3. Monitor the patient's blood pressure, notifying the physician about increases and decreases beyond desired ranges.
  4. Avoid bending the knee and hip of the affected limb.
  5. Monitor for signs and symptoms at or around the graft and incision sites, such as hardness, tenderness, redness, or warmth.
- Thrombectomy (removal of the clot) is the most common treatment for acute graft occlusion; thrombolytic therapy may be used.
- Compartment syndrome occurs when tissue pressure within a confined body space becomes elevated and restricts blood flow.
- Use sterile technique when in contact with the incision and observe for symptoms of infection.

> ▨ **Critical Rescue** ◆ Inform the vascular surgeon if assessment of the operative extremity includes worsening pain, swelling or tenseness, absent pulse, demarcations of color or temperature distal to revascularization, or loss of sensation.

Community-Based Care
- The patient benefits from a case manager who can follow the patient across the continuum of care.
- Patient and family education includes:
  1. Reinforcing the need for individualized positioning and an exercise plan

2. Teaching the patient to avoid raising the legs above the level of the heart unless he or she also has venous stasis
3. Providing written and oral foot care instructions, instructing the patient to:
   a. Keep the feet clean by washing with a mild soap in room-temperature water.
   b. Keep the feet dry, especially between the toes and ankles.
   c. Avoid injury or extended pressure to the feet and ankles.
   d. Always wear comfortable, well-fitting shoes.
   e. Keep the toenails clean, and cut the nails straight across.
   f. Prevent dry, cracked skin.
   g. Prevent exposure to extreme heat or cold.
   h. Avoid heating pads.
   i. Avoid constricting garments.
4. Providing dressing change and incision care instructions, if necessary
5. Providing instructions concerning discharge medications
6. Encouraging the patient to avoid smoking and to limit daily intake of fat to less than 30% of total calories
- Identify the need for a home care nurse or home health aide.
- Home care assessment of the patient includes:
  1. Assessing tissue perfusion to affected extremity
     a. Distal circulation, sensation, and motion
     b. Presence of pain, pallor, paresthesias, pulselessness, paralysis, coolness
  2. Assessing adherence to therapeutic regimen
     a. Following foot care instructions
     b. Quitting smoking
     c. Maintaining dietary restrictions
     d. Participating in exercise regimen
     e. Avoiding both exposure to cold and constrictive clothing
  3. Assessing patient ability to manage wound care and prevent further injury
  4. Assessing coping ability of patient and family members
  5. Assessing home environment for safety hazards

ARTERIOSCLEROSIS AND ATHEROSCLEROSIS

OVERVIEW

- Arteriosclerosis is a thickening or hardening of the arterial wall of the vascular system.
- Atherosclerosis, a type of arteriosclerosis, involves the formation of a plaque within the arterial wall and is the leading con-

tributor to coronary artery disease (CAD) and cerebrovascular disease, leading to a stroke.
- The exact pathophysiologic mechanism of atherosclerosis is unknown but is thought to occur with inflammation of the vessel.
- Atherosclerosis begins as a fatty streak on the intimal surface of an artery and develops into a fibrous plaque that partially or completely occludes the blood flow of the artery.
- Atherosclerosis progresses as the fatty streak becomes calcified, populated with activated WBC, and enlarges while reducing the lumen of the vessel.
- The rate of progression of this process is thought to be influenced by genetic factors, certain diseases, such as diabetes mellitus, and certain behaviors, including smoking, high-fat and high-caloric diets, and lack of exercise.

PATIENT-CENTERED COLLABORATIVE CARE

- Assess:
  1. Take blood pressure in both arms and note any differences.
  2. Palpate pulses at all major sites and note any differences.
  3. Assess for prolonged capillary refill.
  4. Assess temperature differences in lower extremities.
  6. Assess arterial bruits at carotids and femoral pulses.
  7. Assess for elevated serum cholesterol (elevated LDL and low or normal high-density lipoprotein [HDL]), triglyceride, and homocysteine levels.
- Interventions include:
  1. Teaching the patient to limit cholesterol in collaboration with the dietitian:
     a. Limit dietary fat to 30% of total calories per day (American Heart Association Heart Healthy Diet).
  2. Reinforcing the plan for regular, realistic activity with at least 150 minutes weekly as a goal
  3. Administering cholesterol-lowering agents as prescribed for patients who do not respond to diet therapy and other nondrug measures
  4. Encouraging the patient to stop smoking (cigarette smoking lowers levels of HDL cholesterol), to avoid secondary smoke, and to seek a smoking cessation group such as the American Cancer Society's Fresh Start program if needed:
     a. Patients who smoke may consider behavior therapy, a nicotine substitute, buproprion (Wellbutrin) or varenicline (Chantrix), to aid in smoking cessation.
     b. Other complementary and alternative therapies to stop smoking include acupuncture, hypnosis, biofeedback, and support groups.

5. Developing a plan to exercise for 30 minutes daily most days of the week
6. Planning for follow-up and ongoing care with primary care provider at least annually

ARTHRITIS, RHEUMATOID

OVERVIEW

- Rheumatoid arthritis (RA) is a chronic, progressive, systemic inflammatory autoimmune disease process that damages and destroys synovial joints. It has patterns of natural remissions and exacerbations.
- Onset may be acute and severe or slow and insidious.
- Permanent joint changes may be avoided if RA is diagnosed early. Early, aggressive treatment to suppress synovitis may lead to a remission.
- Other areas of the body can be affected; vasculitis can cause malfunction and eventual failure of an organ or system.
- Genetic factors along with environmental conditions interact to trigger RA.
- Female reproductive hormones may influence the development of RA because the disease affects more women than men.

PATIENT-CENTERED COLLABORATIVE CARE

Assessment

- Assess for early disease manifestations, including:
  1. Joint stiffness, swelling, pain (especially of the upper extremities)
  2. Usually symptoms are bilateral (affect both sides) and symmetric (same joints).
  3. Fatigue, generalized weakness
  4. Anorexia, weight loss
  5. Persistent, low-grade fever
  6. Migrating symptoms known as migratory arthritis
  7. Joint infection may be present (one hot, swollen, joint that has pain out of proportion to the other joints).

> 🆘 **Critical Rescue** ◆ Refer the patient to the health care provider (usually the rheumatologist) immediately if manifestations of joint infection are present.

- Assess for late disease manifestations.
  1. Joints become progressively inflamed, puffy, and quite painful.
  2. Morning stiffness lasts longer than 45 minutes.

A

3. Affected joints have a soft or a spongy feeling.
4. Muscles atrophy above and below affected joints.
5. ROM decreases.
6. Most or all of the synovial joints are eventually affected.
7. Joint deformity
8. Carpal tunnel of the wrists
9. Baker's cysts (enlarged popliteal bursae behind the knee)
10. Bone fractures
11. Tendon ruptures (especially the Achilles tendon)
12. Cervical disease may result in subluxation that may be life threatening.

> **Critical Rescue** ◆ Cervical pain with loss of ROM should be reported to the physician.

- Assess for systemic complications:
    1. Exacerbations, often called *flares*
    2. Increased joint swelling and tenderness
    3. Moderate to severe weight loss
    4. Fever
    5. Extreme fatigue
    6. Subcutaneous nodules along muscles or tendons, which may become open and infected or interfere with ADLs
    7. Inflammation of blood vessels, resulting in vasculitis, particularly of small to medium-sized vessels
    8. Ischemic skin and nail lesions that appear in small groups as small, brownish spots
    9. Larger skin lesions that appear on the lower extremities may lead to ulceration, which heal slowly as a result of decreased circulation
    10. Peripheral neuropathy, causing footdrop and paresthesias
    11. Respiratory complication, including pleurisy, pneumonitis, diffuse interstitial fibrosis, and pulmonary hypertension
    12. Cardiac complications, including pericarditis and myocarditis
    13. Ocular involvement, such as iritis or scleritis
    14. Sjögren's syndrome (eye, mouth, and vaginal dryness)
    15. Felty's syndrome (enlarged liver and spleen, leukopenia)
    16. Caplan's syndrome (presence of rheumatoid nodules in the lungs and pneumoconiosis), which is found mainly in coal miners and asbestos workers
- Assess for psychosocial issues:
    1. Fear of becoming disabled and dependent, uncertainty about the disease process, altered body image, devaluation of self, frustration, and depression are common.

2. Physical limitations may result in role changes in the family and society.
3. Extreme fatigue often causes patients to desire an early bedtime and may result in a reluctance to socialize.
4. Body changes may also cause poor self-esteem and body image.
5. The patient may grieve, experience degrees of depression, or have feelings of helplessness caused by a loss of control over a disease that can "consume" the body.
6. Evaluate the patient's support systems and resources.
- Assess laboratory data (none are specific for RA, but all are associated with it):
  1. Positive rheumatoid factor
  2. Positive antinuclear antibody test (ANA or FANA)
  3. Positive anti-Sjögren's syndrome antibodies, especially anti-SS-A (Ro)
  4. Decreased serum complement
  5. Elevated erythrocyte sedimentation rate
  6. Elevated high-sensitivity C-reactive protein (hsCRP)
  7. Altered CBC and platelet count (low hematocrit and hemoglobin levels, high WBC count)
- Other diagnostic assessments
  1. Joint x-rays
  2. Bone scan or joint scan
  3. MRI
  4. Arthrocentesis, a procedure to aspirate a sample of the synovial fluid to relieve pressure and analyze the fluid for inflammatory cells and immune complexes, including rheumatoid factor

Interventions
- Drug therapy used to treat RA includes:
  1. Disease-modifying antirheumatic drugs (DMARDs) are used to slow the progression of mild rheumatoid disease before it progresses. They include:
     a. Methotrexate (Rheumatrex)
     b. Leflunomide (Arava)
     c. Hydroxychloroquine (Plaquenil)
     d. Sulfasalazine (Azulfidine)
  2. Nonsteroidal anti-inflammatory drugs (NSAIDs) are often the drug of choice to relieve pain and inflammation on a short-term basis.
  3. Biological response modifiers (BRMs) interfere with the action of different inflammatory mediators. They are expensive, and not all insurance companies pay for their use.

Patients with multiple sclerosis and tuberculosis are not prescribed these drugs:

A

  a. Etanercept (Enbrel)
  b. Infliximab (Remicade)
  c. Adalimumab (Humira)
  d. Anakinra (Kineret)
  e. Abatacept (Orencia)
  f. Rituximab (Rituxan)
  g. Tocilizumab (Actemra)
4. Steroidal anti-inflammatory drugs
  a. Prednisone (Deltasone, Medrol)
5. Other immunosuppressive drugs
  a. Azathioprine (Imuran)
  b. Cyclophosphamide (Cytoxan)
6. Analgesic drugs
  a. Acetaminophen (Tylenol, Exdol, Datril)
  b. Propoxyphene (Darvon, Novapropoxyn)
  c. Propoxyphene napsylate (Darvocet-N)
- Nonpharmacologic management
  1. Other pain-relief measures: rest, positioning, ice, and heat
  2. Plasmapheresis (or plasma exchange) to remove the antibodies causing the disease
  3. Some patients achieve pain relief with hypnosis, acupuncture, magnet therapy, imagery, or music therapy.
  4. Stress management
  5. Encourage good nutrition, including foods that contain omega-3 fatty acids (salmon, tuna), fish oil capsules, and antioxidant vitamins A, C, and E.
- Promotion of self-care
  1. Identify assistive devices to allow the patient as much independence as possible.
  2. Help patients acquire household items with handles.
  3. Teach patient to use larger muscle groups to perform tasks usually performed by fine muscle groups (e.g., use the flat of the hand to squeeze toothpaste tubes instead of the fingers).
  4. Refer the patient to an occupational or physical therapist or the Arthritis Foundation for special assistive and adaptive devices.
- Management of fatigue
  1. Identify factors that contribute to fatigue (anemia, muscle atrophy, inadequate rest).
  2. Collaborate with the health care team to alleviate or manage contributing factors.

    a. Anemia
- (1) Administer iron, folic acid, vitamin supplements, or a combination of these
- (2) Assess the patient for drug-related blood loss, such as that caused by salicylate therapy, by testing the stool for occult blood.

    b. Muscle atrophy
- (1) Collaborate with a physical therapist to develop and help the patient implement a personalized daily exercise program.

    c. Inadequate rest
- (1) Arrange for a quiet environment.
- (2) Encourage the patient to drink a warm beverage before bedtime.

3. Teach principles of energy conservation.
    a. Pacing activities
    b. Setting priorities
    c. Planning rest periods
    d. Obtaining assistance when possible; delegating activities to the family

- Enhancement of body image
  1. Identify factors to enhance body image.
  2. Determine the patient's perception of changes and the impact of the reactions of family and significant others.
  3. Communicate acceptance of the patient by establishing a trusting relationship.
  4. Encourage the patient to wear street clothes and his or her own nightclothes or bathrobe.
  5. Assist with grooming, such as shaving and makeup.

> **Clinical Landmine** ◆ The patient may use strategies that range from denial or fear to anger and depression. Avoid labeling the patient as manipulative and demanding, because these behaviors may represent how he or she is trying to cope with the effects of the illness.

- Community-based care considerations for discharge include:
  1. Assisting the patient and family to identify structural changes needed in the home before discharge
  2. Reinforcing information about drug therapy
  3. Teaching the patient to consult with the health care provider before trying any over-the-counter or home remedies
  4. Teaching joint protection measures
  5. Teaching the patient to ask for help to prevent further joint damage and disease progression

6. Reviewing energy conservation measures
7. Reviewing the prescribed exercise program
8. Referring the patient to local and national support groups such as the Arthritis Foundation
9. Referring the patient to the nutritionist, counselor, home health nurse, rehabilitation therapist, financial counselor, and local and state support groups as needed
10. Teaching the patient to check with the Arthritis Foundation for the latest information on arthritis myths and quackery

ASTHMA

OVERVIEW

- *Bronchial asthma* is an intermittent and *reversible* airflow obstruction affecting only the airways, not the alveoli.
- Airway obstruction can occur in two ways:
  1. Inflammation, obstructing the *lumen* (the inside) of airways, occurs in response to the presence of specific allergens; general irritants such as cold air, dry air, or fine airborne particles; microorganisms; and aspirin.
  2. Airway hyperresponsiveness, obstructing airways by constricting bronchial smooth muscle causing a narrowing of the airway from the outside, can occur with exercise, an upper respiratory illness, and for unknown reasons.
- Many people with asthma have both problems at the same time.
- Severe airway obstruction can be fatal.
- Although asthma may be classified into different types based on the events known to trigger the attacks, the pathophysiology is similar for all types of asthma regardless of triggering event.
- Inflammation of the mucous membranes lining the airways is a key event in triggering an asthma attack.
- Asthma can occur at any age. About one half of adults with asthma also had the disease in childhood. Asthma is more common in urban settings than in rural settings.

Considerations for Older Adults

Asthma occurs as a new disorder in about 3% of people older than 55 years. Another 3% of people older than 60 years have asthma as a continuing chronic disorder. Lung and airway changes as a part of aging make any breathing problem more serious in the older adult. One problem related to aging is a change in the sensitivity of beta-adrenergic receptors. When stimulated, these receptors relax smooth muscle and cause bronchodilation. As these receptors become less sensitive, they no longer respond as quickly or as strongly to agonists (epinephrine, dopamine) and beta-adrenergic drugs, which are often used as rescue therapy during an acute asthma attack. Teaching older patients how to avoid asthma attacks and to correctly use preventive drug therapy are nursing priorities.

Women's Health Considerations

The incidence of asthma is about 35% higher among women than men, and the asthma death rates are also higher among women. Obesity and hormonal fluctuations around the menstrual cycle are thought to contribute to the difference in incidence, and under-treatment of the disease is thought to be a factor in the higher death rate. Teaching women with asthma how to be a partner in asthma management and the correct use of preventive and rescue drugs remains a nursing priority in improving the outcomes of the disease.

PATIENT-CENTERED COLLABORATIVE CARE

Assessment

- Obtain the patient's personal history.
  1. Episodes of dyspnea, chest tightness, coughing, wheezing, and increased mucus production
  2. Specific patterns of dyspnea appearance (at night, with exercise, seasonally, or in association with other specific activities or environments)
  3. Other allergic symptoms such as rhinitis, skin rash, or pruritus, and whether other family members have asthma or respiratory problems
- Clinical manifestations during an attack include:
  1. Audible wheeze (at first, louder on exhalation)
  2. Increased respiratory rate
  3. Breathing cycle that is longer and requires more effort
  4. Coughing
  5. Patient may not be able to complete a sentence of more than five words.
  6. Decreased oxygen saturation
  7. Pallor or cyanosis of oral mucous membranes and nail beds
  8. Tachycardia
  9. Changes in level of consciousness
  10. Use of accessory muscles (muscle retraction at the sternum, the suprasternal notch, and between the ribs)
- Physical changes from frequent asthma attacks include:
  1. Increased anteroposterior (AP) chest diameter
  2. Increased space between the ribs

- Laboratory assessment data changes during an asthma attack
  1. Decreased Pao_2
  2. Decreased $Paco_2$ (early in attack)
  3. Elevated $Paco_2$ (later in attack)
- Laboratory assessment data changes from allergic asthma
  1. Elevated serum eosinophil count
  2. Elevated immunoglobulin E (IgE) levels
  3. Sputum containing eosinophils, mucous plugs, and shed epithelial cells (Curschmann spirals)
- Diagnostic assessment
  1. Pulmonary function tests (PFTs) measured using spirometry, especially
     a. *Forced vital capacity* (FVC) (volume of air exhaled from full inhalation to full exhalation)
     b. *Forced expiratory volume in the first second* (FEV_1) (volume of air blown out as hard and fast as possible during the first second of the most forceful exhalation after the greatest full inhalation)
     c. *Peak expiratory flow* (PEF) (fastest airflow rate reached at any time during exhalation)
  2. Chest x-rays
  3. Blood levels of therapeutic drugs (theophylline)

Interventions
- The goals of asthma therapy are to improve airflow, relieve symptoms, and prevent episodes by making the patient an active partner in the management plan.
- Priority patient education focuses on:
  1. Teaching the patient to assess symptom severity at least twice daily with a peak flow meter and adjust drugs to manage inflammation and bronchospasms to prevent or relieve symptoms
  2. Assisting the patient to establish a "personal best" peak expiratory flow (PEF) by measuring his or her PEF twice daily for 2 to 3 weeks when asthma is well controlled and using this value to compare all other readings
  3. Instructing the patient to evaluate when to use a rescue inhaler (when PEF is between 50% and 80% of personal best) and when to seek emergency assistance (when PEF is below 50% of personal best)

> 🔧 **Critical Rescue** ◆ Teach the patient who has a reading in the "red zone" to immediately use the rescue drugs and seek emergency help.

  4. Teaching the patient to keep a symptom and intervention diary to learn his or her triggers of asthma symptoms, early

cues for impending attacks, and personal response to drugs
5. Stressing the importance of proper use of the asthma action plan for any severity of asthma
- Drug therapy focuses on prevention of asthma attacks (preventive therapy) and stopping attacks that have already started (rescue therapy).
- Many preventive and rescue drugs are delivered as dry powder inhalers (DPIs) or as aerosol metered dose inhalers (MDIs). Teach patients the proper ways to use and store these inhalers.
- *Preventive therapy drugs are those used to change airway responsiveness to prevent asthma attacks from occurring. They are used every day, regardless of symptoms.*

> ▧ Critical Rescue ◆ Teach patients using preventive therapy to take the prescribed drugs daily, even when asthma symptoms are not present.

1. Bronchodilators increase bronchiolar smooth muscle relaxation and include beta$_2$ agonists, cholinergic antagonists, and methylxanthines.
   a. Long-acting beta$_2$ agonists (LABAs) are delivered by inhaler directly to the site of action: the bronchioles. They need time to build up an effect, but the effects are longer lasting. The use of LABAs is recommended to be co-administered with inhaled steriods.

> ▨ Clinical Landmine ◆ These drugs are useful in preventing an asthma attack but have no value during an acute attack. Teach patients *not* to use LABAs to rescue them during an attack or when wheezing is getting worse.

   b. Cholinergic antagonists (anticholinergic drugs) are similar to atropine and block the parasympathetic nervous system, causing bronchodilation and decreased pulmonary secretions. Most are used by inhaler.
      (1) Ipratropium (Atrovent)
      (2) Tiotropium (Spiriva)
   c. Methylxanthines are used when other types of management are ineffective.
      (1) Theophylline (Theo-Dur)
      (2) Aminophylline (Truphylline)
      (3) Oxtriphylline (Choledyl)
      (4) Dyphylline (Dilor, Lufyllin)

> 🛟 **Critical Rescue** ◆ Teach the patient who takes these drugs daily to keep all appointments for monitoring blood levels of the drug and not to self-increase the dose. These drugs have narrow safety ranges and have many dangerous side effects, especially cardiac and central nervous system stimulation.

2. Anti-Inflammatory drugs decrease the inflammatory responses in the airways. Some are given systemically and have more side effects. Others are used as inhalants and have few systemic side effects.
   a. Inhaled corticosteroids (ICSs)
      (1) Fluticasone (Flovent)
      (2) Budesonide (Pulmicort)
      (3) Mometasone (Asmanex)
   b. Nonsteroidal anti-inflammatory drugs (NSAIDs)
      (1) Nedocromil (Tilade)
      (2) Cromolyn sodium (Intal)
   c. Leukotriene antagonists
      (1) Montelukast (Singulair)
      (2) Zafirlukast (Accolate)
      (3) Zileuton (Zyflo)
   d. Immunomodulators
      (1) Omalizumab (Xolair)
- Rescue therapy drugs are those used to actually stop an attack once it has started. Short-acting beta$_2$ agonists (SABAs) provide rapid but short-term relief. These inhaled drugs are most useful when an attack begins (rescue drug) or as premedication when the patient is about to begin an activity that is likely to induce an asthma attack.
  1. Albuterol (Proventil, Ventolin)
  2. Bitolterol (Tornalate)
  3. Levalbuterol (Xopenex)
  4. Pirbuterol (Maxair)
  5. Terbutaline (Brethaire)

> 🛟 **Critical Rescue** ◆ Teach the patient to always carry the rescue drug inhaler with him or her and to ensure that there is enough drug remaining in the inhaler to provide a quick dose when needed.

- Regular exercise, including aerobic exercise, is a recommended part of asthma therapy.
  1. Teach patients to examine the conditions that trigger an attack and adjust the exercise routine as needed.

2. Some patients may need to premedicate with inhaled beta agonists (SABAs) before beginning activity.

- Supplemental oxygen with high flow rates or high concentrations is often used during an acute asthma attack. Oxygen is delivered by mask, nasal cannula, or endotracheal tube.
- Heliox, a mixture of helium and oxygen (often 50% helium and 50% oxygen) can help improve oxygen delivery to the alveoli.
- *Status asthmaticus* is a severe, life-threatening acute episode of airway obstruction that intensifies once it begins and often does not respond to usual therapy.
  1. Assess for manifestations, including:
     a. Extremely labored breathing and wheezing
     b. Use of accessory muscles
     c. Distention of neck veins are observed
     d. PEF below 50% of expected for patient's age, size, and gender
     e. Oxygen saturation less than 80%
  2. Apply oxygen.
  3. Immediate drug therapy includes:
     a. IV fluids
     b. Potent systemic bronchodilators
     c. IV steroids
     d. Parenteral epinephrine
  4. Prepare for emergency intubation.
  5. If the condition is not reversed, the patient may develop pneumothorax, and cardiac or respiratory arrest.

AVIAN INFLUENZA ("BIRD FLU")

OVERVIEW

- Viral infections are common among wild and domestic birds, including chickens and ducks, and usually remain a problem only among birds.
- A few times, bird viruses have mutated and became highly infectious to humans, resulting in many millions of deaths worldwide. (These include the 1918 "Spanish" influenza and the 1968 and 1997 "Hong-Kong" influenza strains.)
- A new avian virus is the H5N1 strain that has infected millions of birds, especially in Asia, but did not appear to infect humans. *World health officials are concerned that this strain could mutate to allow bird-to-human infection and then mutate again to allow person-to-person human infection. This possibility is a major concern because humans have essentially no naturally occurring immunity to this virus and the infection could lead to a worldwide pandemic with very high mortality.*

- As of January 2008, 349 cases of H5N1 avian influenza in humans have been reported to the World Health Organization (WHO), with a total of 216 deaths (61% mortality rate) in 14 countries in Asia and the Middle East.
- The virus appears to spread by oral-fecal transmission as a result of bird droppings contaminating ponds, lakes, and rivers.
- The infection is *not* spread by eating the cooked meat of contaminated birds.

HEALTH PROMOTION AND MAINTENANCE

- The prevention of a worldwide pandemic of avian flu is the responsibility of everyone.
- No completely effective vaccine is currently available.
- The recommended approach to disease prevention is early recognition of new cases and the implementation of community and personal quarantine and social-distancing behaviors to reduce exposure to the virus.
- When a cluster of cases is discovered in an area, widespread distribution of the antiviral drugs oseltamivir (Tamiflu) and zanamivir (Relenza) should occur.
- The infected patients should be cared for in strict isolation.
- All non-essential public activities in the area should be stopped. These include public gatherings of any type, attendance at schools, religious services, shopping, and many types of employment.
- People should stay home and use their emergency preparedness supplies (food, water, and drugs) they have stockpiled for at least 2 weeks. Travel to and from this area should be stopped.

PATIENT-CENTERED COLLABORATIVE CARE

- Care of the patient with avian influenza focuses on supporting the patient and preventing spread of the disease.
- The initial manifestations of avian influenza are similar to other respiratory infections: cough, fever, and sore throat. These progress rapidly to shortness of breath, and pneumonia. In addition, diarrhea, vomiting, abdominal pain, and bleeding from the nose and gums occur.
- If avian influenza is suspected, coordinate with the health care team to place the patient in an airborne isolation room with negative air pressure. These isolation precautions remain until the diagnosis of H5N1 is confirmed or ruled out.
- Diagnosis is made based on clinical manifestations and positive testing. The most rapid test that is accurate early in the disease course is the H5 polymerase chain reaction test performed at a WHO-approved laboratory.

- When providing care to the patient with avian influenza, personal protective equipment is essential. Ensure that anyone entering the patient's room for any reason wears a fit-tested respirator.
- Use strict Airborne and Contact Precautions.
- Use the antiviral drug oseltamivir (Tamiflu) or zanamivir (Relenza) within 48 hours of the first contact with the infected patient.
- If a vaccine is available, receive it in the recommended two-step process.
- Provide oxygen when hypoxia or breathlessness is present.
- Respiratory treatments to dilate the bronchioles and move respiratory secretions are used.
- Intubation and mechanical ventilation may be needed. Antibiotics are used to treat a bacterial pneumonia that may occur with H5N1.
- The patient with H5N1 may have severe diarrhea and need fluid therapy.

> **Critical Rescue** ◆ The two most important areas to monitor during rehydration are pulse rate and quality and urine output.

BLEEDING, DYSFUNCTIONAL UTERINE

OVERVIEW

- Dysfunctional uterine bleeding (DUB) is bleeding that is excessive or abnormal in amount or frequency without predisposing anatomic or systemic conditions.
- DUB occurs in the absence of ovulation related to ovarian function.
- DUB is associated with polycystic ovary disease, stress, extreme weight changes, and long-term use of drugs, including anticholinergics, morphine, and oral contraceptives.

PATIENT-CENTERED COLLABORATIVE CARE

Assessment

- Common assessment findings for DUB include:
  1. Menstrual irregularities
  2. Symptoms of systemic disease, such as renal or hepatic disease
  3. Variations in weight, obesity
  4. Undernutrition, extreme weight loss

5. Abnormal hair growth (excessive hair on face and body; chest hair; diamond-shaped pubic hair patch)
6. Abdominal pain or masses
7. Anatomic abnormalities

Interventions

Nonsurgical Management

- Hormone therapy for women with DUB who are anovulatory includes medroxyprogesterone or combination oral contraceptives.
- Hormone therapy for women with DUB who are ovulatory includes progestins (during the luteal phase of the menstrual cycle), oral contraceptives, prostaglandin inhibitors, or danazol.
- Evaluate the patient's knowledge about the effects, dosage, and administration schedule of her prescribed hormone therapy.
- Teach the patient the information she needs to know about her prescribed hormone therapy.

Surgical Management

- Surgical management includes diagnostic dilation and curettage (D&C), which involves scraping the endometrial tissue to assess for possible causes of bleeding or to remove bleeding tissue; laser endometrial ablation; and hysterectomy.
- Interventions for the perioperative period include:
  1. Preparing the patient for surgery and providing routine postoperative care, including assessment of vaginal bleeding
  2. While reviewing postoperative care, provide the patient with instructions:
     a. Avoid sexual intercourse, tub bathing, and the use of tampons for 2 weeks.
     b. Slight bleeding is normal, but if bleeding is as heavy as the normal menstrual period or persists for 2 weeks, the patient should notify the health care provider.
     c. Use a hot water bottle or heating pad to relieve abdominal cramping.
     d. Take mild analgesics such as acetaminophen for abdominal pain.

BLINDNESS

See Visual Impairment (Reduced Vision).

BONE MARROW TRANSPLANTATION

See Hematopoietic Stem Cell Transplantation (Bone Marrow Transplantation).

BREAST DISEASE, FIBROCYSTIC

OVERVIEW

- Fibrocystic breast disease (FBD) consists of fibrotic changes or physiologic nodularity of the breast.
- The first stage commonly occurs between the late teens and early 20s. Symptoms include premenstrual bilateral fullness and tenderness, especially in the outer upper quadrant; symptoms resolve after menstruation and recur before the next menstrual cycle.
- In the second stage, which occurs in women in their late 20s and their 30s, bilateral, multicentric nodular areas appear that feel like small marbles, with fullness and soreness.
- The third stage occurs in patients between 35 and 55 years of age, when microscopic or macroscopic cysts develop. The cysts, which occur suddenly and are associated with pain, tenderness, or burning, are usually three dimensional, smooth, mobile, and well defined.
- The cause of FBD is unknown but appears to be related to normal fluctuations in progesterone and estrogen levels during the menstrual cycle.

PATIENT-CENTERED COLLABORATIVE CARE

- Hormonal manipulation is the main focus of drug therapy and includes oral contraceptives to suppress oversecretion of estrogen and progestins.
- Other interventions include:
  1. Vitamins C, E, and B complex
  2. Diuretics to prevent premenstrual breast engorgement
  3. Mild analgesics
  4. Avoidance of excess salt intake before menses
  5. Avoidance of caffeine (not scientifically proven)
  6. Practice of regular breast self-examination
  7. Application of ice or heat
  8. Use of a supportive bra with well-padded straps to decrease tension on ligaments

BURNS

OVERVIEW

- A burn is an injury to the skin and other epithelial tissues as a result of exposure to temperature extremes, mechanical abrasion, chemical abrasion, radiation, and electrical currents.
- Patients who have burn injuries develop many physiologic, metabolic, and psychological changes.

- Immediate local and systemic problems resulting from burns include fluid and protein losses, sepsis, and changes in metabolic, endocrine, respiratory, cardiac, hematologic, and immune functioning.
- Prevention of infection and closure of the burn wound are vitally important because a lack of or delay in wound healing is a key factor for all systemic problems and a major cause of disability and death among patients who are burned.
- Burns are classified by their wound depth and severity.
  1. *Superficial-thickness wounds* have the least damage because the epidermis is the only part of the skin that is injured. The epithelial cells and basement membrane, needed for total regrowth, remain. Common causes of superficial-thickness wounds are prolonged exposure to low-intensity heat (e.g., sunburn) or short (flash) exposure to high-intensity heat. Redness with mild edema, pain, and increased sensitivity to heat occur as a result. The area heals rapidly in 3 to 5 days without a scar or other complication.
  2. *Partial-thickness wounds* involve the entire epidermis and various depths of the dermis. Depending on the amount of dermal tissue damaged, partial-thickness wounds are further subdivided into superficial partial-thickness and deep partial-thickness injuries.
     a. *Superficial partial-thickness wounds* are caused by heat injury to the upper third of the dermis leaving a good blood supply. Wounds are red, moist, and *blanch* (whiten) when pressure is applied. Blisters often form. Nerve endings are exposed, and any stimulation (touch or temperature change) causes intense pain. With care these burns heal in 10 to 21 days with no permanent scar, but some minor pigment changes may occur.
     b. *Deep partial-thickness wounds* extend deeper into the skin dermis, and fewer healthy cells remain. Blister formation does not usually occur. The wound surface is red and dry, with white areas in deeper parts. Edema is moderate, and the degree of pain is less than experienced with superficial burns because more nerve endings have been destroyed.
  3. *Full-thickness wounds* occur with destruction of the entire epidermis and dermis, leaving no true skin cells to repopulate. The wounded tissue does not regrow, and whatever area of the wound not closed by wound contraction will require grafting. The wound has a hard, dry, leathery eschar that must slough off or be removed from the burn wound before healing can occur. The wound may be waxy white, deep red,

yellow, brown, or black. Sensation is reduced or absent in these areas because of nerve ending destruction. Edema is severe under the eschar in a full-thickness wound.

    a. When the injury is circumferential (completely surrounds an extremity or the chest), blood flow and chest movement for breathing may be reduced by tight eschar.

    b. *Escharotomies* (incisions through the eschar) or *fasciotomies* (incisions through eschar and fascia) may be needed to relieve pressure and allow normal blood flow and breathing.

  4. *Deep full-thickness wounds* extend beyond the skin into underlying fascia and tissues. Muscle, bone, and tendons are damaged and exposed. The wound is blackened and depressed, and sensation is completely absent.

- Common causes of burn injury and emergency interventions to limit injury are:

  1. *Dry heat injuries* from open flames. The patient should stop, drop, and roll to smother the flames.

  2. *Moist heat (scald) injuries* are caused by contact with hot liquids or steam. Clothes that are saturated with hot liquids should be removed immediately.

  3. *Contact burns* occur when hot metal, tar, or grease contact the skin, often leading to a full-thickness injury. Removal of the hot substance limits the injury.

  4. *Chemical burns* occur as a result of accidents in homes or industry. The severity of the injury depends on the duration of contact, the concentration of the chemical, the amount of tissue exposed, and the action of the chemical. Dry chemicals should be brushed off the skin and clothing. Wet clothing is removed. Depending on the specific agent, the skin may be flushed with water or covered with mineral oil.

  5. *Electrical injury burns* occur when an electrical current enters the body. These injuries have been called the *grand masquerader* of burn injuries because the surface injuries may look small, but the associated internal injuries can be huge. The longer the electricity is in contact with the body, the greater the damage. Remove the patient from the source of the electricity without endangering yourself (use a wooden pole, rather than a metal one, to separate the person from the electrical sources). Do not touch the person directly while he or she is in contact with the electrical source!

  6. *Radiation injuries* occur when people are exposed to large doses of radioactive material. The most common type of tissue injury from radiation exposure occurs with therapeu-

tic radiation. More serious injury occurs in industrial settings where radioactive energy is produced or radioactive isotopes are used. Removal of the patient from the source of radiation limits the injury.

- Compensatory responses to the stress of the injury and the direct tissue damage occur through the sympathetic nervous system and inflammatory responses. These result in specific and predictable changes in tissue and organ function:
  1. Inflammation
  2. Vital sign changes (decreased BP, tachycardia, increased respiratory rate and depth)
  3. Capillary leak occurs with a *fluid shift* into the interstitial space. This fluid shift, also known as *third spacing* or *capillary leak syndrome,* is a continuous leak of plasma from the vascular space into the interstitial space. The loss of plasma fluids and proteins decreases blood volume and blood pressure. Leakage of fluid and electrolytes from the vascular space continues, causing extensive edema, even in areas that were not burned. Fluid shift with excessive weight gain usually occurs in the first 12 hours after the burn and can continue for 24 to 36 hours. Fluid returns to the vascular space within 48 to 72 hours.
  4. Decreased urine output
  5. Hemoconcentration (elevated hematocrit and hemoglobin)
  6. Fluid and electrolyte imbalances (most commonly metabolic acidosis), hyperkalemia (high blood potassium levels), and hyponatremia (low blood sodium levels)
  7. Decreased to absent peristalsis, formation of Curling's ulcer
  8. Elevated blood glucose levels
  9. Hypermetabolism and body temperature variation
- Burn recovery occurs over the course of three phases. Each phase has unique manifestations and care requirements.
- **Resuscitation/Emergent Phase**
  1. The *resuscitation/emergent phase* is the first phase of a burn injury. It begins at the onset of injury and continues to about 48 hours.
  2. The goals of management during the resuscitation/emergent phase are to:
     a. Secure the airway.
     b. Support circulation by fluid replacement.
     c. Keep the patient comfortable with analgesics.
     d. Prevent infection through careful wound care.
     e. Maintain body temperature.
     f. Provide emotional support.

PATIENT-CENTERED COLLABORATIVE CARE

Assessment

- During assessment, obtain the following injury-related information:
  1. Time of the injury
  2. Source of heat or injurious agent
  3. Detailed description of how and where the burn occurred
  4. Any interventions or other actions taken
  5. Whether drugs or alcohol may have been a factor
  6. Events occurring from the time of the burn to admission
  7. Any other events that could increase the burn injury or cause another injury or health problem
- Obtain the following personal patient information:
  1. Age
  2. Height and weight
  3. Medical history (especially cardiac or kidney disease, chronic alcoholism, substance abuse, diabetes mellitus)
  4. Use of prescribed, OTC, or street drugs within the past 24 hours
  5. Smoking history
  6. Level of pain
  7. Allergies
  8. Immunization status (especially tetanus)
- Assess for:
  1. Direct airway injury
     a. Changes in the appearance or function of the mouth, nose, or throat
     b. Facial burns; singed hair on the head, eyebrows, eyelids, or nose
     c. Blisters or soot on the lips, on oral mucosa, or in sputum
     d. "Smokey" smell of the breath
     e. Progressive hoarseness, wheezing, crowing, stridor
     f. Decreased oxygen saturation
     g. Drooling (inability to swallow oral secretions)

> **⬛ Critical Rescue ◆** Any of these changes may mean the patient is about to lose his or her airway. Immediately apply oxygen and notify the Rapid Response Team if any of these manifestations are present.

  2. Carbon monoxide poisoning
     a. Headache
     b. Decreased cognitive functioning, confusion, coma

    c. Tinnitus

    d. Nausea

    e. Absence of cyanosis or pallor (lips and mucous membranes may appear bright red)

    f. Elevated carboxyhemoglobin levels

3. Smoke poisoning/inhalation

    a. Atelectasis, pulmonary edema

    b. Hemorrhagic bronchitis (6 to 72 hours after injury)

4. Pulmonary fluid overload

    a. Dyspnea

    b. Hypoxia

    c. Moist breath sounds and crackles

5. Cardiovascular changes

    a. Hypovolemic and cardiogenic shock

    b. Circulatory overload with left-sided congestive heart failure

    c. Rapid, thready pulse

    d. Reduced peripheral pulses

    e. Slow or absent capillary refill

    f. Generalized edema

    g. Weight gain

    h. Baseline and continuous electrocardiographic (ECG) tracings

6. Renal or urinary changes

    a. Decreased urine output (<0.5-1 mL/kg/hr)

    b. High urine specific gravity

    c. Proteinuria

    d. Absence of urine output

7. Skin changes

    a. Depth of injury

    b. Size of injury by the total body surface area (TBSA)

    c. Color and appearance

8. Gastrointestinal changes

    a. Decreased or absent bowel sounds

    b. Nausea, vomiting

    c. Abdominal distention

    d. Ulcer formation

    e. Gross or occult blood in vomitus or stool

- Laboratory assessment

1. Increased WBCs, especially the neutrophil percentage, followed by a rapid drop with a left shift

2. Electrolytes

3. Liver enzyme studies

4. Clotting studies

🌐 Cultural Awareness

For African Americans, a sickle cell test may be appropriate if sickle status is unknown. The trauma of a burn injury often triggers a sickle cell crisis in patients who have the disease and in those who carry the trait.

Planning and Implementation

❖**NDx:** Decreased Cardiac Output; Deficient Fluid Volume; Ineffective Tissue Perfusion

Nonsurgical Management

- Rapid infusion of IV fluids, known as *fluid resuscitation*, is needed to maintain sufficient blood volume for normal cardiac output, mean arterial pressure, and tissue oxygenation. Volumes infused can be massive.
  1. Placement of a large-bore central venous catheter.
  2. The most commonly used fluids for resuscitation are crystalloids, especially lactated Ringer's solution. The optimal amount of fluid is replaced at an hourly volume sufficient to maintain a urine output of 30 to 50 mL/hr.
  3. Fluid replacement formulas are calculated from the time of injury and not from the time of arrival at the hospital. The first 50% of the calculated 24-hour volume is delivered in the first 8 hours immediately after the injury, and the remaining 50% is delivered over the next 16 hours.
- Monitoring for adequacy of fluid resuscitation
  1. Hourly urine output
  2. Adjust IV fluid rate on the basis of urine output and burn unit policy.
  3. Invasive monitoring of cardiac and pulmonary function may be needed.
     a. Central venous pressure
     b. Pulmonary artery pressures
     c. Cardiac output
  4. Continuous electrocardiographic (ECG) activity for dysrhythmias

> 🔲 **Clinical Landmine** ◆ Avoid diuretic therapy (except in electrical injuries) because these drugs do not increase cardiac output; they instead decrease circulating volume and cardiac output by pulling fluid from the circulating blood volume to enhance diuresis. This effect reduces blood flow to other vital organs (especially the heart, lungs, and brain) and greatly increases the risk for severe shock.

Considerations for Older Adults

In older patients, especially those with cardiac disease, a complicating factor in reduced cardiac output may be heart failure or myocardial infarction. Drugs that increase cardiac output, such as dopamine (Intropin), or that strengthen the force of myocardial contraction, such as digoxin (Lanoxin), may be used along with fluid therapy.

Surgical Management
- An escharotomy may be needed when tight eschar impairs tissue perfusion.
- A fasciotomy (a deeper incision extending through the fascia) may be needed to relieve constriction from fluid buildup when a burn completely surrounds an extremity.

❖**NDx:** Ineffective Breathing Pattern

Nonsurgical Management
- Airway maintenance
  1. Chin lift or a head tilt maneuver.
  2. Assess rate and depth of ventilation.
  3. Assess adequacy of respiratory effort by oxygen saturation.
  4. Assess for airway obstruction (crowing, stridor, drooling).
  5. If intubated, assess endotracheal tube hourly for patency and location.
  6. Suction as needed.
- Promoting ventilation
  1. Assess chest movement.
  2. Loosen tight thorax or neck dressings.
- Monitoring gas exchange
  1. Check arterial blood gas and carboxyhemoglobin levels.
  2. Assess for cyanosis, disorientation, and increased pulse rate.
- Oxygen therapy
  1. Administer humidified oxygen by facemask, cannula, or hood.
  2. Keep emergency airway equipment at or near the patient's bedside.
- Assist with bronchoscopy to examine vocal cords, assess condition of the respiratory tract, remove sloughing material, and provide deep lung suctioning.
- Mechanical ventilation
- Positioning and deep breathing
  1. Turn patient frequently.
  2. Assist patient out of bed to a chair.
  3. Teach coughing and deep breathing exercises.
  4. Urge incentive spirometry every 2 hours.
  5. Perform chest physiotherapy (if prescribed).

Surgical Management
- Tracheotomy
- Escharotomy
- Chest tube placement

❖**NDx:** Acute Pain; Chronic Pain

Nonsurgical Management
- Assess the patient's pain level hourly.
- Administer drug therapy with opioid and non-opioid analgesics (e.g., morphine sulfate, hydromorphone [Dilaudid], fentanyl).

> 🔲 Critical Rescue ◆ During the emergent postburn phase, the IV route is used for giving opioid drugs because of problems with absorption from the muscle and stomach. When these agents are given by the intramuscular or subcutaneous route, they remain in the tissue spaces and do not relieve pain. When edema is present, all the doses are rapidly absorbed at once when the fluid shift is resolving. This delayed absorption can result in lethal blood levels of analgesics.

- Provide a quiet environment to promote rest and sleep.
- Coordinate with all members of the health care team to ensure that most procedures are performed during the patient's waking hours.
- Use nonpainful tactile stimulation.
  1. Help the patient change positions every 2 hours.
  2. Massage nonburn areas.
  3. Apply heat and maintain warm room temperatures to prevent shivering.
- For the alert patient, encourage him or her to participate in patient-controlled analgesia (PCA). Give an initial bolus of 5 to 10 mg of morphine (or equivalent drug), increasing the PCA dose as needed to achieve pain relief and planning for a change in dosing regimens at night (e.g., giving a bolus dose at bedtime).

Surgical Management
- Surgical management for pain involves early surgical excision of the burn wound.

❖**Collaborative Problem:** Potential for Pulmonary Edema
- Assess hourly for fluid overload (presence of lung crackles, distended neck veins, decreased cognition, decreased oxygen saturation).
- Administer prescribed inotropic drugs (e.g., digoxin).

❖**Collaborative Problem:** Potential for Acute Respiratory Distress Syndrome
- Interventions are aimed at increasing lung compliance and improving Pao$_2$ (partial pressure of arterial oxygen) levels.

1. Give prescribed positive end-expiratory pressure (PEEP) therapy to provide a continuous positive pressure in the airways and alveoli and enhance the diffusion of oxygen across the alveolar-capillary membrane. PEEP can be combined with intermittent mandatory volume.
2. Assess and document the patient's response:
   a. Monitor oxygen saturation continuously.
   b. Monitor arterial blood gas levels.

> **Critical Rescue** ◆ Immediately report any signs of respiratory distress or change in respiratory patterns to the health care team and the respiratory therapist.

3. Administer prescribed neuromuscular blocking drugs (atracurium) to patients receiving mechanical ventilation to reduce oxygen consumption.

- **Acute phase**
   1. The acute phase of burn injury begins about 36 to 48 hours after injury and lasts until wound closure is complete.
   2. A multidisciplinary approach to care is needed.
   3. Care focuses on continued assessment and maintenance of the cardiovascular and respiratory systems, as well as toward GI and nutritional status, burn wound care, pain control, and psychosocial interventions.
   4. Complications of this phase include pneumonia, malnutrition, loss of musculoskeletal function, infection, and sepsis.

PATIENT-CENTERED COLLABORATIVE CARE

Assessment
- Assess for:
   1. Cardiopulmonary dysfunction
      a. Pneumonia
      b. Respiratory failure
   2. Neuroendocrine dysfunction
      a. Hypothermia
      b. Weight loss, negative nitrogen balance, malnutrition
   3. Immune system dysfunction
      a. Local infection
      b. Systemic infection
      c. Sepsis
   4. Musculoskeletal dysfunction
      a. Muscle atrophy
      b. Contracture formation
      c. Decreased ROM
   5. Wound healing impairment

6. Body image changes
7. Grieving
8. Anxiety and fear

Planning and Implementation

❖**NDx:** Impaired Skin Integrity: Wound Care Management

Nonsurgical Management

- Assess all burn wounds at least daily for:
  1. Adequacy of circulation
  2. Size and depth of injury
  3. Presence of infection
  4. Effectiveness of therapy
- Participate in wound débridement procedures to remove debris and nonliving tissue from the burn wound.
  1. *Mechanical débridement* can be performed one or two times daily with hydrotherapy. The patient can be immersed in a tub, showered on a specially designed shower table, or have only small areas of the wound washed at the bedside. Nurses and skilled technicians use forceps and scissors to remove loose, nonviable tissue during hydrotherapy. Burn areas are washed thoroughly and gently with mild soap or detergent and water.
  2. *Enzymatic débridement* can occur naturally by autolysis or, more commonly, artificially by the application of exogenous agents. Topical enzyme agents, such as collagenase (Santyl), are applied directly to the burn wound in once-daily dressing changes. The enzymes digest collagen in necrotic tissues.
  3. Dressing the burn wound using standard wound dressings, biologic dressings, synthetic dressings, or artificial skin
     a. *Standard wound* dressings involve cleansing the wound, applying a topical antimicrobial agent, and then applying multiple layers of gauze over the topical agents. The number of gauze layers depends on the depth of the injury, amount of drainage expected, area injured, patient's mobility, and frequency of dressing changes. The gauze layers are held in place with roller-type gauze bandages applied in a distal to proximal direction or with circular net fabrics. Dressings are reapplied every 8 to 24 hours.
     b. *Biologic dressings* are skin or membranes obtained from human tissue donors or animals. When applied over open wounds, a biologic dressing rapidly adheres and promotes healing or prepares the wound for permanent skin graft coverage. Types of biologic dressings include:
        (1) *Homografts* (allografts) are human skin obtained from a cadaver and provided through a skin bank.

B

(2) *Heterografts* (xenografts) are skin obtained from another species. Pigskin is the most common heterograft and is compatible with human skin.

(3) *Amniotic membrane* is another form of biologic dressing used on burn wounds. Its large size, low cost, and availability have helped with its success.

(4) *Cultured skin* can be grown from a small specimen of epidermal cells from an unburned area of the patient's body. Cells are grown in a laboratory to produce cell sheets that can be grafted on the patient to generate a permanent skin surface.

(5) *Artificial skin* is an alternative approach to closure of the burn wound. This substance has two layers: a Silastic epidermis and a porous dermis made from beef collagen and shark cartilage.

c. *Biosynthetic wound dressings* are a combination of biosynthetic and synthetic materials. Biobrane is the most common type and is made up of a nylon fabric that is partially embedded into a silicone film. Collagen is incorporated into both the silicone and nylon components. The nylon fabric comes into contact with the wound surface and forms an adherent bond until epithelialization has occurred. The porous silicone film allows exudates to pass through.

d. *Synthetic dressings* are made of solid silicone and plastic membranes (e.g., polyvinyl chloride, polyurethane). They are applied directly to the surface of a clean or surgically prepared wound and remain in place until they fall off or are removed. Many are transparent or translucent, allowing the wound to be inspected without removing the dressing.

Surgical Management
- Surgical management of burn wounds focuses on excision and wound covering. Surgical excision is performed early in the postburn period. Grafting may be performed throughout the acute phase as burn wounds are made ready and donor sites are available. Early grafting reduces the time patients are at risk for infection and sepsis. Wound covering by autografting involves taking healthy skin from an area of the patient's intact skin and transplanting it to an excised burn wound.

❖**NDx:** Risk for Infection
- Burn wound infection occurs through *autocontamination,* in which the patient's own normal flora overgrows and invades other body areas, and *cross-contamination,* in which organisms from other people or environments are transferred to the patient.

Nonsurgical Management

- Drug therapy for infection prevention
  1. Tetanus toxoid, 0.5 mL given IM, is routinely given when the patient is admitted to the hospital. Additional administration of tetanus immune globulin (human) (Hyper-Tet) is recommended when the patient's history of tetanus immunization is not known.
  2. Topical antimicrobial drugs are used at every dressing change or wound cleansing to prevent infection in burn wounds. The goal of this therapy is to reduce bacterial growth into the wound and prevent systemic sepsis. The most commonly used agents are silver sulfadiazine (Silvadene, Flamazine ♣) and mafenide acetate (Sulfamylon).
- Drug therapy for treatment of infection
  1. Systemic broad-spectrum antibiotics are used when burn patients have symptoms of an infection, including septicemia. After results of blood cultures and sensitivity status are available, specific drugs may be changed to those that are effective against the specific organisms causing the infection.
- Providing a safe environment
  1. Ensuring appropriate use of asepsis by all health care team members
     a. Wear gloves during all contact with open wounds.
     b. Do not share equipment among patients.
     c. Use disposable items as much as possible.
     d. Daily cleaning of patient's room and bathroom
  2. Keeping plants or flowers in patient's room
  3. Restricting visitors to healthy adults
  4. Possible isolation therapy (less common)
- Monitoring for early recognition of infection by assessing the burn wounds at each dressing change for:
  1. Pervasive odor
  2. Color changes: focal, dark red, brown discoloration in the eschar
  3. Change in texture
  4. Purulent drainage
  5. Exudate
  6. Sloughing grafts
  7. Redness at the wound edges extending to nonburned skin

Surgical Management

- Infected burn wounds with colony counts of or approaching 10^5 colonies per gram of tissue are life threatening and may require surgical excision to control these infections.

❖**NDx:** Imbalanced Nutrition: Less Than Body Requirements

- Coordinate with a nutritionist to calculate the patient's current daily caloric needs and meet his or her desired nutrition status outcomes.
- Nutritional requirements for a patient with a large burn area can exceed 5000 kcal/day and include a diet high in protein for wound healing.
- Nasoduodenal tube feedings are often started within 4 hours of beginning fluid resuscitation to prevent nutritional deficits.
- Encourage patients who can eat solid foods to ingest as many calories as possible.
- Take the patient's preferences into consideration for diet planning and food selection.
- Encourage patients to request food whenever they feel they can eat, not just according to the hospital's standard meal schedule.
- Offer frequent high-calorie, high-protein supplemental feedings.
- Keep an accurate calorie count for foods and beverages that are ingested by the patient.

❖**NDx:** Impaired Physical Mobility

Nonsurgical Management

- Positioning
  1. Maintain the patient in a neutral body position with minimal flexion.
  2. Use splints and other devices on the joints of the hands, elbows, knees, neck, and axillae to prevent contractures.
- ROM exercises
  1. Work with the patient to perform these actively at least three times daily.
  2. Perform passive ROM exercises for patients who are unable to actively perform them.
  3. For burned hands, urge the patient to perform active ROM exercises for the hand, thumb, and fingers every hour while awake.
- Ambulation
  1. Start ambulation as soon as possible after the fluid shifts have resolved.
  2. Assist patients to ambulate at least twice daily.
  3. Increase ambulation length each time.
- Pressure dressings
  1. Apply pressure dressings after grafts heal to help prevent contractures and tight hypertrophic scars.

2. Urge the patient to wear pressure dressings at least 23 hours every day until the scar tissue is mature (12 to 24 months).

Surgical Management

- Surgical management restores mobility rather than prevents immobility. Surgical release of contractures is most commonly performed in the neck, axilla, elbow flexion areas, and hand. Specific surgical procedures to improve movement vary for each patient.

❖**NDx:** Disturbed Body Image

Nonsurgical Management

- Assess which stage of grief the patient is experiencing, and help interpret his or her behaviors.
- Reassure the patient that feelings of grief, loss, anxiety, anger, fear, and guilt are normal.
- Coordinate with other health care team members (e.g., psychologist, psychiatrist, social worker, clergy or religious leader) in addressing these problems.
- Accept the physical and psychological features of the patient.
- Present patients and families with realistic expected outcomes for the patient's functional capacity and physical appearance.
- Plan and encourage the patient's active participation in self-care activities.
- Urge families to include the patient in family decision making to the same degree that he or she participated in this process before the injury.
- Provide information sessions and counseling for the family to help identify effective patterns of support.
- Facilitate the patient's use of these systems and the development of new support systems.
- Make referrals to support groups.

Surgical Management

- Reconstructive and cosmetic surgery can restore function and improve appearance, often increasing the patient's feelings of self-worth and promoting a positive body image. Teach the patient and family about expected cosmetic outcomes.
- **Rehabilitative phase**
  1. The technical rehabilitative phase begins with wound closure and ends when the patient returns to the highest possible level of functioning.
  2. The emphasis during this phase is the psychosocial adjustment of the patient, the prevention of scars and contractures, and the resumption of preburn activity, including resuming work, family, and social roles.

3. This phase may take years or even last a lifetime as patients adjust to permanent limitations that may not be apparent until long after the initial injury.

PATIENT-CENTERED COLLABORATIVE CARE

Assessment

- Explore the patient's feelings about the burn injury.
- Ask the patient or a family member whether there is a history of psychological problems.
- Assess and document the type of coping mechanisms the patient has used successfully during times of stress to assist with a future plan of care.
- Assess the patient's family unit and the family members' history of interaction.
- Identify cultural and ethnic factors, and take these into consideration when planning psychosocial interventions.

Community-Based Care

- Discharge planning for the patient with a burn injury begins at the time of admission to the hospital or burn center.
- Help the patient adjust to the reaction of others to the sight of healing wounds and disfiguring scars.
- Teach the patient and family:
  1. How to perform dressing changes
  2. Signs and symptoms of infection
  3. Drug regimens
  4. Proper use of prosthetic and positioning devices
  5. Correct application and care of pressure garments
  6. Comfort measures to reduce pruritus
  7. Dates for follow-up appointments
- Additional common discharge needs of the patient with burns include:
  1. Financial assessment
  2. Evaluation of family resources
  3. Psychological referral
  4. Patient and family teaching (home care)
  5. Rehabilitation referral
  6. Home assessment (on-site visit)
  7. Medical equipment
  8. Home care nursing referral
  9. Evaluation of community resources
  10. Visit to referral agency
  11. Re-entry programs for school or work environment
  12. Nursing home placement
  13. Prosthetic rehabilitation

CANCER, BREAST

OVERVIEW

- Breast cancer is the most commonly diagnosed cancer in women and is second only to lung cancer as a cause of cancer death in women. Men account for less than 1% of breast cancers.
- Early detection through regular screening methods of breast self-examination (BSE), clinical breast examination, and mammography is the key to effective treatment and survival.
- Many types of breast cancer arise from different cells in breast tissue. They are divided into two broad categories: noninvasive and invasive.
  1. Noninvasive cancers remain within the breast ducts and make up 20% of breast cancers. *Ductal carcinoma in situ* (DCIS) is a common, early, *noninvasive* breast cancer.
  2. Invasive cancers penetrate the tissue surrounding the ducts and make up 80% of all breast cancers. The most common type of invasive breast cancer is *infiltrating ductal carcinoma*. Other types include:
     a. Lobular carcinoma
     b. Medullary carcinoma
     c. Colloid (mucinous) carcinoma
     d. Inflammatory carcinoma
- Invasive breast cancer grows into tissues as an irregular, poorly defined mass. Skin dimpling may appear with advanced disease as a result of fibrotic changes within the tumor and surrounding tissue.
- When the tumor invades lymphatic channels, skin drainage is blocked, causing skin edema, redness, warmth, and an orange peel appearance of the skin (peau d'orange).
- Invasion of the lymphatic channels carries cancer cells to the axillary lymph nodes. Pathologic examination of these nodes helps determine the stage of the disease.
- Breast cancer spreads through the blood and lymph systems to distant sites, most commonly the bone, lungs, brain, and liver.
- There is no single cause of breast cancer, but many risk factors are associated with its development:
  1. Female gender
  2. Advancing age
  3. Family history, especially first-degree relatives, of breast cancer
  4. Previous exposure to high-dose ionizing radiation to the chest
  5. Early menarche (before 12 years of age) and late menopause (after 50 years of age)

6. History of previous breast cancer
7. Nulliparity (no pregnancies) or first birth after 30 years of age

🧬 Genetic Considerations

- Inherited mutations in several genes are related to hereditary breast cancer. The most common known mutations that increase breast cancer risk are in the *BRCA1* and *BRCA2* genes. Mutations in these genes greatly increase breast cancer risk; however, only about 5% of all breast cancers are hereditary.
- Patients with these mutations have an increased risk for other cancers, including ovarian cancer and possibly colon cancer.
- Children of a patient with a *BRCA1* or *BCRA2* germline mutation have a 50% chance of inheriting that mutation.

🌐 Cultural Awareness

- Euro-American women older than 40 years are at a greater risk than other racial or ethnic groups, but African American women younger than 40 have breast cancer more often than others in that age group.
- African American women have a higher death rate at any age compared with other women with the disease. Research suggests that poverty, less education, and inadequate access to screening are related to higher cancer mortality rates for African Americans.
- The same factors may apply to American Indian women. Although they have a low rate of breast cancer, they have one of the poorest 5-year survival rates of all ethnic groups, especially in the southwestern United States.
- Latino and Hispanic women have a lower incidence of breast cancer than white women but a higher death rate. The differences in survival rates reflect the stage at which the cancer is diagnosed.
- Japanese American women and native Hawaiian women also have a higher than average risk for breast cancer.

PATIENT-CENTERED COLLABORATIVE CARE

Assessment

- Obtain patient information about:
  1. Age and race
  2. Marital status
  3. Height and weight
  4. Personal and family history of breast cancer
  5. Hormonal history (oral contraceptives, hormone replacement therapy)

6. Age at menarche and menopause
7. Number of children
8. Age at first child's birth
9. History of the breast mass or lump (and interventions)
10. Health-promoting behaviors, including practice of BSE, clinical breast examination, and mammography
11. How the mass was discovered and how long ago
12. Whether other body changes have been noticed recently, especially bone or joint pain
13. Brief nutritional history, including intake of fat and alcohol
14. Prescribed and OTC drug use, especially hormone supplements

- Assess for:
  1. Specific information about the mass
     a. Describe its location using the face-of-the-clock method.
     b. Shape, size, consistency
     c. Whether it is mobile or fixed to the surrounding tissues
     d. Skin changes, such as dimpling, orange peel appearance, redness and warmth, nipple retraction, or ulceration
  2. Presence of enlarged axillary or supraclavicular lymph nodes
  3. Pain or soreness in the affected breast
  4. Psychosocial adjustment
     a. Assess the patient's current knowledge and need for information.
     b. Determine her self-image.
     c. Ask about sexuality and current intimate relationships.
     d. Determine how the patient has successfully handled stress in the past.
     e. Explore her feelings about the disease and expectations of treatment.
     f. Dispel myths or misconceptions.
     g. Evaluate the need for additional resources.
  5. Imaging assessment for diagnosis and staging
     a. Mammography or digital mammography
     b. Ultrasonography
     c. Breast-specific gamma imaging (BSGI)
     d. Chest x-ray
     e. Bone, liver, and brain scans
     f. CT of the chest and abdomen
     g. MRI
  6. Pathologic examination of tissue for diagnosis and prognosis

a. Biopsy is the definitive test that proves cancer presence or absence.
b. Presence of estrogen and progesterone receptors (cancers that express receptors have a better treatment response)
c. Gene expression profiling
d. Size and location of tumors
e. Lymph node involvement
f. Presence of distant metastasis

Planning and Implementation

❖ NDx: Anxiety

- The patient with breast cancer is usually admitted to the health care facility with a definitive diagnosis established through an outpatient biopsy of the mass.
- The anxiety for the woman with breast cancer begins the moment the lump is discovered. The level of anxiety may be related to past experiences and personal associations with the disease.
- Assess the patient's perceptions of her or his own situation and personal level of anxiety.
- Allow the patient to ventilate these feelings even if a diagnosis has not been established.
- Accept that different patients choose to deal with a cancer diagnosis in individual ways.
- Adjust your approach to care as the patient's emotional state changes.
- Integrate outside resources in the plan of care.

❖ Collaborative Problem: Potential for Metastasis

- After cancer is diagnosed, the extent and location of metastases determine the overall therapeutic strategy.
- Treatment is tailored specifically to each patient, taking into account other health problems and the patient's ability to tolerate a particular therapy.

Nonsurgical Management

- For patients with late-stage breast cancer, such as stage IV, with the presence of confirmed metastasis or for those who cannot withstand a major surgical procedure, the tumor may be removed with a local anesthetic.
- Follow-up treatment may include hormonal therapy, chemotherapy, and sometimes radiation therapy.

Surgical Management

- To improve survival and to reduce the risk for local recurrence, the mass itself should be removed by one of several types of surgery.
- Removal of the axillary lymph nodes for staging purposes is usually performed for patients with palpable axillary lymph nodes.

- When nodes are not palpable, a sentinel lymph node biopsy (SLNB) may be performed during or before breast surgery. If no cancer cells are found in the sentinel node, it is not necessary to remove other lymph nodes in the chain.
- Large tumors may be treated with chemotherapy (*neoadjuvant therapy*) to shrink the tumor before it is surgically removed.
- Surgical approaches include:
  1. *Breast-conserving surgery*, in which the bulk of the tumor is removed (not the entire breast), is used mostly for stage I and II breast cancers and is usually followed with radiation therapy. Types of breast-conserving surgery include lumpectomy, wide excision, partial or segmental mastectomy, and quadrantectomy.
  2. *Modified radical mastectomy*, in which the affected breast, skin, and axillary nodes are completely removed but the underlying muscles remain intact, is indicated when tumor is present in different quadrants of the breast, when the patient may be unable to have radiation therapy, when the tumor is large and the breast is small, and when the patient prefers this approach.
- Provide preoperative care, including psychological preparation and preoperative teaching:
  1. Review the type of procedure planned.
  2. Assess the patient's current level of knowledge.
  3. Teach about postoperative information, including:
     a. The need for a drainage tube
     b. The location of the incision
     c. Mobility restrictions
     d. Length of hospital stay (if any)
     e. The possibility of adjuvant therapy
     f. Give the patient and family written materials to take home as references.
     g. Address body image issues.
     h. Suggest that patients attend classes before surgery in an ambulatory care setting to promote successful early discharge from the hospital.
- Provide postoperative care, including:
  1. Performing routine postoperative care, including pain management, as described in Part One
  2. Placing a sign over the patient's bed to inform the staff to avoid using the affected arm for taking blood pressure measurements, giving injections, or drawing blood
  3. Assessing vital signs on a schedule of decreasing frequency, such as every 30 minutes for two times, every hour for two times, and then every 4 hours

4. Assessing the dressing for bleeding, and monitoring the amount and color of drainage
5. Performing wound care
   a. Observe the wound for signs of swelling and infection.
   b. Assess drainage tubes for patency.
6. Positioning the patient for best drainage and comfort
   a. Head of the bed up at least 30 degrees
   b. Arm on the same side as the axillary dissection elevated on a pillow while he or she is awake
7. Working with the physical therapist to plan progressive exercises.
   a. Squeezing the affected hand around a soft, round object (a ball or rolled washcloth)
   b. Flexion and extension of the elbow

- Breast reconstruction is common for women without complications from the cancer surgery and may be performed during the cancer surgery or at a later time. It may involve one or more stages using skin flaps or prostheses.
- For patients with breast cancer at a stage for which surgery is the main treatment, follow-up with adjuvant radiation therapy, chemotherapy, hormone therapy, or targeted therapy may also be prescribed.
- The decision to follow the original surgical procedure with adjuvant therapy for breast cancer is based on:
  1. Stage of the disease
  2. Patient's age and menopausal status
  3. Patient's preferences
  4. Pathologic examination results
  5. Hormone receptor status
  6. Presence of a known genetic predisposition
- Radiation therapy is administered after breast-conserving surgery and may be delivered by any one of several methods. General management issues for care of patients undergoing radiation therapy are presented in Part One under Cancer Therapy.
  1. Traditional whole-breast irradiation is delivered by external beam radiation over 5 to 6 weeks.
  2. Interstitial brachytherapy, in which several catheters loaded with a radioactive source are inserted at the lumpectomy cavity and surrounding margin, is given over 4 to 5 days.
  3. Balloon brachytherapy, also known as MammoSite, involves the use of a single balloon-tipped catheter that is surgically placed near the tumor bed. The catheter is loaded with a radiation source and inflated to conform to the total cavity. A total of 10 treatments are given, with at least 6 hours between each treatment.

4. Intraoperative radiation therapy uses a high single dose of radiation delivered during the lumpectomy surgery.

- Chemotherapy for breast cancer is delivered systemically with a combination of agents, usually for patients who have stage II or more advanced breast cancer. General management issues for care of patients undergoing radiation therapy are presented in Part One under Cancer Therapy.

- Targeted therapy for breast cancer involves the use of drugs that target specific features of cancer cells, such as a protein, an enzyme, or the formation of new blood vessels. These agents are useful only for cancers that overexpress a certain protein or enzyme. For breast cancer, targeted therapy drugs include:
  1. Trastuzumab (Herceptin) for cancers that overexpress the *HER2/NEU* gene product
  2. Bevacizumab (Avastin) for cancers that overexpress the VEGF receptor

- Hormonal therapy is used to reduce the estrogen available to breast tumors to stop or prevent their growth. Agents include:
  1. Luteinizing hormone–releasing hormone gene (LH-RH) agonists that inhibit estrogen synthesis
     a. Leuprolide (Lupron)
     b. Goserelin (Zoladex)
  2. Selective estrogen receptor modulators (SERMs) that block the effect of estrogen in women who have estrogen receptor (ER)–positive breast cancer
     a. Tamoxifen
     b. Toremifene (Fareston)
     c. Fulvestrant (Faslodex)
  3. Aromatase inhibitors (AIs) to prevent the conversion of androgen to estrogen in the adrenal gland.
     a. Anastrozole (Arimidex)
     b. Exemestane (Aromasin)

Community-Based Care

- Make the appropriate referrals for care after discharge:
  1. Home care
  2. Reach to Recovery
  3. Social services

- Teach the patient and family about:
  1. Wound care: drains, dressings, avoidance of lotions or ointments in the area, keeping the affected arm elevated if a lymph node dissection was performed
  2. Activity restrictions, especially stretching or reaching for heavy objects
  3. Measures to improve body image
  4. Information about interpersonal relationships and roles

5. Exercises to regain full ROM
6. Measures to prevent infection of the incision
7. Measures to avoid lymphedema
8. Measures to avoid injury, infection, and swelling of the affected arm
- Prepare the patient and partner about psychosocial issues:
  1. Describe the expected postoperative appearance.
  2. Reassure her that scars will fade and edema will lessen with time.
  3. Encourage the woman to look at her incision before she goes home and offer to be present when she does so.
  4. Involve the partner or family in teaching.
  5. Discuss sexual concerns before discharge.
  6. Advise sexually active patients receiving chemotherapy or radiotherapy to use birth control during therapy.
  7. Suggest participation in local support groups or national organizations such as the American Cancer Society, the Susan G. Komen "Race for the Cure", the National Breast Cancer Coalition, Y-Me, Sisters Network, Young Survival Coalition, and Pink Ribbon Girls.

CANCER, CERVICAL
OVERVIEW
- Cervical cancer, a common female reproductive cancer that usually arises from the squamous cells on the outside of the uterine cervix, can be preinvasive or invasive.
- *Preinvasive* cancer is limited to the cervix.
- *Invasive* cancer has spread to other pelvic structures by direct extension to the vaginal mucosa, lower uterine segment, parametrium, pelvic wall, bladder, and bowel.
- It can spread distantly to the liver, lungs, or bones.
- Risk factors include:
  1. Infection with human papillomavirus (HPV)
  2. History of sexually transmitted disease
  3. Multiple sex partners
  4. Younger than 18 years of age at first intercourse
  5. Multiparity (multiple pregnancies)
  6. Smoking
  7. Oral contraceptive use
  8. Obesity, poor diet
- Vaccination with the HPV vaccine (Gardasil), ideally before onset of intercourse, appears to protect against the high risk HPV types that are responsible for most cervical cancers.

- Cervical cancer can be detected at early stages, when cure is most likely, through periodic pelvic examinations and Papanicolaou (Pap) smears to screen. Teach women to avoid having this test during the menstrual period and to avoid these activities at least 48 hours before the test:
  1. Douching
  2. Sexual intercourse
  3. Tampons use
  4. Instillation of vaginal creams, jellies, or other drugs

PATIENT-CENTERED COLLABORATIVE CARE

Assessment

- Assess for early manifestations. The classic symptom of invasive cancer is painless, vaginal bleeding. Ask the patient if she has had or now has bleeding. It may start as spotting between menstrual periods or after sexual intercourse or douching. As the cancer grows, bleeding increases in frequency, duration, and amount, and it may become continuous.
- Assess for later manifestations:
  1. Watery, blood-tinged vaginal discharge that becomes dark and foul smelling (occurs as the disease progresses)
  2. Leg pain (along the sciatic nerve)
  3. Swelling of one leg
  4. Flank pain indicating hydronephrosis from tumor blocking a ureter, backing up the fluid into the kidney
- Assess for other manifestations of recurrence or metastasis:
  1. Unexplained weight loss
  2. Dysuria (painful urination)
  3. Pelvic pain
  4. Hematuria (bloody urine)
  5. Rectal bleeding
  6. Chest pain
  7. Coughing
- Diagnosis is made by cytologic examination of the Pap smear. When Pap results are abnormal, an *HPV-typing DNA test* of the cervical sample can determine the presence of one or more high-risk types of the virus. Colposcopic examination may be performed to view the transformation zone and biopsy many areas of the cervix.

Interventions

Surgical Management: Early Stage

- Surgical management for small, early-stage cervical cancer
  1. Loop electrosurgical excision procedure (LEEP) is a diagnostic procedure and a treatment. A thin loop-wire electrode

that transmits a painless electrical current is used to cut away affected tissue.

2. Laser therapy, in which a laser beam is focused on abnormal tissues, vaporizes cancerous cells without obtaining a tissue specimen for analysis.

3. Cryotherapy, in which the entire cervix is frozen, produces necrosis of all superficial cells, including cancer cells.

- Teach patients who have these procedures to follow restrictions for about 3 weeks:
  1. Refrain from sexual intercourse.
  2. Do not use tampons.
  3. Do not douche.
  4. Take showers rather than tub baths.
  5. Avoid lifting heavy objects.
  6. Report any heavy vaginal bleeding, foul-smelling drainage, or fever.

Surgical Management: Microinvasive Stage

- Surgical management at the microinvasive stage depends on the patient's health, desire for future childbearing, tumor size, stage, cancer cell type, and preferences.
- A *conization*, in which a cone-shaped area of cervix is removed surgically, can remove the affected tissue while preserving fertility.
  1. Potential complications from this procedure include hemorrhage and uterine perforation.
  2. Long-term follow-up care is needed because new cancers can develop.
- A *simple hysterectomy,* in which the cervix and body of the uterus is removed but the fallopian tubes and ovaries are spared, may be performed if fertility is not an issue.

Surgical Management: More Invasive Stage

- A *radical hysterectomy* and *bilateral pelvic lymph node dissection* are used for treating cancer that has extended beyond the cervix but not to the pelvic wall.
- *Pelvic exenteration* is a radical surgical procedure performed for invasive cervical cancer and recurrent cancer if there is no evidence of tumor outside the pelvis and no lymph node involvement.
  1. *Anterior* exenteration is the removal of the uterus, cervix, ovaries, fallopian tubes, vagina, bladder, urethra, and pelvic lymph nodes.
  2. *Posterior* exenteration is the removal of the uterus, cervix, ovaries, fallopian tubes, descending colon, rectum, and anal canal.

3. *Total* exenteration is a combination of anterior and posterior procedures.
4. Postoperatively, the patient is admitted to a critical care unit for the first 1 to 2 days because of the high risk for complications.

- Provide preoperative care:
  1. Assess anxiety, concerns about sexual functioning, and the ability to adjust to an altered body image.
  2. Assist in selection of stoma sites.
  3. Provide extensive bowel preparation.
  4. Provide routine preoperative care, as described in Part One.
- Inform the patient what to expect after surgery with regard to:
  1. Transfer to a critical care unit
  2. Multiple IV lines
  3. Other invasive lines and monitoring, such as an arterial line
  4. Nasogastric tube
- Refer to Cancer, Colorectal for preoperative and postoperative care for the patient undergoing colostomy and to Cancer, Urothelial (Bladder) for preoperative and postoperative care for the patient undergoing ileal conduit.
- After surgery, assess for:
  1. Pain
  2. Cardiovascular complications, such as hemorrhage and shock
  3. Pulmonary complications, such as atelectasis and pneumonia
  4. Fluid and electrolyte imbalances, such as metabolic acidosis or alkalosis and dehydration
  5. Renal or urinary complications
  6. GI complications, such as paralytic ileus
  7. Wound infection, dehiscence, or evisceration
- Provide postoperative care, including:
  1. Assisting with coughing and deep breathing
  2. Observing for dehydration
  3. Monitoring urine output
  4. Administering analgesics, as prescribed
  5. Administering and monitoring prescribed total parenteral nutrition
  6. Administering prophylactic heparin and applying antiembolism stockings or sequential compression devices, as prescribed, to prevent deep venous thrombosis
  7. Administering antibiotics, as prescribed
  8. Performing perineal irrigations
  9. Providing sitz baths

Nonsurgical Management

- Radiation therapy is reserved for stage II invasive cervical cancer.
  1. Intracavitary and external radiation therapies are used in combination, depending on the extent and location of the lesion.
  2. General management issues for care of patients undergoing intracavitary (brachytherapy) or external (teletherapy) radiation therapy are presented in Part One under Cancer Therapy.
- Combination chemotherapy with radiation therapy may be used for cervical cancer beyond stage II.
  1. Agents frequently used include cisplatin (Platinol), paclitaxel (Taxol), carboplatin, fluorouracil (5-FU), and mitomycin.
  2. General management issues for care of patients receiving combination chemotherapy are presented in Part One under Cancer Therapy.

Community-Based Care

- Community-based care for the patient after a hysterectomy is described under surgical management of Leiomyomas (Uterine Fibroids).
- The patient is usually in the hospital for at least 1 week after pelvic exenteration surgery.
- The patient is discharged to home or to a skilled nursing facility or transitional care unit for continued recovery.
- Physical activities are limited during convalescence, and the patient will need personal and household assistance for up to 6 months.
- Collaborate with the wound and ostomy care nurse to teach the woman who has undergone a pelvic exenteration and her family how to manage her care.
- A home care nurse may be needed to assist with dressing changes, with ostomy care, and to perform general assessment.
- Collaborate with a nutritionist and enterostomal therapist to teach the patient about stoma care, nutritional adjustments for the ostomies, and drug actions, dosages, and side effects.
- Encourage ROM exercises until walking is permitted.
- Remind the patient about keeping all follow-up appointments.
- Provide information about late complications (e.g., infection, bowel obstruction) so that she can seek medical care promptly.
- Support the patient during the grieving process and encourage her to express her feelings and concerns.
- Encourage the patient to look at the wound or stoma sites.

- Monitor for depression.
- Refer the patient and her partner for counseling about alternatives to intercourse and sexual expression.

CANCER, COLORECTAL

OVERVIEW

- Colorectal cancer (CRC), or cancer of the colon or rectum, is a common malignancy of men and women in the U. S.
- Most CRCs are adenocarcinomas arising from the glandular epithelial tissue of the colon and develop as a multistep process, resulting in loss of key tumor suppressor genes and activation of certain oncogenes that alter colonic mucosa cell division.
- The increased proliferation of the colonic mucosa first forms polyps that can transform into malignant tumors.
- Tumors occur in all areas of the colon and can spread by direct invasion and through the lymphatic and circulatory systems.
- The most common sites of metastasis are the liver, lungs, brain, bones, and adrenal glands.
- Complications include bowel perforation with peritonitis, abscess or fistula formation, frank hemorrhage, and complete intestinal obstruction.
- Risk factors include:
  1. Age older than 50 years
  2. Genetic predisposition
  3. Personal or family history of cancer
  4. Personal history of diseases that predispose to cancer (e.g., familial adenomatous polyposis [FAP], hereditary nonpolyposis colorectal cancer [HNPCC])
  5. Personal history of inflammatory bowel diseases (IBDs), such as ulcerative colitis and Crohn's disease
  6. Diets that are high in fats, red meat, refined carbohydrates, fried or grilled food, and low in fiber

Genetic Considerations

- People with a first-degree relative (sister, sibling, or child) diagnosed with colorectal cancer (CRC) have three to four times the risk of developing the disease.
- An autosomal dominant inherited genetic disorder known as familial adenomatous polyposis (FAP) accounts for 1% of CRCs. People who have this mutation develop thousands of adenomatous polyps over the course of 10 to 15 years that have an almost 100% chance of becoming malignant.

- Surgical prophylaxis with a colectomy can be performed for cancer prevention.
- Hereditary nonpolyposis colorectal cancer (HNPCC) is another autosomal dominant disorder caused by mutations in the *MLH1* and *MLH2* genes. People with these mutations have an 80% chance of developing CRC at an average of 45 years of age.
- Genetic testing is available for both of these familial CRC syndromes.

PATIENT-CENTERED COLLABORATIVE CARE

Assessment

- Obtain patient information about:
  1. Age
  2. Diet history
  3. History of ulcerative colitis or Crohn's disease
  4. Personal history of breast, ovarian, or endometrial cancer; ulcerative colitis; familial polyposis; or adenomas
  5. Change in bowel habits with or without blood in stool
  6. Weight loss, pain, and abdominal fullness (late signs)
- Assess for:
  1. Rectal bleeding (the most common manifestation)
  2. Change in stool
  3. Anemia (low hemoglobin level and hematocrit; stool positive for occult blood)
  4. Cachexia (late sign)
  5. Guarding or abdominal distention (late sign)
  6. Abdominal mass (late sign)
- Diagnostic assessment includes:
  1. Fecal occult blood test (FOBT)
  2. Carcinoembryonic antigen (CEA) blood test
  3. Double-contrast barium enema
  4. Colonoscopy
  5. CT or MRI of the chest, abdomen, pelvis, lungs, or liver

Planning and Implementation

❖**NDx:** Grieving

- Observe and identify:
  1. The patient's and family's current method of coping
  2. Effective sources of support used in the past
  3. The patient's and family's present perceptions of the patient's health problem
  4. Signs of anticipatory grief such as crying, anger, sadness, and withdrawal from usual relationships

- Encourage the patient to verbalize feelings about the diagnosis, treatment, and anticipated changes in body image if an ostomy is planned.
- Instruct the patient what to expect about the appearance and care of the colostomy.
- When the patient is physically able, encourage the patient to look at the ostomy (if performed), and to participate in colostomy care.
- Facilitate grief work by identifying the nature of and reaction to the loss. Encourage the patient to verbalize feelings and identify fears to help move him or her through the appropriate phases of the grief process.
- Invite the patient, family, social worker, or religious leader to participate in the discussion and decisions concerning potential lifestyle modifications, treatment, prognosis, and end-of-life decisions.
- Refer patients who are at risk for or have familial CRC for genetic counseling.

❖**Collaborative Problem:** Potential for Metastasis
Nonsurgical Management
- Radiation therapy
  1. Preoperative radiation therapy is effective in providing local or regional control of the disease.
  2. Radiation is also used postoperatively as a palliative measure to reduce pain, hemorrhage, bowel obstruction, or metastasis.
  3. General management issues for care of patients undergoing radiation therapy are presented in Part One under Cancer Therapy.
- *Chemotherapy* is used after surgery to interrupt cancer cell division and improve survival.
  1. Common drugs include:
     a. 5-Fluorouracil (5-FU)
     b. Leucovorin (LV) (folinic acid)
     c. Capecitabine (Xeloda)
     d. Oxaliplatin (Eloxatin)
     e. Irinotecan (Camptosar)
  2. Common side effects of this therapy are:
     a. Diarrhea
     b. Mucositis
     c. Leukopenia
     d. Mouth ulcers
     e. Peripheral neuropathy
  3. General management issues for care of patients undergoing chemotherapy are presented in Part One, under Cancer Therapy.

- *Targeted therapy* approved for colorectal cancer may include:
  1. Bevacizumab (Avastin)
  2. Cetuximab (Erbitux)

Surgical Management

- In a colon resection, the bowel segment containing the tumor is resected (removed) along with several inches of bowel beyond the tumor margin and regional lymph nodes, and an end-to-end anastomosis is performed. This procedure may be performed by the traditional open method or as minimally invasive surgery by laparoscopy.
- A colectomy (colon removal) with temporary or permanent colostomy may be needed.
- In an abdominal peritoneal (A-P) resection, the sigmoid colon and rectum are removed, the anus is closed, and a permanent colostomy is formed.
- Provide preoperative care:
  1. Implement routine preoperative care as presented in Part One.
  2. Reinforce the surgeon's explanation of the procedure.
  3. If a colostomy is planned, consult the enterostomal therapist (ET) to assist in identifying optimal placement of the ostomy and to instruct the patient about the rationale and general principles of ostomies.
  4. Instruct the patient to consume only clear liquids for a day or more before bowel surgery to minimize colonic contents.
  5. Administer laxatives, enemas, or an oral, liquid, large-volume laxative if ordered, the morning of surgery or the day before surgery to mechanically clean the bowel ("bowel prep").
  6. Give oral or IV antibiotics preoperatively, as prescribed.
- Provide postoperative care, including:
  1. Implementing routine postoperative care as described in Part One
  2. Providing nasogastric tube care, if needed
  3. Providing pain management
  4. Managing the colostomy, if present
     a. If an ostomy pouch is not in place, cover the stoma with petroleum gauze to keep it moist, followed by a dry, sterile dressing.
     b. Place a pouch system on the stoma as soon as possible and in collaboration with the enterostomal therapist.
     c. Observe the stoma for:
        (1) Necrotic tissue
        (2) Unusual amount of bleeding

(3) Color changes (The normal color is red-pink, which indicates high vascularity; pale pink indicates low hemoglobin and hematocrit levels; purple-black indicates compromised circulation.)

   d. Check the pouch system for proper fit and signs of leakage.

   e. Assess for colostomy functioning 2 to 4 days after surgery; stool is liquid immediately after surgery but becomes more solid.

   f. Empty the pouch when excess gas has collected or when it is one-third to one-half full of stool.

5. Irrigating the perineal wound, if present
6. Changing the perineal wound dressing, as directed
7. Assessing perineal wound (Copious serosanguineous drainage is expected.)
8. Providing comfort measures for perineal itching and pain, such as antipruritic drugs (benzocaine) and sitz baths
9. Assessing for signs of infection, abscess, or other complications
10. Instructing the patient about activities such as assuming a side-lying position, avoiding sitting for long periods, and using a foam pad or pillow when in a sitting position

Community-Based Care

- Provide the patient with these verbal and written instructions:
  1. Avoid lifting heavy objects or straining on defecation to prevent tension on the anastomosis site.
  2. Avoid driving for 4 to 6 weeks.
  3. Note the frequency, amount, and character of the stool.
  4. For colon resection, watch for and report manifestations of bowel obstruction and perforation (cramping, abdominal pain, nausea, and vomiting).
  5. Resume a normal diet, but avoid gas-producing foods and carbonated beverages.
- Teach the patient and family colostomy care, including:
  1. Normal appearance of a stoma
  2. Signs and symptoms of complications
  3. How to measure the stoma
  4. How to protect the skin adjacent to the stoma
  5. Dietary measures to control gas and odor
- Other discharge preparation includes:
  1. Inspection of the abdominal incision (and perineal wound if an A-P resection was performed) for redness, tenderness, swelling, and drainage
  2. Pain management, including drug therapy

3. Tips on how to resume normal activities, including work, travel, and sexual intercourse
4. Psychosocial preparation
- Provide these contacts for community and health resources, as needed:
    1. Social services
    2. Enterostomal therapist
    3. United Ostomy Association
    4. American Cancer Society
    5. Home health services
    6. Pharmacy or other medical supply source

CANCER, ENDOMETRIAL (UTERINE)

OVERVIEW

- Endometrial cancer (cancer of the uterus) is the most frequently occurring reproductive organ cancer.
- It is a slow-growing tumor associated with menopause and arises from the glandular component of the endometrial mucosa.
- Its initial growth is within the uterine cavity, followed by extension into the myometrium and cervix.
- Spread occurs through the lymphatics to the ovaries and parametrial, pelvic, inguinal, and para-aortic lymph nodes; by hematogenous metastasis to the lungs, liver, or bone; and by transtubal or intra-abdominal spread to the peritoneal cavity.
- Risk factors associated with endometrial cancer include:
    1. Obesity
    2. Diabetes mellitus
    3. History of uterine polyps
    4. History of infertility
    5. Nulliparity
    6. Polycystic ovarian disease
    7. Estrogen stimulation, including unopposed menopausal estrogen replacement therapy (ERT)
    8. Late menopause
    9. Family history of uterine cancer or hereditary nonpolyposis colon cancer (HNPCC)

PATIENT-CENTERED COLLABORATIVE CARE

Assessment

- Obtain patient information about:
    1. Age and ethnicity
    2. Family history of endometrial cancer or HNPCC
    3. History of diabetes, and hypertension

4. History of obesity
5. Childbearing status, pregnancies, births, infertility
6. Prolonged estrogen use

- Assess for:
  1. Postmenopausal bleeding (the primary symptom)
  2. Watery, serosanguineous vaginal discharge
  3. Low back pain
  4. Abdominal pain
  5. Low pelvic pain
  6. Enlarged uterus

Interventions

Nonsurgical Management

- Radiation therapy (external and internal) is used alone or in combination with surgery, depending on the stage of the cancer.
- When intracavitary radiation therapy (IRT) (brachytherapy) is performed, an applicator is positioned within the uterus through the vagina. Implement these interventions for radiation safety and to prevent dislodgement of either the applicator or the radiation source:
  1. Maintain strict isolation and radiation precautions.
  2. Provide bedrest, laying the patient on her back, with her head flat or elevated less than 20 degrees.
  3. Restrict active movement to prevent dislodgment.
  4. Insert a Foley catheter.
  5. Assess daily for skin breakdown.
  6. Provide a low-residue diet.
  7. Encourage fluid intake.
  8. Administer antiemetics, broad-spectrum anti-infectives, tranquilizers, analgesics, heparin, and antidiarrheal drugs, as prescribed.
  9. Restrict visitors.
- Nurses who are pregnant or attempting pregnancy are usually not assigned patients undergoing intracavitary radiation therapy (IRT).
- Instruct the patient undergoing external radiation (teletherapy) to:
  1. Observe for signs of skin breakdown.
  2. Avoid sunbathing.
  3. Avoid bathing over the markings that outline the treatment site.
  4. Recognize the complications of treatment, including cystitis, diarrhea, and nutritional alterations.
  5. Recognize that reactions to radiation therapy vary among patients and that some may feel unclean or radioactive after treatments.

- General management issues for care of patients undergoing intracavitary (brachytherapy) or external (teletherapy) radiation therapy are presented in Part One under Cancer Therapy.
- Chemotherapy is used as an adjuvant treatment when the risk for distant spread exceeds 20%.
  1. Chemotherapeutic agents frequently used include doxorubicin (Adriamycin), cisplatin (Platinol), and paclitaxel (Taxol).
  2. General management issues for care of patients receiving combination chemotherapy are presented in Part One under Cancer Therapy.
- Hormone therapy may be used for stage I and II cancers that are estrogen dependent, and for stage IV cancer as palliative treatment. Hormones commonly used are medroxyprogesterone (Depo-Provera) and megestrol acetate (Megace).
- Tamoxifen citrate (Nolvadex, Tamofen), an antiestrogen, is also used.

Surgical Management
- Total abdominal hysterectomy and bilateral salpingo-oophorectomy are performed for stage I tumors; a radical hysterectomy with node dissection is performed for stage II and higher-stage tumors.
- For the patient undergoing hysterectomy, refer to preoperative and postoperative care under Cancer, Cervical.
- Nursing interventions include:
  1. Providing emotional support
  2. Creating an atmosphere that encourages the patient to ask questions and express fears and concerns

Community-Based Care
- Provide verbal and written instructions on:
  1. Side effects that should be reported to the physician, including vaginal bleeding, rectal bleeding, foul-smelling discharge, abdominal pain or distention, and hematuria
  2. Dosages, scheduling, and side effects of prescribed drugs
- Inform the patient:
  1. High-dose radiation causes sterility.
  2. Vaginal shrinkage occurs.
  3. Sexual partners cannot "catch" cancer.
  4. The patient is not radioactive (after the intracavitary radiation source is removed).
  5. Vaginal douching may decrease inflammation.
  6. A normal diet may be resumed.
- After an abdominal hysterectomy, give the instructions and information to the patient as discussed under Leiomyomas (Uterine Fibroids).

- Refer the patient to the local chapter of the American Cancer Society.

CANCER, HEAD AND NECK

OVERVIEW

- Head and neck cancers occur in structures within the larynx, the trachea, the throat, the oral cavity, or on the tongue, and they usually arise from the skin or mucosa as squamous cell carcinomas.
- Other origins of head and neck cancers include the salivary glands, the thyroid, and other structures.
- These cancers are slow growing, with the tissue changes occurring in several stages.
  1. Premalignant lesions appear when the mucosa is chronically irritated, changing into tougher mucosa (squamous metaplasia), followed by mucosal thickening (*acanthosis* or hyperplasia) and the development of a keratin layer (keratosis). The chronic irritation damages genes controlling cell growth, allowing enhanced growth of these abnormal cells, leading to:
     a. Leukoplakia, a thickened, white, firmly attached plaque
     b. Erythroplakia, a red, velvety patch
  2. With time, the premalignant lesions become cancerous and may spread (metastasize first into nearby structures, such as lymph nodes, muscle, and bone, and then to more distant sites, usually the lungs or liver).
  3. Degree of malignancy is determined by cellular analysis.
     a. Early-stage cancers are carcinoma in situ and well differentiated.
     b. Cancers that have progressed are moderately differentiated.
     c. Advanced cancers are poorly differentiated.
- The cause of head and neck cancers is unknown, but the two greatest risk factors are tobacco and alcohol use, especially in combination.
- Other risk factors include voice abuse, chronic laryngitis, exposure to industrial chemicals or hardwood dust, poor oral hygiene, and long-term or severe gastroesophageal reflux disease (GERD).

PATIENT-CENTERED COLLABORATIVE CARE

Assessment

- Obtain patient information about:
  1. Tobacco and alcohol use (quantify these)

2. History of recurrent acute or chronic laryngitis or pharyngitis, oral sores, and lumps in the neck
3. Exposure to environmental or occupational pollutants
- Assess for physical manifestations:
  1. Problems related to risk factors
  2. Dietary habits
  3. Weight loss
  4. Hoarseness
  5. Lumps on the head or in the neck
  6. Mouth sores
  7. Laryngeal abnormalities by laryngeal examination using a laryngeal mirror (physician or advanced practice nurse)
- Assess for psychosocial issues:
  1. Patient or family feelings of denial, guilt, blame, or shame
  2. Adequacy of support systems and coping mechanisms
  3. Social and family support systems
  4. Level of education or literacy of the patient and family to plan teaching before and after surgery
  5. Patient's use of speech for employment
- Diagnostic assessment may include:
  1. Laboratory tests, CBC, bleeding times, urinalysis, blood chemistries, protein levels, albumin levels, renal and liver function tests
  2. X-rays of the skull, sinuses, neck, and chest
  3. CT of the head and neck, with or without contrast media
  4. MRI
  5. Brain, bone, and liver scans
  6. Positron emission tomography (PET) scans
  7. Direct and indirect laryngoscopy
  8. Panendoscopy (laryngoscopy, nasopharyngoscopy, esophagoscopy, and bronchoscopy)
  9. Biopsy

Planning and Implementation

❖**Collaborative Problem:** Potential for Respiratory Obstruction

- The goal of treatment is to remove or eradicate the cancer while preserving as much normal function as possible. The specific treatment depends on the extent and location of the lesion.

Nonsurgical Management

- *Radiation therapy* for treatment of small cancers involves external beam delivery of 5000 to 7500 rad (radiation absorbed dose), usually over 6 weeks and in daily or twice-daily doses.
  1. Radiation therapy may be used alone or in combination with surgery. Because radiation therapy slows tissue healing, it may not be performed before surgery.

2. Complications of radiation therapy for head and neck cancer include increased hoarseness, dysphagia, skin problems, and dry mouth (leading to halitosis, taste changes, increased risk for dental caries and dental infection).

3. Dry mouth (xerostomia) is a long-term complication and may be permanent. Interventions include:
   a. Heavy fluid intake, particularly water
   b. Room humidification
   c. Use of artificial saliva (Salivart)
   d. Use of saliva stimulants (Salagen and cevimeline)
   e. Chewing gum and sucking hard candy

4. General management issues for care of patients undergoing radiation therapy are presented in Part One under Cancer Therapy.

- *Chemotherapy* can be used alone or in addition to surgery or radiation for head and neck cancer.
   1. Specific treatment regimens and drug combinations vary but the most commonly used agents for head and neck cancer include cisplatin (Platinol), fluorouracil (5-FU), and gemcitabine (Gemzar).
   2. General management issues for care of patients undergoing chemotherapy are presented in Part One under Cancer Therapy.

- *Targeted therapy* for advanced head and neck cancers may include cetuximab (Erbitux).

Surgical Management

- Tumor size and location (TNM classification) determines the type of surgery needed for the specific head and neck cancer.
- Very small, early-stage tumors may be removed by laser therapy or photodynamic therapy; however, few head and neck tumors are found at this stage, and most require extensive traditional surgery.
- Traditional surgical procedures for head and neck cancers include:
   1. Laryngectomy (total and partial): removal of the larynx
   2. Tracheotomy: creation of a new artificial airway by opening the wall of the trachea
   3. Oropharyngeal cancer resections
   4. Cordectomy: vocal cord removal
   5. Radical neck dissection, which is removal of the primary tumor along with lymph node dissection. It may involve removing skin, muscle, bone, and other structures.
   6. Composite resections are a combination of surgical procedures, including partial or total glossectomies, partial mandibulectomies, and, if needed, nodal neck dissections.

- Provide preoperative care:
  1. Give routine preoperative care, as described in Part One.
  2. Teach the patient about the probable location of the surgical incision, self-care of the airway, alternate methods of communication, suctioning, pain control methods, the critical care environment (including ventilators and critical care routines), nutritional support, feeding tubes, and goals for discharge.
  3. Help the patient to practice the use of an alternate form of communication (e.g., pen and pencil, "magic slate," picture or alphabet board, or computerized word generator).
  4. Determine the communication method most preferred by the patient.
  5. Encourage the patient to express fears and concerns.
  6. Reinforce the surgeon's explanation of the surgical procedure.
- Provide postoperative care:
  1. Routine postoperative care, as described in Part One
  2. Airway maintenance and ventilation
     a. Ventilator management
     b. Suctioning
     c. Oxygen therapy
     d. Humidification
     e. Coughing and deep breathing
     f. Laryngectomy or tracheostomy care (if surgery included tracheotomy or laryngectomy)

> ⚙ **Critical Rescue** ◆ Secretions may remain blood-tinged for 1 to 2 days. Report any increase in bleeding to the surgeon.

  3. Wound management
     a. Evaluate all grafts and flaps hourly for the first 72 hours.
     b. Monitor capillary refill, color, drainage, and Doppler activity of the major feeding vessel.
     c. Position the patient so that the side of the head and neck with the flaps is not dependent.
     d. Monitor drainage and record its amount and character.
     e. Report changes to the surgeon immediately because surgical intervention may be needed.
  4. Hemorrhage prevention
     a. Observe for carotid artery leakage or rupture.

    (1) Rupture results in large amounts of bright red blood spurting quickly.

    (2) Leakage shows as oozing of bright red blood.

> **Critical Rescue** ◆ If a carotid artery leak is suspected, call the Rapid Response Team, and do not touch the area because additional pressure could cause an immediate rupture. If the carotid artery ruptures because of drying or infection, immediately place constant pressure over the site, and secure the airway. Maintain direct manual, continuous pressure on the carotid artery and immediately transport the patient to the operating room for carotid resection. Do not leave the patient. Carotid artery rupture has a high risk of stroke and death. Nursing response can save the patient's life.

5. Nutritional support
   a. Collaborate with the nutritionist to provide the patient with at least 35 to 40 kcal/kg of body weight daily.
   b. IV fluids or parenteral nutrition is used until the intestinal tract is functioning.
   c. Tube feeding by nasogastric, gastrostomy, or jejunostomy tube (usually remains in place for 7 to 10 days after surgery).
   d. Assess the patient's ability to swallow before removing the feeding tube.
6. Speech and language rehabilitation
   a. Collaborate with the speech and language pathologist.
   b. Work with the patient and family toward developing an acceptable communication method.
      (1) Writing
      (2) Picture board
      (3) Computer
      (4) Artificial larynx
      (5) Esophageal speech
   c. Take time to understand the patient's communication.
   d. Celebrate every success.
   e. Arrange for a visit from a laryngectomee (a person who has had a laryngectomy).

❖**NDx:** Risk for Aspiration
- Aspiration is not a problem for the patient who has had a total laryngectomy and a permanent tracheostomy.
- Observe the patient who has had a subtotal, vertical, or supraglottic laryngectomy for aspiration.

- Use these precautions for the patient with a feeding tube in place:
  1. Elevate the head of the bed 30-40 degrees.
  2. Strictly adhere to tube feeding procedure.
  3. Check residual violence before each bolus feeding (or every 4 hours with continuous feeding and abdominal assessment).
  4. Evaluate the patient's tolerance of the tube feeding.
  6. If residual volume is high for 2 consecutive hours (i.e., >200-250 mL), withhold the feeding and notify the physician.

> **Clinical Landmine** ◆ Do not give bolus feedings at night or anytime the patient must remain in a flat, supine position.

- Use these precautions to prevent aspiration when feeding the patient or assisting him or her with eating:
  1. Avoid having meals when the patient is fatigued.
  2. Provide smaller and more frequent meals.
  3. Provide adequate time; do not hurry the patient.
  4. Provide close supervision if the patient is self-feeding.
  5. Keep emergency suctioning equipment close at hand and turned on.
  6. Avoid water and other "thin" liquids.
  7. Thicken all liquids, including water.
  8. Avoid foods that generate thin liquids during the chewing process, such as fruit.
  9. Position the patient in the most upright position possible.
  10. When present, completely (or at least partially) deflate the tube cuff during meals.
  11. Suction before and after initial cuff deflation to clear the airway and allow maximum comfort during the meal.
  12. Feed each bite or encourage the patient to take each bite slowly.
  13. Encourage the patient to "dry swallow" after each bite to clear residue from the throat.
  14. Avoid consecutive swallows of liquids.
  15. Provide controlled, small volumes of liquids using a spoon.
  16. Encourage the patient to "tuck" his or her chin down and forward while swallowing.
  17. Allow the patient to indicate when he or she is ready for the next bite.
  18. If the patient coughs, stop the feeding until the patient indicates the airway has been cleared.
  19. Continuously monitor tolerance to oral food intake by assessing respiratory rate, ease, pulse oximetry, and heart rate.

- Teach the patient the supraglottic method of swallowing:
    1. Inhaling and holding his or her breath (to close the vocal folds)
    2. Placing food or liquid in swallow position
    3. Swallowing while holding breath
    4. Coughing after swallowing and before inhaling (to clear any residue that may have entered the larynx)

❖**NDx:** Anxiety

- Explore the reason for anxiety (e.g., fear of the unknown, lack of teaching, fear of pain, fear of airway compromise, fear of hospitalization, loss of control).
- Encourage the patient and family to express their feelings about the cancer diagnosis and uncertainty of treatment outcome.
- Dispel myths and correct misconceptions.
- Accept that different patients choose to deal with a cancer diagnosis in individual ways.
- Adjust your approach to care as the patient's emotional state changes.
- Integrate outside resources into the plan of care.
- Give prescribed antianxiety drugs.

❖**NDx:** Disturbed Body Image

- The patient with head and neck cancer may have a permanent change in body image because of deformity, the presence of a stoma or artificial airway, speech changes, and a change in the method of eating.
- Help the patient set realistic goals, starting with involvement in self-care.
- Teach the patient alternate communication methods.
- Teach the family to ease the patient into a normal social environment.
- Use positive reinforcement and encouragement while demonstrating acceptance and caring behaviors.
- Refer the patient and family for counseling, as needed.
- Teach the patient tips for an enhanced appearance, including:
    1. The use of loose-fitting, high-collar shirts or sweaters, scarves, and jewelry to cover the laryngectomy stoma, tracheostomy tube, and other changes related to surgery
    2. The use of cosmetics to cover scars and skin disfigurement

Community-Based Care

- Ensure that the patient and family are able to perform tracheostomy or stoma care and participate in nutrition, wound care, and communication methods.
- Coordinate the efforts of the health care team in assessing the specific discharge needs and making the appropriate referrals to home care agencies.

- Coordinate the scheduling for chemotherapy or radiation therapy with the patient and family.
- Ensure that the home environment is assessed for general cleanliness, ease of patient access to toileting and living areas, need for increased humidity, and transportation.
- Teach the patient and family about:
  1. Stoma or tracheostomy or laryngectomy care
  2. Incision and airway care
  3. Safety
  4. Wearing a medical alert (Medic Alert) bracelet and carrying a special identification card
  5. Smoking cessation
  6. Community support agencies

CANCER, LUNG

OVERVIEW

- Lung cancer is a leading cause of cancer-related deaths worldwide.
- The overall 5-year survival rate for all patients with lung cancer is only 14% because most lung cancers are diagnosed at a late stage, when metastasis is present.
- Lung cancers are classified by cell type as small cell lung cancer (SCLC) and non–small cell lung cancer (NSCLC), which includes epidermoid (squamous cell) cancer, adenocarcinoma, and large cell cancer.
- Metastasis (spread) of lung cancer occurs by direct extension, through the blood, and by invading lymph glands and vessels. Common sites of metastasis for lung cancer are the bone, liver, brain, and adrenal glands.
- Lung cancers occur as a result of repeated exposure to inhaled substances that cause chronic tissue irritation or inflammation. Cigarette smoking is the major risk factor and is responsible for 85% of all lung cancer deaths.
- Nonsmokers exposed to *passive*, or *secondhand*, smoke also have a greater risk for lung cancer.
- Additional causes of lung cancer are chronic exposure to asbestos, beryllium, chromium, coal distillates, cobalt, iron oxide, mustard gas, petroleum distillates, radiation, tar, nickel, uranium, benzopyrenes, and hydrocarbons.

Genetic Considerations

- Variation is seen in lung cancer development among people with similar smoking histories, suggesting that genetic factors can influence susceptibility.

- Differences in a gene product that activates carcinogens (a cancer susceptibility gene) and another gene product that clears carcinogens from the body (a cancer resistance gene) are associated with differences in personal susceptibility to lung cancer.
- Differences in a gene that regulates cell division, the *Tp53* gene, may be the most important genetic susceptibility link for lung cancer development. Mutations in the alleles of this gene are known to increase the susceptibility to a wide variety of cancers with and without exposure to environmental risks, including lung cancer development among smokers and nonsmokers.
- Lung cancer interferes with oxygenation and tissue perfusion by a variety of ways, including bronchial obstruction, airway compression, compression of alveoli, and compression of blood vessels.
- Common manifestations of lung cancer are associated with respiratory problems and include dyspnea, pallor to cyanosis, tachycardia, bloody sputum, and cough.
- Pain is common when lymph nodes are enlarged and press on nerves.

PATIENT-CENTERED COLLABORATIVE CARE

Assessment

- Obtain patient information about:
  1. Risk factors, including smoking, hazards in the workplace, and warning signals
  2. Pack-year smoking history
  3. Cough
     a. Timing
     b. Productivity
  4. Sputum
     a. Amount
     b. Color
     c. Character
  5. Chest pain, tightness, or pressure
     a. Location
     b. Severity
     c. Duration
     d. Quality
     e. Radiation
  6. Dyspnea
     a. Duration
     b. Change in endurance
- Assess for pulmonary manifestations:
  1. Hoarseness
  2. Wheezing

   3. Decreased or absent breath sounds
   4. Breathing pattern abnormalities
      a. Prolonged exhalation alternating with periods of shallow breathing
      b. Rapid, shallow breathing
   5. Areas of tenderness or masses palpated on the chest wall
   6. Increased fremitus (vibration) in areas of tumor
   7. Decreased or absent fremitus on side with bronchial obstruction
   8. Tracheal deviation
   9. Pleural friction rub
   10. Asymmetry of diaphragm movement
   11. Use of accessory muscles
   12. Retraction between ribs or at sternal notch
- Assess for nonpulmonary manifestations:
   1. Weight loss
   2. Muffled heart sounds
   3. Dysrhythmias
   4. Cyanosis of the lips and fingertips
   5. Clubbing of the fingers
   6. Bone pain
   7. Fever and chills, related to pneumonitis, bronchitis, or pneumonia
- Assess for late manifestations, including fatigue, weight loss, anorexia, dysphagia, nausea and vomiting, lethargy, confusion, and personality changes.
- Assess for psychosocial issues of fear, anxiety, guilt, or shame.
   1. Convey acceptance, and interact with the patient in a non-judgmental way.
   2. Encourage the patient and family to express their feelings about the possible diagnosis of lung cancer.
- Diagnosis of lung cancer is made on the basis of:
   1. Direct examination of cancer cells obtained by biopsy
   2. Chest x-rays
   3. CT scan
   4. Fiberoptic bronchoscopy
   5. Thoracoscopy or thoracentesis
   6. MRI
- Other tests used to determine extent of metastasis include radionuclide scans of the liver, spleen, brain, and bone and positron emission tomography (PET) scanning.

Nonsurgical Management
- *Chemotherapy* is often the treatment of choice for lung cancers, and it may be used alone or as adjuvant therapy in combination with surgery.

- The exact combination of drugs used depends on the response of the tumor and the overall health of the patient; however, most include platinum-based agents.
- Side effects that occur with chemotherapy for lung cancer include:
  1. Chemotherapy-induced nausea and vomiting (CIN)
  2. Alopecia
  3. Mucositis
  4. Immunosuppression
  5. Anemia
  6. Thrombocytopenia
  7. Peripheral neuropathy (PN)
- General management issues for care of patients undergoing radiation therapy are presented in Part One under Cancer Therapy.
- *Targeted therapy* is common in the treatment of later stage lung cancer and involves the use of drugs that target specific features of cancer cells, such as a protein, an enzyme, or the formation of new blood vessels. These agents are useful only for cancers that overexpress a certain protein or enzyme. For lung cancer, targeted therapy drugs include:
  1. Erlotinib (Tarceva), an oral drug
  2. Bevacizumab (Avastin), which is given IV
- *Radiation therapy* may be used for locally advanced lung cancers confined to the chest. It is used in addition to surgery or chemotherapy and is most commonly given by external beam daily over 5 to 6 weeks.
- Common side effects of radiation therapy for lung cancer are:
  1. Chest skin irritation and peeling
  2. Fatigue and taste changes
  3. Wheezing from inflamed airways
  4. Esophagitis
- General management issues for care of patients undergoing radiation therapy are presented in Part One under Cancer Therapy.
- *Photodynamic therapy* (PDT) may be used to remove small bronchial tumors when they are accessible by bronchoscopy. The patient is first injected with an agent that sensitizes cells to light. This drug enters all cells but leaves normal cells more rapidly than cancer cells, allowing it to concentrate in cancer cells. At about 48 hours, the patient goes to the operating room and is placed under anesthesia and intubated. A laser light is focused on the tumor. The light activates a chemical reaction within the cells retaining the sensitizing drug that induces irreversible cell damage. Some cells die and slough immediately; others continue to slough for several days.

- The photosensitizing drug has many effects that require special patient teaching and care both before and after the laser treatment. General management issues for care of patients undergoing PDT are presented in Part One under Cancer Therapy.
- When PDT is used in the airways, the patient usually requires a stay in the ICU for airway management.

Surgical Management
- Surgery is the main treatment for stage I and stage II NSCLC. Total removal of a non–small cell primary lung cancer is undertaken in hope of achieving a cure. If complete resection is not possible, the surgeon removes the bulk of the tumor.
- The specific surgery depends on the stage of the cancer and the patient's overall health and functional status. Surgeries include:
  1. Removal of the tumor only
  2. Removal of a lung segment (segmentectomy)
  3. Removal of a lobe (lobectomy)
  4. Removal of an entire lung (pneumonectomy)
- These procedures can be performed by open thoracotomy or by thoracoscopy with minimally invasive surgery in selected patients.
- Provide preoperative care:
  1. Administer routine preoperative care, as described in Part One.
  2. Teach the patient about the probable location of the surgical incision or thoracoscopy openings, shoulder exercises, and about the chest tube and drainage system (except after pneumonectomy).
  3. Encourage the patient to express fears and concerns.
  4. Reinforce the surgeon's explanation of the surgical procedure.
- Provide postoperative care, as described in Part One:
  1. Pain management
  2. Respiratory management with mechanical ventilation for the first 24 hours)
  3. Respiratory management for patients breathing on their own after the first 24 hours
     a. Maintain a patent airway.
     b. Assess respiratory status at least every 2 hours.
        (1) Check the alignment of the trachea.
        (2) Assess oxygen saturation.
        (3) Assess the rate and depth of respiration.
        (4) Listen to breath sounds in all remaining lobes.
        (5) Assess the oral mucous membranes for cyanosis and the nail beds for rate of capillary refill.
     c. Perform oral suctioning, as necessary.
     d. Provide oxygen therapy, as prescribed

    e. Assist the patient to a semi-Fowler position or up in a chair as soon as possible.

    f. Encourage the patient to use the incentive spirometer every hour while awake.

    g. If coughing is permitted, help the patient cough by splinting any incision and ensuring that the chest tube does not pull with movement.

4. Apply closed chest drainage (see closed chest drainage and chest tubes in Appendix 9, "The Patient Requiring Chest Tubes").

Interventions

- Several interventions are available for palliation.
- Oxygen therapy with humidification is prescribed when the patient is hypoxemic or to relieve dyspnea and anxiety.
- Drug therapy includes:
  1. Bronchodilators and corticosteroids, for the patient with bronchospasm
  2. Mucolytics to ease removal of thick mucus and sputum
  3. Antibiotics when bacterial infection is present
- Radiation therapy is used to help relieve hemoptysis, obstruction of the bronchi and great veins, dysphagia, and pain resulting from bone metastasis. Usually, radiation for palliation uses higher doses for shorter periods. Skin care issues and fatigue are the same as those occurring with radiation therapy for cure.
- Thoracentesis and pleurodesis for pleural effusion
  1. *Thoracentesis* is fluid removal by suction from the placement of a large needle or catheter into the intrapleural space.
  2. *Pleurodesis* is the deliberate development of an inflammation in the pleural space to cause the pleura to stick to the chest wall and prevent formation of effusion fluid. Agents such as liquid sclerosing chemicals or talc are instilled in the chest by thoracentesis after the effusion fluid has been removed.
  3. *Dyspnea management* is needed because the patient with lung cancer tires easily and is often most comfortable resting in a semi-Fowler position. Dyspnea is reduced with oxygen, use of a morphine drip, and positioning for comfort. The severely dyspneic patient may be most comfortable sitting in a lounge chair or reclining chair.
- Pain management may be needed for chest pain and pain radiating to the arm. The goal is to keep the patient as comfortable as possible.
  1. Drugs include opioid drugs as oral, parenteral, or transdermal preparations.
  2. Analgesics are given around-the-clock and PRN (for breakthrough pain).

3. Additional nonpharmacologic measures may include positioning, hot or cold compresses, distractions, and guided imagery.
4. Perform ongoing pain assessment, as described in Part One.
5. Evaluate the patient's response to the management strategies and collaborate with the health care team to make adjustments as necessary for improved patient comfort.

- Refer the terminal patient to Hospice or other palliative care programs.
- Refer the family to the American Cancer Society and other community agencies, as needed, for support groups or the use of home care equipment.

CANCER, OVARIAN

OVERVIEW

- Ovarian cancer is the leading cause of death from female reproductive cancers.
- Most ovarian cancers are epithelial tumors that form on the surface of the ovaries.
- These tumors grow rapidly, spread quickly, and are often bilateral.
- Ovarian cancers metastasize by direct extension into nearby organs and through blood and lymph circulation to distant sites. Free-floating cancer cells also spread through the abdomen to seed new sites, usually accompanied by ascites.
- Women who have a mutation in the *BRCA1* gene are at high risk for developing ovarian cancer, although the actual number of women with the mutation for this hereditary form of ovarian cancer is relatively small.
- Survival rates are low because ovarian cancer is so often not detected until its late stages.

PATIENT-CENTERED COLLABORATIVE CARE

Assessment

- Obtain patient information about risk factors for ovarian cancer:
  1. Family history of ovarian cancer
  2. *BRCA1* mutation status
  3. History of breast, bowel, or endometrial cancer
  4. History of infertility
  5. Nulliparity
  6. History of dysmenorrhea or heavy bleeding
  7. Diet history, including intake of animal fat

- Ask the patient about manifestations of ovarian cancer:
  1. Abdominal pain, swelling, or bloating
  2. Vague GI disturbances such as dyspepsia (indigestion) and gas
  3. Urinary frequency or incontinence
  4. Unexpected weight loss
  5. Vaginal bleeding
- Assess for complications of advancing metastatic cancer:
  1. Pleural effusion
  2. Ascites
  3. Lymphedema
  4. Intestinal obstruction
  5. Malnutrition
- Diagnosis and staging are performed by surgical exploration and biopsy analysis.
- Other assessment techniques helpful in staging the cancer and monitoring therapy progress include the CA 125 cancer antigen test, transvaginal ultrasonography, chest x-ray, and CT.

Interventions

- Nursing care of the patient with ovarian cancer is similar to that for endometrial or cervical cancer.
- Treatment options depend on the extent of the cancer and usually include surgery first, followed by chemotherapy. Radiation therapy is used for more widespread cancers.

Surgical Management

- Total abdominal hysterectomy and bilateral salpingo-oophorectomy (BSO) are the surgical procedures for all stages of ovarian cancer.
- When cancer has spread to other abdominal organs or lymph nodes, the tumors can be removed during the surgery.
- After surgery, nursing care is similar to that of the patient undergoing a hysterectomy for uterine leiomyomas:
  1. Assess vital signs.
  2. Assess pain.
  3. Assess catheter and drain function.
  4. Apply antiembolism stockings or compression devices.
  5. Teach the use of incentive spirometry.
  6. Monitor for complications.

Nonsurgical Management

- For all stages of ovarian cancer, cisplatin (Platinol), carboplatin, and paclitaxel (Taxol) are the most common chemotherapeutic drugs used, and they may be given IV or intraperitoneally.
- External radiation therapy (teletherapy) is used only if the disease has progressed after surgery and chemotherapy.

- General management issues for care of patients receiving combination chemotherapy and external radiation therapy are presented in Part One under Cancer Therapy.

CANCER, PANCREATIC

OVERVIEW

- Pancreatic tumors are highly malignant and originate in the epithelial cells of the pancreatic ductal system.
- Primary tumors usually are adenocarcinomas and grow in well-defined, glandular patterns.
- These cancers grow rapidly and spread to surrounding organs (stomach, duodenum, gallbladder, and intestine) by direct extension and invasion of the lymphatic and vascular system.
- Pancreatic cancer may result from metastasis from cancer of the lung, breast, thyroid, or kidney or from skin melanoma.
- The most common area of the pancreas in which cancer develops is the head of the pancreas.
- The exact cause of pancreatic cancer is unknown, but risk factors include:
  1. Advancing age
  2. Smoking
  3. Genetic predisposition with mutation in the *BRCA2* gene, *PALLD* gene, or a history of hereditary nonpolyposis colorectal cancer (HNPCC)
  4. Chronic pancreatitis
  5. Liver cirrhosis
- Other risk factors appear to include:
  1. Diabetes mellitus
  2. High intake of red meat, especially processed meat like bacon
  3. Long-term exposure to chemicals such as gasoline and pesticides
  4. Obesity
- Most pancreatic cancers are not diagnosed until the disease is advanced and overall survival is low.

PATIENT-CENTERED COLLABORATIVE CARE

Assessment

- Obtain patient information about:
  1. Jaundice (yellow discoloration) and pruritus (itching)
  2. Clay-colored stool and dark, frothy urine
  3. Abdominal pain described as a vague, constant dullness in the upper abdomen and nonspecific in nature; pain related to eating or activity; or back pain

4. Weight loss (unplanned)
5. Anorexia accompanied by early satiety, nausea, flatulence, and vomiting
- Assess for:
  1. High blood glucose levels
  2. Splenomegaly
  3. GI bleeding
  4. Leg or calf pain (from thrombophlebitis)
  5. Fatigue and weakness
  6. Dull sound on abdominal percussion indicating ascites
- Diagnostic assessment may include:
  1. Elevated levels of serum amylase, serum lipase, alkaline phosphatase, and bilirubin
  2. Elevated level of carcinoembryonic antigen (CEA)
  3. Elevated levels of CA 19-9 and CA 242
  4. Abdominal ultrasound
  5. Spiral or helical CT
  6. Endoscopic retrograde cholangiopancreatography (ERCP)
  7. Aspiration of pancreatic ascitic fluid

Interventions
- Management of the patient with pancreatic cancer is geared toward preventing tumor spread and decreasing pain. These measures are palliative, not curative. The cancers are often metastatic and recur despite treatment.

Nonsurgical Management
- Drug therapy includes:
  1. High doses of opioid analgesia; dependency is not a consideration because of the poor prognosis
  2. *Chemotherapy*, which has limited success
     a. Specific treatment regimens and drug combinations vary, but the most commonly used agents for pancreatic cancer include 5-fluorouracil (5-FU), gemcitabine (Gemzar), capecitabine (Xeloda), and docetaxel (Taxotere).
     b. General management issues for care of patients undergoing chemotherapy are presented in Part One under Cancer Therapy.
  3. *Targeted therapy* for pancreatic cancer may include erlotinib (Tarceva).
- *External beam radiation therapy* to shrink pancreatic tumor cells, alleviating obstruction and improving food absorption may provide pain relief but has not increased survival rates.
- Implantation of radon seeds in combination with systemic or intra-arterial administration of floxuridine (FURD) has also been used.
- Biliary stents may be inserted to relieve biliary obstruction.

Surgical Management
- Surgery is the most effective form of management for pancreatic cancer.
- The classic surgery, the Whipple procedure, entails extensive surgical manipulation, including resection of the proximal head of the pancreas, the duodenum, a portion of the jejunum, the stomach (partial or total gastrectomy), and the gallbladder, with anastomosis of the pancreatic duct (pancreatojejunostomy), the common bile duct (choledochojejunostomy), and the stomach (gastrojejunostomy) to the jejunum. The spleen may also be removed (splenectomy). This surgery may be performed by the traditional open abdominal method or by laparoscopic minimally invasive surgery (in select cancers).
- Palliative measures to relieve obstruction, such as cholecystojejunostomy, may be performed as a bypass procedure.
- Preoperative care and monitoring includes:
  1. Inserting the nasogastric (NG) tube for decompression
  2. Starting IV fluids or total parenteral nutrition to improve the patient's nutritional status before surgery
- Postoperative care and monitoring includes:
  1. Providing routine postoperative care as described in Part One
  2. Monitoring the drainage tubes placed during surgery to remove drainage and secretions from the area and to prevent stress on the anastomosis site
  3. Assessing the tubes and drainage devices for undue stress or kinking and maintaining tubes in a dependent position
  4. Monitoring drainage for color, consistency, and amount
  5. Observing for fistula formation (Drainage of pancreatic fluids are corrosive and irritating to the skin, and internal leakage causes peritonitis.)
  6. Placing the patient in a semi-Fowler position to reduce stress on the incision and anastomosis and to optimize lung expansion
  7. Maintaining fluid and electrolyte balance
  8. Closely monitoring vital signs for decreased blood pressure and increased heart rate, decreased vascular pressures, decreased hemoglobin levels and hematocrit, and electrolyte imbalances
  9. Assessing blood glucose levels for transient hyperglycemia or hypoglycemia resulting from surgical manipulation of the pancreas
  10. Monitoring the patient for pitting edema of the extremities and dependent edema in the sacrum and back

- Enteral feeding with a commercially prepared tube feeding is used while intestinal function is intact.
- A jejunostomy tube is inserted for late stages of pancreatic carcinoma; this method is preferred for lessening reflux and facilitating absorption.
- Hyperalimentation by TPN to optimize nutrition may be used as a single measure or in combination with tube feedings; a Hickman or other type of tunnelled catheter may be required for long-term use.

Community-Based Care

- Many of the care measures are palliative and aimed at providing symptom relief.
- Many patients are diagnosed just a few months before death occurs.
- Special home care preparations depend on the patient's physical condition and activity limitations.
- Regular home care nursing and assistive nursing personnel are scheduled to assist the patient and family.
- Help the patient identify what needs to be done to prepare for death, such as write a will, see family members and friends, and make requests for memorial service or funeral known.
- Refer the patient and family to religious leader or support services.

CANCER, PROSTATIC

OVERVIEW

- Prostate cancer is the most common type of cancer and the second leading cause of cancer deaths in men in North America.
- Most prostate tumors are adenocarcinomas arising from epithelial cells located in the posterior lobe or outer portion of the gland, and most are androgen sensitive (need testosterone to grow).
- These cancers are usually slow growing and metastasize first into nearby lymph nodes and then to bones of the pelvis, sacrum, and lumbar spine.
- In advanced stages of the disease, additional metastatic sites may include the lungs, liver, adrenals, and kidneys.
- In some men, prostate tissue grows very rapidly, leading to noncancerous, high-grade prostatic intraepithelial neoplasia (HGPIN), creating a high risk for developing more aggressive prostate cancer.
- Many men with prostate cancer can be cured of the disease, and others may live 10 years or more with the disease.

- Most men with prostate cancer are being diagnosed at earlier stages as a result of the introduction of the prostate-specific antigen (PSA) serum biomarker to diagnose the disease.
- The exact cause of prostate cancer remains unclear, but known risk factors include:
  1. Advancing age
  2. An intact hypothalamic-pituitary-testicular pathway
  3. Eating a diet high in animal fat (e.g., red meat)
  4. Viral infections
  5. Family history of prostate cancer
  6. Genetic predisposition
  7. Tobacco use
  8. Alcohol consumption

Genetic Considerations

- Specific gene mutations may increase the risk for prostate cancer, including alterations in the *EPHB2* gene and *BCRA2* gene.

PATIENT-CENTERED COLLABORATIVE CARE

Assessment

- Obtain patient information about:
  1. Age
  2. Race and ethnicity
  3. Family history of prostate cancer
  4. Nutritional habits
  5. Problems with urination
     a. Difficulty in starting urination
     b. Frequent bladder infections
     c. Urinary retention
  6. Pain during intercourse, especially when ejaculating
  7. Any other pain (particularly bone pain)
- Assess for:
  1. Gross blood in the urine (hematuria)
  2. Pain in the pelvis, spine, hips, or rib
  3. Swollen lymph nodes, especially in the groin areas
- Assess for psychosocial issues:
  1. Anxiety and fear
  2. Assess the reaction of the patient to the diagnosis and observe how his family or significant others react to the illness.
  3. Expect that patients will go through the grieving process and may be in denial or depressed.
  4. Determine what support systems the patient has, such as family, spiritual leaders, or community group support, to help him through diagnosis, treatment, and recovery.

5. Refer the patient with concerns related to sexuality and erectile dysfunction to his surgeon (urologist), sex therapist, or intimacy therapist, if available.
- Diagnostic assessment for cancer and metastasis may include:
  1. Digital rectal examination (DRE) (A prostate that is found to be stony hard and have palpable irregularities or indurations is suspected to be malignant.)
  2. Elevated levels of complexed prostate-specific antigen (cPSA) (greater than 3.4 ng/mL)
  3. Elevated levels of serum acid phosphatase
  4. Transrectal ultrasound (TRUS) of the prostate
  5. Prostate tissue biopsy
  6. Lymph node biopsy
  7. CT of the pelvis and abdomen
  8. MRI

> Clinical Landmine ◆ Prostate-specific antigen (PSA) analysis should never be used as a screening test without a digital rectal examination (DRE). Because other prostate problems also increase the PSA level, it is not specifically diagnostic for cancer, and some patients with prostate cancer have PSA levels *less than* 4 ng/mL. The PSA should be drawn before the DRE is performed because the examination can increase the PSA level due to prostate irritation.

Planning and Implementation
❖**NDx:** Impaired Urinary Elimination
- Patients are faced with several treatment options, depending on the stage of the disease and their overall health. A urologist and an oncologist are needed to help them make the best decision.
- Because prostate cancer is slow growing with late metastasis, older men who are asymptomatic and have other illness may choose observation without immediate active treatment, an option known as *watchful waiting*, or expectant therapy.
- Active treatment options are classified as local and systemic therapies. Local therapies include surgery and radiation. A variety of drugs is used for systemic therapy. Specific management is based on the extent of the disease and the patient's physical condition.

Surgical Management
- Surgery is the most common intervention for a cure. Minimally invasive surgery (MIS) or an open surgical technique for radical

prostatectomy (prostate removal) is most often performed. Other surgeries for palliation may include:
1. Transurethral resection of the prostate (TURP) to promote urination
2. Bilateral orchiectomy (removal of both testicles) to slow the spread of cancer by removing the main source of testosterone

- *Laparoscopic radical prostatectomy* (LRP) is an MIS for cure for patients who have a PSA less than 10 ng/mL and have no previous hormone therapy or abdominal surgeries. Advantages are:
  1. Decreased hospital stay (1 to 2 days)
  2. Minimal bleeding
  3. Smaller incisions and less scarring
  4. Less postoperative discomfort
  5. Decreased time for the urinary catheter
  6. Fewer complications
  7. Faster recovery and return to usual activities
- *Traditional open radical prostatectomy* can be performed through a retropubic or perineal approach, but the retropubic method is done most often to preserve perineal nerves needed for penile erection.
- Provide preoperative care, including:
  1. Routine preoperative care, as described in Part One
  2. Teaching the patient about the probable location of the surgical incision, the use of an indwelling urinary catheter, placement of drains, and the possibility of temporary erectile dysfunction (ED)
  3. Encouraging the patient to express fears and concerns
  4. Reinforcing the surgeon's explanation of the surgical procedure
- Provide postoperative care, including:
  1. Routine postoperative care, as described in Part One
  2. Encouraging him to use patient-controlled analgesia (PCA), as needed
  3. Helping him to get out of bed in a chair on the night of surgery, and ambulate the next day
  4. Maintaining the sequential compression device until he begins to ambulate
  5. Monitoring for deep vein thrombosis and pulmonary embolus
  6. Keeping an accurate record of intake and output, including drainage device drainage
  7. Keeping the urinary meatus clean using soap and water
  8. Avoiding rectal procedures or treatments

9. Teaching the patient how to care for the urinary catheter because he will be discharged with the catheter in place
10. Teaching the patient how to use a leg bag
11. Emphasizing the importance of not straining during bowel movement and advising the patient to avoid suppositories or enemas
12. Reminding the patient about the importance of follow-up appointments with the physician to monitor progress

Nonsurgical Management

- Nonsurgical management is usually an adjunct to surgery but may be done as an alternative intervention if the cancer is widespread or the patient's condition or age prevents surgery.
- *External or internal radiation therapy* may be used in the treatment of prostate cancer or for palliation of late-stage symptoms.
  1. *External beam radiation therapy (EBRT)* comes from a source outside the body. Patients are usually treated 5 days each week for 6 to 9 weeks.
  2. Complications of EBRT may include:
     a. Erectile dysfunction
     b. Acute radiation cystitis
     c. Radiation proctitis
  3. *Internal radiation therapy (brachytherapy)* can be delivered by implanting low-dose radiation seeds directly into and around the prostate gland.
  4. General management issues for care of patients undergoing radiation therapy are presented in Part One under Cancer Therapy.
- Hormone therapy is often used for prostate tumors because many are hormone dependent, and these tumors can be reduced or have their growth slowed through androgen deprivation. Manipulating the patient's hormones may be accomplished in two ways:
  1. The testosterone influence can be removed by a bilateral orchiectomy (surgery).
  2. Luteinizing hormone-releasing hormone (LH-RH) agonists or antiandrogens can be given (drugs).
     a. LH-RH agonists include:
        (1) Leuprolide (Lupron)
        (2) Goserelin (Zoladex)
        (3) Triptorelin (Trelstar)
     b. Antiandrogen drugs include:
        (1) Flutamide (Eulexin, Euflex)
        (2) Bicalutamide (Casodex)
        (3) Nilutamide (Nilandron)

3. Side effects of hormone therapy may include:
   a. Hot flashes
   b. *Gynecomastia* (breast development)
- *Systemic cytotoxic chemotherapy* is an option for patients whose cancer has spread and for whom other therapies have not worked.
  1. Specific treatment regimens and drug combinations vary, but the most commonly used agents for prostate cancer include docetaxel (Taxotere), cisplatin (Platinol), and etoposide (VP-16, VePesid).
  2. General management issues for care of patients undergoing chemotherapy are presented in Part One under Cancer Therapy.
- *Cryotherapy* (cryoablation) is a minimally invasive procedure for patients whose disease is known to be confined to the prostate gland. Transrectal cryoprobes are positioned around the prostate gland. Liquid nitrogen freezes the gland and results in prostate cell death.

Community-Based Care
- Include the patient's sexual partner in any teaching and discharge planning.
- Assess and address the patient's physical and psychosocial needs before hospital discharge and ensure their continued management in the community setting.
- Home care management of the patient after a radical prostatectomy includes:
  1. Collaborating with the case manager to coordinate the efforts of various health care providers, surgical unit nursing staff, and possibly a home care nurse
  2. Ensuring continuity of care during the weeks or months of therapies
  3. Health teaching about:
     a. Indwelling urinary catheter care, including:
        (1) Caring for the catheter
        (2) Using a leg bag
        (3) Identifying manifestations of infection and other complications
     b. Exercise by walking short distances
     c. Restricting lifting to no more than 15 pounds for up to 6 weeks
     d. Maintaining an upright position and not walking bent or flexed
     e. Avoiding vigorous exercise such as running or jumping for at least 12 weeks
     f. Avoiding straining at defecation

g. Showering rather than soaking in a bathtub for the first 2 to 3 weeks

h. Inspecting the incision site daily for signs of infection

i. Keeping follow-up appointments

- Refer the patient and partner to agencies or support groups such as the American Cancer Society's Man to Man program, Us TOO International (*www.ustoo.com*) sponsored by the Prostate Cancer Education and Support Network, the Prostate Cancer Foundation (*www.porstatecancerfoundation.org*), or the National Prostate Cancer Coalition (*www.fightprostatecancer.org*). Other personal and community support services, such as spiritual leaders or churches and synagogues, are also important to many patients.

- Refer men with erectile dysfunction (ED) to a specialist who can help with this problem.

- Refer patients with urinary incontinence to a urologist who specializes in this area.

CANCER, UROTHELIAL (BLADDER)

OVERVIEW

- Urothelial cancers are malignant tumors of the urothelium, which is the lining of transitional cells in the kidney, renal pelvis, ureters, urinary bladder, and urethra.

- Most urothelial cancers occur in the bladder; the term *bladder cancer* is the general term used to describe this condition.

- Most bladder cancers are transitional cell carcinomas of the bladder and are easily controlled.

- After the cancer spreads beyond the bladder's transitional cell layer, they are highly invasive and can spread beyond the bladder, with recurrence happening up to 10 years after being cancer free. If untreated, the tumor invades surrounding tissues, spreads to distant sites (liver, lung, and bone), and ultimately leads to death.

- Causes of urothelial cancers include tobacco use; exposure to chemicals used in the hairdressing, rubber, paint, electric cable, and textile industries; *Schistosoma haematobium* (a parasite) infection; excessive use of drugs containing phenacetin; and long-term use of cyclophosphamide (Cytoxan, Procytox ♦).

PATIENT-CENTERED COLLABORATIVE CARE

Assessment

- Obtain patient information about:
  1. Age and gender
  2. Patient's perception of general health
  3. Active and passive exposure to cigarette smoke

4. Occupation
5. Description of any change in the color, frequency, or amount of urine
6. Presence of any abdominal discomfort
7. Presence of dysuria, frequency, or urgency

- Assess for:
  1. Overall appearance of the patient, especially skin color and general nutritional status
  2. Abdomen for asymmetry, tenderness, and bladder distention
  3. Urine for color, clarity, presence of blood (first sign of bladder cancer)
  4. Anxiety or fear
  5. Patient's methods of coping and the degree of support from family members
- Diagnostic assessment includes:
  1. Urinalysis
  2. Cystoscopy with retrograde urography
  3. Biopsy of visible bladder tumor
  4. Excretory urography
  5. CT scans
  6. Ultrasonography
  7. MRI for deep, invasive tumors

Interventions

Nonsurgical Management

- Prophylactic immunotherapy with intravesical instillation of bacille Calmette-Guérin (BCG) is used to prevent recurrence of superficial bladder cancers.
- Multiagent chemotherapy is successful in prolonging life after distant metastasis has occurred but rarely results in a cure.
- Radiation therapy is also useful in prolonging life.

Surgical Management

- The type of surgery for bladder cancer depends on the type and stage of the cancer and the patient's general health.
- Transurethral resection of the bladder tumor (TURBT) or partial cystectomy is performed for small, early, superficial tumors and only a portion of the bladder is removed.
- Complete bladder removal (cystectomy) with additional removal of surrounding muscle and tissue offers the best chance of a cure for large, invasive bladder cancers. The ureters are diverted into one of several types of collecting reservoirs or a ureterostomy. The common types of alternative bladders are ileal conduit, continent pouch, bladder reconstruction also known as neobladder, and ureterosigmoidostomy.
  1. *Ureterostomy* (or a ureteroureterostomy) results in the ureters placed on the skin surface as one or two stomas that

drain urine into an external pouching system. This system is now less common.

2. *Ileal conduit* results in the ureters surgically placed in the ileum, which is brought to the skin surface as a stoma. Urine is collected in a pouch on the skin around the stoma.

3. *Ureterosigmoidostomy* results in the ureters surgically placed into a specially constructed segment of the sigmoid colon. No external pouching is needed.

4. *Continent pouches* (e.g., Kock's pouch) are internal pouches constructed from an ileal segment. Although these pouches open to the outside of the abdomen, a fold prevents urine leakage. Urine is drained with intermittent catheterization, and an external pouch is not needed.

5. *Neobladder* is the reconstruction of the bladder from bowel tissue and connecting it to the patient's urethra. Many patients learn to control voiding from the neobladder and neither external pouching nor intermittent catheterization is needed.

- Provide preoperative care, including:
  1. Implementing routine preoperative care as presented in Part One
  2. Reinforcing the surgeon's explanation of the procedure
  3. Ensuring educational counseling about the specific urinary diversion and postoperative care requirements for self-care practices, methods of pouching, control of urine drainage, and management of odor
  4. Coordinating with the surgeon and enterostomal therapist (ET) for selection of the stoma

- Provide postoperative care, including:
  1. Implementing routine postoperative care as described in Part One
  2. Monitoring urine output and urine characteristics
  3. Working with the ET to focus care on the wound, the skin, and urinary drainage
  4. Managing external pouching systems for patients with cutaneous ureterostomy or ureteroureterostomy
  5. Managing the Penrose drain and plastic Medena catheter for patients who have had construction of a continent reservoir
  6. Performing initial irrigation and intermittent catheterization of the neobladder
  7. Teaching the patient with a neobladder how to use new cues to know when to void, such as voiding at prescribed times or noticing a feeling of neobladder pressure

Community-Based Care

- Provide health teaching to the patient and family about:
  1. Drugs, diet and fluid therapy, the use of external pouching systems, and the technique for catheterizing a continent reservoir
  2. Electrolyte replacement
  3. Avoiding foods that are known to produce gas (if the urinary diversion uses the intestinal tract)
  4. External pouch application, local skin care, pouch care, methods of adhesion, and drainage mechanisms
  5. Intermittent catheterization (with a continent reservoir)
- Assist the patient to prepare for the impact of urinary diversion on self-image, body image, sexual functioning, and self-esteem.
- Discuss issues related to sexuality.
- Refer patients and families to community support and information organizations such as The United Ostomy Association, the American Cancer Society, and The Wound, Ostomy, and Continence Nurses Society.

CARDITIS, RHEUMATIC (RHEUMATIC ENDOCARDITIS)

- Rheumatic carditis (rheumatic endocarditis) is a sensitivity response that develops after an infection with group A beta-hemolytic streptococci.
- Inflammation is evident in all layers of the heart and results in impaired contractile function of the myocardium, thickening of the pericardium, and valvular damage.
- Common manifestations include:
  1. Tachycardia
  2. Cardiomegaly
  3. Development of a new murmur or change in existing murmur
  4. Pericardial friction rub
  5. Precordial pain
  6. Electrocardiogram (ECG) changes (prolonged PR interval)
  7. Indications of heart failure
  8. Evidence of an existing streptococcal infection
  9. Elevated serum findings: Antideoxyribonuclease B titer, antistreptolysin O titer, complement assay, C-reactive protein
- Treatment includes:
  1. Giving antibiotics, usually penicillin or erythromycin (Eryc, Erythromid)

2. Managing fever by maintaining hydration, administering antipyretics
3. Encouraging the patient to obtain adequate rest
4. Teaching the patient that antibiotic prophylaxis to prevent infective endocarditis must be considered for dental and invasive procedures throughout life

CARDIOMYOPATHY

OVERVIEW

- Cardiomyopathy is a subacute or chronic heart muscle disease of unknown cause.
- Cardiomyopathy is divided into three categories on the basis of abnormalities in structure and function:
  1. Dilated cardiomyopathy (DCM), the most common type, involves extensive damage to the myofibrils and interference with myocardial metabolism; it is characterized by dilation of both ventricles and impairment of systolic function.
  2. Asymmetric ventricular hypertrophy and disarray of the myocardial fibers are cardinal features of hypertrophic cardiomyopathy (HCM). Left ventricular (LV) hypertrophy leads to a stiff left ventricle that results in diastolic filling abnormalities. In about 50% of patients, HCM is transmitted as a single-gene autosomal dominant trait.
  3. Restrictive cardiomyopathy (RCM), the least common of the three cardiomyopathies, results in restriction of filling of the ventricles. It is caused by endocardial or myocardial disease and produces a clinical picture similar to that of constrictive pericarditis.
- Sudden death may be the first and only manifestation of cardiomyopathy.

PATIENT-CENTERED COLLABORATIVE CARE

Assessment

- Assess for clinical manifestations of DCM:
  1. Left ventricular (LV) failure at onset of disease, progressing to biventricular failure
  2. Progressive dyspnea on exertion
  3. Orthopnea
  4. Palpitations
  5. Activity intolerance
  6. Atrial fibrillation
- Assess for clinical manifestations of HCM:
  1. Exertional dyspnea
  2. Angina

3. Syncope
4. Atypical chest pain that occurs at rest, is prolonged, has no relation to exertion, and is not relieved by nitrates
5. Ventricular dysrhythmias
- Assess for clinical manifestations of RCM:
  1. Exertional dyspnea
  2. Weakness
  3. Exercise intolerance
  4. Palpitations
  5. Syncope

Interventions
Nonsurgical Management
- Care of the patient with DCM or RCM is the same as that for patients with heart failure (see Heart Failure).
- Treatment includes:
  1. Administering an angiotensin-converting enzyme inhibitor or angiotensin receptor blocker and a beta blocker to block the neurohormonal contributions to cardiomyopathy. Diuretics, vasodilators, and cardiac glycosides may be used as substitutes or as adjuncts as the disease progresses.
  2. Anticipating procedure to implant automatic cardiac defibrillator to promote synchronous ventricular emptying and control ventricular dysrhythmias
  3. Teaching the patient to abstain from alcohol because of its cardiac depressant effects
  4. Teaching the patient to report any palpitations, dizziness, or fainting, which may indicate a dysrhythmia
- Management of HCM includes beta-adrenergic blocking agents (carvedilol); strenuous exercise is prohibited.

Surgical Management
- The type of surgery performed depends on the type of cardiomyopathy.
- The most commonly performed surgery for HCM is excision of a portion of the hypertrophied ventricular septum to create a widened outflow tract.
- Cardiomyoplasty is used when cardiac transplantation is not an option and the patient is asymptomatic at rest.
- Heart transplantation is the treatment of choice for patients with severe DCM; a donor heart from a person with a comparable body weight and ABO compatibility is transplanted into a recipient within 6 hours of procurement.
- Criteria for candidates for heart transplantation include:
  1. Life expectancy less than 1 year
  2. Age younger than 65 years (variable)
  3. New York Heart Association class III or IV (poor functional status)

4. Normal or only slightly increased pulmonary vascular resistance
5. Absence of active infection
6. Stable psychosocial status
7. No evidence of drug or alcohol abuse

- Nursing interventions include:
  1. Providing postoperative care similar to that provided for patients having open-heart surgery (see surgical management of Coronary Artery Disease)
  2. Monitoring carefully for occult bleeding into the pericardial sac with the potential for cardiac tamponade
  3. Teaching the patient to change positions slowly due to the potential of orthostatic hypotension
  4. Monitoring closely for infection and respiratory distress.
- Provide discharge teaching:
  1. Teach the patient to report signs and symptoms of rejection, such as hypotension, dysrhythmias, weakness, fatigue, dizziness, respiratory distress, weight gain, or edema (initial episode of acute rejection usually occurs in the first 3 months after transplantation).
  2. Inform the patient that the surgeon will perform endomyocardial biopsy at regularly scheduled intervals to detect rejection.
  3. Teach the patient the importance of taking immunosuppressants for life to prevent transplant rejection.
  4. Encourage the patient to follow a lifestyle similar to that of patients with coronary artery disease.
  5. Encourage the patient to participate in an exercise program, allowing at least 10 minutes of warm-up and cool-down for the denervated heart to adjust to changes in activity level.
  6. Provide information about discharge drugs and diet.

> **Clinical Landmine** ♦ Avoid fluid overload in patients with cardiomyopathy, and use daily weights to assess fluid balance. A gain of 1 kg is equivalent to an extra liter of fluid.

CARPAL TUNNEL SYNDROME

OVERVIEW

- Carpal tunnel syndrome (CTS) is a condition in which the median nerve in the wrist becomes compressed, causing pain and numbness.
- Risk factors include common repetitive strain injury (RSI), synovitis, excessive hand exercise, edema or hemorrhage into

the carpal tunnel, or thrombosis of the median artery, Colles' fracture of the wrist, and hand burns.

- People at risk are those whose jobs require repetitive hand activities involving pinch or grasp during wrist flexion, such as factory workers, computer operators, and jackhammer operators.
- CTS most often occurs in women between the ages of 30 and 60 years.

PATIENT-CENTERED COLLABORATIVE CARE

Assessment

- Assess for:
  1. Nature, location, and intensity of patient-reported hand pain and numbness and whether symptoms are worse at night
  2. Presence of *paresthesia* (painful tingling) in the hand or hands
  3. Positive results for *Phalen's maneuver*, producing paresthesia in the palmar side of the thumb, index, and middle finger and radial half of the ring finger within 60 seconds (patient is asked to relax the wrist into flexion or place the back of the hands together and flex both wrists simultaneously)
  4. Positive results for Tinel's sign, which is the same response as for Phalen's maneuver elicited by tapping lightly over the area of the median nerve in the wrist
  5. Weak pinch, clumsiness, and difficulty with fine movements that progresses to muscle weakness
  6. Muscle wasting in the affected hand
  7. Wrist swelling
  8. Autonomic changes such as skin discoloration, nail brittleness, and increased or decreased palmar sweating
- Diagnostic assessment may include any of these: standard x-rays, electromyography (EMG), MRI, and ultrasonography.

Interventions

Nonsurgical Management

- Drug therapy
  1. NSAIDs
  2. Corticosteroid injections
- Wrist immobilization with temporary splinting in a neutral position or slight extension during the day, during the night, or both

Surgical Management

- Surgery is performed to relieve the pressure on the median nerve by providing nerve decompression through either open carpal tunnel release (OCTR) or endoscopic carpal tunnel release (ECTR).

- When CTS is a complication of rheumatoid arthritis, a *synovectomy* (removal of excess synovium) through a small inner-wrist incision may be performed.
- Provide preoperative care, including:
  1. Reinforcing the teaching provided by the surgeon regarding the nature of the surgery
  2. Reviewing postoperative care so that the patient knows what to expect
- Provide postoperative care, including:
  1. Monitoring vital signs
  2. Checking the dressing for drainage and tightness
  3. Checking the neurovascular status of the digits every hour during the immediate postoperative period
  4. Encouraging the patient to move all fingers of the affected hand at least every hour
  5. Administering pain medication, as needed
  6. Teaching patients who had the endoscopic procedure to keep the hand and arm elevated above heart level for several days
  7. Explaining that certain hand movements, including lifting heavy objects, may be restricted and a wrist-hand splint worn for 4 to 6 weeks after surgery
  8. Reminding the patient that weakness and discomfort may last for weeks or months
  9. Teaching the patient how to assess neurovascular status
  10. Ensuring that assistance is available in the home for routine daily tasks and ADLs

CATARACTS

OVERVIEW

- A cataract is an opacity of the lens that distorts the image projected onto the retina.
- Types of cataracts include:
  1. *Age-related cataracts:* Most common and usually affect people older than 65 years
  2. *Traumatic cataracts:* Caused by blunt trauma to or around the eye, penetrating eye injury, and exposure to excessive heat, x-rays, or radioactive material
  3. *Toxic cataracts:* Occur after long-term exposure to drugs, such as corticosteroids, phenothiazide-based drugs, and miotic drugs
  4. *Associated cataracts:* Occur with other diseases, such as diabetes mellitus, hypoparathyroidism, Down syndrome, and atopic dermatitis

5. *Complicated cataracts:* Develop as a complication of other eye disorders, such as retinitis pigmentosa, glaucoma, and retinal detachment

PATIENT-CENTERED COLLABORATIVE CARE

Assessment

- Assess patient information about:
  1. Age
  2. Recent or past trauma to the eye
  3. Exposure to radioactive materials, x-rays, or ultraviolet light
  4. Systemic disease (e.g., diabetes mellitus, hypoparathyroidism, Down syndrome, or atopic dermatitis)
  5. Prolonged use of corticosteroids, chlorpromazine, or miotic drugs
  6. Intraocular disease (e.g., recurrent uveitis)
- Ask the patient to describe his or her vision, specifically about:
  1. Blurred vision
  2. Decreased color perception
  3. Double vision
  4. Reduced visual acuity
- Assess the eye for:
  1. Loss of red reflex
  2. Presence of white pupil (late stage)

Planning and Implementation

❖**NDx:** Disturbed Sensory Perception: Visual Related to Altered Sensory Reception

- Surgery is the only cure for cataracts. However, patients often live with reduced vision for years before the cataract is removed.
- Interventions for enhanced communication, safety, and independence before surgery are described later in Visual Impairment (Reduced Vision) on p. 676.
- The most common surgical procedure is removal of the lens by phacoemulsification and replacement with a clear plastic lens for specific vision correction.
- Provide preoperative care:
  1. Assess how the patient's vision affects ADLs, especially dressing, eating, and ambulating.
  2. Reinforce the information provided by the ophthalmologist, and teach about the nature of cataracts, their progression, and their treatment.
  3. Stress that care after surgery requires the instillation of different types of eyedrops several times each day for 2 to 4 weeks.

4. Assess the patient's ability to evaluate eye appearance and instill eyedrops.
5. If the patient is unable to perform these tasks, help him or her make arrangements for this care.

- Provide postoperative care:
  1. Teach him or her to wear dark glasses outdoors or in brightly lit environments until the pupil responds to light.
  2. Teach the patient and family members how to instill the prescribed eyedrops.
  3. Create a written schedule for the timing and the order of eyedrops administration.
  4. Stress the importance of keeping all follow-up appointments.
  5. Teach the patient and family about expected manifestations (mild eye itching, a "bloodshot" appearance, slightly swollen eyelid, creamy white, dry, crusty drainage on the eyelids and lashes).
  6. Suggest the use of cool compresses and a mild analgesic such as acetaminophen (Abenol ♣, Tylenol) for control of discomfort.
  7. Remind him or her to avoid aspirin because of its effects on blood clotting.
  8. Instruct the patient to notify the ophthalmologist if there is significant swelling or bruising around the eye; pain occurring with nausea or vomiting; increasing redness of the eye, a change in visual acuity, tears, and photophobia; and yellow or green drainage.

> ⬛ Critical Rescue ◆ Teach the patient to report any reduction in vision immediately to the ophthalmologist.

  9. Teach the patient to avoid activities that can increase intraocular pressure, including:
     a. Bending from the waist
     b. Lifting objects weighing more than 10 lbs
     c. Sneezing, coughing
     d. Blowing the nose
     e. Straining to have a bowel movement
     f. Vomiting
     g. Having sexual intercourse
     h. Keeping the head in a dependent position
     i. Wearing tight shirt collars

Community-Based Care

- If the patient has difficulty instilling eyedrops, a supportive neighbor, friend, or family member can be taught the procedure. Eyedrops are often prescribed for 2 to 4 weeks after cataract surgery.

- Remind the patient that he or she may wash his or her hair 1 or 2 days after surgery, but only with the head tilted back, such as in a beauty salon or barber shop, to avoid getting water in the eye. Teach the patient to stand in the shower with the face away from the showerhead for the first week after surgery.
- Teach the patient about activity restrictions. Cooking and light housekeeping are permitted, but vacuuming should be avoided for several weeks because of the forward flexion involved and the rapid, jerky movements required.
- Advise him or her to refrain from operating machinery, and participating in certain sports, such as golf, until given specific permission from the ophthalmologist.

CELIAC DISEASE

- Celiac sprue is thought to be due to a genetic immune hypersensitivity response to gluten or its breakdown products or to result from the accumulation of gluten in the diet with peptidase deficiency.
- Celiac disease causes a disruption to the gut mucosa and can result in inflammation and malabsorption.
- The xylose absorption test can be diagnostic if malabsorption in the small intestine is present; a biopsy is performed for diagnostic confirmation.
- Gluten-free diets are available for those with celiac sprue.
- Steroids are sometimes given in celiac disease to decrease inflammation.

CHLAMYDIAL INFECTION

OVERVIEW

- *Chlamydial trachomatis* is an intracellular bacterium that causes genital chlamydial infection, which is the most common sexually transmitted disease (STD) in the U. S.
- Manifestations are similar to those of gonorrheal infections and the incubation period ranges from 1 to 3 weeks, but the pathogen may be present in the genital tract for months without producing symptoms.
- The main manifestation in men is urethritis with dysuria, frequent urination, and a watery, mucoid discharge. Complications include epididymitis, prostatitis, infertility, and Reiter's syndrome.

- Many women may have no symptoms or have a mucopurulent cervicitis that occurs with a change in vaginal discharge, easily induced cervical bleeding, urinary frequency, and abdominal discomfort or pain. Complications include salpingitis, pelvic inflammatory disease (PID), ectopic pregnancy, and infertility.

PATIENT-CENTERED COLLABORATIVE CARE

Assessment
- Obtain patient information about:
  1. Personal medical history
  2. Menstrual history (from women)
  3. History of sexual activity, including age at onset, number of sexual partners, recent new sexual partner, use of a nonbarrier method of birth control
  4. Personal history of STDs
  5. Sexual partner history of STDs
  6. Presence of symptoms, including vaginal or urethral discharge, dysuria (painful urination), pelvic pain, irregular bleeding
- Diagnostic assessment requires sampling cells from the endocervix and/or urethra and testing for:
  1. Gram staining (to rule out gonorrhea)
  2. Tissue culture for *Chlamydia*
  3. Gene amplification tests or DNA amplification tests (ligand chain reaction [LCR] and polymerase chain reaction [PCR])
  4. Enzyme-linked immunoassay (ELISA)
  5. Direct fluorescent antibody (DFA)

Interventions
- Drug therapy includes any one of the following regimens:
  1. Azithromycin (Zithromax): 1 g orally in a single dose
  2. Doxycycline (Monodox, Doxy-Caps, Doxycin ♣): 100 mg orally two times each day for 7 days
  3. Erythromycin base (E-Mycin, Eramycin, Erythromid ♣): 500 mg orally four times each day for 7 days
  4. Erythromycin ethylsuccinate (EES, Apo-Erythro ♣): 800 mg orally four times each day for 7 days
  5. Oflaxcin (Floxin): 300 mg orally two times each day for 7 days
  6. Levofloxacin (Levoquin): 500 mg orally daily for 7 days
- Testing and treatment of sexual partners
- Patient education, teach about:
  1. The mode of disease transmission
  2. The incubation period
  3. Manifestation, including the possibility of asymptomatic infections

4. Treatment of infection with antibiotics
5. The need for abstinence from sexual intercourse until the patient and partner have completed treatment
6. No test of cure is required, but all women should be rescreened 3 to 4 months after treatment because of the high risk for PID if reinfection occurs.
7. The need for the patient and partner to return for evaluation if symptoms recur or new symptoms develop
8. Possible complications of untreated or inadequately treated infection, such as PID, ectopic pregnancy, or infertility

CHOLECYSTITIS

OVERVIEW

- Cholecystitis is an inflammation of the gallbladder that can occur as an acute or chronic process.
- Acute cholecystitis (inflammation) usually develops in association with cholelithiasis (gallstones). About one half of the adult U. S. population have asymptomatic gallstones.
- Acalculous cholecystitis occurs in the absence of gallstones and is associated with biliary stasis caused by any condition that affects the regular filling or emptying of the gallbladder such as decreased blood flow to the gallbladder or anatomic problems such as kinking of the gallbladder neck or cystic duct that can result in pancreatic enzyme reflux into the gallbladder and cause inflammation.
- Chronic cholecystitis results when repeated episodes of cystic duct obstruction results in chronic inflammation, and the gallbladder becomes fibrotic and contracted, resulting in decreased motility and deficient absorption.
- Complications of cholecystitis include pancreatitis and cholangitis (inflammation and inflection of the common bile ducts).
- Cholangitis is usually associated with choledocholithiasis (common bile duct stones).
- Jaundice (yellow discoloration of body tissues) and icterus (yellow discoloration of the sclera) can occur in acute disease but are most commonly seen in the chronic phase of cholecystitis. Jaundice results from increased bilirubin in the body that collects in the skin and sclera. Itching and a burning sensation result.

PATIENT-CENTERED COLLABORATIVE CARE

Assessment
- Record patient information:
  1. Height and weight

2. Sex, age, race, and ethnic group
3. Food preferences, including fat and cholesterol intake
4. Food intolerances and related GI symptoms, including flatulence, dyspepsia (indigestion), eructation (belching), anorexia, nausea, vomiting, and abdominal pain in relation to fatty food intake
5. Exercise routine or daily activities
6. Family history of gallbladder disease
7. In women, history of estrogen replacement therapy

- Assess for:
  1. Abdominal pain of varying intensity in the right upper abdominal quadrant, including radiation to the right upper shoulder; ask the patient to describe the intensity, duration, precipitating factors, and relief measures
  2. Other GI symptoms, including nausea, vomiting, dyspepsia, flatulence, eructation, and feelings of abdominal heaviness
  3. With right subcostal palpation, increasing pain with deep inspiration (Murphy's sign)
  4. Guarding, rigidity, and rebound tenderness (Blumberg's sign)
  5. Sausage-shaped mass in the right upper quadrant
  6. Late symptoms seen in chronic cholecystitis, such as jaundice, clay-colored stools, and dark urine
  7. Steatorrhea (fatty stools)
  8. Elevated temperature with tachycardia and dehydration from fever and vomiting
  9. Results of serum liver enzyme and bilirubin tests (may be elevated)
  10. Increased WBC count
  11. Elevated serum and urine amylase levels (if pancreas is affected)

⧼ Considerations for Older Adults

- Older adults and patients with diabetes mellitus have atypical manifestations, including the absence of pain and fever. Localized tenderness may be the only presenting sign.
- The older adult may become acutely confused.
- Older adults should not be given meperidine (Demerol) for pain because it can cause acute confusion and nausea.

Planning and Implementation
Nonsurgical Management
- Patients with chronic cholecystitis are encouraged to consume frequent, small, low-fat meals.

- If gallstones are causing an obstruction of bile flow, fat-soluble vitamins and bile salts may be prescribed to facilitate digestion and vitamin absorption.
- Food and fluids are withheld during nausea and vomiting episodes; nasogastric (NG) decompression is initiated for severe vomiting.
- Drug therapy includes:
  1. Opioid analgesics to relieve pain and reduce spasm
  2. Antispasmodic agents or anticholinergics to relax the smooth muscle
  3. Antiemetics to provide relief from nausea and vomiting

Surgical Management

- A percutaneous transhepatic biliary catheter may be inserted to decompress obstructed extrahepatic ducts so bile can flow.
- Cholecystectomy (removal of the gallbladder) is the usual surgical treatment. One of two procedures may be performed:
  1. Laparoscopic laser procedure (performed more often than the traditional surgical approach)
  2. Traditional open surgical approach for complicated or infected sites.
     a. A T-tube drain is surgically inserted when the common bile duct is explored to ensure patency of the duct.
- Provide preoperative care:
  1. Stress the importance of deep breathing, coughing, and turning, as well as early ambulation after surgery.
  2. Teach how to use a folded blanket or pillow as a splint for the abdomen to prevent jarring during coughing.
- Laparoscopic laser cholecystectomy is commonly performed by making several small punctures, through which the laparoscope is inserted. A laser dissects the gallbladder before removal through a puncture site. This procedure is less invasive than traditional surgery and is performed on an outpatient (ambulatory) basis.
- Provide postoperative care for laparoscopic patients:
  1. Teach the patient the importance of early ambulation to absorb the carbon dioxide that is retained in the abdomen.
  2. Inform the patient that he or she can return to usual activities 1 to 3 weeks after the procedure.
- Provide postoperative care for traditional surgery patients:
  1. Administer IV (by patient-controlled analgesia [PCA]) for pain relief, as ordered.
  2. Administer antiemetics for relief of postoperative nausea and vomiting, as ordered.
  3. Advance the diet from clear liquids to solid foods, as tolerated by the patient.

4. Maintain the patient's T-tube:
   a. Keep the drainage system below the level of the gallbladder.
   b. Assess the amount, color, consistency, and odor of drainage (bile output is approximately 400 mL/day).
   c. Administer synthetic bile salts such as dehydrocholic acid (Decholin), as ordered.
   d. Report to the physician sudden increases or output of more than 1000 mL in 24 hours in bile output.
   e. Assess for foul odor and purulent drainage and report changes in drainage to the physician.
   f. Inspect the skin around the T-tube insertion site for signs of inflammation.
   g. Never irrigate, aspirate, or clamp the T-tube without a physician's order.
   h. Assess the drainage system for pulling, kinking, or tangling of the tubing.
   i. Place the patient in a semi-Fowler position when in bed.
   j. Assist the patient with early ambulation.
   k. Teach patient to observe stools for brown color 7 to 10 days postoperatively.

◤**National Patient Safety Goal**

Before the start of any invasive procedure, conduct a final verification process using active communication to confirm the correct patient, procedure, and site.

Community-Based Care
- If traditional surgery is performed, give the patient written postoperative instructions on:
  1. Inspection of the abdominal incision for redness, tenderness, swelling, and drainage
  2. Dressing change, wound care, and T-tube drain care instructions
  3. Pain management, including prescriptions
  4. Signs and symptoms of infection, including when to call the physician (elevated temperature and increased pain)
  5. Activity limitations include avoiding lifting a weight greater than 25 pounds and restricting driving for 2 to 4 weeks
- Provide diet therapy instructions based on the patient's tolerance of fats. Instruct the patient to add one food at a time to trial tolerance and weight reduction after healing from surgery, if indicated.
- Provide information to the patient and family about the potential for postcholecystectomy syndrome manifested by jaundice

of the skin or sclera, darkened urine, light-colored stools, pain, fever, and chills.
- Refer to home health nursing if needed.

CHRONIC OBSTRUCTIVE PULMONARY DISEASE (COPD)

OVERVIEW

- *Chronic obstructive pulmonary disease* (COPD) is an irreversible chronic lung disease that includes both emphysema and chronic bronchitis.
- The major features of *emphysema* that lead to dyspnea are:
  1. Loss of lung elasticity
  2. Hyperinflation of the lung (air trapping)
- Emphysema is classified as panlobular, centrilobular, or paraseptal depending on the pattern of destruction and dilation of the gas-exchanging units (acini). Each type can occur alone or in combination in the same lung. Most are associated with smoking or chronic exposure to other inhalation irritants.
- *Bronchitis* is an inflammation of the bronchi and bronchioles caused by chronic exposure to irritants, especially tobacco smoke. It affects only the airways.
- The major features of chronic bronchitis are:
  1. Increased number and size of mucous glands, which produce large amounts of thick mucus
  2. Thickening of bronchial walls that impairs airflow
  3. Poor gas exchange with decreased Pao_2 (hypoxemia) and increased $Paco_2$ (respiratory acidosis)
- Risk factors for COPD include cigarette smoking, alpha$_1$-antitrypsin (AAT) deficiency, and air pollution.

Cultural Awareness

The prevalence of smoking remains higher among African Americans, blue-collar workers, and less-educated people than the overall population of the U. S. Smoking prevalence is highest among northern plains American Indians and Alaskan Natives. The overall prevalence of smoking for men and women has decreased over the past 2 decades, but the decrease for women has been less than it has been for men. Development of culturally appropriate smoking cessation programs and research examining barriers to cessation in these populations may help reduce this disparity.

Genetic Considerations

The gene for AAT has many known mutations, some of which increase the risk for emphysema. Variation of mutations (polymorphisms) results in different levels of AAT deficiency. This variation is one reason why the disease is more severe for some people than for others. The most serious mutation for an increased risk for emphysema is the Z mutation, although others also increase the risk but to a lesser degree.

- Complications of COPD include:
  1. Hypoxemia
  2. Acidosis
  3. Respiratory infection
  4. Pneumothorax
  5. Cardiac failure
  6. Dysrhythmias

PATIENT-CENTERED COLLABORATIVE CARE

Assessment

- Obtain and record patient information:
  1. Age, gender, occupational history, ethnic-cultural background, and family history
  2. Smoking history, including the length of time the patient has smoked and the number of packs smoked daily
  3. Current breathing problems:
     a. Does the patient have difficulty breathing while talking? Can he or she speak in complete sentences, or is it necessary to take a breath between every one or two words?
     b. Ask about the presence, duration, or worsening of wheezing, coughing, and shortness of breath, and what activities trigger these problems.
     c. If the cough is productive, what is the sputum color and amount, and has the amount increased or decreased?
     d. What is the relationship between activity tolerance and dyspnea? How is the patient's activity level and shortness of breath now compared with a month earlier and a year earlier? Is he or she having any difficulty with eating, sleeping, or performing ADLs?
  4. Weight and general appearance: The patient with increasingly severe COPD is thin, with loss of muscle mass in the extremities, enlarged neck muscles, has a barrel-shaped chest, and is slow moving and slightly stooped.
- Assess for:
  1. Respiratory changes
     a. Breathing rate and pattern, especially rapid, shallow respirations, paradoxical respirations, or use of accessory muscles
     b. Abnormal chest retractions and asymmetric chest expansion

   c. Limited diaphragmatic movement (excursion) and diaphragm position

   d. Hyperresonant chest sounds on percussion

   e. Wheezes and other abnormal sounds

   f. Degree of dyspnea using a Visual Analog Dyspnea Scale (VADS)

2. Cardiovascular changes
   a. Heart rate and rhythm
   b. Swelling of feet and ankles
   c. Cyanosis, or blue-tinged, dusky appearance
   d. Delayed capillary refill
   e. Clubbing of the fingers

3. Psychosocial issues
   a. Social isolation
   b. Exposure to smoke or crowded living conditions
   c. Work, family, social, and sexual roles that may change and affect self-esteem
   d. Anxiety and fear related to dyspnea that may reduce the patient's ability to participate in a full life
   e. Encourage the patient and family to express their feelings about the limitations on lifestyle and disease progression.
   f. Assess patient and family awareness and use of support groups and services.

4. Economic issues
   a. The patient may not be able to work or might have had to change jobs, resulting in reduced income or changes in health insurance coverage.
   b. Drugs, especially the metered dose inhalers (MDIs) and dry powder inhalers (DPIs), are expensive, and many patients with limited incomes may use them only during exacerbations and not as prescribed.

5. Diagnostic and laboratory tests
   a. Serial arterial blood gas (ABG) values for hypoxemia and hypercarbia
   b. Oxygen saturation by pulse oximetry
   c. Sputum cultures
   d. Hematocrit and hemoglobin for polycythemia
   e. Serum electrolyte levels for hypophosphatemia, hyperkalemia, hypocalcemia, and hypomagnesemia, which reduce muscle strength
   f. Serum AAT levels in patients with a family history of COPD
   g. Chest x-rays
   h. Pulmonary function test (PFT) changes

i. Peak expiratory flow rates

j. Carbon monoxide diffusion test

Planning and Implementation

❖**NDx:** Impaired Gas Exchange

Nonsurgical Management

- Maintain a patent airway:
  1. Keep the patient's head, neck, and chest in alignment.
  2. Assist patient to clear the airway of secretions.
- Monitor for changes in respiratory status in the hospitalized patient with COPD at least every 2 hours.
- Enhance coughing effectiveness:
  1. Assist the patient to a sitting position with head slightly flexed, shoulders relaxed, and knees flexed.
  2. Teach the patient to take a deep breath, hold it for 2 seconds, and cough two or three times in succession.
  3. Teach the patient to follow coughing with several maximal inhalation breaths.
- Oxygen therapy
  1. Provide oxygen as prescribed, usually a flow rate of 2 to 4 L/min by nasal cannula or up to 40% by Venturi mask.
  2. Ensure that there are no open flames or other combustion hazards in rooms where oxygen is in use.

> 📷 Critical Rescue ◆ Assess the respiratory status of the patient with COPD who is receiving oxygen therapy at least hourly for respiratory depression. A low arterial oxygen level is this patient's primary drive for breathing.

- Drug therapy includes:
  1. Inhaled bronchodilator drugs, such as albuterol (Proventil, Ventolin), ipratropium (Atrovent, Apo-Ipravent ♣), tiotropium bromide (Spiriva), theophylline (Elixophyllin, Theo Dur, Uniphyl, Theolair, many others)
  2. Inhaled or systemic anti-inflammatory drugs, such as fluticasone (Flovent), prednisone (Deltasone, Predone)
  3. Mucolytic drugs, such as acetylcysteine (Mucosil, Mucomyst ♣) or dornase alfa (Pulmozyme)
  4. Stepped therapy is recommended for patients with chronic bronchitis or emphysema who are aware of their disease and are able to participate in symptom management.
  5. Teach patients and family members the correct techniques for using inhalers and to care for them properly.
- Pulmonary rehabilitation can improve function and endurance in patients with COPD.

1. Teach patients about the need for exercise training to prevent general and pulmonary muscle deconditioning.
2. Collaborate with the physical therapist and patient to plan an individualized exercise program.
3. Remind the patient to perform planned exercises at least two or three times each week.
4. Teach patients whose symptoms are severe to modify the exercise by using a walker with wheels or, if needed, to use oxygen therapy during the exercise period.

Surgical Management

- Lung transplantation may be performed for select patients with end-stage COPD.
- Lung reduction surgery can improve gas exchange through removal of the hyperinflated lung tissue areas that are useless for gas exchange.
- Preoperative care includes:
    1. Pulmonary rehabilitation to maximize lung and muscle function
    2. Testing with pulmonary plethysmography, gas dilution, or perfusion scans to determine the location of greatest lung hyperinflation and poorest lung blood flow
    3. Standard preoperative care and teaching, as described in Part One
- Postoperative care includes:
    1. Routine postoperative care, as described in Part One
    2. Pain management
    3. Close monitoring for continuing respiratory problems
    4. Chest tube management
    5. Maintenance of bronchodilator and mucolytic therapy
    6. Pulmonary hygiene with incentive spirometry 10 times per hour while awake, chest physiotherapy starting on the first day after surgery, and hourly pulmonary assessment

❖**NDx:** Ineffective Breathing Pattern

- Assess the patient to determine the breathing pattern, especially the rate, rhythm, depth, and use of accessory muscles.
- Identify factors that may contribute to the increased work of breathing, such as respiratory infection.
- Interventions aim to improve the patient's breathing efforts and decrease the work of breathing.
    1. Teach breathing techniques.
        a. Diaphragmatic or abdominal breathing
        b. Pursed-lip breathing
    2. Patient positioning
        a. Assist the patient to an upright position.
        b. Elevate the head of the bed.

3. Teach energy conservation techniques to plan and pace activities for maximal tolerance and minimal discomfort.
   a. Work with the patient to develop a personal daily schedule for activities and rest periods.
   b. Encourage the patient to avoid working with the arms raised or reaching above the head.
   c. Teach the patient to adjust work heights to reduce back strain and fatigue.
   d. Remind him or her to keep arm motions smooth and flowing to prevent jerky motions that waste energy.
   e. Teach about the use of adaptive tools for housework, such as long-handled dustpans, sponges, and dusters, to reduce bending and reaching.
   f. Suggest how to organize work spaces so that items used most often are within easy reach.
   g. Teach the patient not to talk when engaged in other activities that require energy, such as walking.
   h. Teach him or her to avoid breath-holding while performing any activity.

❖**NDx:** Ineffective Airway Clearance

- Excessive secretions lead to compromised breathing, poor oxygenation and tissue perfusion, and increase the risk for respiratory infections.
- Assess breath sounds and oxygen saturation routinely as part of physical assessment and before and after interventions.
- Teach the patient to cough effectively on arising in the morning, before mealtimes, and before bedtime. Instruct the patient to:
  1. Sit in a chair or on the side of a bed with feet placed firmly on the floor.
  2. Position himself or herself with shoulders turned inward, bend the head slightly downward, and hug a pillow against the stomach.
  3. Take a few deep breaths in through the nose, out through pursed lips, and then bend forward slowly while coughing two or three times from the same breath.
  4. Observe the color, consistency, odor, and amount of secretions.
  5. Repeat the entire coughing procedure at least twice.
- Perform suctioning only when abnormal breath sounds are present, not on a routine schedule.
  1. Assess the patient for dyspnea, tachycardia, and dysrhythmias during the procedure.
  2. Assess for improved breath sounds after suctioning.
- Assist patients who can tolerate sitting in a chair out of bed for 1-hour periods two to three times each day.

- Unless hydration needs to be avoided for other health problems, teach the patient with COPD to drink at least 2 to 3 L of water daily.
- Teach patients how to use flutter valve mucous clearance devices to remove airway secretions.

❖**NDx:** Imbalanced Nutrition: Less Than Body Requirements

- The patient with COPD often has food intolerance, nausea, early satiety, loss of appetite, and meal-related dyspnea.
- The increased work of breathing raises calorie and protein needs and leads to protein-calorie malnutrition.
- Malnourished patients have reduced effective breathing because of loss of total body mass, ventilatory muscle mass and strength, lung elasticity, and alveolar-capillary surface area.
- Identify patients at risk for or who have this complication and request nutritional consultation.
- Monitor patient weight and other indicators of nutrition, such as skin condition and serum prealbumin levels.
- Manage dyspnea to reduce the shortness of breath that interferes with eating.
  1. Urge the patient to rest before meals.
  2. Teach the patient to plan the biggest meal of the day for the time when he or she is most hungry and well rested. Four to six small meals each day may be preferred to three larger ones.
  3. Teach the patient to use pursed-lip and abdominal breathing to alleviate dyspnea.
  4. Suggest the use of a bronchodilator 30 minutes before the meal.
- Collaborate with the patient and nutritionist for food selection to prevent weight loss and improve appetite (foods that are easy to chew, high in calories and protein, and not gas forming).
  1. Teach the patient to avoid dry foods, which stimulate coughing, and foods such as milk and chocolate, which increase the thickness of saliva and secretions.
  2. Suggest that he or she avoid caffeinated beverages because they increase urine output and may lead to dehydration.
  3. Urge the patient to eat high-calorie, high-protein foods.
  4. Suggest dietary supplements, such as Pulmocare, that provide nutrition with reduced carbon dioxide production.
  5. If early satiety is a problem, advise the patient to avoid drinking fluids before and during meals.

❖**NDx:** Anxiety

- Patients with COPD often have increased anxiety during acute dyspneic episodes, especially if they feel as though they are choking on excessive secretions. Anxiety has been shown to cause dyspnea.

- Help the patient develop a written plan that states exactly what to do if symptoms flare.
- Stress the use of pursed-lip and diaphragmatic breathing techniques during periods of anxiety or panic.
- Recommend professional counseling, if needed, as a positive suggestion. Stress that talking with a counselor can help identify techniques to maintain control over the dyspnea and feelings of panic.
- Explore other approaches to control dyspneic episodes and panic attacks, such as progressive relaxation, hypnosis therapy, and biofeedback.

❖**NDx:** Activity Intolerance

- Assist with ADLs of eating, bathing, and grooming based on assessment of the patient's needs and fatigue level.
- Encourage the patient to pace activities and not to rush.
- Assess the patient's response to activity by noting skin color changes, pulse rate and regularity, blood pressure, and work of breathing.
- Suggest the use of supplemental oxygen during periods of high energy use, such as bathing or walking.

❖**Collaborative Problem:** Potential for Pneumonia or Other Respiratory Infections

- Patients with COPD who have excessive secretions or who have artificial airways are at increased risk for respiratory tract infections.
- Teach patients to avoid large crowds and anyone who is ill.
- Stress the importance of receiving a pneumonia vaccination and a yearly influenza vaccination.

Community-Based Care

- Coordinate with all members of the health care team to individualize plans for the patient to be discharged to home.
- Determine what equipment and assistance will be needed in the home setting.
- Teach the patient and family about:
  1. The disease and its course
  2. Drug therapy
  3. Manifestations of infection
  4. Avoidance of respiratory irritants
  5. Nutrition therapy regimen
  6. Activity progression
  7. The need to identify and avoid stressors that can worsen the disease

8. Breathing techniques
9. Energy conservation measures
10. Relaxation therapy
11. Effective coughing techniques
- Collaborate with the care manager and social worker to obtain needed home services:
  1. Oxygen and nebulizer
  2. Hospital-type bed
  3. Home health nurse or aide
  4. Financial assistance
- Provide appropriate referrals, as needed:
  1. Home care visits
  2. Meals on Wheels
  3. Support groups
  4. Smoking cessation programs

CIRRHOSIS

OVERVIEW

- Cirrhosis is a chronic, progressive liver disease characterized by diffuse fibrotic bands of connective tissue that distort the normal architectural anatomy of the liver, resulting in disturbed metabolic processes and circulatory pathology.
- Cirrhosis is essentially an irreversible reaction to hepatic inflammation and necrosis.
  1. In compensated cirrhosis, the liver has significant scarring but is still able to perform essential functions without causing significant symptoms.
  2. In decompensated cirrhosis, liver function is significantly impaired, with obvious signs and symptoms of liver failure.
- The main causes of cirrhosis are:
  1. Alcohol
     a. Alcohol has a direct toxic effect on liver cells, causing liver inflammation (alcoholic hepatitis).
     b. The liver becomes enlarged with cellular infiltration by fat, leukocytes, and lymphocytes.
     c. Early scar formation is caused by fibroblast infiltration and collagen formation.
     d. Damage to the liver progresses, and widespread scar tissue forms with fibrotic infiltration of the liver as a result of cellular necrosis.
  2. Viral hepatitis
     a. Inflammation caused by hepatitis infection over time leads to progressive scarring of the liver.

      b. Alcohol accelerates the process in the presence of hepatitis C; hepatitis B causes low-grade damage over decades that can lead to cirrhosis.

3. Autoimmune hepatitis: Immune system produces autoantibodies to hepatocytes, causing inflammation of the liver.

4. Steatohepatitis
   a. Fat and cholesterol deposits in the liver cause chronic inflammation.
   b. Risk factors are obesity and an elevated lipid profile.

5. Drugs and toxins
   a. Prescriptive, OTC, and illicit drugs; herbal supplements; mushrooms; and environmental exposure to toxins may damage the liver so significantly that cirrhosis occurs.

6. Biliary disease
   a. Chronic biliary obstruction, bile stasis, and inflammation result in severe obstructive jaundice.
   b. Primary biliary cirrhosis (PBC) results from intrahepatic bile stasis.
   c. Primary sclerosing cholangitis (PSC) is characterized by diffuse inflammation and fibrosis that involves the biliary system.

7. Cardiovascular disease
   a. Severe right-sided congestive heart failure results in an enlarged, edematous, congested liver.
   b. The liver serves as a reservoir for a large amount of venous blood that the failing heart is unable to pump into circulation.
   c. The liver becomes anoxic, resulting in liver cell necrosis and fibrosis.

8. Various metabolic and genetic disorders can cause cirrhosis.

- Complications of cirrhosis include:
  1. Portal hypertension: A persistent increase in pressure within the portal vein develops as a result of increased resistance or obstruction to flow. Blood flow backs into the spleen, causing splenomegaly. Veins in the esophagus, stomach, intestines, abdomen, and rectum become dilated.
  2. Ascites: Free fluid containing almost pure plasma accumulates within the peritoneal cavity. Increased hydrostatic pressure from portal hypertension results in venous congestion of the hepatic capillaries, causing plasma to leak directly from the liver surface and portal vein. Other contributing factors include reduced circulating plasma protein and increased hepatic lymphatic formation.

3. Bleeding esophageal varices: Fragile, thin-walled, distended esophageal veins become irritated and rupture. Varices occur most frequently in the lower esophagus.

4. Coagulation defects: Decreased synthesis of bile fats in the liver prevents the absorption of fat-soluble vitamins. Without vitamin K and clotting factors II, VII, IX, and X, the patient is susceptible to bleeding and easy bruising.

5. Jaundice is caused by one of two mechanisms:
   a. In hepatocellular jaundice, the liver is unable to effectively excrete bilirubin.
   b. In intrahepatic obstruction, edema, fibrosis, or scarring of the hepatic bile duct channels and bile ducts interferes with normal bile and bilirubin excretion.

6. Portal systemic encephalopathy (also known as hepatic encephalopathy and hepatic coma): End-stage hepatic failure and cirrhosis is manifested by neurologic symptoms and characterized by altered level of consciousness, impaired thinking processes, and neuromuscular disturbances, e.g., "liver flap".

7. Hepatorenal syndrome: Progressive, oliguric kidney failure is associated with hepatic failure, resulting in functional impairment of kidneys with normal anatomic and morphologic features. It is manifested by a sudden decrease in urinary flow and elevated serum urea nitrogen and creatinine levels, with abnormally decreased urine sodium excretion and increased urine osmolarity.

8. Spontaneous bacterial peritonitis manifestations include fever, chills, and abdominal pain and tenderness.

PATIENT-CENTERED COLLABORATIVE CARE

Assessment
- Record patient information:
  1. Age, sex, and race
  2. Employment history, including working conditions exposing the patient to harmful chemical toxins
  3. History of individual and family alcoholism
  4. Previous medical conditions, including jaundice, acute viral hepatitis, biliary tract disease, viral infections, blood transfusions, autoimmune disorders, and history of heart disease or respiratory disorders
  5. Sexual history
  6. History of or present substance use
  7. Family history of liver disease
- Assess for:
  1. Generalized weakness, fatigue

2. Weight changes (loss or gain)
3. GI symptoms, including loss of appetite, early morning nausea and vomiting, dyspepsia, flatulence, and changes in bowel habits
4. Abdominal pain or tenderness
5. Jaundice of the skin and sclera
6. Dry skin, rashes, pruritus
7. Petechiae or ecchymosis
8. Palmar erythema
9. Spider angiomas on the nose, cheeks, upper thorax, and shoulders
10. Hepatomegaly palpated in the right upper quadrant
11. Ascites revealed by bulging flanks and dullness on percussion of the abdomen
12. Protruding umbilicus
13. Dilated abdominal veins (caput medusae)
14. Presence of blood in vomitus or nasogastric (NG) drainage
15. Fetor hepaticus: the fruity, musty breath odor of chronic liver disease
16. Amenorrhea in women
17. Testicular atrophy, gynecomastia, and impotence in men
18. Changes in mentation and personality
19. Asterixis (liver flap), a coarse tremor characterized by rapid, nonrhythmic extension and flexions in the wrist and fingers
20. Elevated serum liver enzyme and serum bilirubin levels
21. Decreased total serum protein and albumin levels
22. Elevated serum globulin level
23. Altered coagulation factors; prolonged bleeding times
24. Elevated serum ammonia level
25. Enlarged liver

Planning and Implementation

❖**NDx:** Excess Fluid Volume, Risk for Imbalanced Fluid Volume

Nonsurgical Management

- Provide diet therapy:
  1. Provide a low-sodium diet initially, restricting sodium to 500 mg to 2 g/day.
  2. Suggest alternatives to salt, such as lemon, vinegar, parsley, oregano, and pepper.
  3. Collaborate with the dietitian to explain purpose of diet and meal planning; suggest elimination of table salt, salty foods, canned and frozen vegetables, and salted butter and margarine.

4. Restrict fluid intake to 1000 to 1500 mL/day if the serum sodium level falls.
5. Supplement vitamin intake with thiamine, folate, and multivitamin preparations.

- Provide drug therapy:
    1. Give diuretics to reduce intravascular fluid and to prevent cardiac and respiratory impairment.
    2. Monitor intake and output carefully.
    3. Weigh the patient daily.
    4. Measure abdominal girth daily.
    5. Monitor serum electrolytes.
    6. Administer low-sodium antacids.
- Paracentesis may be indicated if dietary restrictions and drug administration fail to control ascites.
    1. Explain the procedure and verify informed consent obtained.
    2. Obtain vital signs and weight, and check allergies.
    3. Assist the patient to an upright position at the side of the bed.
    4. Monitor vital signs every 15 minutes during the procedure; rapid, drastic removal of ascitic fluid leads to decreased abdominal pressure, which may contribute to vasodilation and shock.
    5. Measure and record drainage; send samples to laboratory if ordered.
    6. Position the patient in a semi-Fowler position in bed, and maintain bedrest until vital signs are stable.
- Provide comfort measures:
    1. Elevate the head of the bed to minimize shortness of breath.
    2. Encourage the patient to sit up in a chair with his or her feet elevated.

Surgical Management

- A peritoneovenous shunt may be placed for severe ascites. Ascites are drained through a one-way valve into a silicone rubber tube that terminates in the superior vena cava.
- Preoperative care is aimed at optimizing the patient's physical state.
- Provide preoperative care by treating underlying medical conditions:
    1. Treat abnormal coagulation with fresh-frozen plasma or vitamin K.
    2. Correct electrolyte imbalances.
    3. Ensure that packed RBCs are available for surgery.
    4. Provide routine preoperative care.

- Provide postoperative care:
  1. Provide routine postoperative care.
  2. Auscultate breath sounds for the presence of crackles, indicating excessive lung fluid.
  3. Assess for excess fluid volume and hemodilution.
  4. Administer diuretics for volume excess.
  5. Monitor coagulation study results.
  6. Perform daily abdominal girth measurements.
  7. Record accurate fluid intake and output daily.
  8. Weigh the patient daily.

❖**Collaborative Problem:** Potential for Esophageal or Gastric Hemorrhage

- Portal hypertension causes bulging and weakening of venules and veins along the esophagus and antrum of the stomach.
- Esophageal bleeding is controlled by:
  1. Gastric intubation to lavage the stomach until the fluid returned is clear
  2. Esophagogastric balloon tamponade to compress bleeding vessels with a tube called a tamponade tube
     a. The tube is inserted through the nose and into the stomach. The large esophageal balloon compresses the esophagus; a smaller gastric balloon helps anchor the tube and exerts pressure against bleeding varices at the distal esophagus and the cardia of the stomach; a third limen terminates in the stomach and is connected to suction, allowing the aspiration of gastric contents and blood.
     b. Check balloons for integrity and leaks; label each lumen to prevent errors in adding or removing pressure and volume.
     c. Keep tube taped and secure.
     d. Keep an extra tube and scissors at the bedside.
     e. Monitor the patient for respiratory distress caused by obstruction from the esophageal balloon or aspiration; if distress occurs, cut both balloon ports to allow for rapid balloon deflation and tube removal.
  3. Administering blood products (RBCs and fresh-frozen plasma) and IV fluids
  4. Giving vasopressin intra-arterially or IV to lower pressures in the portal venous system to decrease bleeding
  5. Injection sclerotherapy, which may be performed during endoscopy to sclerose bleeding esophageal varices
     a. Monitor the patient's vital signs and assess for chest pain.
     b. Administer pain drug and report severe pain to the physician.

C

    c. Assess lung sounds to determine presence of pneumonia or pleural effusion.
6. Endoscopic band ligation procedure, which uses bands to ligate the bleeding varices
7. Transjugular intrahepatic portal-systemic shunt, a nonsurgical procedure whereby the physician implants a shunt, passed through a catheter, between the portal vein and the hepatic vein to reduce portal venous pressure and therefore control the bleeding

> **Clinical Landmine** ◆ Avoid placing or manipulating the nasogastric or orogastric tube in a patient who is at high risk for or diagnosed with esophageal varices because tube movement can injure a dilated vessel, causing it to rupture and bleed.

Surgical Management
- Surgical management of portal hypertension and esophageal varices is a last resort intervention associated with high mortality from coagulation abnormalities, infection, poor tolerance to anesthesia, and ascites.

❖**Collaborative Problem:** Potential for Portal-Systemic Encephalopathy (PSE)

Nonsurgical Management
- Provide diet therapy:
  1. Patient has increased nutritional requirements: high-carbohydrate, moderate-fat, and high-protein foods.
  2. Patients with PSE usually have protein intake limited in the diet to reduce excess protein breakdown by intestinal bacteria leading to ammonia formation.
  3. Patients with cirrhosis who have GI bleeding are given nothing orally (NPO), and a nasogastric (NG) tube may be inserted. Insertion of a nasogastric (NG) tube should be performed by an experienced provider who can intervene if esophageal varices are damaged and leak or bleed with passage of the polyvinyl tube.
  4. Total parenteral nutrition may be needed if NPO status persists more than 3 days.
- Provide drug therapy:
  1. Administer lactulose to promote excretion of fecal ammonia.
     a. When giving lactulose orally, dilute it with fruit juice to help the patient tolerate the sweet taste.
     b. The desired effect of lactulose is two to five soft stools per day; watery diarrheal stools may signify excessive lactulose administration.

2. Neomycin sulfate acts as an intestinal antiseptic to destroy normal flora in the bowel, diminishing protein breakdown, and decreasing ammonia production.

3. Metronidazole (Flagyl, Novonidazol) is a broad-spectrum antibiotic with similar action to neomycin but has less potential for kidney toxicity.

4. Administer stool softeners, as ordered, to prevent constipation in long-term therapy.

5. Be aware of reduced metabolism of many drugs, especially opioids, sedatives, and other central nervous system (CNS) agents.

Community-Based Care

- Health teaching is individualized for the patient, depending on the cause of the disease.
- Identify if the patient needs a family member or friend to help with drugs, a home health care nurse or aide.
- Teach the patient and family to:
  1. Follow the prescribed diet.
  2. Restrict sodium intake if ascites occur.
  3. Restrict protein intake if susceptible to encephalopathy.
  4. Take diuretics as prescribed, report symptoms of hypokalemia, and consume foods high in potassium.
  5. Take H_2-receptor antagonist agent or proton pump inhibitor for GI bleeding.
  6. Avoid all nonprescription drugs.
  7. Avoid alcohol (refer to Alcoholics Anonymous if patient is an alcoholic).
  8. Recognize signs and symptoms of PSE.
  9. Notify their health care provider immediately in case of GI bleeding or PSE.
  10. Keep follow-up visits with the physicians.

COLITIS, ULCERATIVE

OVERVIEW

- Ulcerative colitis is a chronic inflammatory process affecting the mucosal lining of the colon or rectum. It can affect absorption of vital nutrients.
- Classified as an inflammatory bowel disease, ulcerative colitis is characterized by diffuse inflammation of the intestinal mucosa, resulting in loss of surface epithelium, causing ulceration and abscess formation.
- Ulcerative colitis typically begins in the rectum and proceeds in a uniform, continuous manner proximally toward the cecum.
  1. Epithelial cell damage and loss, areas of ulceration, redness, and bleeding occur in the acute stage.

2. Chronic changes in the colon lead to fibrosis and retraction of the bowel resulting in muscle hypertrophy, deposits of fat and fibrous tissue, and a narrower and shorter colon.
- Complications of the disease include intestinal perforation with peritonitis and fistula formation, toxic megacolon, hemorrhage, increased risk for colon cancer, abscess formation, bowel obstruction, malabsorption, and extraintestinal clinical manifestations.

PATIENT-CENTERED COLLABORATIVE CARE

Assessment
- Record patient information:
  1. Family history of inflammatory bowel disease
  2. Previous and current therapy for illnesses
  3. Diet history, including usual patterns and intolerances of milk products and greasy, fried, or spicy foods
  4. History of weight loss
  5. Presence of abdominal pain, cramping, urgency, and diarrhea
  6. Bowel elimination patterns; color, consistency, and character of stools and the presence or absence of blood
  7. Relationship between the occurrence of diarrhea and the timing of meals, pain, emotional distress, and activity
  8. Extraintestinal symptoms such as arthritis, mouth sores, vision problems, and skin disorders
- Assess for:
  1. Abdominal cramping, pain, and distention
  2. Bloody diarrhea, tenesmus (uncontrollable straining)
  3. Low-grade fever, tachycardia
  4. Patient's understanding of the disease process
  5. Psychosocial impact of the disease
     a. Relationship of life events to disease exacerbations
     b. Stress factors that produce symptoms
     c. Family and social support systems
     d. Concerns regarding the possible genetic basis and associated cancer risks of the disease
  6. Abnormal laboratory values: hematocrit, hemoglobin, WBC count, erythrocyte sedimentation rate, electrolytes

Planning and Implementation
❖**NDx:** Diarrhea

Nonsurgical Management
- Management of ulcerative colitis is aimed at relieving the symptoms and reducing intestinal motility, decreasing inflammation, and promoting intestinal healing.
- At the onset of treatment, activity is restricted to promote comfort and intestinal healing.

- Diarrhea management
  1. Record the color, volume, frequency, and consistency of stools.
  2. Monitor the skin in the perianal area for irritation and ulceration resulting from loose, frequent stools.
  3. Stool cultures may be ordered.
- Drug therapy
  1. Salicylate compounds may be prescribed.
     a. Sulfasalazine (Azulfidine, PMS-Sulfasalazine) is used to prevent recurrence and to treat acute exacerbations; the drug should be taken after meals with a full glass of water.
     b. Oral mesalamine (Asacol, Pentasa, Salofalk) is used for its anti-inflammatory effect.
     c. Olsalazine (Dipentum) is used for maintenance therapy.
  2. Corticosteroids may be prescribed during acute exacerbations.
  3. Immunosuppressants in combination with steroids may be given; observe for side effects such as thrombocytopenia, leukopenia, anemia, kidney failure, infection, headache, GI ulceration, stomatitis, and hepatotoxicity.
  4. Antidiarrheal drugs are given to provide symptomatic management of diarrhea; they are given cautiously because they can precipitate colonic dilation and toxic megacolon.
  5. Infliximab (Remicade) may be given for refractory disease or for severe complications, such as toxic megacolon.
- Diet therapy may include:
  1. NPO status for the patient with severe symptoms
  2. Total parenteral nutrition (TPN) while NPO
  3. Elemental formulas, which are absorbed in the upper bowel, thereby minimizing bowel stimulation
  4. Low-fiber diet; teach patient to avoid foods such as whole-wheat grains, nuts, and fresh fruits or vegetables
  5. Avoidance of caffeinated beverages, pepper, and alcohol
- Encourage the patient to avoid smoking.
- Ensure that the patient has easy access to the bedside commode or bathroom.
- Complementary and alternative therapies used as a supplement to traditional therapies may include herbs such as flaxseed, selenium, vitamin C, biofeedback, yoga, acupuncture, and Ayurveda (combination of diet, herbs, breathing exercises).

Surgical Management
- The need for surgery is based on the patient's response to medical interventions.

- Surgical procedures include
  1. Total proctocolectomy with permanent ileostomy: The colon, rectum, and anus are removed and the anus closed. The end of the terminal ileum forms the stoma, which is located in the right lower quadrant. Postoperatively, the nurse provides skin and ostomy care.
     a. Oral or parenteral antibiotics may be given preoperatively as a bowel antiseptic.
     b. Usually, the patient wears an ostomy pouch at all times.
     c. Initial output from the ileostomy is a loose, dark green liquid; over time, the volume decreases, becomes thicker, and turns yellow-green or yellow-brown.
     d. Any foul or unpleasant odor may be a symptom of some underlying problem (blockage or infection).
  2. Total colectomy with a continent ileostomy (Kock ileostomy) or ileal reservoir: An intra-abdominal pouch or reservoir is constructed from the terminal ileum where stool can be stored until the pouch is drained by the nurse or patient. The pouch is connected to the stoma with a nipple-like valve constructed from an intussuscepted portion of the ileum; the stoma is flush with the skin.
     a. Immediately postoperatively, a Foley catheter is placed in the pouch and connected to low intermittent suction and irrigated, as ordered.
     b. Monitor the character and quality of drainage.
     c. Teach the patient to drain the stoma. When the pouch needs to be emptied, the patient experiences a sense of fullness.
  3. Total colectomy with ileoanal anastomosis (two stages): In the first stage, the surgeon excises the rectal mucosa, performs an abdominal colectomy, constructs the reservoir or pouch to the anal canal, and creates a temporary loop ileostomy. After 3 to 4 months, the loop ileostomy is closed.
  4. Creation of an ileoanal reservoir, also known as a J-pouch: The colon is removed, and the ileum is sutured into the rectal stump to form a reservoir.
  5. If the procedure involves an ostomy, an enterostomal therapist is consulted for recommendations on the location.
  6. Specific nursing care interventions are determined by the procedure performed, including ostomy or perineal wound care.

❖**NDx:** Chronic Pain
- Pain management includes:
  1. Assessing the patient for changes in complaints and responses to pain that may indicate disease complications, such as

increased inflammation, obstruction, hemorrhage, or peritonitis

2. Assessing for pain, including its character, pattern of occurrence (such as before or after meals, during the night, or before or after bowel movements), and duration
3. Assisting the patient to reduce or eliminate factors that can precipitate or increase the pain
4. Using antidiarrheal drugs with caution to control diarrhea; toxic megacolon can develop
5. Giving anticholinergic drugs, if prescribed, before meals to provide relief from the pain and cramping that may occur with diarrhea
6. Referring to a dietitian for diet teaching and meal planning
7. Taking measures to relieve irritated skin caused by frequent contact with diarrheal stool
8. Assisting the patient to use other pain relief measures such as biofeedback and music therapy

❖**Collaborative Problem:** Potential for Gastrointestinal (GI) Bleeding

- Monitor the patient for signs and symptoms of internal bleeding.
- Check all stools for blood, using gross and occult examinations.
- Monitor hemoglobin, hematocrit, and electrolyte levels.
- Observe for fever, tachycardia, fluid volume depletion, severe abdominal pain, and change in mental status (especially in older adults).
- Notify the health care provider immediately of GI bleeding, because surgical interventions may be necessary.

> 🔲 Critical Rescue ◆ Monitoring intake and output, especially in a high-output ostomy, can prevent severe hypovolemia and related complications.

Community-Based Care

- Health teaching includes:
  1. Providing information on the nature of the disease, including acute episodes, remissions, and symptom management
  2. Teaching dietary measures to reduce bloating and cramping
  3. Providing information on drug actions and doses
  4. Teaching the patient and family members symptoms that should be reported immediately to the health care provider
  5. Teaching the patient to include adequate amounts of salt and water in their diet because the ileostomy promotes the loss of these elements

6. Teaching the necessity for using caution in situations that promote profuse sweating or fluid loss, such as:
   a. During strenuous physical activities
   b. In high environmental temperature
   c. During episodes of diarrhea or vomiting
7. Providing additional information for the patient with an ostomy regarding:
   a. Ostomy care
   b. Pouch care
   c. Skin care
   d. Special issues related to drugs (e.g., to avoid taking enteric-coated drugs and capsule drugs); the patient should inform health care providers and the pharmacist that he or she has an ostomy.
   e. Symptoms to watch for, such as increased or no drainage; stomal swelling; color of stoma
   f. Activity limitations, including avoidance of heavy lifting
- Refer the patient to home heath care ostomy outpatient clinics if needed.
- Refer the patient to support groups such as the United Ostomy Association and the Crohn's and Colitis Foundation of America.

COMPARTMENT SYNDROME

OVERVIEW

- Compartments are areas in the body where muscles, blood vessels, and nerves are contained within fascia, especially in extremities.
- Fascia is an inelastic tissue that surrounds groups of muscles, blood vessels, and nerves in the body.
- Acute compartment syndrome (ACS) is a serious condition in which increased pressure from tissue swelling as a result of blood or fluid collection within one or more compartments causes massive compromise of circulation to the area.
- It is usually a complication of musculoskeletal trauma in the lower leg and forearm, but it can be seen with severe burns, extensive insect bites, or massive infiltration of IV fluids.
- Pressure to the compartment can also occur from an external source, such as tight, bulky dressings and casts.
- If the condition is not treated, cyanosis, tingling, numbness, pain, paresis, and permanent tissue damage can occur.
- Complications of ACS can include infection, persistent motor weakness in the affected extremity, contracture, and myoglobinuric renal failure.
- In extreme cases, amputation becomes necessary.

PATIENT-CENTERED COLLABORATIVE CARE

- Nursing care includes:
  1. Identifying patients who may be at risk
  2. Monitoring for early signs of ACS, by assessing for the "six Ps", which include:
     a. Pain
     b. Pressure
     c. Paralysis
     d. Paresthesia
     e. Pallor
     f. Pulselessness
  3. Invasive monitoring of compartment pressure in patients at especially high risk for ACS using a handheld device with a digital display
  4. When external conditions are causing the syndrome, implementing interventions to relieve the pressure
     a. Loosening tight bulky dressings
     b. Following agency protocol about cutting a tight cast

> 🔲 Critical Rescue ◆ When manifestations indicate compartment syndrome, notify the surgeon immediately, because irreversible damage can occur within a few hours.

- Surgical intervention is a fasciotomy (opening in the fascia) made by incising through the skin and subcutaneous tissues into the fascia of the affected compartment to relieve the pressure and restore circulation to the affected area.
- After fasciotomy, the open wound is packed and dressed on a regular basis until secondary closure occurs.
- Débridement and skin grafting may be required.

CORNEAL ABRASION, ULCERATION, AND INFECTION

OVERVIEW

- A *corneal abrasion* is a painful scrape or scratch of the cornea that disrupts the integrity of this structure, most commonly caused by the presence of a small foreign body, trauma, and contact lens use.
- The abrasion provides a portal of entry for organisms leading to *corneal infection,* which can lead to corneal ulceration
- *Corneal ulceration* is a deeper disruption of the corneal epithelium, often occurring with bacterial, fungal, or viral infection. *This problem is an emergency and can lead to permanently impaired vision.*

PATIENT-CENTERED COLLABORATIVE CARE

Assessment

- Assess for these problems in the affected eye:
  1. Severe pain
  2. Reduced vision
  3. Photophobia
  4. Eye secretions
  5. Cloudy or purulent fluid on eyelids or eyelashes
  6. Hazy, cloudy cornea with a patchy area of ulceration
  7. Damaged areas appear green with fluorescein stain

Interventions

- Drug therapy delivered as eyedrops
  1. Antibiotics, antifungals, and antivirals are prescribed to reduce or eliminate the organisms. Usually, a broad-spectrum antibiotic is prescribed first, and it may be changed when culture results are known.
  2. Steroids may be used with antibiotics to reduce the inflammatory response in the eye.
  3. Usually the anti-infective therapy involves instilling eyedrops *every hour* for the first 24 hours.
  4. Teach the patient how to apply the eyedrops correctly.
  5. Teach the patient to not use the drug in the unaffected eye.
  6. Teach the patient to wash hands after touching the affected eye and before touching or doing anything to the healthy eye.
  7. If both eyes are infected, separate bottles of drugs are needed for each eye and are clearly labeled *right eye* and *left eye*.
  8. Teach the patient to completely care for one eye, then wash the hands, and using the drugs for the remaining eye, care for that eye.
  9. Teach the patient to not wear contact lenses during the entire time that these drugs are being used.

> 🛟 Critical Rescue ♦ Stress the importance of applying the drug as often as prescribed, even at night. Stopping the infection at this stage can save the patient's vision in the infected eye.

CORNEAL OPACITIES, KERATOCONUS, AND CORNEAL TRANSPLANTATION

OVERVIEW

- The cornea can permanently lose it shape, become scarred or cloudy, or become thinner, reducing refraction and interfering with useful vision.

- Keratoconus is the degeneration of the corneal tissue resulting in abnormal corneal shape that can occur with trauma or may occur as part of an inherited disorder.

PATIENT-CENTERED COLLABORATIVE CARE

- Management for a permanent corneal disorder that obscures vision is a *keratoplasty* (corneal transplant), the surgical removal of diseased corneal tissue and replacement with tissue from a human donor cornea.
- Provide preoperative care:
  1. Assess the patient's knowledge of the surgery and of expected care before and after surgery.
  2. Examine the eyes for signs of infection and report any redness, drainage, or edema to the ophthalmologist.
  3. Instill antibiotic drops into the eye.
  4. Obtain IV access.
  5. Inform the patient that local anesthesia usually is used.
- Provide postoperative care:
  1. The eye is covered with a pressure patch and a protective shield. This dressing is left in place until the next day, when the patient returns to the surgeon.
  2. Notify the ophthalmologist of changes in vital signs or of drainage on the dressing.
  3. Perform patient and family teaching about:
     a. Applying an eye patch
     b. Wearing an eye shield at night and whenever around small children or pets
     c. Instilling eyedrops
     d. Examining the eye daily for the presence of infection or graft rejection
     e. Reporting immediately to the surgeon the presence of purulent discharge, a continuous leak of clear fluid from around the graft site (not tears), or excessive bleeding
     f. Reporting manifestations of graft rejection to the surgeon that include redness starting in the donor cornea near the graft edge and moving toward the center, reduced vision, and corneal clouding
     g. Avoiding jogging, running, dancing, and any other activity that promotes rapid or jerky head motions for several weeks after surgery
     h. Avoiding activities that can increase intraocular pressure, including:
        (1) Bending from the waist
        (2) Lifting objects weighing more than 10 lbs
        (3) Sneezing, coughing

(4) Blowing the nose
(5) Straining to have a bowel movement
(6) Vomiting
(7) Having sexual intercourse
(8) Keeping the head in a dependent position
(9) Wearing tight shirt collars

CORONARY ARTERY DISEASE
OVERVIEW

- Coronary artery disease (CAD) is a broad term that includes chronic angina and acute coronary syndromes.
- CAD affects the arteries that provide blood, oxygen, and nutrients to the myocardium.
- CAD causes ischemia when insufficient oxygen is supplied to meet the requirements of the myocardium. Infarction (necrosis or cell death) occurs when severe ischemia is prolonged, resulting in irreversible damage to tissue.
- The most common cause of CAD is atherosclerosis, which is characterized by a lesion that narrows the vessel lumen or obstructs blood flow (see Atherosclerosis).
- The most common symptom of CAD is angina. Angina, also known as angina pectoris, is a sign of myocardial ischemia, a temporary imbalance between the ability of the coronary arteries to supply oxygen and the demand of the myocardium for it.
  1. Stable angina is chest discomfort that occurs with exertion in a pattern that is familiar to the patient and that has not increased in frequency, duration, or intensity of symptoms during the past several months; it is usually associated with a stable atherosclerotic plaque.
  2. Unstable angina is chest pain or discomfort that is new or newly occurs at rest or with minimal exertion or an increase in the number of episodes ("attacks") or an increase in the quality or intensity of pain.

Women's Health Considerations

- Many women experience atypical angina, described as a choking sensation that occurs with exertion, indigestion, pain between the shoulders, or an aching jaw.
- Angina is more likely to be the primary presenting symptom of CAD in women than in men.
- Angina is twice as common as myocardial infarction (MI) in women.
- Women have higher morbidity and mortality rates after MI than men do.

- MI occurs when coronary blood flow is stopped and the myocardial muscle is abruptly and severely deprived of oxygen. Ischemia and necrosis (infarction) of the myocardial tissue result if blood flow is not restored. Generally, an MI is caused by an unstable plaque that initiates the inflammatory cascade and leads to thrombus formation. The clot is the cause of coronary artery blood flow cessation. The patient's response to an MI depends on which coronary arteries were obstructed and which part of the left ventricular wall was damaged: anterior, lateral, septal, inferior, or posterior.
  1. Patients with obstruction of the left anterior descending artery have anterior or septal MIs, or both; patients with anterior MIs are most likely to experience left ventricular heart failure and ventricular dysrhythmias.
  2. Patients with obstruction of the circumflex artery may experience a posterior wall or a lateral wall MI and sinus dysrhythmias.
  3. Patients with obstruction of the right coronary artery often have inferior MIs; these patients are likely to experience bradydysrhythmias or atrioventricular conduction defects, especially transient second-degree heart block.
- Nonmodifiable risk factors that contribute to the onset and progression of CAD include age, gender, family history, and ethnic background.
- Modifiable risk factors include elevated serum cholesterol levels, cigarette smoking, hypertension, impaired glucose tolerance, obesity, physical inactivity, and stress.

PATIENT-CENTERED COLLABORATIVE CARE

Assessment

- Collection of historical data is delayed until interventions for pain, vital sign instability, and dysrhythmias are initiated and the discomfort resolves.
- Record the patient's family history and risk factors.
- Assess for clinical manifestations of angina and MI:
  1. Quality, onset, duration, and alleviating and aggravating factors related to chest pain
  2. Nausea and vomiting
  3. Diaphoresis
  4. Dizziness
  5. Weakness
  6. Palpitations
  7. Shortness of breath
  8. Diminished or absent pulses

C

9. Dysrhythmias: tachycardia, premature beats, irregular rhythm
10. Abnormal blood pressure
11. S_3 gallop or S_4 heart sound
12. Increased respiratory rate
13. Crackles or wheezes (if concurrent heart failure occurs)
14. Elevated temperature
15. Denial (early reaction to chest discomfort)
16. Fear and anxiety
17. Elevated serum cardiac enzyme levels
    a. Myoglobin
    b. Troponin
    c. Creatine kinase (CK-MB isoenzyme)
18. Electrocardiography (ECG) changes
    a. In angina, ST depression or elevation or T-wave inversion that manifests on the ECG
    b. In MI, ST elevation, T-wave inversion, and abnormal Q wave in two or more contiguous leads
19. Results of exercise tolerance test (stress test), thallium scan, contrast-enhanced magnetic resonance (CMR), multigated acquisition (MUGA) scan, and cardiac catheterization, if performed

Considerations for Older Adults

- About 25% of older adults and patients with diabetes who experience MI complain primarily of shortness of breath; chest discomfort may be mild or absent.
- Many older patients do not typically experience chest discomfort but have disorientation or confusion as the primary manifestation.

Women's Health Considerations

- Chest discomfort is often not the initial symptom.
- Women may initially have atypical symptoms such as heart "flutters" without pain, shortness of breath, fatigue, and depression.
- As the MI progresses, women usually report atypical chest discomfort: arm and shoulder pain, back pain, or an aching jaw, neck, or tooth.

Cultural Awareness

- Modifiable risk factors vary for people of different racial and ethnic backgrounds. Some of the differences may be explained by lack of access to health care or genetic factors. American

Indians, for example, have limited access to care or language barriers in a predominantly English-speaking, Euro-American health care system. Nutritional preferences may explain some of the differences. For instance, high cholesterol is more common in African American and Hispanic populations. Diets higher in fat and cholesterol are often less expensive and may be a factor in explaining differences, and obesity is more common in these groups. Genetic factors may also contribute to the differences among ethnic groups.

> ▨ Clinical Landmine ◆ Do not delay in reporting the patient's chest pain. Prompt diagnostic testing and treatment can lead to reperfusion of the myocardium and optimal outcomes.

Planning and Implementation
- For the patient with CAD, planning and intervention focus on restoring perfusion through the coronary arteries.

❖**NDx:** Acute Pain
- Management of acute pain related to an imbalance between myocardial oxygen supply and demand drug therapy includes:
  1. Supplemental oxygen to provide additional oxygen to the ischemic myocardium; a nasal canula at 2 to 4 L is usually sufficient.
  2. Nitroglycerin (sublingually), used for angina, to increase collateral blood flow, redistributing blood flow toward the subendocardium; if three repeated doses given 5 minutes apart do not relieve discomfort, the patient may be experiencing an MI and needs immediate evaluation in a heart center.
  3. Nitroglycerin (IV), administered in a specialized unit to carefully monitor the patient's blood pressure; hypotension is a serious side effect of this drug.
  4. Morphine sulfate (IV) for patients unresponsive to nitroglycerin
  5. Aspirin (325 mg, chewed), which may be administered immediately to reduce platelet aggregation
  6. Metoprolol, a beta-blocker to reduce sympathetic stimulation of the compromised myocardium and prevent life-threatening dysrhythmias
  7. Initiating heparin IV continuously to prevent clot extension in the coronary arteries until the patient can be transported to the cardiac catheterization laboratory for definitive treatment

- Other interventions include:
  1. Obtaining a 12-lead ECG to determine the location of compromised coronary artery blood flow
  2. Placing the patient in a semi-Fowler position for comfort
  3. Maintaining a quiet, calm environment to the extent possible
  4. Providing acetaminophen (Tylenol, Exdol) for headaches caused by nitroglycerin

> 🦅 Clinical Landmine ♦ Heparin is one of 10 medications most commonly associated with adverse events in the hospital setting. If you are unsure about calculations or dosage, ask the pharmacist for verification.

❖**NDx:** Ineffective Tissue Perfusion (Cardiopulmonary) Related to Interruption of Arterial Blood Flow

Definitive treatment is percutaneous intervention (PCI), which typically involves placement of a stent to open the clotted coronary artery.

- If an interventional radiologist is not available to place a stent, then thrombolytic agents are given IV or by intracoronary route during cardiac catheterization to dissolve thrombi in the coronary arteries and to restore myocardial blood flow. Examples include tissue plasminogen activator (tPA; Alteplase, Activase), anisoylated plasminogen-streptokinase activator complex (APSAC), reteplase (Retavase), and tenecteplase (TNKase).
- Fibrinolytic agents are most effective when used within 6 hours of a coronary event.
- Interventions after administration of fibrinolytic agents include monitoring the patient for signs of obvious and occult bleeding and reporting indications of bleeding immediately to the physician (most common in women who receive thrombolytic therapy).
  1. Monitor the patient for indications of cerebrovascular bleeding.
  2. Observe all IV sites for bleeding and patency.
  3. Monitor clotting studies.
  4. Observe for signs of internal bleeding (watching hematocrit and hemoglobin).
  5. Test stool, urine, and emesis for occult blood.
- Glycoprotein (GP) IIb/IIIa inhibitors prevent fibrin from attaching to activated platelets at the site of a thrombus after PCI or fibrinolysis.
  1. GP IIb/IIIa is used particularly in unstable angina and non–Q-wave MI and before and during percutaneous coronary

intervention (PCI) to ensure patency of the newly opened artery.

2. If GP IIb/IIIa inhibitors are used with fibrinolytic agents, then the dose of the thrombolytic should be reduced.

- Monitor for indications of coronary artery reperfusion, including abrupt cessation of chest pain or discomfort, sudden onset of ventricular dysrhythmias, and resolution of ST segment depression, and reduction of markers of myocardial damage over a period of 12 hours.
- IV heparin and aspirin may be given after thrombolytic therapy to reduce additional clot formation; monitor activated partial thromboplastin time (aPTT).

❖**NDx:** Activity Intolerance Related to Fatigue Caused by Imbalance Between Oxygen Supply and Demand

- Promote rest and provide assistance in ADLs to minimize oxygen demands during episodes of chest pain.
- Progress patient mobility gradually, starting with having the patient dangle the legs at the side of the bed and proceeding to ambulation.
- Assess the patient's vital signs and level of fatigue with each higher level of activity.
- Notify the health care provider if there are indications of activity intolerance: decreases greater than 20 mm Hg in the systolic blood pressure, changes of 20 beats/min in the pulse rate, or complaints of dyspnea, chest pain, or dizziness.
- Consider initiating cardiac rehabilitation if the patient has not participated previously. Cardiac rehabilitation is divided into three phases:
  1. Phase 1 begins with acute illness and ends with discharge from the hospital.
  2. Phase 2 begins after discharge and continues through convalescence at home.
  3. Phase 3 involves long-term conditioning.

❖**NDx:** Ineffective Coping Related to Effects of Acute Illness and Major Changes in Lifestyle

- Direct interventions toward assisting the patient to take personal actions to manage lifestyle stressors related to CAD:
  1. Assess the patient's understanding of the disease process.
  2. Assess the patient's coping mechanisms (commonly denial, anger, and depression) and level of anxiety.
  3. Provide simple, repeated explanations of therapies, expectations, and surroundings.
  4. Help the patient identify the information that is most important to obtain.

5. Denial that results in a patient's "acting out" and refusing to follow treatment regimen can be harmful.
   a. Remain calm and avoid confronting the patient.
   b. Clearly indicate when a behavior is not acceptable and is potentially harmful.
6. Anger may be the result of a patient's attempt to regain control of his or her life.
   a. Encourage patient to verbalize frustrations.
   b. Provide opportunities for decision making and control.
7. Depression may be a patient's response to grief.
   a. Listen to the patient, and do not offer false or general reassurances.
   b. Acknowledge depression, but expect the patient to perform ADLs and other activities within restrictions.

- For the patient who experiences an MI, planning and interventions focus on identifying and treating complications from the damage to the heart. After an MI, the following drugs are often prescribed:
  1. Aspirin daily to prevent platelet aggregation at the site of obstruction
  2. Beta-adrenergic agents to prevent pathologic cardiac remodeling and prevent dysrhythmias
     a. Monitor heart rate rhythm, and blood pressure.
  3. Angiotensin-converting enzyme (ACE) inhibitor to prevent ventricular remodeling and the development of heart failure
     a. Monitor for decreased urinary output, hypotension, cough, and changes in serum potassium, creatinine, and blood urea nitrogen.
  4. Statin (antilipemic) to reduce serum cholesterol, which contributes to plaque formation, and to provide anti-inflammation
     a. Monitor liver enzymes and serum cholesterol.
  5. Calcium channel blockers for patients with variant angina or for those who are hypertensive and continue to have angina despite therapy with beta blockers

❖**Collaborative Problem:** Potential for Dysrhythmias
- If a dysrhythmia occurs, the following actions are taken:
  1. Identify the dysrhythmia.
  2. Assess the patient's hemodynamic status: blood pressure and peripheral with level of consciousness.
  3. Evaluate the patient for chest discomfort.
- Dysrhythmias are treated when they are causing hemodynamic compromise, are increasing myocardial oxygen requirements,

or are predisposing to lethal ventricular dysrhythmias (see Dysrhythmias).

❖**Collaborative Problem:** Potential for Heart Failure
- Heart failure is a relatively common complication after MI; the most severe form of heart failure, cardiogenic shock, accounts for most in-hospital deaths after MI.

Nonsurgical Management
- Decreased cardiac output related to heart failure is a common complication after MI.
- Assess the patient with left ventricular failure and pulmonary edema by auscultating for crackles and identifying their location within the lungs.
- Assess for:
  1. Decreased peripheral oxygenation
  2. Crackles or adventitious breath sounds
  3. Tachypnea, wheezing, frothy sputum
  4. Change in patient's orientation or mental status
  5. Urine output of less than 30m L/hr
  6. Cold, clammy skin with poor peripheral pulses
  7. Unusual fatigue
  8. Recurrent chest pain
  9. Changes in right atrial pressure, pulmonary artery pressure, systolic and diastolic pressures, pulmonary wedge pressure, systemic vascular resistance, cardiac output, and cardiac index
- Classification of post-MI heart failure follows the New York Heart classification and American College of Cardiology/ American Heart Association Guidelines.
  1. Mild post-MI heart failure often responds well to reduction in preload with IV nitrates and diuretics. Monitor hourly the urine output and vital signs; review serum potassium levels; and assess for signs of heart failure.
  2. Moderate post-MI heart failure may require diuresis and more aggressive medical intervention such as reduction of afterload (IV nitroglycerin or nitroprusside) or enhancement of cardiac contractility (dopamine, dobutamine, or milrinone).
  3. Severe heart failure in cardiogenic shock is manifested by tachycardia, hypotension, blood pressure less than 90 mm Hg systolic or 30 mm Hg less than the patient's baseline, cold and clammy skin with poor peripheral pulses, agitation, pulmonary congestion, and continued chest pain.
- Medical management includes:
  1. IV morphine to decrease pulmonary congestion and relieve pain

2. Oxygen therapy (intubation and mechanical ventilation may be necessary)
3. Information from hemodynamic monitoring, which is used to titrate drug therapy
4. Diuretics, nitroglycerin, or nitroprusside to reduce preload

- Patients who do not respond to drug therapy may require an intra-aortic balloon pump (IABP) or left ventricular assistive device, which is used to improve myocardial perfusion, reduce afterload, and facilitate ventricular emptying.
- Immediate reperfusion may be performed on patients with cardiogenic shock. A left-sided cardiac catheterization is performed. If the patient has a treatable lesion, the surgeon performs a PCI or the patient undergoes a coronary artery bypass graft (CABG).
- The goal of medical management of right-sided heart ventricular failure is to improve right ventricular stroke volume.
  1. Provide IV fluids (as much as 200 mL/hr) to increase right atrial pressure (central venous pressure [CVP]) to 20 mm Hg.
  2. Monitor pulmonary artery wedge pressure (goal is maintaining values of 15 to 20 mm Hg).
  3. Auscultate the lungs to detect early left-sided heart failure.
  4. Monitor cardiac output to ensure that fluid administration has the desired effect.

❖**Collaborative Problem:** Potential for Recurrent Symptoms and Extension of Injury

- Recurrent chest pain despite medical therapy is a major indicator of surgery.

Surgical Management

- Percutaneous coronary interventions (PCI), an invasive but technically nonsurgical technique, is performed to provide symptom reduction for patients with chest discomfort without a significant risk of complications. PCI is performed by introducing a balloon-tipped catheter into the area of the coronary artery occlusion. When the balloon is inflated, it presses the atherosclerotic plaque against the vessel wall to reduce or eliminate the occlusion.
- Techniques used to ensure patency of the vessel are laser angioplasty, stents, and atherectomy devices.
- Nursing interventions include:
  1. Monitoring for potential problems after the procedure, including acute closure of the vessel, bleeding from the insertion site, reaction to the dye used in angiography, hypotension, hyperkalemia, and dysrhythmias

2. Instructing the patient to report the development of chest pain immediately
3. Frequently monitoring pulses, skin color, and warmth of the limb where the catheter was inserted and reporting changes immediately to the physician
4. Maintaining immobilization of the affected limb for at least 6 hours
5. Maintaining pressure dressing
6. Elevating the head of the bed slowly, per hospital protocol
7. Instructing the patient to:
   a. Return to usual activities in 1 to 2 weeks or when instructed by the physician.
   b. Avoid heavy lifting for several weeks.
   c. Apply manual pressure if there is bleeding from the insertion site and notify the physician if the bleeding is extensive or if oozing persists for more than 15 minutes.
   d. Take nitrates, aspirin, beta blockers, ACE inhibitors, and statin, as prescribed.

- Coronary artery bypass graft (CABG) surgery is indicated when other treatments have been unsuccessful. This procedure is performed while the patient is under general anesthesia and undergoing cardiopulmonary bypass. The graft to the saphenous vein or the internal mammary artery bypasses the occluded vessel to restore blood supply to the myocardium.
- Preoperative care includes:
  1. If surgery is performed as an elective procedure, familiarizing the patient and family with the cardiac surgical critical care environment
  2. Teaching the patient how to splint the chest incision, cough and deep breathe, perform arm and leg exercises, what to expect during the postoperative period, and how pain will be managed
- Provide immediate postoperative care in a specialized unit:
  1. Maintain mechanical ventilation for 3 to 6 hours.
  2. Monitor chest tube drainage system.
  3. Monitor pulmonary artery and arterial pressures.
  4. Frequently assess vital signs and cardiac rate and rhythm.
  5. Ensure that pain is appropriately managed.
  6. Treat symptomatic dysrhythmias according to unit protocols or physician's order.
  7. Monitor for complications of open heart surgery, including:
     a. Fluid and electrolyte imbalances
     b. Hypotension
     c. Hypothermia
     d. Hypertension

   e. Bleeding
   f. Cardiac tamponade
   g. Altered cerebral perfusion
- Provide continued postoperative care:
  1. Encourage deep breathing and coughing every 2 hours while splinting incision after extubation.
  2. Assist the patient in slowly resuming activity and ambulation.
  3. Monitor for dysrhythmias, especially atrial fibrillation.
  4. Assess for wound or sternal infection (mediastinitis), such as prolonged fever (more than 4 days), reddened sternum, purulent incisional drainage, and elevated WBC.
  5. Observe for indications of postpericardiotomy syndrome: pericardial and pleural pain, pericarditis, friction rub, elevated temperature and WBC count, and dysrhythmias; problem may be self-limiting or may require treatment for pericarditis.
- Minimally invasive direct coronary arterial bypass (MIDCAB) is indicated for patients with a lesion of the left anterior descending artery. Cardiopulmonary bypass is not required.
  1. Assess the patient for postoperative chest pain and electrocardiographic changes because occlusion of the internal mammary artery graft occurs acutely in 10% of patients.
  2. Encourage the patient to cough and deep breathe (chest tube and thoracotomy incision).
- Transmyocardial laser revascularization, for patients with unstable angina and inoperable CAD with area of reversible myocardial ischemia, involves the creation of 20 to 24 long, narrow channels through the left ventricular muscle to the left ventricle, which eventually allows oxygenated blood to flow.
- Robotic heart surgery allows surgeons to operate endoscopically through 8- to 10-mm long incisions in the chest wall, eliminating tremors that can exist with human hands, increasing the ability to reach inaccessible sites, and improving depth perception and visual acuity.

> ▣ **Critical Rescue** ◆ Monitoring the ECG and using the bedside alarms to notify about changes in ST from baseline can provide an early warning of coronary artery occlusion after any of the radiologic or surgical interventions for CAD. Immediately notify the physician about new-onset dysrhythmias, ST elevation, and other changes in the ECG indicating ischemia, injury, or infarct.

Community-Based Care

- The patient should be assigned to a case manager at the beginning of the hospitalization to provide constant care and assist with the transition to home or subacute care center.
- Most patients are still recovering from their illness or surgery when discharged from the hospital; home health services may be required.
- Teach the patient and family about:
  1. The pathophysiology of angina and MI
  2. Risk factor modification
     a. Smoking cessation
     b. Dietary changes (decreasing fat intake)
     c. Blood pressure control
     d. Blood glucose control
  3. Gradual increase in physical and sexual activity, according to cardiac rehabilitation protocol
  4. Cardiac drugs
  5. Occupational considerations, if any
  6. Complementary and alternative therapies such as progressive relaxation, guided imagery, music therapy, pet therapy
- Teach the patient to seek medical assistance if they experience:
  1. Pulse rate that remains 50 or less while awake
  2. Wheezing or difficulty breathing
  3. Weight gain of 3 pounds in 1 week, or 1 to 2 pounds overnight
  4. Slow, persistent increase in nitroglycerin use
  5. Dizziness, faintness, or shortness of breath with activity
- Patients should call for emergency transportation to the hospital if they experience the following:
  1. Chest discomfort that does not improve after 20 minutes or after taking three nitroglycerin tablets
  2. Extremely severe chest or epigastric discomfort with weakness, nausea, or fainting
  3. Other angina symptoms that are particular to the patient, such as fatigue or nausea
- Other important discharge plans include:
  1. Referring the patient to the American Heart Association for information
  2. Referring the patient for continued cardiac rehabilitation
  3. Referring the patient who has had CABG surgery to Mended Hearts, a nationwide program that provides education and support to patients and their families

CROHN'S DISEASE

OVERVIEW

- Crohn's disease, or regional enteritis, is an idiopathic inflammatory disease that occurs anywhere in the GI tract but most often affects the terminal ileum with patchy lesions that extend through all bowel layers.
- Chronic nonspecific inflammation of the entire intestinal tract occurs, and eventually deep fissures and ulcerations develop and often extend through all bowel layers, predisposing the patient to development of bowel fistulas.
- Chronic pathologic changes include thickening of the bowel wall, resulting in narrowing of the bowel lumen and strictures.
- Complications of Crohn's disease include malabsorption, fistulas, hemorrhage, abscess formation, bowel obstruction, and cancer (usually after the patient has the disease for 15 to 40 years).

PATIENT-CENTERED COLLABORATIVE CARE

Assessment

- Assess for:
  1. Fever, abdominal pain, loose stools
  2. Frequency, consistency, and presence of blood in the stool
  3. Periumbilical pain before and after bowel movements
  4. Weight loss (indicates serious nutritional deficiencies)
  5. Family history of the disease
  6. Distention, masses, or visible peristalsis
  7. Ulcerations or fissures of the perianal area
  8. Bowel sounds diminished or absent in the presence of severe inflammation
  9. High-pitched or rushing sounds over the areas of narrowed bowel loops
  10. Diarrhea with steatorrhea (the stool does not usually contain blood) but is fatty, frothy, and foul smelling
  11. Psychosocial issues related to coping skills and support systems
  12. Results of barium enema and upper GI series that show narrowing, ulcerations, strictures, and fistulas consistent with Crohn's disease
  13. Results of laboratory studies, especially WBC count and electrolytes

Interventions

- The care of the patient with Crohn's disease is similar to care for the patient with ulcerative colitis (see Colitis, Ulcerative).

- Drug therapy includes:
  1. Sulfasalazine, used as an anti-inflammatory
  2. Metronidazole (Flagyl, Novonidazol), used for patients with fistulas
  3. Immunosuppressive therapy, used for patients with refractory disease or fistulas
  4. Infliximab (Remicade), an antitumor necrosis factor, used for active disease and fistulas
- Malnutrition can result in poor fistula and wound healing, loss of lean muscle mass, decreased immune system response, and increased morbidity and mortality.
  1. Monitor tolerance to diet.
  2. Assist the patient to select high-calorie, high-protein, high-vitamin, low-fiber meals.
  3. Offer oral supplements such as Ensure and Vivonex.
  4. Record food intake and accurate calorie count.
  5. Total parenteral nutrition (TPN) may be needed for severe exacerbations while the patient is NPO.
- Electrolyte therapy includes:
  1. Fluid and electrolyte replacement by oral liquids and nutrients, as well as IV fluids
  2. Cautious use of antidiarrheal agents to decrease fluid loss
  3. Strict monitoring of intake and output
- Impaired skin integrity results from fistula formation. The degree of associated problems is related to the location of the fistula, the patient's general health status, and the character and amount of fistula drainage.
  1. In collaboration with the enterostomal therapist, apply a pouch to the fistula to prevent skin irritation and to measure the drainage.
  2. Cover the area around the fistula with skin barriers, such as Stomahesive or DuoDerm, and apply a wound drainage system over the fistula, securing it to the protective barriers.
  3. Clean adjacent skin and keep it dry. The wound drainage should never be allowed to have direct skin contact without prompt cleaning because intestinal fluid enzymes are caustic.
  4. Observe for subtle signs of infection or sepsis such as fever, abdominal pain, or change in mental status.
- Some patients with Crohn's disease require surgery such as a bowel resection and anastomosis with or without a colon resection to improve the quality of life (see Surgical Management under Cancer, Colorectal).
- Stricturoplasty may be performed for bowel strictures.

Community-Based Care
See Community-Based Care under Colitis, Ulcerative.

CYSTIC FIBROSIS

C

OVERVIEW

- Cystic fibrosis (CF) is a genetic disease present from birth that affects many organs and lethally impairs pulmonary function.
- The underlying problem of CF is blocked chloride transport in cell membranes, causing the formation of thick, sticky, mucus.
- This mucus plugs up glands in the lungs, pancreas, liver, salivary glands, and testes, causing atrophy and organ dysfunction.
- Nonpulmonary problems include pancreatic insufficiency with malnutrition and intestinal obstruction, poor growth, male sterility, and cirrhosis of the liver.
- The primary cause of death in the patient with CF is respiratory failure.
- The disorder is most common among white individuals, and about 4% are carriers. It is very rare among African Americans or Asians. Males and females are affected equally.

Genetic Considerations

- CF is an autosomal recessive disorder in which both gene alleles must be mutated for the disease to be expressed. The CF gene is located on chromosome 7 and produces a protein that controls chloride movement across cell membranes.
- There is great variation in the severity of CF; however, life expectancy is always considerably reduced, with an average of 32 years.
- People with one mutated allele are carriers and have few or no symptoms of CF but can pass the abnormal allele on to their children.
- More than 1200 different mutations have been identified. The inheritance of different mutations is responsible for the wide variation in disease severity.

PATIENT-CENTERED COLLABORATIVE CARE

Assessment

- The major diagnostic test is sweat chloride analysis, and additional genetic testing can be performed to determine which specific mutation a person may have.
- Assess for these nonpulmonary manifestations: abdominal distention, gastroesophageal reflux, rectal prolapse, foul-smelling

stools, steatorrhea (excessive fat in stools), small stature, and underweight for height.

- Assess for these common pulmonary manifestations: frequent or chronic respiratory infections, chest congestion, limited exercise tolerance, cough, sputum production, use of accessory muscles, and decreased pulmonary function (especially FVC and FEV_1).

Interventions

Nonsurgical Management

- Nutritional management focuses on weight maintenance, vitamin supplementation, diabetes management, and pancreatic enzyme replacement.
- Pulmonary management is focused on preventive maintenance and management of pulmonary exacerbation.
  1. Preventive or maintenance therapy involves the use of a regimen of chest physiotherapy, positive expiratory pressure, active cycle breathing technique, and an individualized regular exercise program. Drug therapy includes bronchodilators, anti-inflammatory agents, mucolytics, and antibiotics.
  2. Exacerbation therapy is needed when the patient with CF has a change in manifestations from baseline. Management focuses on airway clearance, increased oxygenation, and antibiotic therapy.
     a. Supplemental oxygen
     b. Heliox delivery of 50% oxygen and 50% helium
     c. Airway clearance techniques (ACTs) four times each day
     d. Intensified bronchodilator and mucolytic therapies; steroidal anti-inflammatory agents or IV antibiotics

> 🛡️ Critical Rescue ◆ A serious bacterial infection for patients with CF is *Burkholderia cepacia,* which is spread by casual contact from one CF patient to another. Special infection control measures that limit close contact between persons with CF are needed, which include separating CF patients on hospital units and seeing them in the clinic on different days. Strict procedures approved by the Cystic Fibrosis Foundation should be used when cleaning clinic rooms, pulmonary function laboratories, and respiratory therapy equipment to reduce the risk of contamination.

  3. Teach patients about protecting themselves by avoiding direct contact of bodily fluids such as saliva and sputum. Teach them not to routinely shake hands or kiss people in

social settings. Handwashing is critical because the organism also can be acquired indirectly from contaminated surfaces such as sinks and tissues.

Surgical Management

- The surgical management of the patient with CF involves lung and/or pancreatic transplantation.
- Lung transplant procedures include two lobes or a single lung transplantation, as well as double-lung transplantation. Most often the patient with CF has a bilateral lobe transplant from a cadaver donor or living-related donor.
- Provide preoperative care:
  1. Teach the patient the expected regimen of pulmonary hygiene to be used in the period immediately after surgery.
  2. Assist the patient in a pulmonary muscle strengthening and conditioning regimen.
- Provide postoperative care:
  1. The patient is intubated for at least 48 hours and has chest tubes and arterial lines in place. Much of the care needed is the same as that for any thoracic surgery.
  2. Assess for bleeding, infection, and transplant rejection.
  3. Anti-rejection drug regimens must be started immediately after surgery, which increases the risk for infection. The drugs generally used for routine long-term rejection suppression after organ transplantation are combinations of:
     a. Very specific immunosuppressants (cyclosporine [Sandimmune])
     b. Less specific immunosuppressants (azathioprine [Imuran] or mycophenolate mofetil [CellCept])
     c. One of the corticosteroids (prednisone [Apo-Prednisone ✤, Deltasone ✤] or prednisolone [Delta-Cortef]).

CYSTITIS (URINARY TRACT INFECTION)

OVERVIEW

- Cystitis is an inflammation of the urinary bladder with both infectious and noninfectious causes. Infectious causes are bacteria, viruses, fungi, and parasites. Noninfectious causes are chemical exposure and radiation therapy.
- Interstitial cystitis is a chronic inflammation of the entire lower urinary tract (bladder, urethra, and adjacent pelvic muscles) that is not the result of infection and can lead to pyelonephritis and sepsis.
- Urosepsis is the spread of infection from the urinary tract to the bloodstream.

- Coliform bacteria, especially *Escherichia coli* normally found in the GI tract, account for most cases of bacterial cystitis.
- Other factors that contribute to the development or recurrence of cystitis, or urinary tract infections (UTIs), include:
  1. Structural or functional abnormalities of the urinary tract
  2. Use of indwelling urinary catheters
  3. Sexual intercourse, diaphragm use, and pregnancy in women
  4. Prostate disease

Considerations for Older Adults

- UTIs occur more often in older adults than in younger adults, with women more commonly affected than men.
- Elderly patients are at greater risk than others of having an overwhelming and generalized infection, known as urosepsis.

National Patient Safety Goal

Timely reporting of abnormal CBC results (especially an elevated WBC count), abnormal urinalysis results (especially positive nitrogen and leukoesterase), and positive urine culture reports are essential to initiating and evaluating effective antibiotic treatment.

> **Critical Rescue** ◆ A decrease in mental status or increase in heart rate combined with a decrease in blood pressure can indicate clinical instability or urosepsis requiring immediate intervention.

> **Clinical Landmine** ◆ Avoid use of indwelling urinary catheters for longer than 3 days if possible to reduce nosocomial UTIs.

PATIENT CENTERED COLLABORATIVE CARE

Assessment

- Record patient information:
  1. History of UTIs
  2. History of renal or urologic problems, such as kidney stones, structural disease, or functional problems with voiding
  3. History of health problems, such as diabetes mellitus or impaired immunity
- Assess for:
  1. Increased frequency in voiding
  2. Urgency to void
  3. Pain or discomfort on urination

4. Change in urine color, clarity, or odor; presence of WBCs or RBCs
5. Presence of nitrogen or leukoesterase with urinalysis
6. Positive urine culture
7. Elevated plasma WBC (occasional)
8. Abdominal or back pain
9. Bladder distention
10. Feelings of incomplete bladder emptying
11. Voiding in small amounts
12. Difficulty in initiating urination
13. Complete inability to urinate
14. Urinary meatus inflammation
15. Prostate gland changes or tenderness

Considerations for Older Adults

- The only symptoms may be as vague as increasing mental confusion or frequent unexplained falls.
- Sudden onset of or worsening of incontinence may be an early symptom.
- Fever, tachycardia, tachypnea, and hypotension even without any urinary symptoms may be signs of urosepsis.
- Loss of appetite, nocturia, and dysuria are common symptoms.

Planning and Implementation
- Drug therapy includes:
  1. Antibiotics: In simple, acute bacterial cystitis in healthy, ambulatory patients, a 1- to 3-day course of oral antibiotic treatment may be adequate. A 7- to 14-day course of oral or parenteral antibiotics may be needed for complex, chronic, or recurring infections and for urosepsis.
  2. Analgesics or antipyretics to promote comfort
  3. Urinary antiseptics such as nitrofurantoin (Macrodantin, Nephronex) and trimethoprim (Proloprim, Trimpex)
  4. Antispasmodics to decrease bladder spasm and promote complete bladder emptying
  5. Antifungal agents such as amphotericin B in daily bladder instillations and ketoconazole (Nizoral) in oral form
- Diet therapy includes:
  1. Ensuring that the patient maintains an adequate caloric intake
  2. Ensuring sufficient fluid intake to maintain clear or light yellow urine (about 2 to 3 L/day), unless contraindicated
- Other therapy includes providing warm sitz baths to relieve perineal discomfort.

Surgical Management

- Surgical interventions for management of cystitis include urologic procedures for structural abnormalities or endourologic procedures to manipulate or pulverize kidney stones if these conditions are associated with cystitis.

▼ National Patient Safety Goal

Implement a fall-reduction program for older patients to reduce the risk of patient harm when confusion accompanies cystitis.

Community-Based Care

- Teach the patient to:
  1. Self-administer drugs and complete all of the prescribed drug.
  2. Expect changes in color of urine as appropriate.
  3. Use appropriate techniques to prevent discomfort with sexual activities and how to prevent postcoital infections.
  4. Consume liberal fluid intake to maintain urine color as clear or light yellow.
  5. Clean the perineum after urination.
  6. Empty the bladder as soon as the urge is felt.
  7. Obtain adequate rest, sleep, and nutrition.
  8. Avoid known irritants such as caffeine, bubble baths, nylon underwear, and scented toilet tissue.
  9. Wear cotton underwear.
  10. Seek prompt medical care if symptoms recur.
  11. Pregnant women with cystitis require prompt and aggressive antibiotic treatment because this infection can lead to preterm labor and premature birth.
- Refer patients to the National Kidney Foundation as appropriate.
- Refer patients with interstitial cystitis to the Interstitial Cystitis Foundation.

CYSTOCELE

- A *cystocele* is a protrusion of the bladder through the vaginal wall resulting from weakened pelvic structures.
- Causes include obesity, advanced age, childbearing, or genetic predisposition.
- Assess for:
  1. Difficulty in emptying the bladder
  2. Urinary frequency and urgency
  3. Urinary tract infection
  4. Stress urinary incontinence (loss of urine during activities)

5. Bulging of the anterior vaginal wall when the woman is asked to bear down during a pelvic examination

- Diagnostic tests may include cystography, measurement of residual urine, IV urogram (IVU), voiding cystourethrography (VCUG), cystometrogram, and uroflowmetry.
- Management of patients with mild symptoms is conservative and may include:
  1. Use of a pessary for bladder support
  2. Estrogen cream therapy to prevent atrophy and weakening of vaginal walls
  3. Kegel exercises to strengthen perineal muscles
- Surgical intervention for severe symptoms is usually an anterior colporrhaphy (anterior repair) to tighten the pelvic muscles for better bladder support.
- Teach the patient after surgery to use these precautions for 6 weeks:
  1. Limit her activities.
  2. Not lift anything heavier than 5 pounds.
  3. Avoid strenuous exercises.
  4. Avoid sexual intercourse.
  5. Notify her health care provider if she has signs of infection, such as fever, persistent pain, or purulent, foul-smelling discharge.

DEHYDRATION

OVERVIEW

- Dehydration is a state in which fluid intake is less than what is needed to meet the body's fluid needs, resulting in a fluid volume deficit.
- It may be an *actual* decrease in total body water caused by either too little intake of fluid or too great a loss of fluid; or it can occur as a *relative* dehydration, without an actual loss of total body water, such as when water shifts from the plasma into the interstitial space.

Considerations for Older Adults

Older patients are at high risk for dehydration because they have less total body water than younger adults. Many older adults have decreased thirst sensation and may have difficulty with walking or other motor skills needed for ingesting fluids. They also may take drugs such as diuretics, antihypertensives, and laxatives that increase fluid excretion.

- Isotonic dehydration is the most common type of fluid volume deficit, in which fluid is lost only from the extracellular fluid

(ECF) space, including both the plasma and the interstitial spaces.
- Circulating blood volume is decreased (hypovolemia) and leads to inadequate tissue perfusion.
- Causes include:
  1. Hemorrhage
  2. Vomiting, diarrhea
  3. Profuse salivation
  4. Fistulas, draining abscesses
  5. Profuse diaphoresis
  6. Burns and other severe wounds
  7. Long-term NPO status
  8. Diuretic therapy
  9. Continuous GI or nasogastric (NG) suctioning

PATIENT-CENTERED COLLABORATIVE CARE

Assessment
- Obtain and record patient information:
  1. Nutritional history
  2. Fluid history
     a. Intake and output volumes
     b. Weight (A weight change of 1 pound corresponds to a fluid volume change of about 500 mL.)
  3. Presence of excessive sweating, diarrhea
  4. Drug therapy (especially diuretics and laxatives)
  5. Medical history
     a. Diabetes
     b. Kidney disease
  6. Level of consciousness and mental status
  7. Amount of strenuous physical activity
  8. Exposure to high environmental temperatures
  9. Dizziness or light-headedness when standing
- Assess for:
  1. Cardiovascular changes
     a. Heart rate increases
     b. Weak peripheral pulses
     c. Decreased blood pressure
     d. Decreased pulse pressure
     e. Orthostatic (postural) hypotension
     f. Flat neck and hand veins in dependent position
  2. Respiratory changes
     a. Increased respiratory rate
     b. Increased respiratory depth
  3. Skin changes
     a. Dry mucous membranes

  b. Tongue has a pastelike coating or fissures
  c. Dry, flaky skin
  d. Poor skin turgor (skin "tents" when pinched)

Considerations for Older Adults

Assess skin turgor in an older adult by pinching the skin over the sternum or on the forehead, rather than the back of the hand, because these areas more reliably indicate hydration. As a person ages, the skin loses elasticity and tents on hands and arms even when the person is well hydrated.

  4. Neurologic changes
     a. Alterations of mental status (especially confusion)
     b. Low-grade fever
  5. Renal changes
     a. Decreased output
     b. Increased urine concentration (specific gravity greater than 1.030, dark amber, strong odor)

> **Critical Rescue** ♦ Urine output below 500 mL/day for any patient without kidney disease is cause for concern and should be reported to the health care provider.

- Diagnostic assessment: No single laboratory test result confirms or rules out dehydration. Instead, it is determined by laboratory findings along with clinical manifestations. Common laboratory findings for dehydration include:
  1. Elevated levels of hemoglobin and hematocrit
  2. Increased serum osmolarity, glucose, protein, blood urea nitrogen, and various electrolytes

> **Clinical Landmine** ♦ Hemoconcentration is not present when dehydration is from hemorrhage. Therefore, do not rely only on laboratory values to identify dehydration.

Interventions
- Management of dehydration aims to prevent injury, prevent further fluid losses, and increase fluid compartment volumes to normal ranges.
  1. Patient safety issues (to prevent falls)
     a. Monitor vital signs, especially heart rate and blood pressure.
     b. Assess muscle strength, gait stability, and level of alertness.
     c. Instruct the patient to get up slowly from a lying or sitting position and to immediately sit down if he or she feels light-headed.
     d. Implement the falls precautions.

D

2. Fluid replacement
   a. Oral fluid replacement is used for correction of mild to moderate dehydration if the patient is alert enough to swallow and can tolerate oral fluids. Commercial solutions for adults include Equalyte, Oralyte, and Rehydralyte.
   b. IV fluid replacement is used when dehydration is severe and when the patient is not alert enough to swallow or cannot tolerate oral fluids.
   c. Measure fluid intake.
   d. Monitor pulse rate and quality.
   e. Monitor urine output.
3. Drug therapy may correct some causes of the dehydration.
   a. Antidiarrheal drugs
   b. Antiemetics
   c. Antipyretics

DEMENTIA

OVERVIEW

- Dementia, also known as Alzheimer's disease (AD) and dementia, Alzheimer's type (DAT), is a chronic, progressive, degenerative disease that accounts for 60% of the dementias occurring in persons older than 65 years.
- Dementia is also seen in people in their 40s and 50s, which is referred to as early dementia, or presenile dementia, Alzheimer's type.
- Alzheimer's dementia is characterized by memory loss and progressive cognitive impairment caused by neurofibrillary tangles and senile plaques in the brain.
- The exact cause of AD is unknown; genetic predisposition, chemical changes, environmental agents, and immunologic alterations have been implicated in the pathology.
- The use of ibuprofen and other nonsteroidal anti-inflammatory drugs has been demonstrated to reduce the risk of developing AD if taken years before symptoms develop. However, the long-term use of these agents may result in significant gastrointestinal (GI) or kidney complications.

PATIENT-CENTERED COLLABORATIVE CARE

Assessment

- Record patient information:
  1. Age
  2. Current employment status and work history

3. Self-management skills for daily living
4. Ability to complete independent activities: grocery shopping, laundry, meal planning, and financial transactions
5. Driving ability
6. Oral and written communication skills
7. Behavior
8. Family history of AD
9. Medical history, with particular attention to head trauma, viral illness, or exposure to metal or toxic waste

- Assess for:
  1. Indicators of the stages of the disease
     a. Early (stage I) AD is characterized by forgetfulness, misplacing household items, mild memory loss, short attention span, decreased performance, loss of judgment, subtle changes in personality and behavior, and the inability to travel alone to new destinations. There are no associated social or employment problems.
     b. Middle (stage II) AD is characterized by severe impairments in all cognitive functions; gross intellectual impairments; complete disorientation to time, place, and event; physical impairment; loss of ability to care for self; visual-spatial deficits; speech-language problems; and incontinence.
     c. Late (stage III) AD is characterized by lost motor and verbal skills and by severe physical and cognitive deterioration and total dependence for the ADLs.
  2. Cognitive changes, such as changes in attention, concentration, judgment, perception, learning, and short-term memory
  3. Alterations in communication and language skills
  4. Changes in behaviors and personality, such as aggressiveness, paranoia, inappropriate social interactions, rapid mood swings, and increased confusion at night or when fatigued
  5. Changes in self-management requiring assistance in hygiene, dressing, following directions, or completing familiar activities

- Genetic testing specifically for apolipoprotein E (apo-E) may be helpful as an ancillary test (not a predictive test) for the differential diagnosis of AD.
- A variety of laboratory or radiographic tests are performed to rule out other treatable causes of dementia or delirium.

Planning and Implementation

❖**NDx:** Chronic Confusion

- Collaborate with the health care team to prevent overstimulation and provide a structured and orderly environment.

1. Assess the room for pictures on the wall that could be misinterpreted as people, animals, or events that could harm the patient.
2. Ensure that the room has adequate, nonglare lighting and no potentially frightening shadows.
3. Place the patient in a quiet area of the unit, away from obvious exits and within easy view of the staff, preferably in a private room.
4. Arrange the patient's schedule to provide as much uninterrupted sleep at night as possible. Fatigue increases confusion and behavioral problems such as agitation and aggression.
5. Establish a daily routine, explaining changes in routine before they occur and again immediately before they take place.
6. Place familiar objects, clocks, and single-date calendars in easy view of the patient. Encourage the family to provide pictures of family members and close friends that are labeled with the person's name on the picture.
7. Keep the environment free of distractions; provide an unobstructed environment.
8. Regularly reorient the patient to the environment (during early stages).
9. Use validation therapy for later stages of the disease to prevent agitation.
10. Collaborate with the physical and occupational therapist to assist the patient to maintain independence in ADLs as long as possible through the use of assistive devices (grab bars in the bathroom) and exercise programs.
11. Develop an individualized bowel and bladder program for the patient.
12. Attract the patient's attention before conversing.
13. Speak slowly and distinctly in short, clear sentences.
14. Allow sufficient time for the patient to respond.
15. In the home environment, place complete outfits on a single hanger for the patient to choose from; encourage the family to include the patient in meal planning, grocery shopping, and other household routines as able.
16. Provide drug therapy:
    a. Cholinesterase inhibitors are approved for symptomatic treatment of AD.
    b. Selective serotonin reuptake inhibitors are used to treat depression; tricyclic antidepressants should not be used because of their anticholinergic effect.

c. Psychotropic drugs, also called antipsychotic and neuroleptic drugs, should be reserved for a patient with emotional and behavioral health problems that may accompany dementia, such as hallucinations and delusions.

d. Many drugs are being studied for use in patients with AD.

17. Use art, massage, dance, and music therapy in the long-term care setting to minimize agitation.

❖**NDx:** Risk for Injury Related to Wandering, Elder Abuse, or Mistreatment

- The following nursing planning and implementation is used to decrease the risk for injury.

1. Ensure that the patient always wears an identification bracelet or badge that cannot be removed by the patient.
2. Ensure that alarms or other barriers to outside doors are working properly at all times.
3. Check on the patient frequently.
4. Take the patient for walks several times each day, and encourage the patient to participate in activities to decrease his or her restlessness.
5. Talk calmly and softly, redirecting the patient as needed and using diversion.
6. Keep the patient busy with structured activities such as puzzles, board games, and music and art activities.
7. Remove and secure all sharp objects and medications.
8. Implement seizure precautions if there is a history of seizures.
9. Keep an updated photograph of the patient that can be used if the patient wanders away.
10. Inform the patient's family about the Safe Return program, a national government-funded program of the Alzheimer Association that assists in the identification and safe, timely return of individuals with AD and related dementias who wander off and become lost.

❖**NDx:** Sleep Deprivation Related to Changes in Sleep Phases, Anxiety, or Depression

- To promote a day-night pattern:

1. Establish a pre-bedtime ritual.
   a. Personal hygiene
   b. Quiet environment
   c. Backrub or small snack
2. Keep the patient active during the day with a balance between active and passive activities; if possible, discourage the patient from taking a nap.

❖**NDx:** Compromised Family Coping or Caregiver Role Strain

- The following nursing planning and implementation is used to increase family coping and decrease caregiver role strain:
    1. Advise the family to seek legal counsel regarding the patient's competency and the need to obtain guardianship or durable power of attorney.
    2. Refer the family to a local support group affiliated with the Alzheimer's Disease Association.
    3. Assess the family and other caregivers for signs of stress, such as anger, social withdrawal, anxiety, depression and lack of concentration, sleepiness, irritability, and health problems; refer them to their health care provider.
    4. Encourage the family to maintain its own social network and to obtain respite care periodically.
    5. Assist the family to identify and develop strategies to cope with the long-term consequences of the disease.

🛡 National Patient Safety Goal

Maintain the timeliness of reporting critical laboratory values so that reversible causes of delirium receive effective interventions, such as hemoglobin or electrolyte replacement therapy.

Community-Based Care

- When possible, the patient should be assigned to a case manager who can assess the patient's need for health care resources and facilitate appropriate placement throughout the continuum of care.
- The patient is usually cared for in the home until late in the disease process. Therefore, teach the patient and family:
    1. How to assist the patient with ADLs
    2. How to use adaptive equipment
    3. With dietary consultation, how to select and prepare food that the patient is able to chew and swallow
    4. How to prevent the patient from wandering
    5. What to do if the patient has a seizure
    6. How to protect the patient from injury
    7. Drug information (if drugs are prescribed) and how to secure drugs so patient does not take them inappropriately
    8. How to implement the diversion, including activity or exercise
    9. How to obtain respite services
    10. Strategies that caregivers can use to reduce their stress, including:
        a. Maintaining realistic expectations for the person with AD

b. Taking one day at a time
c. Trying to find positive aspects of each incident or situation
d. Using humor with the person who has AD
e. Setting aside time each day for rest or recreation, away from caregiving duties if possible
f. Seeking respite care periodically
g. Exploring alternative care settings early in the disease process for possible use later
h. Establishing advance directives with the person who has AD early in the disease process
i. Taking care of themselves by watching their diet, exercising, and getting plenty of rest
j. Being realistic about what they can do, and getting and accepting help from family, friends, and community resources

- Refer the patient's family and significant others to the local chapter of the Alzheimer's Disease Association.

DIABETES INSIPIDUS

OVERVIEW

- Diabetes insipidus (DI) is a water metabolism problem caused by an antidiuretic hormone (ADH) deficiency (a decrease in ADH synthesis or an inability of the kidneys to respond to ADH). ADH deficiency results in the excretion of large volumes of dilute urine.
- DI is classified into four types depending on whether the problem is caused by too little ADH or an inability of the kidneys to respond to ADH.
  1. *Nephrogenic*: an inherited disorder in which the renal tubules do not respond to the actions of ADH, which results in inadequate water absorption by the kidney
  2. *Primary*: results from a problem in the hypothalamus or pituitary gland resulting in lack of ADH production or release
  3. *Secondary*: results from tumors in or near the hypothalamus or pituitary gland, head trauma, infectious processes, surgical procedures, or metastatic tumors (usually from the lung or breast)
  4. *Drug-related*: most often caused by lithium (Eskalith, Lithobid, Carbolith ✢) and demeclocycline (Declomycin), which can interfere with the kidney response to ADH

PATIENT-CENTERED COLLABORATIVE CARE

Assessment

- Assess patient information:
  1. History of known causes, such as recent surgery, head trauma, or drugs
  2. Excretion of large amounts of dilute urine (more than 4 L in 24 hours) in excess of fluid intake
  3. Dehydration manifestations (e.g., poor skin turgor, dry mucous membranes, weight loss in excess of 1 pound/day)
  4. Increased or excessive thirst
  5. Low urine specific gravity (below 1.005) and urine osmolality (50 to 200 mOsm/kg)
  6. Indications of circulatory collapse, shock (low blood pressure; rapid, thready pulse; increased respiratory rate; decreased pulse pressure)
  7. Neurologic changes such as irritability, lethargy, or decreased cognition

Interventions

- Drug therapy may include:
  1. Desmopressin acetate (DDAVP), a synthetic form of vasopressin given intranasally in a metered spray or as an oral tablet; frequency of dosing depends on the patient's response
  2. Aqueous vasopressin for short-term therapy or when the dosage must be changed frequently; given parenterally
  3. Chlorpropamide (Diabinese, Insulase), an antidiabetic drug that also decreases urine output by an unknown mechanism; given orally
- Nursing interventions include:
  1. Replacing fluids by encouraging the patient to drink fluids equal to the amount of urinary output (If the patient is unable to do so, provide IV, as prescribed.)
  2. Monitoring accurately intake and output
  3. Monitoring for vital sign changes indicating circulatory collapse (e.g., low blood pressure; rapid, thready pulse)
  4. Monitoring for indications of dehydration: dry skin, poor skin turgor, and dry or cracked mucous membranes
  5. Measuring urine specific gravity at least once daily
  6. Monitoring therapy effectiveness by weighing the patient every day
- Patient education includes:
  1. Teaching the patient that polyuria and thirst are signals for the need for another drug dose
  2. Teaching the patient to weigh himself or herself daily to identify weight gain as a manifestation of possible water intoxication

3. Teaching about the side effects of nasal sprays, including ulceration of the mucous membranes, allergy, sensation of chest tightness, and inhalation of the spray into the lungs, which precipitates pulmonary problems

4. Teaching what to do if side effects occur or if an upper respiratory infection develops

5. Teaching the patient going home on vasopressin how to self-inject the drug

6. Encouraging the patient with chronic DI to wear a medical alert bracelet or necklace at all times

DIABETES MELLITUS

OVERVIEW

- Diabetes mellitus (DM) is a metabolic disease that results from either the loss of the ability to make insulin or the loss of receptor sensitivity to the presence of insulin. The first result of either of these problems is higher than normal blood glucose levels (hyperglycemia). Fat, protein, and energy metabolism also are affected.

- Insulin, a hormone made in the beta cells of the pancreas, enables body cells to store and use carbohydrates, fat, and protein. It binds to insulin receptors on select cell membranes, allowing glucose in the blood to move into cells to make energy. As glucose from the blood enters the cells, the blood glucose level goes back to normal (euglycemia). The glucose in the cell can be used immediately to make adenosine triphosphate (ATP) if the cell needs more chemical energy. If the cell already has enough ATP, the glucose is made into glycogen and stored for later use in the liver and muscle.

- The lack of insulin in diabetes from a lack of production or a problem with insulin use at its cell receptor prevents some cells from using glucose for energy. Without insulin, the body enters a serious state of cellular starvation, breaking down body fat and protein.

- Obvious clinical features of DM are chronic hyperglycemia (elevated blood glucose levels), polyuria (excessive urination), polydipsia (excessive thirst and drinking), and polyphagia (hunger).

- Without proper management, DM results in energy and vascular changes that adversely affect every body system.

- Diabetes is classified according to the cause of the disease and the severity of insulin lack. The three most common types of DM are type 1, type 2, and gestational diabetes.

1. *Type 1 diabetes* is an autoimmune disorder in which beta cells of the pancreas are destroyed in a genetically susceptible person and no insulin is produced. Type I diabetes:
   a. Is abrupt in onset
   b. Requires insulin injections to prevent hyperglycemia and ketosis and to sustain health
   c. Represents less than 10% of all people who have diabetes
   d. Occurs primarily in childhood or adolescence but can occur at any age
   e. Causes patients to be thin and underweight
   f. May follow a viral infection
   g. Can lead to ketoacidosis
2. *Type 2 diabetes* is a problem resulting from a reduction in the ability of most cells to respond to insulin (insulin resistance), poor control of liver glucose output, and decreased beta cell function. Type 2 diabetes:
   a. Is generally slow in onset
   b. May require oral antidiabetic drug therapy or insulin to correct hyperglycemia
   c. Is usually found in middle-aged and older adults but may occur in younger obese people
   d. May be part of the *metabolic syndrome*
   e. Often occurs in families in an autosomal dominant pattern of inheritance
   f. Occurs more frequently among obese people
   g. Is usually not associated with ketoacidosis
   h. Represents about 90% of all people who have diabetes
   i. May be present for years before it is diagnosed
3. Gestational diabetes mellitus (GDM)
   a. Carbohydrate intolerance noted during pregnancy and confirmed by an oral glucose tolerance test
   b. Is suspected when a first baby weighs more than 9 lbs
   c. Patients are at high risk for type 2 diabetes after pregnancy.
- Acute complications of diabetes mellitus (DM) include:
  1. Diabetic ketoacidosis (DKA)
     a. DKA occurs in people with type 1 diabetes and is most often precipitated by illness, especially infection.
     b. Patients have acidosis and severe dehydration.
     c. Laboratory diagnosis is based on serum glucose level equal to or greater than 300 mg/dL (16.7 mmol/L), arterial pH less than 7.35, arterial bicarbonate level less than 15 mEq/L, blood urea nitrogen level greater than 20 mg/dL, creatinine level greater than 1.5 mg/dL, and ketonuria.

    d. Clinical manifestations of dehydration and acidosis include decreased skin turgor, dry mucous membranes, hypotension, tachycardia, tachypnea, Kussmaul respirations, abdominal pain, nausea, and vomiting; central nervous system depression results in changes in consciousness varying from lethargy to coma.

    e. Death occurs in 1% to 10% of these cases even with appropriate treatment. Mortality is highest for older patients who also have infection, stroke, myocardial infarction (MI), vascular thrombosis, intestinal obstruction, or pneumonia.

2. Hyperglycemic-hyperosmolar state (HHS)

    a. HHS is a hyperosmolar state caused by hyperglycemia of any origin; it differs from DKA by the absence of ketosis and by much higher blood glucose levels (may exceed 600 mg/dL) and blood osmolarity levels (may exceed 320 mOsm/L).

    b. Dehydration is the most common cause of HHS and becomes worse with the disorder.

    c. HHS occurs almost exclusively in patients with type 2 diabetes.

    d. It occurs most often in older adults and those who are unaware of their diabetic condition.

    e. Conditions such as silent myocardial infarction (MI), sepsis, pancreatitis, and stroke and drugs such as glucocorticoids, diuretics, phenytoin sodium, propranolol, and calcium channel blockers may precipitate HHS.

Considerations for Older Adults

- Older adults with diabetes are at the greatest risk for dehydration and subsequent HHS. The onset of HHS is slow and may not be recognized. The older patient often seeks medical attention later and is sicker than younger patients. The mortality rate for HHS is as high as 40% to 70% among older adults.

> **Clinical Landmine ◆** HHS does not occur in people who are adequately hydrated. Take steps to avoid dehydration in susceptible patients.

3. Hypoglycemia

    a. Hypoglycemia is a blood glucose level lower than 70 mg/dL.

    b. It can be caused by excessive insulin, some oral antidiabetic drugs, insufficient food intake, and increased physical activity.

    c. Neurogenic symptoms of hypoglycemia, which result from autonomic nervous system stimulation triggered by hypoglycemia, include hunger, diaphoresis, weakness, and nervousness. These symptoms occur when there is an *abrupt* decrease in the blood glucose level.

    d. Neuroglycopenic symptoms, which result directly from brain glucose deprivation, including headache, confusion, slurred speech, behavioral changes, and coma, occur with a more *gradual* decline in blood glucose level.

    e. If not managed properly, hypoglycemia can lead to brain damage and death.

- The classic signs and symptoms of hypoglycemia may not appear in older diabetic patients; changes in levels of consciousness may be slow and progress through confusion and bizarre behavior. Coma may come without warning.
- Chronic complications of diabetes result from blood vessel changes related to hyperglycemia. These changes lead to serious health problems and early death. Although nothing prevents the complications, they can be slowed significantly by tight control of blood glucose levels. The chronic complications can be divided into macrovascular (large vessel) and microvascular (small vessel) problems.

    1. Macrovascular complications include:

        a. Coronary heart disease

        b. Peripheral vascular disease (often leading to amputation)

        c. Cerebrovascular disease

    2. Microvascular complications include:

        a. Ocular complications (can lead to blindness): diabetic retinopathy, retinal detachment, macular degeneration, myopia, cataracts, and glaucoma

        b. Diabetic neuropathy (damage to peripheral and autonomic nerves)

        c. Diabetic nephropathy (renal failure)

        d. Male erectile dysfunction

Cultural Awareness

- Diabetes is a significant problem for African Americans, American Indians, and Mexican Americans.
- In all populations, prevalence of type 2 diabetes rises with age and obesity.
- Minority group members have a higher risk for complications such as hypertension, retinopathy, neuropathy, and nephropathy, than whites, even after adjusting for differences in blood glucose control.

PATIENT-CENTERED COLLABORATIVE CARE

Assessment

- Ask about and record patient information:
  1. Age
  2. Birth weight of children
  3. Weight change
  4. Occurrence of a recent illness or extreme stress
  5. Omission of insulin or oral antidiabetic drugs if the patient is a known diabetic
  6. Change in eating habits
  7. Change in exercise schedule or activity level
  8. Presence and duration of polyuria, polydipsia, polyphagia, and loss of energy
  9. History of small skin injuries becoming infected more easily or taking a longer time to heal
  10. In women, frequency and duration of vaginal infections
  11. Presence of cardiovascular disease such as dysrhythmias, heart failure, hypertension, or stroke
  12. Presence of diabetes in a parent or sibling
  13. History of higher than normal fasting blood glucose levels
- Assess for:
  1. Elevated fasting blood glucose level (higher than 126 mg/dL) or random blood glucose level (greater than 200 mg/dL)
  2. Abnormal oral glucose tolerance test
  3. Glycosylated hemoglobin assay (HbA_{1c}) results greater than 7.5%
  4. Positive results for urinary ketones; presence of albumin and glucose in the urine
  5. Abdominal pain, nausea, and vomiting (in DKA)
  6. Dehydration (e.g., poor skin turgor, dry mucous membranes, hemoconcentration with elevated hematocrit and hemoglobin levels, decreased urine output, dark and strong-smelling urine)

Planning and Implementation

❖**NDx:** Risk for Injury Related to Hyperglycemia

Nonsurgical Management

- Drug or insulin therapy is indicated when a patient with type 2 diabetes cannot achieve blood glucose control with dietary modification, regular exercise, and stress management.
  1. *Sulfonylureas:* The most common drugs in this class are glipizide (Glucotrol) and glyburide (DiaBeta). These oral drugs are used for patients who still have some pancreatic beta cell function; hypoglycemia is the most serious complication; other side effects include hematologic reactions, allergic skin reactions, and GI effects.

2. *Meglitinide analogues*: Repaglinide (Prandin) and nateglinide (Starlix) are oral drugs that have actions and side effects similar to sulfonylurea agents. Adverse effects include hypoglycemia, GI disturbances, upper respiratory infections, arthralgia, back pain, and headache.

3. *Biguanides*: Metformin (Glucophage) is the major drug in this class. This drug does not cause hypoglycemia.

> **Clinical Landmine** ◆ Metformin can cause lactic acidosis in patients with renal insufficiency and should not be used by anyone with kidney disease. To prevent kidney damage, the drug should be withheld for 48 hours before and after using contrast material or any surgical procedure requiring anesthesia.

4. *Alpha-glucosidase inhibitors*: These oral drugs include acarbose (Precose) and miglitol (Glyset). They reduce hyperglycemia after meals by slowing digestion and absorption of carbohydrate within the intestine. Drugs in this class do not cause hypoglycemia. Side effects include abdominal discomfort related to undigested carbohydrate in the intestinal tract.

5. *Thiazolidinediones (TZDs)*: These oral drugs include rosiglitazone (Avandia) and pioglitazone (Actos). They work by increasing the sensitivity of insulin receptors, promoting glucose utilization in peripheral tissues. Liver function studies should be done at the start of therapy and at regular intervals while on therapy.

> **Clinical Landmine** ◆ Rosiglitazone has been associated with an increased risk for heart-related deaths and should not be used in patients with serious cardiac problems.

6. *Combination agents*: These are combinations from two different classes of drugs, such as Glucovance, which combines glyburide with metformin. Remember that the side effects of combination agents include those of all drugs contained in the combination.

7. *Amylin analogues*: The drug in this class is pramlintide (Symlin), which is similar to amylin, a naturally occurring hormone produced by beta cells in the pancreas, that works with and is co-secreted with insulin in response to blood glucose elevation. It works in at least 3 different ways to reduce blood glucose levels and is injected subcutaneously. This drug can be used for patients with either type 1 or type 2 diabetes.

> 🔯 Critical Rescue ◆ Assess the patient for severe hypoglyc-
> emia because this drug can lower blood glucose levels below
> normal.

8. *Incretin analogues*: The drug in this class is exenatide (Byetta)
   and is injected subcutaneously. It is a natural "gut" hormone
   that works with insulin to lower plasma glucose levels. This
   drug is approved for use only in combination with a sulfonylurea, metformin, or both in patients with type 2 diabetes.

> 🔯 Critical Rescue ◆ When this drug is used with a sulfony-
> lurea, assess the patient for hypoglycemia.

9. *DPP-IV inhibitors*: The drug in this class is sitagliptin
   (Januvia). It is an oral drug that increases the body's natural
   incretin hormone levels and reduces high blood glucose
   levels. Side effects include stuffy or runny nose, sore throat,
   upper respiratory infection, GI disturbances, and renal
   insufficiency.
- Insulin therapy is necessary for type 1 diabetes and for moderate to severe type 2 diabetes.
  1. Insulin is available in rapid-, short-, intermediate-, and long-
     acting forms, which may be injected separately, and some can
     be mixed in the same syringe.
  2. Insulin regimens try to duplicate the normal release pattern
     of insulin from the pancreas, including single daily injec-
     tions, two-dose protocol, three-dose protocol, four-dose
     protocol, combination therapy, and intensified insulin
     regimens.
  3. Teach the patient that insulin type, injection techniques, site
     of injection, and individual response can all affect absorp-
     tion, onset, degree, and duration of insulin activity and rein-
     force that changing insulin may affect blood glucose
     control.
  4. Complications of insulin therapy include:
     a. Hypoglycemia
     b. *Dawn phenomenon,* a fasting hyperglycemia thought to
        result from nocturnal release of growth hormone secre-
        tion that may cause blood glucose elevations around 5 to
        6 AM and is managed or prevented by providing more
        insulin for the overnight period
     c. *Somogyi phenomenon,* a morning hyperglycemia resulting
        from effective counterregulatory response to nighttime
        hypoglycemia, that is managed or prevented by ensuring

adequate dietary intake at bedtime and evaluating the insulin dose and exercise program

d. Hypertrophic lipodystrophy, a spongy swelling at or around injection sites

e. Lipoatrophy, a loss of subcutaneous fat in areas of repeated injection that is treated by injection of human insulin at the edges of the atrophied area

f. Lipohypertrophy, an increased swelling of fat that occurs at the site of repeated injections and is prevented by rotating injection sites

5. Insulin may be administered by:

   a. Subcutaneous injection

   b. Continuous subcutaneous infusion of insulin using an externally worn pump containing a syringe and reservoir with rapid or short-acting insulin connected to the patient by an infusion set

   c. Insulin pumps implanted into the peritoneal cavity where insulin can be absorbed in a more physiologic manner

   d. Injection devices, whereby the needle is replaced by an ultrathin liquid stream of insulin forced through the skin under high pressure

6. Teach the patient about storage, dose preparation, injection procedures, and complications associated with drug therapy.

7. Instruct the patient to always buy the same type of syringes and use the same gauge and needle length; short needles are not used for an obese patient.

- The patient needs to know how to perform all aspects of self-monitoring of blood glucose (SMBG) and understand several issues:

  1. Accuracy of the results depends on the accuracy of the specific blood glucose meter, operator proficiency, and test strip quality.

  2. Results are influenced by the amount of blood on the strip, the calibration of the meter to the strip currently in use; environmental conditions of altitude, temperature, and moisture; and patient-specific conditions of hematocrit, triglyceride level, and presence of hypotension.

  3. Teach the patient how to clean the equipment and how to prevent infection.

  4. Instruct the patient *not* to use alternative site testing (forearm, upper arm, abdomen, thigh, and calf) in the following situations:

     a. When patient is hypoglycemic or susceptible to hypoglycemia (at time of peak activity of basal insulin)

  b. After exercise
  c. During an illness
  d. When blood glucose levels are changing rapidly
  e. Before driving
- Diet therapy
  1. Collaborate with the patient, physician, and nutritionist to formulate an individualized meal plan for the patient.
  2. Day-to-day consistency in the timing and amount of food eaten helps control blood glucose. Patients taking insulin need to eat at consistent times that are coordinated with the timed action of insulin.
  3. Base meal plan on blood glucose monitoring results, total blood lipid levels, and glycosylated hemoglobin.
  4. Dietary guidelines are based on individual needs of the patient.
     a. Protein intake: 15% to 20% of total daily calories is appropriate for patients with normal kidney function. In patients with microalbuminuria, reduction of protein to 10% of calories may slow progression of kidney failure.
     b. Less than 10% of total daily calories should be from saturated fat and up to 10% should be from polyunsaturated fat.
     c. Foods high in *trans*-fatty acids are avoided or severely restricted.
     d. Remaining calories are from monounsaturated fat and carbohydrates.
     e. High-fiber diets improve carbohydrate metabolism and lower cholesterol levels. High-fiber foods are added to the patient's diet gradually to prevent cramping, loose stools, and flatulence.
     f. Suggest artificial sweeteners such as sucralose, saccharin, aspartame, and acesulfame K, instead of sugar to enhance dietary compliance.
     g. Warn patients that fat replacers may increase carbohydrate content in foods.
  5. Teach the patient that alcohol may be taken in moderation only if diabetes is well controlled.
  6. Explain and reinforce how to read food labels.
  7. Reinforce dietary teaching such as how to follow the exchange system for meal planning and how to perform carbohydrate counting.
  8. Support and reinforce information provided by the nutritionist regarding how to make adjustments in nutritional intake during illness, planned exercises, and social occasions.

Considerations for Older Adults

- A realistic approach to diet therapy is essential for older diabetic patients.
- Attempts to change long-time eating habits may be difficult.
- Patients who live alone, do their own food preparation, and have physical limitations may have difficulty following the diet recommended by the American Diabetes Association.
- Socioeconomic factors may also affect a patient's ability to prepare the proper foods.

- Regular physical exercise is a recommended component of a comprehensive diabetes treatment plan.
  1. Collaborate with the patient and rehabilitation specialist to develop an exercise program.
  2. Instruct the patient to have a complete physical examination before starting an exercise program at home.
  3. Instruct the patient to wear proper footwear with good traction and cushioning and to examine the feet after exercise.
  4. Discourage exercise in extreme heat or cold or during periods of poor glucose control.
  5. Advise the patient to stay hydrated.
  6. Patients with type 1 diabetes should perform vigorous exercise only if blood glucose levels are between 80 and 250 mg/dL and no ketones are present in the urine.
  7. Teach the patient about the risks and complications related to exercise such as prolonged alterations in blood glucose levels, vitreous hemorrhage, or retinal detachment in patients with proliferative retinopathy, and increased proteinuria and foot and joint injury in patients with peripheral neuropathy.

Surgical Management

- Whole-pancreas transplantation can be performed in one of three ways: pancreas transplantation alone (PTA) in the preuremic patient, pancreas transplantation after successful kidney transplantation (PAK), and simultaneous pancreas-kidney (SPK) transplantation.
  1. Immunosuppressive therapy is needed for life to prevent rejection of the transplanted pancreas.
  2. Complications include venous thrombosis, rejection, and infection.

❖**NDx:** Delayed Surgical Recovery

- Surgery is a physical and emotional stressor, making the diabetic patient more at risk for intraoperative and postoperative complications.

- Provide preoperative care:
  1. Discontinue antidiabetic drugs.
     a. Chlorpropamide (Diabinese) 36 hours before surgery
     b. Metformin (Glucophage) 48 hours before surgery
     c. All other oral antidiabetic drugs on the day of surgery
  2. Restart oral antidiabetic drugs only after renal function has been re-evaluated and found to be normal.
  3. Start IV fluids to maintain hydration when the patient is admitted.
  4. Monitor blood glucose results and administer insulin as ordered.
- Intraoperative IV administration of short-acting insulin in 5% to 10% glucose is recommended for all insulin-treated patients and for drug-treated or diet-treated patients who are undergoing general anesthesia and whose diabetes is poorly controlled.
- Provide postoperative care:
  1. Monitor vital signs, especially temperature; hypothermia may cause high blood glucose levels.
  2. Monitor fluid and electrolyte balance; patients with azotemia may have problems with fluid management.
  3. Continue glucose and insulin infusions until the patient is stable and able to tolerate oral feedings.
  4. May need to administer short-acting insulin until the patient's usual drug regimen can be restarted.
  5. Provide pain management, ideally with patient-controlled analgesia (PCA) pump.
  6. Monitor for postoperative complications, including:
     a. Myocardial infarction (MI)
     b. Hypoglycemia
     c. Hyperkalemia or hypokalemia
     d. Uncontrolled blood glucose
     e. Impaired wound healing or wound infection
     f. Renal dysfunction

❖**NDx:** Risk for Injury Related to Disturbed Sensory Perception

- Nonhealing foot wounds cause more inpatient hospital days than any other complication of diabetes.
- Loss of pain, pressure, and temperature sensation in the foot increases the risk for injury and ulceration.
- Foot deformities common in diabetic neuropathy may lead to callus formation, ulceration, and increased areas of pressure.
- Foot care education includes:
  1. Teaching preventive foot care to the patient; sensory neuropathy, ischemia, and infection are the leading causes of foot disease.

2. Recommending that the patient have shoes fitted by an experienced shoe fitter such as a certified podiatrist, and instructing the patient to change shoes at midday and in the evening and to wear socks or stockings with shoes

3. Instructing the patient on how to care for wounds

- Refer the patient to a specialist for orthotic devices to eliminate pressure on infected or open wounds of the foot.

- Topical application of growth factors may be used to accelerate tissue healing for long-standing foot ulcers.

- Wound care for diabetic ulcers includes a moist wound environment, débridement of necrotic tissue, and offloading or elimination of pressure.

❖ **NDx:** Chronic Pain

- Drug therapy may include:
  1. Anticonvulsants for pain secondary to diabetic neuropathy
  2. Tricyclic antidepressants, particularly amitriptyline (Elavil, Levate ❧), nortriptyline (Pamelor), or selective serotonin and norepinephrine reuptake inhibitors, such as duloxetine (Cymbalta), as prescribed, to alleviate peripheral neuropathic pain
  3. Capsaicin cream, 0.075% (e.g., Axsain ❧, Zostrix-HP) topically to relieve neuropathic pain

- Use other nondrug pain management techniques as appropriate, such as bed cradles, warm baths, and backrubs.

❖ **NDx:** Risk for Injury Related to Disturbed Sensory Perception (Visual)

- Encourage all patients to have a baseline ophthalmic examination and yearly follow-up examinations.

- Advise the patient to seek a retinal specialist if problems are present.

- Collaborate with the rehabilitation specialist to recommend strategies to improve the patient's visual abilities; strategies include improving lighting, placing dark equipment against a white background, coding objects such as insulin vials with bright colors or felt-tip markers, and using large-type books and newspapers.

- Various stages of diabetic retinopathy can be treated with laser therapy or surgery.

- Teach the patient with limited vision the following strategies for using adaptive devices to self-administer insulin:
  1. Ensuring proper placement of the device on the syringe
  2. Holding the insulin bottle upright when measuring insulin
  3. Avoiding air bubbles in the syringe by pulling a small amount of insulin into the syringe, moving the plunger in and out three times, and measuring insulin on the fourth draw

❖ **NDx:** Ineffective Tissue Perfusion, Renal

- Stress the importance of maintaining a normal blood glucose level, maintaining a blood pressure level below 130/85 mm Hg, and being screened annually for microalbuminuria.

- Teach the patient to limit protein to 0.8 g/kg of body weight per day if he or she has overt nephropathy.
- Teach the patient about the signs and symptoms of urinary tract infection.
- Adjustment by the health care provider of the insulin dosage for patients undergoing dialysis.
- Advise the patient not to take any OTC drugs, especially NSAIDs, without checking with the health care provider.

❖**Collaborative Problem:** Potential for Hypoglycemia

- Monitor glucose levels before administering hypoglycemic agents, before meals, at bedtime, and when the patient is symptomatic.
- Treat the patient with *mild* hypoglycemia (hungry, irritable, shaky, weak, headache, fully conscious, blood glucose less than 60 mg/dL [3.4 mmol/L]) who is able to swallow with *one* of these:

    2 to 3 glucose tablets
    4 oz of fruit drink
    4 oz of regular soft drink
    8 oz of skim milk
    6 saltines
    3 graham crackers
    6 to 10 hard candies
    4 cubes of sugar
    2 teaspoons of sugar

- Blood glucose level should be tested after 15 minutes.
- Treat the patient with *moderate* hypoglycemia (cold and clammy skin, pale, rapid pulse, rapid shallow respirations, marked changes in mood, drowsiness, blood glucose less than 40 mg/dL [2.2 mmol/L]) with 15 to 30 g of rapidly absorbed carbohydrates and additional food such as low-fat milk or cheese after 10 to 15 minutes.

> 🛟 Critical Rescue ◆ For the patient with *severe* hypoglycemia (unable to swallow, unconscious or convulsing, blood glucose usually less than 20 mg/dL [1.0 mmol/L]), treat by this approach:
>
> - Administer glucagon, 1 mg subcutaneously or IM.
> - Repeat the dose in 10 minutes if the patient remains unconscious.
> - Notify the primary health care provider immediately, and follow instructions.
> - If still unconscious, transport the patient to the nearest emergency department.
> - Provide a small meal when the patient wakes and is no longer nauseated.

- Teach the patient to prevent the four common causes of hypoglycemia: excess exercise, excess insulin, alcohol use, and deficient food intake.
- Encourage the patient to wear an identification (Medical Alert) bracelet.

❖**Collaborative Problem:** Potential for Diabetic Ketoacidosis

- Monitor for signs and symptoms of diabetic ketoacidosis (DKA).
- Give insulin bolus as indicated, followed by a continuous drip.
- Check the patient's blood pressure, pulse, and respirations every 15 minutes until stable.
- Monitor the patient for hypokalemia (symptoms are muscle weakness, abdominal distention or paralytic ileus, hypotension, and weak pulse); before administering potassium, ensure that the patient's urine output is at least 30 mL/hr.
- Replace both fluid volume and ongoing losses, monitoring for congestive heart failure and pulmonary edema if large volume of IV fluid is administered.
- Record urine output, temperature, and mental status every hour.
- Assess the patient's level of consciousness, hydration status, fluid and electrolyte balance, and blood glucose levels every hour until stable; once stable, assess every 4 hours.
- Instruct the patient about how to prevent future episodes of DKA by contacting the primary health care provider when the blood glucose is greater than 250 mg/dL, when ketonuria is present for more than 24 hours, when unable to take food or fluids, and when illness persists for more than 1 to 2 days.

❖**Collaborative Problem:** Potential for Hyperglycemic-Hyperosmolar State (HHS)

- Administer IV fluids and insulin as indicated, and monitor and assess the patient's response to therapy.
- Assess for signs of cerebral edema and immediately report change in level of consciousness; change in pupil size, shape, or reaction to light; or seizure activity to the physician.

Community-Based Care

- Discharge planning includes:
  1. Ensuring that the patient understands the significance, symptoms, causes, and treatment of hypoglycemia and hyperglycemia
  2. Assisting the patient to identify the items needed for the administration of insulin and for glucose monitoring
  3. Teaching the patient how to monitor blood sugar level

4. Teaching the patient how to administer drugs and prevent hypoglycemia
5. In collaboration with the nutritionist, teaching the patient basic survival skills associated with drugs, diet, exercise, and complications
6. Referring the patient to a diabetes educator for the necessary education
7. Helping the patient adapt to diabetes, including teaching stress management techniques and identifying coping mechanisms
8. Referring the patient to the American Diabetes Association and its resources
9. Providing information about community resources, such as diabetic education programs

DIVERTICULA, ESOPHAGEAL

- Diverticula are sacs resulting from the herniation of esophageal mucosa and submucosa into surrounding tissue.
- Patients with esophageal diverticula are at risk for esophageal perforation.
- The most common form of diverticulum is Zenker's diverticulum, which is usually located near the hypopharynx and occurs most often in older adults.

PATIENT-CENTERED COLLABORATIVE CARE

Assessment
- Assessment findings include:
  1. Dysphagia
  2. Regurgitation
  3. Feelings of fullness or pressure
  4. Halitosis
  5. Nocturnal cough

Interventions
- Diet therapy and positioning are the primary interventions for controlling symptoms related to diverticula.
- Nursing interventions include:
  1. Collaborating with the dietitian to determine the size and frequency of meals and the texture and consistency that can best be tolerated by the patient
  2. Elevating the head of the bed for sleep to avoid reflux of gastric contents onto diverticula
  3. Teaching the patient to avoid the recumbent position and vigorous exercising for at least 2 hours after eating to prevent reflux

4. Teaching the patient to avoid restrictive clothing at the abdomen and thorax and to minimize stooping or bending to reduce reflux
- Surgical management is aimed at excision of the diverticula.
- Postoperative care
  1. Monitor for bleeding and perforation.
  2. Maintain the patient on NPO status for several days to promote healing.
  3. Do not irrigate the nasogastric (NG) tube used for decompression unless specifically ordered by the physician.
  4. Maintain hydration and nutrition through IV fluids and enteral feedings until oral intake is permitted.
  5. Manage the patient's postoperative pain.
  6. Teach the patient to observe for complications such as infection or poor wound healing.
  7. Teach the patient measures to take to reduce reflux (elevating head of bed, avoiding recumbent position).

DIVERTICULAR DISEASE

OVERVIEW

- Diverticular disease includes diverticulosis and diverticulitis.
  1. Diverticulosis is pouchlike herniations of the mucosa through the muscular wall of any portion of the gut, but it most commonly refers to diverticula of the colon. They can occur in any part of the intestine but are most common in the sigmoid colon. High intraluminal pressure forces the formation of a pouch in the weakened area of the mucosa, commonly near blood vessels. Without inflammation, diverticula are asymptomatic.
  2. Diverticulitis, or inflammation of one or more diverticula, results when the diverticulum retains undigested food, which compromises the blood supply to that area and facilitates bacterial invasion of the diverticular sac, which may then perforate. A perforated diverticulum can progress to intra-abdominal perforation with generalized peritonitis.

PATIENT-CENTERED COLLABORATIVE CARE

Assessment

- Patients with diverticulosis are usually asymptomatic; a minor history of left quadrant pain or constipation may be reported.
  1. Diverticula may be identified on colonoscopy, barium enema (rectal), or upper gastrointestinal (GI) tract series (small intestine).

- Assess for clinical manifestations of diverticulitis:
  1. Abdominal pain may begin as intermittent and may progress to continuous. Pain may be localized to the left lower quadrant and increase with coughing, straining, or lifting. Generalized abdominal pain is a sign of perforation and peritonitis.
  2. Fever
  3. Nausea and vomiting
  4. Abdominal distention
  5. Palpable, tender abdominal or rectal mass
  6. Blood in the stool (microscopic to larger amounts)
  7. Elevated WBC; reduced hematocrit and hemoglobin if bleeding occurs
  8. Hypotension and dehydration occurs if massive bleeding occurs (see Hypovolemic Shock).
  9. Signs of septic shock occur if peritonitis has occurred.
  10. Flat plate x-ray to evaluate for free air and fluid outside the GI tract
  11. CT scan to diagnose abscess or thickening of lumen due to repeated inflammation and injury
  12. Monitor serum electrolytes.
  13. Monitor intake, output, and patient fluid status.
  14. If a nasogastric tube is used for gastric decompression or to manage vomiting, assess output for amount and quality or color.

Interventions
- Drug therapy
  1. Administer broad-spectrum antibiotics such as metronidazole (Flagyl) plus trimethoprim/sulfamethoxazole (Bactrim, Septra), or ciprofloxacin (Cipro).
  2. Implement management for mild or moderate pain; if pain is severe, use opioids.
  3. Laxatives and enemas are not given because they increase intestinal motility.
- Report the appearance of blood in the nasogastric (NG) output if decompressive NG tube is used.
- Recommend rest.
- Teach the patient to refrain from lifting, straining, coughing, stooping or bending to avoid increased intra-abdominal pressure.
- Diet therapy
  1. Provide IV fluids for hydration during the acute phase of the disease or when NPO.
  2. When taking oral food, diet may be restricted to clear liquids or low fiber.

3. Introduce a fiber-containing diet gradually when symptoms have resolved.
4. Consult with a nutritionist to promote healthy food choices.
5. Keep a food diary.

Surgical Management

- Patients with diverticulitis need emergent surgery if one of the following occurs:
  1. Rupture of the diverticulum with subsequent peritonitis
  2. Pelvic abscess
  3. Bowel obstruction
  4. Fistula
  5. Persistent fever or pain after 4 days of medical treatment
  6. Uncontrolled bleeding
- Surgical management includes a colon resection with an end-to-end anastomosis or temporary or permanent colostomy.
- Preoperative care includes:
  1. Reinforcing physician teaching about the possible need for a temporary or permanent colostomy
  2. Administering IV fluids, antibiotics, and pain medications, if prescribed
  3. Maintaining NPO status with an nasogastric (NG) tube in place for patients having emergency surgery
- Postoperative care includes:
  1. Maintaining drainage system at the abdominal incision site
  2. If a colostomy was created, monitoring colostomy stoma for color and integrity
  3. Maintaining the nasogastric (NG) tube for several days until peristalsis returns
  4. Introducing clear liquids slowly after bowel sounds return (usually 2 to 3 days) and gradually advancing the diet as tolerated
  5. Providing the patient with an opportunity to express feelings about the colostomy
  6. Consulting with the wound or ostomy specialist
  7. Providing written postoperative instructions on:
     a. Inspection of the incision for redness, tenderness, swelling, and drainage
     b. Dressing change procedures, if necessary
     c. Avoidance of activities that increase intra-abdominal pressure, including straining at stool, bending, lifting heavy objects, and wearing restrictive clothing
     d. Pain management, including prescriptions

- Teach the patient and family:
  1. To follow dietary considerations for diverticulosis, which include consultation with the nutritionist and:
     a. Eating a diet high in cellulose and hemicellulose, which are found in wheat bran, whole grain breads, and cereals
     b. Eating fruits and vegetables with high-fiber content (unless diverticulitis occurs)
     c. If the recommended fiber requirements cannot be tolerated, a bulk-forming laxative such as psyllium (Metamucil) can be used to increase fecal size and consistency.
     d. Encouraging fluids to prevent bloating that may accompany a high-fiber diet
     e. Avoiding alcohol, which has an irritant effect on the bowel
     f. Advising that fat intake should not exceed 30% of the total daily caloric intake
     g. Avoiding all fiber when the symptoms of diverticulitis are present
  2. To monitor for signs and symptoms of diverticulitis (see earlier) (fever, abdominal pain, and bloody stools are common symptoms)
  3. To avoid enemas and laxatives other than bulk-forming laxatives such as psyllium hydrophilic mucilloid (Metamucil)

DYSRHYTHMIAS, CARDIAC

OVERVIEW

- Cardiac dysrhythmias are abnormal rhythms of the heart's electrical system that are caused by disturbances of cardiac electrical impulse formation or conduction, or both.
- Many cardiac diseases cause dysrhythmia: congenital heart disease, myocardial injury or infarction, cardiomyopathy, left or right ventricular dysfunction.
- Contributing factors can also cause and worsen dysrhythmias: electrolyte imbalance, hypoxemia, serum acidosis and alkalosis, and drug toxicity are the most common contributing factors.
- Tachydysrhythmias are heart rates greater than 100 beats/min.
  1. Signs and symptoms include palpitations, chest discomfort; pressure or pain from myocardial ischemia or infarction; restlessness; anxiety; pale, cool skin; and syncope from hypotension.
  2. They may cause heart failure as indicated by dyspnea, orthopnea, pulmonary crackles, distended neck veins, fatigue, and weakness.

- Bradydysrhythmias are characterized by a heart rate less than 60 beats/min.
  1. The patient may tolerate a low heart rate if blood pressure is adequate.
  2. Symptomatic bradydysrhythmias lead to hypotension, myocardial ischemia or infarction, other dysrhythmias, and heart failure.
- Premature complexes are early complexes that occur when a cardiac cell or group of cells other than the sinoatrial (SA) node becomes irritable and fires an impulse before the next sinus impulse is generated.
  1. Bigeminy: when normal complexes and premature complexes occur alternately in a repetitive two-beat pattern, with a pause occurring after each premature complex so that complexes occur in pairs
  2. Trigeminy: a repetitive three-beat pattern, usually occurring as two sequential normal complexes followed by a premature complex and a pause, with the same pattern repeating itself in triplets
  3. Quadrigeminy: a repetitive four-beat pattern, usually occurring as three sequential normal complexes followed by a premature complex and a pause, with the same pattern repeating itself in a four-beat pattern
- Escape complexes and rhythms may occur when the sinoatrial (SA) node fails to discharge or is blocked or when a sinus impulse fails to depolarize the ventricles.
- Dysrhythmias are further classified according to their site of origin.
- Sinus dysrhythmias include:
  1. Sinus tachycardia occurs when the SA node discharge exceeds 100 beats/min. Treatment is based on identifying the underlying cause (e.g., angina, fever, hypovolemia, pain); beta-adrenergic blocking agents may be prescribed.
  2. Sinus bradycardia, a decreased rate of SA node discharge of less than 60 beats/min. If the patient is symptomatic, treatment includes atropine, a pacemaker, and avoidance of parasympathetic stimulations such as prolonged suctioning.
- Atrial dysrhythmias
  1. Premature atrial complex (PAC) occurs when atrial tissue becomes irritable. This ectopic focus fires an impulse before the next sinus impulse is due.
     a. No intervention is generally needed except to treat the cause, such as heart failure or valvular disease.

2. Supraventricular tachycardia (SVT) involve the rapid stimulation of atrial tissue at a rate of 100 to 280 beats/min with a mean of 170 beats/min.
   a. No intervention is generally needed except to treat the cause.
   b. Sustained SVT may need to be treated with radiofrequency catheter ablation.
   c. Oxygen therapy, antidysrhythmic drugs, or synchronized cardioversion may also be needed.
3. Atrial flutter is a rapid arterial depolarization occurring at a rate of 250 to 350 times/min.
   a. Drug treatment includes ibutilide (Covert), amiodarone (Cordarone), and diltiazem (Cardizem).
   b. Synchronized cardioversion is done if the patient is hemodynamically compromised.
   c. Rapid atrial overdrive pacing or radiofrequency catheter ablation may be needed if none of the mentioned treatments are successful.
4. Atrial fibrillation (AF) consists of rapid atrial impulses at a rate of 350 to 600 times/min.
   a. Treatment is the same as for atrial flutter.
   b. Anticoagulants are given as this rhythm places the patient at high risk for emboli formation in the atrial appendage. The clot can break off and travel through major arteries causing stroke, myocardial infarction (MI), pulmonary emboli, deep vein thrombosis, and other thrombotic disease.

- Junctional dysrhythmias may occur when the cells in the atrioventricular (AV) junctional node generate an impulse. Junctional rhythms usually are an escape rhythm and do not persist beyond the acute disease that caused slowing or absence of SA pacemaker function.
  1. If treatment is needed, generally atropine is used to speed up the junctional rhythm (ACLS bradycardic algorithm).
  2. A pacemaker is used for definitive treatment.
- Ventricular dysrhythmias
  1. Idioventricular rhythm (ventricular escape rhythm) occurs when the ventricular cells became the pacemakers of the heart.
     a. This bradycardic rhythm is often symptomatic, with hypotension or decreased or absent peripheral pulses.
     b. Immediate resuscitation measures are required (ACLS bradycardic algorithm).
  2. Premature ventricular complexes (PVCs) result from increased irritability of the ventricular cells. PVCs are early

ventricular complexes followed by a pause and often occur in repetitive rhythms.

   a. The patient may be asymptomatic or may experience palpitations, chest discomfort, or diminished or absent peripheral pulses.

   b. If there is no underlying heart disease, PVCs are not treated other than by eliminating any contributing cause.

   c. In the presence of myocardial ischemia or infarction, symptomatic PVCs are treated with oxygen and amiodarone (Cordarone); other drugs are prescribed if an MI occurs.

3. Ventricular tachycardia (VT), or "V tach," occurs with repetitive firing of an irritable ventricular ectopic focus, usually at a rate of 140 to 180 beats/min.

   a. Symptoms depend on ventricular rate; the patient may be hemodynamically compromised and in cardiac arrest.

   b. Sustained VT is treated with oxygen, amiodarone, lidocaine, or magnesium sulfate.

   c. Unstable VT is treated with emergency cardioversion followed by oxygen and antidysrhythmic therapy.

   d. With pulseless VT, immediately begin cardiopulmonary resuscitation (CPR) and defibrillate as soon as possible. If the patient remains pulseless, continue CPR and other resuscitative measures.

   e. After the patient has been successfully converted, attention is given to treating the reversible causes of VT.

4. Ventricular fibrillation (VF), sometimes called "V-fib," is the result of electrical chaos in the ventricles.

   a. The patient immediately loses consciousness, becoming pulseless and apneic. Within minutes, death occurs unless there is prompt restoration of an organized rhythm.

   b. Immediate defibrillation is performed and Advanced Cardiac Life Support (ACLS) algorithm is followed.

5. Ventricular asystole, the complete absence of any ventricular rhythm. The patient is in full cardiac arrest and is treated with CPR and by following the ACLS algorithm.

- Atrioventricular (AV) conduction blocks exist when supraventricular impulses are excessively delayed or totally blocked in the AV node or intraventricular conduction system.

1. First-degree AV block: All sinus impulses eventually reach the ventricles; conduction is slowed.

   a. The patient usually has no symptoms, and no treatment is needed.

 b. If due to drug therapy, the offending drug is withheld and the health care provider notified.

 c. If associated with symptomatic bradycardia, oxygen is administered.

2. Second-degree AV block type I (AV Wenckebach or Mobitz type I): Each successive sinus impulse takes a little longer to conduct through the AV node, until one impulse is completely blocked and fails to depolarize the ventricles. The symptomatic patient is treated with oxygen and atropine; a pacemaker may be needed.

3. Second-degree AV block type II (Mobitz type II): The block is infranodal, occurring below the His bundle, and involves a constant block in one of the bundle branches; the impulse fails to reach the ventricle.

 a. Symptoms depend on the frequency of the dropped rate.

 b. If the patient is symptomatic, he or she is treated with prophylactic pacing to avert the threat of sudden third-degree heart block.

 c. A permanent pacemaker may be required.

4. Third-degree heart block (complete heart block): None of the sinus impulses conducts to the ventricles.

 a. Clinical manifestations depend on the overall ventricular rate and cardiac output and may have hemodynamic consequences such as light-headedness, confusion, syncope, seizures, hypotension, or cardiac arrest.

 b. Oxygen and atropine are given to the patient who is symptomatic; prophylactic pacing may be initiated.

5. Bundle branch block: A conduction delay or block occurs within one of the two main bundle branches below the bifurcation of the His bundle.

 a. There are no clinical manifestations and no specific interventions.

 b. A new bundle branch block may be an indicator of a recent MI; be alert to symptoms of acute coronary syndrome.

PATIENT-CENTERED COLLABORATIVE CARE

❖**NDx:** Decreased Cardiac Output and Ineffective Tissue Perfusion
Interventions

- The major interventions are to assess for complications and monitor the patient for response to treatment.

 1. Monitor the patient's electrocardiograph (ECG) and assess for signs and symptoms of dysrhythmias.

2. Assess apical and radial pulses for a full minute for any irregularity.
3. Management includes:
   a. Drug therapy
   b. Vagal maneuvers such as carotid sinus massage and Valsalva maneuvers
   c. Cardioversion
   d. Temporary or permanent pacing
   e. CPR or ACLS
   f. Defibrillation
   g. Radiofrequency catheter ablation
   h. Aneurysmectomy
   i. Coronary artery bypass grafting
   j. Insertion of an implantable cardioverter-defibrillator (ICD)

> 🔲 Critical Rescue ◆ Call the Rapid Response Team for an increase or onset in irregular pulses or rhythm when it is associated with a deterioration in consciousness or blood pressure. It may be an early sign of electrolyte disturbance, drug toxicity, or new myocardial injury.

Community-Based Care

- A case manager or care coordinator identifies the need for health care resources at home and coordinates access to the services.
- Discharge planning and health care resources:
  1. Provide information on lifestyle modifications including activity restrictions.
  2. Teach the patient and family the name, dosage, schedule, and side effects of drugs.
  3. Teach and observe the patient and family taking a pulse.
  4. Stress the importance of reporting chest discomfort, shortness of breath, and change in heart rhythm and rate to the health care provider.
  5. Post emergency numbers.
  6. Encourage the patient to follow diet instructions.
  7. Instruct the patient to keep all appointments with the health care provider.
  8. Encourage family members to learn CPR.
  9. Refer to the American Heart Association (AHA) or the provincial affiliate of the Heart and Stroke Foundation in Canada and other community agencies.

D

- Give the following special instructions to a patient with a pacemaker or ICD device:
  1. Give instructions on how to care for the pacemaker or ICD and how it functions (if appropriate) and the importance of reporting any fever or any redness, swelling, or drainage at the pacemaker or ICD insertion site.
  2. Keep your ICD identification card in your wallet and consider wearing a medical alert bracelet.
  3. Do not wear tight clothing or belts that could cause irritation over the site.
  4. Keep handheld cellular phones at least 6 inches away from the generator, with the handset on the ear opposite the side of the generator.
  5. Avoid sources of strong electromagnet fields such as large electrical generators and radio or television transmitters and radar.
  6. If you feel symptoms when you are near any device, move 5 to 10 feet away from it and check your pulse.
  7. Notify all health care providers, including your dentist, that you have a pacemaker or ICD device.
  8. Notify airport security personnel before passing through a metal detector (screening device) that you have a pacemaker or ICD, and show them your identification card.
  9. MRI is contraindicated.
- Give the following special instructions to a patient with a pacemaker:
  1. Take your pulse for 1 minute at the same time each day, and record the rate in your pacemaker diary.
  2. Take your pulse any time you feel symptoms of possible pacemaker failure, and report your heart rate and symptoms to your health care provider.
  3. Know the rate at which your pacemaker is set, and know the rate changes to report to your physician.
  4. Know the indications of battery failure, and report these findings to your health care provider.
  5. Check your pulse, and report any of the following symptoms to your health care provider: difficulty breathing, dizziness, fainting, chest pain, weight gain, and prolonged hiccupping.
  6. Do not operate electrical appliances directly over your pacemaker site because they may cause it to malfunction. Be sure electrical appliances are properly grounded.
  7. Do not lean over electrical or gasoline engines or motors.

- Give the following special instructions to a patient with an ICD:
  1. Sit or lie down immediately if you feel dizzy, faint, or light-headed.
  2. Avoid activities that involve rough contact with the ICD implantation site.
  3. Avoid sources of strong electromagnet fields such as large electrical generators and radio or television transmitters because they may inhibit tachydysrhythmia detection and therapy or may cause inadvertent antitachycardial pacing or shocks. If beeping tones are heard coming from the device, move away from the electromagnetic field immediately before the inactivation sequence is completed, and notify the health care provider.
  4. Report symptoms such as fainting, nausea, weakness, black-out, and rapid pulse to your health care provider.
  5. Know how to perform cough CPR as instructed.
  6. Notify your health care provider if your ICD device discharges.
  7. Avoid strenuous activities that may cause your heart rate to meet or exceed the rate cutoff of your ICD device because this causes the device to discharge inappropriately.

> 🔲 Critical Rescue ◆ Teach the patient to keep all appointments to assess the function and to interrogate any implanted cardioversion-defibrillator (ICD) device. Many of these devices also maintain records that can be accessed at the cardiology visit; the record can be used to understand the type, frequency, and duration of dysrhythmias and to adjust the device or medications.

> 🔲 Clinical Landmine ◆ Many antidysrhythmic drugs have a narrow safety range and dangerous side effects, and many interact with other medications. Avoid adding OTC or pre-scribed drugs to the patient's regimen without first ensuring that the prescriber is aware of the antidysrhythmic drug used.

ECTASIA, DUCTAL

- Ductal ectasia is a benign breast problem in women approaching menopause, caused by thickening and dilation of breast ducts.

- The ducts are blocked, becoming distended and filled with cellular debris, which activates an inflammatory response.
- Manifestations are a hard and tender mass with irregular borders; greenish brown nipple discharge; enlarged axillary nodes; and redness and edema over the mass.
- Ductal ectasia does increase breast cancer risk, but the mass may be difficult to distinguish from breast cancer.
- Because the risk for breast cancer is increased among women in the menopause age group, accurate diagnosis is vital.
- Nipple discharge is examined microscopically for any atypical or malignant cells.
- Warm compresses and antibiotics may be helpful in relieving symptoms and improving drainage.
- The affected area may be excised.
- Nursing interventions focus on reducing the anxiety and providing support through the diagnostic and treatment procedures.

ENCEPHALITIS

OVERVIEW

- Encephalitis, an inflammation of the brain parenchyma (brain tissue) and often the meninges, is most often caused by infective organisms:
  1. Arboviruses transmitted through the bite of an infected tick or mosquito
  2. Enteroviruses associated with mumps and chickenpox
  3. Herpes simplex virus type 1, which is the most common nonepidemic type
  4. Amoebae such as *Naegleria* and *Acanthamoeba*, found in warm freshwater, may also be involved.

PATIENT-CENTERED COLLABORATIVE CARE

Assessment

- Assessment findings include:
  1. Fever
  2. Nausea and vomiting
  3. Stiff neck; nuchal rigidity
  4. Decreased level of consciousness and impaired cognition
  5. Motor dysfunction
  6. Focal neurologic deficits
  7. Symptoms of increased intracranial pressure
  8. Ocular palsies
  9. Facial weakness

10. Abnormal cerebrospinal fluid analysis
11. Elevated WBC count

> 🔲 **Critical Rescue** ◆ Level of consciousness is the most sen-
> sitive indicator of neurologic status. Inform the physician of
> worsening cognition or decreased arousal, because this may
> mean worsening of acute neurologic disease.

Interventions
- The treatment for encephalitis is similar to that for
  meningitis.
  1. Maintain a patent airway; avoid aspiration.
  2. Encourage and assist the patient to reposition, and
     deep breathe frequently; suction if respiratory status is
     compromised.
  3. Monitor vital signs and neurologic signs, such as level of
     consciousness, orientation, pupil responses, and motor
     movement.
  4. Elevate the head of the bed 30 to 45 degrees.
  5. Administer acyclovir (Zovirax) for herpes encephalitis; no
     specific drug therapy is available for infection by arboviruses
     or enteroviruses.
  6. If there are permanent neurologic disabilities, the patient is
     discharged to a rehabilitation setting or a long-term care
     facility.

ENDOCARDITIS, INFECTIVE

OVERVIEW
- Infective endocarditis (previously called bacterial endocarditis)
  refers to a microbial infection (virus, bacterium, fungus) involving the endocardium.
- Infective endocarditis occurs primarily in patients who are
  IV drug abusers, have had cardiac valve replacements, have
  experienced systemic infection, or have structural cardiac
  defects.
- Portals of entry for infecting organisms include:
  1. Oral cavity, especially if dental procedures have been
     performed
  2. Skin rashes, lesions, or abscesses
  3. Infections (cutaneous, genitourinary or gastrointestinal,
     systemic)
  4. Surgical or invasive procedures, including IV line
     placement

PATIENT-CENTERED COLLABORATIVE CARE

Assessment

- Assessment findings include:
  1. Signs of infection, including fever, chills, malaise, night sweats, and fatigue
     a. Older adults may remain afebrile.
  2. Heart murmurs, usually regurgitant in nature
  3. Right-sided heart failure, evidenced by:
     a. Peripheral edema
     b. Weight gain
     c. Anorexia
  4. Left-sided heart failure, evidenced by:
     a. Fatigue
     b. Shortness of breath
     c. Crackles
  5. Evidence of arterial embolization from fragments of vegetation on valve leaflets, which may travel to other organs and compromise function
  6. Manifestations of acute embolization include:
     a. Splenic emboli: sudden abdominal pain and radiation to the left shoulder
     b. Kidney infarction: flank pain that radiates to the groin and is accompanied by hematuria or pyuria
     c. Mesenteric emboli: diffuse abdominal pain, often after eating and abdominal distention
     d. Brain emboli: signs of stroke, confusion, reduced concentration, and difficulty speaking
     e. Pulmonary emboli: pleuritic chest pain, dyspnea, and cough
  7. Petechiae of the neck, shoulders, wrists, ankles, mucous membranes, or conjunctivae
  8. Splinter hemorrhages, or black longitudinal lines or small red streaks in the nail bed
  9. Osler's nodes (reddish, tender lesions with a white center on the pads of the fingers, hands, and toes)
  10. Janeway's lesion (nontender hemorrhagic lesion found on the fingers, toes, nose, and earlobes)
  11. Positive blood culture
  12. Low hemoglobin level and hematocrit
  13. Abnormal transesophageal echocardiography

Interventions

- Interventions include:
  1. Administering IV antimicrobial therapy
  2. Monitoring the patient's tolerance to activity

3. Protecting the patient from contact with potentially infective organisms

4. Monitoring for signs of embolization, particularly decreased oxygenation, changes in mentation, and signs of acute coronary syndromes

- Surgical intervention includes removal of the infected valve, repair or removal of congenital shunts, repair of injured valves and chordae tendineae, and draining abscesses in the heart or elsewhere.

- Preoperative and postoperative care for the patient having surgery involving the valves is similar to that described for patients undergoing a coronary artery bypass grafting or valve replacement.

Community-Based Care

- Teach the patient and family:

1. Information on the cause of the disease and its course, drug regimens, signs and symptoms of infection, and practices to prevent future infections

2. How to administer IV antibiotic and care for the IV site, ensuring that all supplies are available to the patient discharged to home

3. The importance of good personal and oral hygiene, such as using a soft toothbrush, brushing the teeth twice each day, and rinsing the mouth with water after brushing

4. To avoid the use of dental irrigation devices and dental floss

5. To inform health care providers and dentists about the history of endocarditis so that prophylactic antibiotics are given before treatment

ENDOMETRIOSIS

OVERVIEW

- Endometriosis is a benign problem in which the endometrial (inner uterine) tissue implants *outside* the uterine cavity, most commonly on the ovaries and the cul-de-sac (posterior rectovaginal wall) and less commonly on other pelvic organs and structures.

- This tissue responds to cyclic hormonal stimulation just as if it were in the uterus.

- Monthly cyclic bleeding occurs at the site of implantation, where it is trapped, causing pain, irritation, scarring, and adhesion formation in the surrounding tissue.

- When endometriosis is on an ovary, a *chocolate cyst* can form.

- The cause of endometriosis is unknown.
- The disorder is most often found in women during their reproductive years and can lead to infertility.

PATIENT-CENTERED COLLABORATIVE CARE

Assessment
- Obtain patient information about:
  1. Menstrual history, sexual history, and bleeding characteristics
  2. Pain, which is the most common symptom of endometriosis
  3. Dyspareunia (painful sexual intercourse)
  4. Painful defecation
  5. Low backache
  6. Infertility
  7. GI disturbances
- Assess for and document:
  1. Pelvic tenderness
  2. Tender nodules in the posterior vagina and limited movement of the uterus
  3. Anxiety, because of uncertainty about the diagnosis and potential infertility
- Diagnostic studies may include:
  1. Tests to rule out pelvic inflammatory disease (PID) caused by chlamydia or gonorrhea
  2. Serum cancer antigen CA 125
  3. Transvaginal ultrasound
  4. Laparoscopy and biopsy

Interventions
Nonsurgical Management
- Hormonal contraceptives for cycle control
- NSAIDs to reduce prostaglandins secretion
- Hormonal suppressive therapy
  1. Gonadotropin-releasing hormone (GnRH) agonists (e.g., leuprolide [Lupron Depot])
  2. Androgenic agents (e.g., danazol [Danocrine])
  3. Antiestrogenic aromatase inhibitors

Surgical Management
- Surgical management of endometriosis with laser therapy through laparoscopy removes the implants and adhesions, allowing the woman to remain fertile.
- In women with intractable pain, severing a pelvic nerve may provide relief.
- If the patient does not wish to have children, the uterus and ovaries may be removed.

EPIDIDYMITIS

OVERVIEW

- *Epididymitis* is an inflammation of the epididymis, which may result from an infectious or noninfectious source such as trauma.
- Bacterial infection is the most common cause.
- It can be a complication of a sexually transmitted disease (STD), such as gonorrhea or chlamydia.
- Less often, it can be a complication of long-term use of an indwelling urinary catheter, prostatic surgery, or a cystoscopic examination.
- The major causative organism for men younger than 35 years is *Chlamydia trachomatis*.
- Main manifestations include pain along the inguinal canal and along the vas deferens, followed by pain and swelling in the scrotum and the groin.
- If untreated, the infection can spread and an abscess may form, requiring an orchiectomy (removal of one or both testes). If both testes are affected, sterility may result.

PATIENT-CENTERED COLLABORATIVE CARE

- Obtain patient information about:
  1. Pain along the inguinal canal
  2. Pain and swelling of the scrotum and groin
- Assess for and document:
  1. Pyuria
  2. Bacteruria
  3. Fever and chills
- Diagnosis is made on the basis of manifestations and a smear or culture of the urine or prostate secretions to identify the causative organism.
- Interventions include:
  1. Drug therapy
     a. Appropriate antibiotics
     b. NSAIDs to decrease inflammation and promote comfort
  2. Comfort measures, including:
     a. Staying in bed with the scrotum elevated
     b. Wearing a scrotal support when ambulating
     c. Applying cold compresses or ice to the scrotum intermittently
     d. Taking sitz baths
     e. Avoiding lifting, straining, or sexual activity until the infection is under control (which may take as long as 4 weeks)

- The sexual partner should be treated if the infection is caused by an STD.
- An epididymectomy (excision of the epididymis from the testicle) may be needed if the problem is recurrent or chronic.
- An ultrasound study often is done to rule out an abscess or tumor.

ERECTILE DYSFUNCTION

E

OVERVIEW

- Erectile dysfunction (ED) is the inability to achieve or maintain an erection for sexual intercourse.
- Organic ED is a gradual deterioration of function. The man first notices diminishing firmness and a decrease in frequency of erections. Causes include:
  1. Inflammation of the prostate, urethra, or seminal vesicles
  2. Surgical procedures such as prostatectomy
  3. Pelvic fractures
  4. Lumbosacral injuries
  5. Vascular disease, including hypertension
  6. Chronic neurologic conditions, such as Parkinson's disease or multiple sclerosis
  7. Endocrine disorders, such as diabetes mellitus or thyroid disorders
  8. Smoking and alcohol consumption
  9. Drugs
  10. Poor overall health that prevents sexual intercourse
- Functional ED usually has a psychologic cause. Men with functional ED have normal nocturnal (nighttime) and morning erections. Onset is usually sudden and preceded by a period of high stress.

PATIENT-CENTERED COLLABORATIVE CARE

- Assess the medical, social, and sexual history; determine if there is a medical or organic cause.
- Hormone testing is used for patients who have a poor libido, small testicles, or sparse beard growth.
- Serum levels of testosterone and gonadotropins are also measured.
- Duplex Doppler ultrasonography may be performed to determine the adequacy of arterial and venous blood flow to the penis.
- Functional ED is managed by sexual counseling and drugs that increase penile blood flow.

Nonsurgical Management
- Nonsurgical management of organic ED may include:
  1. Drug therapy to improve penile blood flow
     a. Sildenafil (Viagra)
     b. Vardenafil (Levitra)
     c. Tadalafil (Cialis)
     d. Instruct patients to abstain from alcohol before sexual intercourse because it may impair the ability to have an erection.
     e. Common side effects of these drugs include headaches, facial flushing, and diarrhea.
  2. Vacuum devices
     a. A vacuum device is a cylinder that fits over the penis, and a vacuum is created with a pump. The vacuum draws blood into the penis to maintain an erection.
     b. The advantage of this procedure is that the device is easy and safe to use regardless of what drugs the patient may be taking.
  3. Intracorporal injections
     a. Vasoconstrictive drugs can be injected directly into the penis to reduce blood outflow and make the penis erect.
     b. Common agents are papaverine, phentolamine (Regitine), and alprostadil.
     c. Adverse effects include priapism (prolonged erection), penile scarring, fibrosis, bleeding, bruising at the injection site, pain, infection, and vasovagal responses.
  4. Intraurethral applications
     a. Prostaglandin E (alprostadil [Muse]) is a self-administered suppository that is placed in the urethra and causes an erection in about 10 minutes.
     b. Advantages include the simplicity of the procedure and noninvasiveness.
     c. Disadvantages are a decrease in spontaneity, syncope, and burning of the urethra after the application.

Surgical Management
- Penile implants can be surgically placed when other modalities fail. Devices include semirigid, malleable, or hydraulic inflatable and multicomponent or one-piece instruments.
- Advantages include the man's ability to control his erections.
- The major disadvantages include device failure and infection.

FATIGUE SYNDROME, CHRONIC (CFS)

- Chronic fatigue syndrome (CFS), also known as chronic fatigue and immune dysfunction syndrome (CFIDS), is a chronic illness. Patients have severe fatigue for 6 months or longer, usually following flu-like symptoms.

- For a diagnosis of CSF, four or more of the following criteria must be met:
  1. Sore throat
  2. Substantial impairment in short-term memory or concentration
  3. Tender lymph nodes
  4. Muscle pain
  5. Multiple-joint pain with redness or swelling
  6. Headaches of a new type, pattern, or severity (not familiar to the patient)
  7. Unrefreshing sleep
  8. Postexertional malaise lasting more than 24 hours
- There is no test to confirm the disorder, and the cause is unknown.
- Management is supportive and focuses on alleviation or reduction of symptoms:
  1. NSAIDs for body aches and pain
  2. Low-dose antidepressants for promoting sleep and preventing or treating depression
  3. Teaching the patient to follow healthy practices:
     a. Adequate sleep
     b. Proper nutrition
     c. Regular exercise (but not excessive enough to increase fatigue)
     d. Stress management
     e. Energy conservation
  4. Use of complementary and alternative therapies
     a. Acupuncture
     b. Tai chi
     c. Massage
     d. Herbal supplements
- Refer the patient to the National Chronic Fatigue Syndrome and Fibromyalgia Association for information and support groups (*www.ncfsfa.org*).

FIBROMYALGIA SYNDROME

OVERVIEW

- Fibromyalgia is manifested by pain and tenderness at specific sites in the back of the neck, upper chest, trunk, low back, and extremities.
- The tender points (trigger points) can be palpated to elicit pain in a predictable, reproducible pattern.

- Other symptoms include:
  1. Mild to severe fatigue
  2. Sleep disturbances
  3. Numbness or tingling in the extremities
  4. Sensitivity to noxious odors, loud noises, and bright lights
  5. Headache and jaw pain
  6. GI manifestations: abdominal pain, diarrhea, constipation, and heartburn
  7. Genitourinary manifestations: dysuria, urinary frequency, urgency, and pelvic pain
  8. Cardiovascular manifestations: dyspnea, chest pain, and dysrhythmias
  9. Visual manifestations: blurred vision and dry eyes
- Interventions include:
  1. Antidepressive agents to promote sleep and reduce pain or muscle spasms
     a. Amitriptyline (Elavil, Apo-Amitriptylin ✤)
     b. Nortriptyline (Pamelor)
     c. Trazodone (Desyrel)
  2. Selective serotonin reuptake inhibitors for depression
     a. Sertraline (Zoloft)
     b. Escitalopram oxalate (Lexapro)
  3. NSAIDs
  4. Physical therapy
  5. Regular exercise, which includes stretching, strengthening, and low-impact aerobic exercise
  6. Complementary and alternative therapies such as tai chi, acupuncture, hypnosis, and stress management
- Refer the patient to the National Chronic Fatigue Syndrome and Fibromyalgia Association for additional information.

FISSURE, ANAL

- An anal fissure is a superficial erosion of the anal canal.
- Acute anal fissures are superficial and heal spontaneously with conservative treatment.
- Pain during and after defecation is the most common symptom, but bleeding may also occur.
- Other symptoms associated with chronic fissures are pruritus, urinary frequency or retention, dysuria, and dyspareunia.
- Diagnosis is made by physical examination.
- Nonsurgical interventions include local, symptomatic relief measures such as warm sitz baths, analgesics, and bulk-forming agents.

- Topical anti-inflammatories or opiate suppositories are helpful if spasms are severe.
- Surgical excision of the fissure may be necessary if the fissures do not respond to medical management.

FISTULA, ANAL

- An anal fistula, or fistula in ano, is an abnormal tract leading from the anal canal to the perianal skin.
- Most anal fistulas result from anorectal abscesses, but they can be associated with tuberculosis, Crohn's disease, cancer, or AIDs.
- Symptoms include pruritus, purulent discharge, and tenderness or pain aggravated by bowel movements.
- Because fistulas do not heal spontaneously, surgery (fistulotomy) is necessary.
- Pain relief measures, such as sitz baths, flushable wipes, analgesics, and stool softeners, are used to reduce tissue trauma and discomfort.
- Hygiene is important; clean the anal area after each bowel movement.
- Avoid constipation and straining with stool.

FLAIL CHEST

OVERVIEW

- Flail chest is the inward movement of the thorax during inspiration, with outward movement during expiration, usually involving only one side of the chest.
- It results from multiple rib fractures or ribs fractured in more than one place caused by blunt chest trauma leaving a segment of the chest wall loose.
- Flail chest often occurs in high-speed vehicular crashes. Another cause is bilateral separations of the ribs from their cartilage connections without an actual rib fracture during cardiopulmonary resuscitation (CPR).
- Gas exchange, the ability to cough, and the ability to clear secretions are impaired.

PATIENT-CENTERED COLLABORATIVE CARE

- Assess the patient for and document:
  1. Paradoxical chest movement ("sucking inward" of the loose chest area during inspiration and a "puffing out" of the same area during expiration)

  2. Pain
  3. Dyspnea
  4. Cyanosis
  5. Tachycardia
  6. Hypotension
- Interventions include:
  1. Humidified oxygen
  2. Pain management
  3. Promotion of lung expansion through deep breathing and positioning
  4. Secretion clearance by coughing and tracheal aspiration
  5. Psychosocial support
  6. Intubation with mechanical ventilation and positive end-expiratory pressure (PEEP)
  7. Surgical stabilization (only in extreme cases of flail chest)
- Monitor the patient's:
  1. Vital signs
  2. Oxygen saturation and arterial blood gases
  3. Fluid and electrolyte balance
  4. Central venous pressure (CVP)

FLUID OVERLOAD

OVERVIEW

- Fluid overload, also called overhydration, is an excess of body fluid, not a disease. It is a clinical sign of a problem in which fluid intake or retention is greater than the body's fluid needs.
- Fluid overload may be an actual excess of total body fluid or a relative fluid excess.
- The most common type of fluid overload is hypervolemia because the problems result from excessive fluid in the extracellular fluid (ECF) space.
- Most problems caused by fluid overload are related to fluid volume excess in the vascular space or to dilution of specific electrolytes and blood components.
- Causes of fluid overload are related to excessive intake or inadequate excretion of fluid and include:
  1. Excessive fluid replacement
  2. Kidney failure (late phase)
  3. Heart failure
  4. Long-term corticosteroid therapy
  5. Syndrome of inappropriate antidiuretic hormone (SIADH)
  6. Psychiatric disorders with polydipsia
  7. Water intoxication

PATIENT-CENTERED COLLABORATIVE CARE

Assessment

- Assess for and document:
  1. Cardiovascular changes
     a. Bounding pulse quality
     b. Peripheral pulses full
     c. Elevated blood pressure
     d. Decreased pulse pressure
     e. Elevated central venous pressure
     f. Distended neck and hand veins
     g. Engorged varicose veins
     h. Weight gain
  2. Respiratory changes
     a. Respiratory rate increased
     b. Shallow respirations
     c. Dyspnea increases with exertion or in the supine position
     d. Moist crackles present on auscultation
  3. Skin and mucous membrane changes
     a. Pitting edema in dependent areas
     b. Skin pale and cool to touch
  4. Neuromuscular changes
     a. Altered level of consciousness
     b. Headache
     c. Visual disturbances
     d. Skeletal muscle weakness
     e. Paresthesias
  5. Gastrointestinal changes
     a. Increased motility
     b. Enlarged liver
- Diagnosis of fluid overload is based on assessment findings and the results of laboratory tests. Usually, serum electrolyte values are normal, but decreased hemoglobin, hematocrit, and serum protein levels may result from excessive water in the vascular space (hemodilution).

Interventions

- Management of patients with fluid overload aims to ensure patient safety, restore normal fluid balance, provide supportive care until the imbalance is resolved, and prevent future fluid overload.
  1. Patient safety to prevent fluid overload from becoming worse, leading to pulmonary edema and heart failure
     a. Monitor for indicators of increased fluid overload at least every 2 hours.

> 🔄 **Critical Rescue** ◆ Pulmonary edema can occur very
> quickly and can lead to death. Notify the health care provider
> of any change that indicates the fluid overload is not respond-
> ing to therapy or is becoming worse.

    b. Use a pressure-reducing or pressure-relieving overlay on
the mattress.

    c. Assess skin pressure areas, especially the coccyx, elbows,
hips, and heels, daily for signs of redness or open areas.

    d. Assist the patient to change positions every 2 hours.

2. Drug therapy focuses on removing the excess fluid (diuretics,
conivaptan [Vaprisol]).

    a. Monitor the patient's response to drug therapy.

       (1) Weight loss

       (2) Increased urine output

    b. Observe for manifestations of electrolyte imbalance.

       (1) Changes in electrocardiographic (ECG) patterns

       (2) Changes in sodium and potassium values

3. Nutritional therapy

    a. Sodium restriction

    b. Fluid restriction

FOOD POISONING

- Food poisoning is caused by ingestion of infectious organisms
in food.
- Prevention occurs with hand washing, properly handling, and
processing food.
- There are three common types of food poisoning.

1. Staphylococcal food poisoning

    a. *Staphylococcus* grows in meats and dairy products and can
be transmitted by human carriers.

    b. Symptoms of staphylococcal infection include abrupt
onset of vomiting, diarrhea, and abdominal cramping,
usually 2 to 4 hours after the ingestion of contaminated
food.

    c. The diagnosis is made when stool culture yields 100,000
enterotoxin-producing staphylococci.

    d. Treatment includes oral or IV fluids if the fluid volume is
grossly depleted.

2. *Escherichia coli* infection

    a. Increasingly, *E. coli* is associated with food poisoning.

    b. Symptoms include vomiting, diarrhea, abdominal cramp-
ing, and fever.

    c. Treatment includes IV fluids and antibiotic therapy.

3. Botulism
  a. Botulism is a severe, life-threatening food poisoning associated with a high mortality rate; it is most commonly acquired from improperly processed canned foods.
  b. The incubation period is 18 to 36 hours, and the illness may be mild or severe.
  c. *Clostridium botulinum* enters the bloodstream from the intestines and causes symptoms of diplopia, dysphagia, dysphonia, respiratory muscle paralysis, nausea, vomiting, and diarrhea or constipation.
  d. The diagnosis is made by the history and stool culture revealing *C. botulinum*; the serum may be positive for toxins.
  e. Treatment of botulism includes trivalent botulism antitoxin (ABE), stomach lavage, IV fluids, and tracheostomy with mechanical ventilation if respiratory paralysis occurs.
  f. To prevent botulism, discard cans of food that are punctured, are swollen, or have defective seals. Discard glass containers with visible air bubbles in liquid.

- *Salmonellosis* is a bacterial infection that is classified as a food poisoning or gastroenteritis.
  1. Incubation is 8 to 48 hours after ingestion of contaminated food or drink.
  2. Fever, nausea, vomiting, cramping abdominal pain, and severe diarrhea, which may be bloody, last 3 to 5 days.
  3. Diagnosis is made by stool culture.
  4. Treatment is based on symptoms.
  5. Salmonellosis can be transmitted by the *five Fs*: flies, fingers, food, feces, and fomites; strict handwashing is essential to avoid transmission.

FRACTURE, NASAL

OVERVIEW

- A nasal fracture often results from injuries received during falls, sports activities, motor vehicle accidents, or physical assaults.
- Bone or cartilage displacement can cause airway obstruction or cosmetic deformity and is a potential source of infection.

PATIENT-CENTERED COLLABORATIVE CARE

Assessment

- Assess for and document:
  1. Deviation or malalignment of the nasal bridge
  2. Change in nasal breathing

3. Crackling of the skin (crepitus) on palpation
4. Midface bruising and pain
5. Blood or clear cerebrospinal fluid (CSF) draining from one or both nares

> **⬛ Critical Rescue** ◆ CSF drainage may indicate a skull fracture. CSF can be differentiated from normal nasal secretions because CSF contains glucose that tests positive with a dipstick. When CSF dries on a piece of filter paper, a yellow halo appears as a ring at the dried edge of the fluid. Immediately report positive findings to the health care provider.

Interventions

- Management for a simple fracture is usually a closed reduction performed by the health care provider, using local or general anesthesia, within the first 24 hours after injury.
- Teach the patient to use cold compresses for pain relief and to reduce swelling.
- Management of more severe fractures may require surgery.
  1. Rhinoplasty, a surgical reconstruction of the nose for cosmetic purposes and to improve airflow
     a. Packing is in place with a "moustache" dressing (or drip pad) under the nose.
     b. A splint or cast may cover the nose for better alignment and protection.
     c. Nursing care involves:
        (1) Observing for edema and bleeding
        (2) Checking vital signs every 4 hours until the patient is discharged
        (3) Assessing how often the patient swallows
        (4) Examining the throat with a penlight for bleeding
        (5) Teaching the patient to:
           (i)   Stay in semi-Fowler position.
           (ii)   Move slowly.
           (iii) Rest.
           (iv)   Use cool compresses on the nose, eyes, or face.
           (v)   Drink at least 2500 mL/day.
           (vi)   Limit Valsalva maneuvers (e.g., forceful coughing, straining during a bowel movement).
           (vii) Not to sniff upward or blow the nose.
           (viii) Avoid aspirin and NSAIDs.
  2. Nasoseptoplasty or submucous resection (SMR) straightens a deviated septum. Nursing care is similar to that for a rhinoplasty.

FRACTURES

OVERVIEW

- A fracture is a break or disruption in the continuity of a bone.
- Fractures are classified as complete or incomplete.
  1. *Complete fracture:* The break is across the entire width of the bone in such a way that the bone is divided into two distinct sections.
  2. *Incomplete fracture:* The fracture does not divide the bone into two portions because the break is through only part of the bone.
- Fractures can also be described by the extent of associated soft-tissue damage.
  1. A *simple fracture* does not extend through the skin and therefore has no visible wound.
  2. An *open (compound) fracture* has a disrupted skin surface that causes an external wound. These fractures are often graded to define the extent of tissue damage.
     a. Grade I is the least severe injury, and skin damage is minimal.
     b. Grade II is accompanied by skin and muscle contusions.
     c. Grade III has damage to skin, muscle, nerve tissue, and blood vessels.
- Fractures are also defined by their cause.
  1. *Pathologic (spontaneous) fractures* occur after minimal trauma to a bone that has been weakened by disease.
  2. *Fatigue (stress) fractures* result from excessive strain and stress on the bone.
  3. *Compression fractures* are produced by a loading force applied to the long axis of cancellous bone.
- Bone healing occurs in five stages.
  1. Stage 1 occurs within 24 to 72 hours after the injury with hematoma formation at the site of the fracture.
  2. Stage 2 occurs in 3 days to 2 weeks when granulation tissue begins to invade the hematoma, stimulating the formation of fibrocartilage.
  3. Stage 3 of bone healing usually occurs within 2 to 6 weeks as a result of vascular and cellular proliferation. The fracture site is surrounded by new vascular tissue known as a callus that begins the nonbony union.
  4. Stage 4 usually takes 3 to 6 months and results in gradual resorption of the callus with transformation into bone.
  5. Stage 5 consists of bone consolidation and remodeling. This stage may start as early as 6 weeks after fracture and can continue for up to 1 year.

Considerations for Older Adults

- Bone formation and strength rely on adequate nutrition, especially calcium, phosphorus, vitamin D, and protein.
- For women, the loss of estrogen after menopause is detrimental to the body's ability to form new bone tissue.
- Other diseases, such as arteriosclerosis, reduce arterial circulation to bone. The bone receives less oxygen and reduced amounts of nutrients, both of which are needed for repair.
- Acute complications of fractures
  1. *Acute compartment syndrome* (ACS) is a serious condition in which increased pressure within one or more tissue compartments causes massive compromise of circulation to the area. The most common sites for the problem in patients experiencing musculoskeletal trauma are the compartments in the lower leg and forearm. Edema fluid forms and is trapped within the compartment pressing on nerves (causing pain) and blood vessels, preventing adequate tissue perfusion and oxygenation. Without treatment, ACS can lead to infection, loss of motor function, contracture formation, and release of myoglobin leading to renal failure. Treatment is by surgical fasciotomy.

> **Critical Rescue** ◆ Monitor for early signs of ACS by assessing for the *six Ps*: pain, pressure, paralysis, paresthesia, pallor, and pulselessness. Report these findings to the surgeon immediately.

  2. *Crush syndrome* (CS) results from an external crush injury that compresses one or more compartments in the leg, arm, or pelvis. It is a potentially life-threatening, systemic complication that results from hemorrhage and edema after a severe fracture injury. Management involves early recognition and adequate IV fluids, diuretics, and low-dose dopamine to enhance renal perfusion. When not managed, results of this syndrome include:
     a. Acute compartment syndrome
     b. Hypovolemia
     c. Hyperkalemia
     d. Rhabdomyolysis (myoglobulin released from skeletal muscle into the bloodstream)
     e. Acute tubular necrosis (ATN) and kidney failure
     f. Dark brown urine
     g. Muscle weakness and pain

3. *Hypovolemic shock* may occur with a fracture as a result of damage to bone blood vessels or the severing nearby arteries.

4. *Fat embolism syndrome* (FES) is a serious complication in which fat globules are released from the yellow bone marrow into the bloodstream within 12 to 48 hours after an injury. These emboli clog small blood vessels that supply vital organs, most commonly the lungs, and impair organ perfusion. FES usually results from long bone fractures and pelvic bone or fracture repair, but it is occasionally seen in patients who have a total joint replacement. Manifestations include decreased level of consciousness (LOC), anxiety, respiratory distress, tachycardia, tachypnea, fever, hemoptysis, and petechiae, a macular, measles-like rash that may appear over the neck, upper arms, or chest and abdomen.

5. *Venous thromboembolism* (VTE) includes deep vein thrombosis (DVT) and its major complication, pulmonary embolism (PE). It is the most common complication of lower extremity surgery or trauma and the most common fatal complication of musculoskeletal surgery.

6. Infection is possible with fractures because the trauma disrupts the body's defense system. Wound infections may range from superficial skin infections to deep wound abscesses. Bone infection, or *osteomyelitis*, is most common with open fractures in which skin integrity is lost and after surgical repair of a fracture.

- Chronic complications of fractures
  1. *Ischemic necrosis*, sometimes referred to as *aseptic* or *avascular necrosis* (AVN) or *osteonecrosis,* can occur when the blood supply to the bone is disrupted and bone death follows.
  2. *Delayed union* is a fracture that has not healed within 6 months of injury. Some fractures never achieve union; that is, they never completely heal (*nonunion*). Others heal incorrectly (*malunion*).

PATIENT-CENTERED COLLABORATIVE CARE

Assessment

- Assess pain level and if the patient is in severe pain, delay the interview until he or she is more comfortable.
- Obtain patient information about:
  1. Cause of the fracture
  2. Events leading to the fracture and the immediate postinjury care
  3. Drug history, including substance abuse (recreational drug use) and alcohol abuse

    4. Medical history
    5. Occupation and recreational activities
    6. Nutritional history
- Assess for and document:
    1. Life-threatening complications of the respiratory, cardiovascular, and neurologic systems (priority assessment)
    2. Fracture site
        a. Change in bone alignment
        b. Shortening of change in bone shape
        c. ROM
        d. Presence of increased pain on movement, crepitus, bruising or bleeding, subcutaneous emphysema, swelling

> 📋 Critical Rescue ◆ If pain occurs when the patient moves the body part or area below the injury, stop the movement immediately.

    3. Neurovascular function on the affected and unaffected extremity
        a. Skin color and temperature
        b. Sensation
        c. Mobility
        d. Pain
        e. Pulses distal to the fracture site
        f. Nail beds for capillary refill
    4. Degree of soft-tissue damage
    5. Amount of overt bleeding
    6. Muscle spasm
- Special assessment considerations include:
    1. Factures of the shoulder and upper arm are assessed with the patient in a sitting or standing position, if possible, so that shoulder drooping or other abnormal positioning can be seen.
    2. More distal areas of the arm are assessed with the patient in a supine position so that the extremity can be elevated to reduce swelling.
    3. Place the patient in a supine position for assessment of the lower extremities and pelvis.
    4. Pelvic fractures can cause internal organ damage resulting in hemorrhage. When a pelvic fracture is suspected, assess vital signs, skin color, and the level of consciousness for indications of shock. Check the urine for blood, which indicates damage to the urinary system, often the bladder.
- Psychosocial assessment depends on the extent of the injury and other complications.

- Stresses that result from a chronic condition affect relationships between the patient and family members or friends, body image, sexuality, and financial resources.
- Diagnostic tests for fractures may include:
  1. Standard x-rays and tomograms
  2. CT scans
  3. MRI

Planning and Implementation

❖**NDx:** Risk For Peripheral Neurovascular Dysfunction

> 🔲 Critical Rescue ◆ For any patient who experiences trauma, first assess for respiratory distress, bleeding, and head injury. If any of these conditions is present, provide lifesaving care before being concerned about the fracture. In the community setting, provide emergency interventions until medical treatment in a hospital is available, or call 911 for the emergency team (first responders).

- After lifesaving care is completed, provide emergency fracture care.
  1. Assess the fracture.
  2. Control bleeding.
  3. Check vital signs.
  4. Place the patient in a supine position.
  5. Keep the patient warm.
  6. Immobilize the area of the fracture by splinting.
  7. Place sterile gauze loosely over the open area of a compound fracture.
  8. Recheck neurovascular status after splinting.

Nonsurgical Management
- Fracture management begins with reduction (realignment of the bone ends for proper healing) and immobilization of the fracture.
  1. *Closed reduction* is the manipulation of the bone ends for realignment while applying a manual pull, or traction, on the bone.
  2. *Bandages, splints, or commercial immobilizers* may be used to immobilize certain areas of the body, such as the scapula and clavicle.
  3. *Casts* are rigid devices that immobilize the affected body part while allowing other body parts to move. They are used to hold bone fragments in place after reduction for more complex fractures or fractures of the lower extremity. A cast allows early mobility, correction of deformity, prevention of deformity, and reduction of pain.

- Cast materials include:
  1. Plaster-of-Paris
     a. Requires application of a well-fitted stockinette under the padding material
     b. Takes 24 to 72 hours to dry
     c. Feels warm or hot immediately after application
     d. Is heavy and may have rough edges that require "petaling"
     e. Can be misshaped if handled incorrectly while drying
        (1) Do not cover casts until dry.
        (2) Handle cast with palms of hands rather than fingers until dry.
        (3) Turn patient every 1 to 2 hours to facilitate cast drying.
     f. Can bear more weight than synthetic cast materials
  2. Fiberglass, which is lightweight, dries in 10 to 15 minutes, and can bear weight 30 minutes after application, is most often used on upper extremities.
  3. Polyester-cotton knit casts, which take 7 minutes to dry and can withstand weight bearing in about 20 minutes, are most often used on upper extremities.
- Types of casts include:
  1. Arm cast
     a. When a patient is in bed, elevate the arm above the heart to reduce swelling; the hand should be higher than the elbow.
     b. When the patient is out of bed, support the arm with a sling placed around the neck so that the weight is distributed over a large area of the shoulders and trunk, not just the neck.
  2. Leg cast
     a. Leg casts allow mobility and require the patient to use ambulatory aids such as crutches.
     b. A cast shoe, sandal, or boot that attaches to the foot or a rubber walking pad attached to the sole of the cast assists in ambulation (if weight bearing is allowed) and helps prevent damage to the cast.
     c. Elevate the affected leg on pillows when the patient is in bed or in a chair to reduce swelling.
  3. Cast brace
     a. This device enables the patient to bend unaffected joints while the fracture is healing. The fracture must show signs of healing and minimal tissue edema before application of this cast.

b. As healing occurs, the cast may be removed and replaced with a soft brace.
4. Body and spica cast
   a. A body cast encircles the trunk of the body, whereas a spica cast encases a portion of the trunk and one or two extremities.
   b. The patient is at risk for skin breakdown, pneumonia or atelectasis, constipation, and joint contractures.
   c. *Cast syndrome* (superior mesenteric artery syndrome) is a serious complication in which partial or complete upper intestinal obstruction can occur and cause abdominal distention, epigastric pain, nausea, and vomiting. Placing a window in the abdominal portion of the cast or bivalving the cast may be sufficient to relieve pressure on the duodenum.

- Cast care involves:
  1. Handling a wet cast carefully with the palms of the hands to prevent indentations and resultant pressure areas on the patient's skin
  2. Preventing skin irritation from rough cast edges by petaling the cast with the placement of small strips of tape over the rough edges
  3. Cutting a window (done by the health care provider, orthopedic technician, or specially trained nurse) into the cast over a wound so that the wound can be observed and cared for
  4. Ensuring that the cast is not too tight by inserting a finger between the cast and the skin
  5. Notifying the health care provider when the cast is too tight so that it can be cut with a cast cutter to relieve pressure or allow tissue swelling. The cast may be bivalved (cut lengthwise into two equal pieces) if bone healing is almost complete. Either half of the cast can be removed for inspection or for provision of care. The two halves are then held in place by an elastic bandage wrap.
  6. Protecting the cast in the perineal area from becoming contaminated with urine or feces by encasing the area in plastic before the patient uses the urinal or bedpan
  7. Assisting the patient in a body cast or long-leg cast to use a fracture bedpan
  8. Monitoring the patient's neurovascular status distal to the cast every hour for the first 24 hours
  9. Inspecting the cast daily (after it is dry) for drainage, cracking, crumbling, alignment, and fit

    a. Describing and documenting any drainage on the cast in the medical record

    b. Notifying the health care provider immediately about any sudden increases in the amount of drainage or change in the integrity of the cast

10. Smelling the cast for foul odor and palpating it for hot areas every shift

11. Assessing for and reporting complications from casting:
    a. Infection
    b. Circulation impairment
    c. Peripheral nerve damage
    d. Skin breakdown
    e. Pneumonia or atelectasis
    f. Thromboembolism
    g. Joint contracture
    h. Muscle atrophy

- Traction is the application of a pulling force to a part of the body to provide reduction, alignment, and rest. It is also used to decrease muscle spasm and prevent or correct deformity and tissue damage.

1. Categories of traction
    a. *Running traction* provides a pulling force in one direction, and the patient's body acts as countertraction. Moving the body or bed position can alter the countertraction force.

    b. *Balanced suspension* provides the countertraction so that the pulling force of the traction is not altered when the bed or patient is moved. This allows for increased movement and facilitates care.

2. Types of traction
    a. *Skin traction* involves the use of a Velcro boot (Buck's traction), belt, or halter, securely placed around a body part to decrease painful muscle spasms. Weight is limited to 5 to 10 pounds (2.3 to 4.5 kg) to prevent injury to the skin.

    b. *Skeletal traction* uses pins, wires, tongs, or screws that are surgically inserted directly into bone to allow the use of longer traction time and heavier weights usually 15 to 30 pounds (6.8 to 13.6 kg). It aids in bone realignment.

    c. *Plaster traction* combines skeletal traction and a plaster cast.

    d. *Brace traction* is a device that exerts a pull for correction of alignment deformities.

    e. *Circumferential traction* uses a belt around the body, such as pelvic traction for low back problems.

3. Care for the patient in traction includes:
   a. Maintaining correct balance between traction pull and countertraction force

> **Clinical Landmine** ◆ Do not remove weights without a prescription. Do not lift them manually or allow them to set on the floor. Weights should be freely hanging at all times, with the ropes knotted securely.

   b. Inspecting the skin at least every 8 hours for signs of irritation or inflammation
   c. Removing (when possible) the belt or boot that is used for skin traction every 8 hours to inspect under the device
   d. Inspecting the points of entry of pins and wires or pin sites for signs of inflammation or infection at least every 8 hours
   e. Following agency policy for how to clean the pin site areas and ensure that it follows the evidence-based guidelines from the National Association of Orthopaedic Nurses
   f. Checking traction equipment to ensure its proper functioning and inspecting all ropes, knots, and pulleys at least every 8 to 12 hours for loosening, fraying, and positioning
   g. Checking the weight for consistency with the health care provider's prescription
   h. Replacing the weights if they are not correct and notifying the health care provider or orthopedic technician
   i. Reporting patient complaints of severe pain from muscle spasm to the health care provider when body realignment fails to reduce the discomfort
   j. Assessing neurovascular status of the affected body at least every 4 hours, or more often if indicated

Surgical Management

- *Open reduction with internal fixation* (ORIF) permits early mobilization. Open reduction allows direct visualization of the fracture site, and internal fixation uses metal pins, screws, rods, plates, or prostheses to immobilize the fracture during healing. An incision is made to gain access to the broken bone and allow implanting one or more devices into bone tissue.
- *External fixation* involves fracture reduction and the percutaneous implantation of pins may into the bone. The pins are then held in place by an external metal frame to prevent bone movement.
  1. Advantages of external fixation include:
     a. Minimal blood loss
     b. Early ambulation and exercise of the affected body

    c. Maintaining alignment in closed fractures that will not maintain position in a cast

    d. Stabilization of comminuted fractures that require bone grafting

  2. A disadvantage of external fixation is the increased risk for pin site infection and osteomyelitis.

- Provide preoperative care, including:
  1. Routine preoperative care as described in Part One
  2. Teaching the patient about what to expect during and after the surgery
  3. Applying Buck's traction before surgery for a fractured hip
  4. Teaching the patient and family about alterations to clothing that may be required when a large, external fixator is in place

- Provide postoperative care, including:
  1. Routine postoperative care as described in Part One
  2. Monitoring neurovascular status at least every hour for the first 24 hours after surgery and then as often as agency policy, surgeon preference, and patient condition indicate
  3. Assessing for and reporting complications

- Additional procedures may be needed when surgical repairs are not successful and the bone does not heal (nonunion).
  1. *Electrical bone stimulation* may be noninvasive or invasive. It involves using electrical current simulators near or into a fracture site. This procedure, when used for about 6 months, has resulted in bone healing for some patients.
  2. *Bone grafting* is the use of bone chips from the patient, a cadaver donor, or a living donor and packing or wiring the chips between the bone ends to facilitate union.
  3. *Low-intensity pulsed ultrasound (Exogen therapy)* involves the application of ultrasound treatments for about 20 minutes each day to the fracture site.

❖**NDx:** Acute Pain
- Drug therapy
  1. Opioid and non-opioid analgesics

> 🦟 **Clinical Landmine** ◆ Meperidine should never be used for older adults because it has toxic metabolites that can cause seizures and other complications.

  2. Anti-inflammatory drugs
  3. Muscle relaxants
  4. Complementary and alternative therapies
    a. Ice or heat
    b. Elevation of the affected body part

  c. Supporting the extremity with pillows
  d. Rest and quiet
  e. Music
  f. Massage
  g. Warm, soothing bath
  h. Therapeutic touch
  i. Distraction
  j. Imagery
  5. More interventions for pain are presented in Part One.

❖**NDx:** Risk for Infection

- When caring for a patient with an open fracture, use strict aseptic technique for dressing changes and wound irrigations.
- Immediately notify the health care provider if you observe inflammation and purulent drainage.
- Monitor the patient's vital signs every 4 to 8 hours because increases in temperature and pulse often indicate systemic infection.

> 🔧 **Critical Rescue** ◆ Older adults may not have a temperature elevation, even in the presence of severe infection. Use other indicators of infection.

- Administer prescribed prophylactic or indicated antibiotics.
- Perform vacuum-assisted closure (VAC) technique, if prescribed.

❖**NDx:** Impaired Physical Mobility

- Nursing interventions to prevent complications of impaired mobility focus on assessing for complications in immobilized patients with fractures.
- Nursing interventions to increase mobility include:
  1. Reinforcing the teaching provided by the physical therapist regarding the use of ambulatory aids
  2. Evaluating whether the patient is using the ambulatory aid correctly
- Types of ambulatory aids include:
  1. *Crutches*, which require strong arms, balance, and coordination
     a. To prevent pressure on the axillary nerve, there should be two to three fingerbreadths between the axilla and the top of the crutch when the crutch tip is at least 6 inches (15 cm) diagonally in front of the foot.
     b. The crutch is adjusted so that the elbow is flexed no more than 30 degrees when the palm is on the handle.
     c. The most common gait for crutch walking after musculoskeletal injury is the three-point gait, which allows minimal weight bearing on the affected leg.

2. *Walkers*, which are most often used by the older patient who needs additional support for balance
3. *Canes*, which are used when only minimal support is needed for an affected leg
   a. The cane is placed on the *unaffected* side.
   b. It should create no more than 30 degrees of flexion of the elbow.
   c. The top of the cane should be parallel to the greater trochanter of the femur.

❖**NDx:** Imbalanced Nutrition: Less Than Body Requirements

- Collaborate with the nutritionist to focus on meeting the patient's nutritional needs.
  1. Assess the patient's food likes and dislikes.
  2. Work with the nutritionist to plan meals that are both appealing and nutritional (high-protein, high-calorie diet).
  3. Administer supplements of vitamins B, C, and D, as prescribed.
  4. Urge the patient to increase the intake of foods high in calcium, particularly milk and milk products to reduce the risk for hypocalcemia.
  5. Urge the patient to increase intake of foods high in iron content to prevent anemia. A daily multivitamin with iron supplement may be prescribed.

Community-Based Care

- Collaborate with the case manager or the discharge planner in the hospital to plan care for the patient with a fracture who is being discharged.

🛡 National Patient Safety Goal

Be sure to communicate the plan of care to the health care agency receiving the patient.

- Provide continuity of care, including:
  1. Identifying structural barriers to mobility in the home
  2. Ensuring the patient has easy access to the bathroom
  3. Assessing for environmental factors contributing to falls
     a. Scatter rugs
     b. Waxed floors
     c. Walkway areas
  4. Assessing the patient's ability to safely use a wheelchair or ambulatory aid
  5. Arranging for a home health care nurse to make one or two visits to check that the home is safe and that the patient and family are able to follow the interdisciplinary plan of care
  6. Providing verbal and written instructions on the care of bandages, splints, casts, or external fixators

7. Referring the patient and family for assistance with financial issues, understanding the long-term nature of the recovery period, job counseling, possible professional counseling
8. Emphasizing the importance of follow-up visits with the health care provider and other therapists

- Teach the patient and family about:
  1. Care of the extremity after removal of the cast
     a. Remove scaly, dead skin carefully by soaking; do not scrub.
     b. Move the extremity carefully. Expect discomfort, weakness, and decreased ROM.
     c. Support the extremity with pillows or your orthotic device until strength and movement return.
     d. Exercise slowly as instructed by your physical therapist.
     e. Wear support stockings or elastic bandages to prevent swelling (for lower extremity).
  2. Wound assessment and dressing
  3. Recognition of complications
  4. When and where to seek professional health care if complications occur

FRACTURES OF SPECIFIC SITES

- *Clavicular, self-healing*: A splint or bandage is used for immobilization.
- *Scapular*: Immobilization with a commercial immobilizer is used until the fracture heals, usually in 2 to 4 weeks.
- *Proximal humerus*: When impacted, the injury is usually treated conservatively with a sling for immobilization; when displaced, the fracture often requires open reduction with internal fixation (ORIF) with pins or a prosthetic device.
- *Humeral shaft*: Correction is achieved by closed reduction and application of a hanging-arm cast or splint.
- *Elbow (olecranon)*: Is corrected by closed reduction and application of a cast. ORIF is performed for displaced fractures, and a splint is worn during the healing phase.
- *Forearm*: The ulna without accompanying injury is corrected with closed reduction and casting. If it is displaced, ORIF with intramedullary rods or plates and screws is required.
- *Wrist and hand:* Injury is most commonly to the carpal scaphoid bone, which is corrected by closed reduction and casting for 6 to 12 weeks. If the bone does not heal, ORIF with bone grafting is performed.
- *Colles' (wrist) fracture*: Fracture of the last inch of the distal radius is managed by casting for 6 to 8 weeks.

- *Metacarpals and phalanges (fingers)*: Metacarpal fractures are immobilized for 3 to 4 weeks. Phalangeal fractures are immobilized in finger splints for 10 to 14 days.
- *Hip-intracapsular*: Involves the upper third of the femur within the joint capsule. Hip-extracapsular: involves the upper third of the femur outside of the joint capsule. Injury is managed by surgical repair, depending on the exact location of the fracture; ORIF may include an intramedullary rod, pins, prostheses (for femoral head or neck fractures), or a compression screw. Buck's traction may be applied before surgery.

Considerations for Older Adults

- Older adults are at risk for hip fracture because of physiologic aging changes, reduced vision, disease processes, drug therapy, and environmental hazards.
- These fractures occur most often in older women with osteoporosis.
- Other disease processes, such as foot disorders and changes in cardiac function, increase the risk for hip fracture.
- Drugs such as diuretics, cardiac drugs, antidepressants, sedatives, opioids, and alcohol are factors that increase the risks for falling in older adults. Use of three or more drugs at the same time drastically increases the risk for falls.
- The older adult is more likely to have complications from the fracture and its management.
- Although older patients recover fully from hip fracture repair and regain their functional ability, some patients are not able to return to their pre-fracture ADLs and mobility level.

- *Lower two thirds of the femur:* Usually managed surgically by ORIF with nails, rods, or a compression screw. When extensive bone fragmentation or severe tissue trauma is found, external fixation may be employed.
- *Patellar* (knee cap): Usually repaired by closed reduction and casting or internal fixation with screws
- *Tibia and fibula*: Corrected with closed reduction with casting for 8 to 10 weeks; internal fixation with nails or a plate and screws, followed by a long leg cast for 4 to 6 weeks; or external fixation for 6 to 10 weeks followed by application of a cast
- *Ankle*: May require a combination of closed and open techniques, depending on the severity and extent of the fracture. An arthrodesis (fusion) may be needed if the bone does not heal.
- *Foot or phalanges*: Managed with closed or open reduction. Crutches are used for ambulation.

- *Ribs and sternum*: Have the potential to puncture the lungs, heart, or arteries by bone fragments or ends. Fractures of the lower ribs may damage underlying organs, such as the liver, spleen, or kidneys. These fractures tend to heal spontaneously without surgical intervention.
- *Pelvis*: Pelvic fractures are the second most common cause of death from trauma. The major concern related to pelvic injury is venous oozing or arterial bleeding. Loss of blood volume leads to hypovolemic shock. When a non–weight-bearing part of the pelvis is fractured, management can be as minimal as bedrest on a firm mattress or bed board. A weight-bearing pelvis fracture requires external fixation or open reduction with internal fixation (ORIF), or both. Progression to weight bearing depends on the stability of the fracture after fixation. Some patients can fully bear weight within days of surgery, whereas others managed with traction may not be able to bear weight for as long as 12 weeks.
- *Compression fractures of the vertebrae* (spine) are associated with severe pain, deformity (kyphosis), and possible neurologic compromise. Nonsurgical management includes bedrest, analgesics, nerve blocks, and physical therapy to maintain muscle strength. Compression fractures that remain painful and impair mobility may be surgically treated with vertebroplasty or kyphoplasty, in which bone cement is injected through the skin (percutaneously) directly into the fracture site to provide stability and immediate pain relief. Kyphoplasty also includes the insertion of a small balloon into the fracture site and inflating it to contain the cement and to restore height to the vertebra.

FROSTBITE

OVERVIEW

- Frostbite is a significant cold-related injury that occurs as a result of inadequate insulation against cold weather.
- Contributors to frostbite include wearing wet clothing, fatigue, dehydration, poor nutrition, smoking, alcohol consumption, and impaired peripheral circulation.

PATIENT-CENTERED COLLABORATIVE CARE

Assessment

- Severity of frostbite is related to the degree of tissue freezing and the resultant damage it produces.
  1. *Frostnip* is a superficial cold injury with initial pain, numbness, and pallor of the affected area. It is easily remedied with application of warmth and does not induce tissue damage.

2. *First-degree frostbite* is the least severe type of frostbite, with hyperemia of the involved area and edema formation.
3. *Second-degree frostbite* has large, fluid-filled blisters that develop with partial-thickness skin necrosis.
4. *Third-degree frostbite* is a full-thickness injury that appears as small blisters containing dark fluid and an affected body part that is cool, numb, blue, or red and does not blanch.
5. *Fourth-degree frostbite* is severe, with no blisters or edema; the part is numb, cold, and bloodless. Full-thickness necrosis extends into the muscle and bone.

Interventions for First Aid

- Recognize frostbite by observing for a white, waxy appearance of exposed skin, especially on the nose, cheeks, and ears.
- Seek shelter from the wind and cold.
- Use body heat to warm up superficial frostbite-affected areas by placing warm hands over the affected areas on the face or placing cold hands under the arms in the axillary region.

Interventions: Hospital Care

- Rapidly rewarm in a water bath at a temperature range of 40° C to 42° C (104° F to 108° F) or by using hot towels.
- Provide analgesic agents, especially IV opiates, and IV rehydration.

> **Clinical Landmine** ♦ Dry heat should never be applied, nor should the frostbitten areas be rubbed or massaged as part of the warming process. These actions produce further tissue injury.

- Handle the injured areas gently, and elevate them above heart level if possible to decrease tissue edema.
- Use splints to immobilize extremities during the healing process.
- Assess the patient at least hourly for the development of compartment syndrome.
- Immunize the patient for tetanus prophylaxis.
- Apply only loose, nonadherent, sterile dressings to the damaged areas.
- Avoid compression of the injured tissues.
- Topical and systemic antibiotics may be prescribed.
- Management of severe, deep frostbite requires the same types of surgical intervention as deep or severe burns.

GASTRITIS

OVERVIEW

- Gastritis is inflammation of the gastric mucosa.
- Mucosal injury occurs and is worsened by histamine release and vagal nerve stimulation.

- Hydrochloric acid diffuses into the mucosa and injures small vessels, resulting in edema, hemorrhage, and erosion of the gastric lining.
- Gastritis can be classified as acute or chronic.
  1. Acute gastritis, the inflammation of gastric mucosa or submucosa, may result from the onset of infection (*H. pylori*, *Escherichia coli*) after exposure to local irritants such as alcohol or aspirin, NSAIDs, bacterial endotoxins, ingestion of corrosive substances, or from the lack of stimulation of normal gastric secretions. It occurs in various degrees of mucosal necrosis and inflammation, with complete regeneration and healing usually occurring within a few days and complete recovery with no residual damage usually ensuing.
  2. Chronic gastritis is a diffuse chronic inflammatory process involving the mucosal lining of the stomach that usually heals without scarring but can progress to hemorrhage and ulcer formation. It may be caused by chronic local irritation from alcohol, drugs, smoking, radiation, infectious agents (e.g., *H. pylori*), and environmental agents. Of patients with gastric ulcers, 50% have associated chronic gastritis.
- Three subtypes of chronic gastritis
  1. Type A is associated with the presence of antibodies to parietal cells. An autoimmune pathogenesis has been proposed. Type A accompanies pernicious anemia.
  2. Type B usually is caused by *H. pylori* infection.
  3. Atrophic gastritis is found most often in older adults after exposure to toxic substances in the workplace or *H. pylori* infection, or it can be related to autoimmune factors.

PATIENT-CENTERED COLLABORATIVE CARE

Assessment

- Acute gastritis, assess for:
  1. Abdominal tenderness and bloating
  2. Anorexia, cramping, nausea, and vomiting
  3. Hematemesis, melena
  4. In stress-induced gastritis, possible symptoms of intravascular volume depletion
  5. Aspirin-related gastritis may result in dyspepsia
- Chronic gastritis, assess for:
  1. Vague complaints or periodic epigastric distress, which may be relieved by food
  2. Anorexia
  3. Pain that worsens with intake of food, especially spicy or fatty food
  4. Weight loss

Interventions

- Acute gastritis is treated symptomatically and supportively. If the patient experienced a GI bleed with severe hemorrhage, a blood transfusion may be needed. Fluid replacement is indicated for severe fluid loss.
- Treatment of chronic gastritis varies with the cause.
- Drug therapy
  1. Proton pump inhibitors are used to reduce gastric acid secretion.
  2. H_2 histamine blockers may be used instead of proton pump inhibitors.
  3. Antacids are used as buffering agents.
  4. Vitamin B_{12}, as ordered, is used for patients with pernicious anemia.
  5. Bismuth subsalicylates, metronidazole (Flagyl, Novonidazole ✦), tetracycline, or ampicillin (Amcill, Ampicin) is used if *H. pylori* is present.
  6. Instruct the patient to avoid using drugs associated with gastric irritation, including steroids, chemotherapeutic agents, and NSAIDs.
- Diet therapy
  1. Instruct the patient to avoid foods and spices that contribute to distress, including tea, coffee, cola, chocolate, mustard, paprika, cloves, pepper, and Tabasco sauce.
  2. Instruct the patient to avoid consuming large, heavy meals.
- Teach techniques to reduce discomfort, such as progressive relaxation, cutaneous stimulation, guided imagery, and distraction.
- Advise the patient to stop smoking, if appropriate, and to avoid alcohol and caffeine.
- Surgery is indicated when conservative measures have failed to control bleeding (see Surgical Management under Peptic Ulcer Disease).

GASTROENTERITIS

OVERVIEW

- Gastroenteritis is an increase in the frequency and water content of stools and vomiting as a result of inflammation of the mucous membranes of the stomach and intestines, primarily affecting the small bowel.
- The disease may be viral or bacterial in origin, causing an inflammatory response in one of three ways:
  1. Release of enterotoxin, causing local inflammation and diarrhea

2. Penetration of the organism into the intestine, causing cellular destruction, necrosis, and ulceration (diarrhea occurs with WBCs or RBCs)
3. Attachment of the organism to the mucosal epithelium, destroying cells of the intestinal villi with resultant malabsorption

- Viral gastroenteritis can be classified as epidemic viral gastroenteritis or rotavirus gastroenteritis (incubation about 48 hours and affecting infants and young children).
  1. Norwalk virus is spread by the oral-fecal route and is a common cause of waterborne epidemics of gastroenteritis.
- Bacterial gastroenteritis can be divided into three general types:
  1. *Campylobacter* enteritis
  2. *Escherichia coli* diarrhea
  3. Shigellosis

PATIENT-CENTERED COLLABORATIVE CARE

Assessment

- The patient's history can provide information about the potential cause.
  1. Onset of diarrhea with accompanying abdominal cramping or pain
  2. Nausea and vomiting
  3. Bloody, mucous, or watery, foul-smelling stool
  4. Fever: temperature may be normal or elevated from 101° F to 103° F (38.2° C to 39.2° C)
  5. Dehydration exhibited by poor skin turgor, dry mucous membranes, orthostatic blood pressure changes, hypotension, and oliguria
  6. Viral symptoms, such as myalgia, headache, and malaise
  7. Positive result of a stool culture

Interventions

- Provide fluid replacement therapy, as ordered.
  1. Administer oral rehydration therapy with commercially prepared products such as Resol.
  2. Administer hypotonic IV fluids for severe dehydration; add potassium if the patient is hypokalemic.
  3. Check vital signs and orthostatic blood pressure, as clinically indicated.
  4. Check weight daily.
  5. Maintain strict intake and output.
  6. Depending on the type of gastroenteritis, notify the local health department.

- Provide diet therapy.
  1. Advise the patient to take small volumes of clear liquids with electrolytes.
  2. Advise the patient not to drink water because it does not contain any electrolytes to replace those lost.
  3. Slowly progress the diet to include small portions of saltine crackers and toast. When this is tolerated, consider adding bland foods (e.g., nonfat soup, custard, yogurt, cottage cheese, baked or mashed potatoes, cooked vegetables), and then progress to the patient's regular diet.
  4. Advise the patient to avoid caffeine.
- Provide drug therapy, as ordered.
  1. Drugs that suppress intestinal motility, such as antiemetics or anticholinergics for bacterial or viral gastroenteritis, are not routinely given.
  2. Antibiotics may be given if gastroenteritis is caused by bacterial infection.
  3. Anti-infective agents, such as trimethoprim/sulfamethoxazole (Septra, Bactrim), are given if the patient has shigellosis.
  4. Diarrhea that continues for 10 days is probably not caused by gastroenteritis, and an investigation for other causes is done.
- Provide skin care.
  1. Teach the patient to avoid toilet paper and harsh soaps and to gently clean the area with warm water and absorbent cotton, followed by thorough drying with absorbent cotton.
  2. Cream, oil, or gel can be applied to a damp, warm washcloth or flushable wipe to remove excrement adhering to excoriated skin.
  3. Hydrocortisone cream or a protective barrier cream should be applied to the skin between stools; witch hazel compresses (e.g., Tucks) and sitz baths can relieve discomfort.
- Teach the patient the following health practices:
  1. Replace lost fluids.
  2. Follow the recommended diet.
  3. Wash hands after each bowel movement to minimize the risk of disease transmission.
  4. Do not share eating utensils, glasses, and dishes, and maintain strict personal hygiene.
  5. Maintain clean bathroom facilities.
  6. Inform the health care provider if symptoms persist beyond 3 days.
  7. Adhere to these precautions for up to 7 weeks after the illness or up to several months if *Shigella* was the causative organism.

8. Follow written instructions for drugs, if ordered, including dosage, schedule of administration, and side effects.

GASTROESOPHAGEAL REFLUX DISEASE

OVERVIEW

- Gastroesophageal reflux disease (GERD) occurs as the result of the backward flow (reflux) of GI contents into the esophagus.
- Reflux produces symptoms by exposing the esophageal mucosa to the irritating effects of gastric or duodenal contents, resulting in inflammation.
- A person with acute symptoms of inflammation is often described as having reflux esophagitis, which may be mild or severe.
- The degree of inflammation is related to the acid concentration of the refluxed material, the number of reflux episodes, and the length of time that the esophagus is exposed to the irritant.

PATIENT-CENTERED COLLABORATIVE CARE

Assessment

- Record patient information related to heartburn or esophageal pain. Dyspepsia (also called heartburn or pyrosis), the primary symptom, is described as a substernal or retrosternal burning sensation that tends to move up and down the chest in a wave-like fashion; severe heartburn may radiate to the neck or jaw or may be felt in the back.
  1. Location, quality, onset, and duration of dyspepsia or esophageal pain
  2. Pain aggravated by bending over, straining, or lying in a recumbent position
- Pain occurs after each meal, and persists for 20 minutes to 2 hours.
- Chest pain may result from esophageal spasm.
- Ask whether he or she has been newly diagnosed with asthma or has experienced morning hoarseness or pneumonia. These symptoms suggest severe reflux reaching the pharynx or mouth or pulmonary aspiration.
- Other symptoms associated with GERD
  1. Water brash (reflex salivary hypersecretion)
  2. Dysphagia (difficulty swallowing) or odynophagia (painful swallowing)
  3. Chronic cough that occurs mostly at night
  4. Belching and a feeling of flatulence or bloating after eating

5. Regurgitation not associated with belching or nausea; warm fluid traveling up the throat, resulting in a sour or bitter taste in the mouth

- Assess results of 24-hour pH monitoring, esophageal manometry (motility testing), and scintigraphy (measure of reflux of radioisotope).

Interventions

Nonsurgical Management

- Explore the patient's meal plan and food preferences, and in collaboration with the nutritionist, meet with the patient and family to plan diet modifications to reduce GERD symptoms. Teach the patient to:
  1. Avoid chocolate, fatty (especially fried) foods and carbonated beverages because they reduce lower esophageal sphincter (LES) pressure or cause local irritation.
  2. Eat four to six small meals a day.
  3. Avoid eating 3 hours before bedtime.
  4. Limit or eliminate alcohol and tobacco.
  5. Remain upright after meals for 1 to 2 hours.
- Teach the patient and family the risk factors that can exacerbate the disease.
- Stress the importance of ongoing monitoring.
- Encourage lifestyle changes.
  1. If the patient is obese, collaborate with the nutritionist and meet with the patient and family to examine approaches to weight reduction.
  2. Explore the possibility and means of smoking cessation and make appropriate referrals.
  3. Instruct the patient to elevate the head of the bed by 6 inches to prevent nighttime reflux.
  4. Instruct the patient to sleep in the left lateral decubitus (side-lying) position.
  5. Encourage the patient to avoid wearing tight-fitting clothing and working in a bent-over or stooped position.
- Drug therapy
  1. Antacids are used for their acid-neutralizing effects.
  2. Proton pump inhibitors are the main treatment for GERD and provide effective, long-acting inhibition of gastric acid secretion.
  3. H_2-histamine receptor blockers are sometimes used instead of proton pump inhibitors to reduce gastric acid production, provide symptom improvement, and support healing of the inflamed esophageal tissue.
  4. Prokinetic drugs are used to accelerate gastric emptying and improve LES pressure and esophageal peristalsis.

- Identify whether the patient is on any drugs that may lower LES pressure and cause reflux, such as oral contraceptives, anticholinergic agents, beta-adrenergic agonists, nitrates, and calcium channel blockers.

Surgical Management
- Noninvasive endoscopic procedures
  1. The Stretta procedure involves the application of radiofrequency energy near the gastroesophageal junction, which inhibits the activity of the vagus nerve, reducing discomfort for the patient.
  2. The Bard EndoCinch Suturing System (BESS) involves suturing near the LES.
- The major surgical procedure for patients who have not responded to aggressive medical management is the laparoscopic Nissen fundoplication.

◤ National Patient Safety Goal

Be sure to use two patient identifiers before starting any procedure.

GLAUCOMA

OVERVIEW

- Glaucoma is a group of ocular diseases resulting in increased intraocular pressure (IOP). IOP is the fluid pressure within the eye.
- A normal IOP of 10 to 21 mm Hg is maintained when there is a balance between production and outflow of aqueous humor.
- If the IOP becomes too high, the extra pressure presses on blood vessels in the eye and prevents blood flow, resulting in poorly oxygenated photoreceptors, which then become ischemic and die. When too many have died, sight is lost, and the person is permanently blind.
- In most types of glaucoma, vision is lost gradually and painlessly from the periphery to the central area, without the person's awareness.
- Types of glaucoma
  1. *Primary*: The structures involved in circulation and reabsorption of the aqueous humor undergo direct pathologic changes from aging, heredity, and central retinal vessel occlusion.
     a. Primary open-angle glaucoma (POAG) has reduced outflow of aqueous humor through the chamber angle. Because the fluid cannot leave the eye at the same rate it is produced, IOP gradually increases.

b. Angle-closure glaucoma (also called closed-angle glaucoma, narrow-angle glaucoma, or acute glaucoma) has a sudden onset and is an emergency.
2. *Secondary*: Glaucoma results from other problems within the eye, such as uveitis, iritis, trauma, and ocular surgeries.
3. *Associated*: Glaucoma results from systemic disease, such as diabetes mellitus and hypertension.

PATIENT-CENTERED COLLABORATIVE CARE

Assessment

- Assess for manifestations of early primary open-angle glaucoma (POAG):
  1. Increased ocular pressure
  2. Reduced accommodation
- Assess for late manifestations of late primary open-angle glaucoma (POAG):
  1. Peripheral visual field losses
  2. Decreased visual acuity not correctable with glasses
  3. Appearance of halos around lights
  4. Increased cupping and atrophy of the optic disc
  5. IOP tonometry reading between 22 and 32 mm Hg

Interventions

Nonsurgical Management

- Drug therapy for glaucoma focuses on reducing IOP with eyedrops:
  1. Prostaglandin agonists
     a. Bimatoprost (Lumigan)
     b. Latanoprost (Xalatan)
     c. Travoprost (Travatan)
     d. Unoprostone isopropyl (Rescula)
  2. Adrenergic agonists
     a. Apraclonidine (Iopidine)
     b. Brimonidine tartrate (Alphagan)
     c. Dipivefrin hydrochloride (Propine)
     d. Epinephryl borate (Epifrin, Epinal, Eppy/N)
  3. Beta-adrenergic blockers
     a. Betaxolol hydrochloride (Betoptic)
     b. Carteolol (Cartrol, Ocupress)
     c. Levobetaxolol (Betaxon)
     d. Levobunolol (Betagan)
     e. Metipranolol (OptiPranolol)
     f. Timolol (Betimol, Timoptic)
  4. Cholinergic agonists
     a. Carbachol (Carboptic, Isopto Carbachol, Miostat)

    b. Echothiophate (Phospholine Iodide)

    c. Pilocarpine (Adsorbocarpine, Akarpine, IsoptoCarpine, Ocu-Carpine, Ocusert, Piloptic, Pilopine, Pilostat)

  5. Carbonic anhydrase inhibitors

    a. Brinzolamide (Azopt)

    b. Dorzolamide (Trusopt)

  6. Combination agents

    a. Brimonidine tartrate and timolol maleate (Combigan)

- Teach the patient:

  1. Stress the importance of instilling the drops on time and not skipping doses.

  2. When more than one drug is prescribed, teach the patient to wait 10 to 15 minutes between drug instillations to prevent one drug from "washing out" or diluting another drug.

  3. Teach the technique of punctal occlusion (placing pressure on the corner of the eye near the nose) immediately after eyedrop instillation to prevent systemic absorption of the drug.

  4. Stress the need for good handwashing, keeping the eyedrop container tip clean, and avoiding touching the tip to any part of the eye.

Surgical Management

- Surgery is used when drugs for the patient with open-angle glaucoma are not effective in controlling IOP. The two most common procedures are laser trabeculoplasty and filtering microsurgery.

- *Laser trabeculoplasty* burns the trabecular meshwork, scarring it and causing the meshwork fibers to shrink. Fiber shrinkage increases the size of the spaces between the fibers, improving outflow of aqueous humor and a reduction in IOP.

- *Filtering microsurgery* creates a drainage hole in the iris between the posterior and anterior chambers.

- When surgical therapies fail, a *shunt* or glaucoma drainage device may be implanted that has a small tube or filament connected to a flat plate positioned on the outside of the eye in the eye orbit. The open part of the fine tube is placed into the front chamber of the eye, just in front of the iris. The fluid then drains into the area around the flat plate, where it collects and is reabsorbed into the bloodstream.

- The most serious complication after glaucoma surgery is choroidal hemorrhage. Manifestations include:

  1. Acute pain deep in the eye

  2. Decreased vision

  3. Vital sign changes

G

GLOMERULONEPHRITIS, ACUTE

OVERVIEW

- Acute glomerulonephritis results from injury to the glomeruli
- Glomerular injury is the result of immune complexes deposited in kidney tissue; an immune complex is made up of antigens and antibodies
- Immune complexes trigger inflammation, which can further damage kidney tissue.

PATIENT-CENTERED COLLABORATIVE CARE

Assessment

- Record patient information:
  1. History of recent infections, particularly skin and upper respiratory infections
  2. Recent travel
  3. Activities with exposure to viruses, bacteria, fungi, or parasites
  4. Recent illnesses, operations, or invasive procedures
  5. Known systemic diseases, especially those associated with inflammation or autoimmunity such as systemic lupus erythematosus
- Assessment findings include:
  1. Skin lesions or incisions, including piercings that could be the source of infection
  2. Edema of the face, eyelids, hands, and peripheral tissue
  3. Fluid overload and circulatory congestion
  4. Difficulty breathing, nocturnal or exertional dyspnea or orthopnea
  5. Crackles in lung fields
  6. S_3 heart sound (gallop rhythm)
  7. Neck vein distention
  8. Changes in patterns of urination
  9. Smoky, reddish brown, or cola-colored urine
  10. Dysuria
  11. Decreased urine output
  12. Mild to moderate hypertension
  13. Changes in weight
  14. Fatigue and malaise
  15. RBCs and protein in the urine
  16. Increased blood urea nitrogen (BUN) and creatinine levels
  17. Decreased urine creatinine clearance
  18. Positive cultures from blood, skin, or throat

19. Serologic testing for antistreptolysin-O titers, C3 complement levels, immunoglobulin G, antinuclear bodies, and circulating immune complexes

- A percutaneous needle biopsy may define the pathologic condition, assist in determining prognosis, and help outline treatment.

Interventions

- Appropriate anti-infective agents such as penicillin, erythromycin, or azithromycin are given to treat infection.
- To prevent infection spread, the health care provider may order anti-infective drugs for persons in close contact with the patient.
- Sodium and water restriction, along with diuretics, may be needed for the patient with hypertension, circulatory congestions, and edema.
  1. Antihypertensive agents are given to treat hypertension.
  2. The usual fluid allowance is equal to the 24-hour urinary output plus 500 to 600 mL for insensible fluid loss.
- Potassium and protein intake may be restricted to prevent hyperkalemia and additional uremic manifestations of the elevated BUN level.
- Plasmapheresis may be attempted.
- Energy management includes:
  1. Encouraging and promoting a restful environment
  2. Teaching and demonstrating energy conservation techniques
  3. Encouraging the patient to practice relaxation techniques
- Health teaching includes:
  1. Reviewing prescribed drug instructions, including purpose, timing, frequency, duration, and side effects
  2. Ensuring that the patient and family understand dietary and fluid modifications
  3. Advising the patient to measure weight and blood pressure daily and to notify the health care provider of any sudden changes
  4. Advising the patient to exercise each day, as tolerated
  5. Teaching the importance of rest
  6. Instructing the patient about peritoneal or vascular access care if short-term dialysis is required to control excess fluid volume or uremic symptoms

GLOMERULONEPHRITIS, CHRONIC

OVERVIEW

- Chronic glomerulonephritis, or chronic nephritic syndrome, is the diagnostic name given to known and unknown causes of kidney deterioration or kidney failure that develop over 20 to 30 years.

- The exact cause is unknown. Changes are thought to result from the effects of hypertension, intermittent or recurrent infections and inflammation, and poor blood flow to the kidneys.
- Kidney tissue atrophies, and the functional mass of nephrons decreases, which alters glomerular filtration.
- Glomerular injury results in proteinuria because of increased permeability of the glomerular basement membrane.
- The process eventually results in chronic kidney injury (CKI) or end-stage kidney disease (ESKD) and uremia, requiring dialysis or transplantation.

PATIENT-CENTERED COLLABORATIVE CARE

Assessment

- Record the patient's history.
- Health problems, including systemic disease, kidney or urologic problems, and infectious diseases, especially streptococcal infections and recent exposure to infection
- Presence of symptoms indicating systemic volume overload: S_3, neck vein engorgement, edema, and crackles in the lungs with tachypnea
- Changes in urinary status, including amount, frequency of voiding, and changes in urine color, clarity, and odor
- Changes in activity tolerance and comfort
- Changes in mental concentration or memory
- Proteinuria
- Decreased creatinine clearance
- Serum electrolyte changes
- Radiographic findings of renal size (usually small)
- Perform a physical assessment.
  1. Inspect the skin for yellow color, ecchymosis, and rashes.
  2. Inspect for evidence of edema in tissues.
  3. Measure blood pressure and weight.
  4. Auscultate the heart for an S_3 sound.
  5. Auscultate the lungs for the presence of rales or crackles.
  6. Observe the rate and depth of breathing pattern.
  7. Inspect neck veins for engorgement.
  8. Inspect urine and evaluate urinalysis results.
  9. Evaluate serum BUN, creatine, and electrolytes.
  10. Assess for uremic symptoms, such as slurred speech, ataxia, tremors, or asterixis (flapping tremor of the fingers or the inability to maintain a fixed posture with the arms extended and wrists hyperextended).

Interventions
- Management of chronic glomerulonephritis is similar to conservative management for ESKD.
- Treatment consists of dietary modification, fluid intake sufficient to prevent reduced blood flow volume to the kidneys, and drug therapy to temporarily control the symptoms of uremia.
- Eventually, the patient requires dialysis or transplantation.

GLOMERULONEPHRITIS, RAPIDLY PROGRESSIVE

- Rapidly progressive glomerulonephritis, a type of acute nephritis, develops over several weeks or months and causes a significant loss of kidney function.
- Manifestations occur rapidly as kidney failure, fluid volume excess, hypertension, oliguria, electrolyte imbalances, and uremic symptoms.
- Kidney deterioration often progresses to end-stage kidney disease (ESKD).

GONORRHEA
OVERVIEW

- Gonorrhea is a sexually transmitted bacterial infection caused by *Neisseria gonorrhoeae,* a gram-negative intracellular diplococcus.
- It is transmitted by direct sexual contact with mucosal surfaces (vaginal intercourse, orogenital contact, or anogenital contact).
- The first symptoms of gonorrhea may appear 3 to 10 days after sexual contact with an infected person, or the disease can be present without symptoms and can be transmitted or progress without warning.
- In women, ascending spread of the organism can cause pelvic infection (pelvic inflammatory disease [PID]), endometritis (endometrial infection), salpingitis (fallopian tube infection), and pelvic peritonitis.
- More drug-resistant strains of the disease have developed.

PATIENT-CENTERED COLLABORATIVE CARE
Assessment
- Obtain patient information about:
  1. Sexual history that includes sexual orientation and sites of intercourse
  2. Allergies to antibiotics

3. Symptoms in men
   a. Dysuria
   b. Penile discharge (profuse, yellowish green fluid or scant, clear fluid)
   c. Urethritis
   d. Pain or discomfort in the prostate, seminal vesicles, or epididymal regions
4. Symptoms in women
   a. Vaginal discharge (yellow, green, profuse, odorous)
   b. Urinary frequency
   c. Dysuria
5. Anal manifestations (in men or women)
   a. Itching and irritation
   b. Rectal bleeding
   c. Diarrhea
   d. Painful defecation
- Assess for and document:
  1. Oral cavity manifestations
     a. Reddened throat
     b. Ulcerated lips
     c. Tender gingivae
     d. Blisters in the throat
  2. Discharge from the urethra, cervix, and rectum
  3. Tenderness of the lower abdomen
  4. Manifestations of disseminated gonococcal infection (DGI)
     a. Fever
     b. Chills
     c. Skin lesions on hands and feet
     d. Joint pain, with or without swelling, heat, or redness
- Diagnostic testing may include:
  1. Nucleic acid amplification tests (NAATs) using samples from urine or vaginal swabs
  2. Gram staining of smears from penile discharge
  3. Cultures of discharge from the female genital tract

> 🔲 Critical Rescue ◆ All patients with gonorrhea should be tested for syphilis, chlamydia, hepatitis B and C, and HIV infection because they may have been exposed to these sexually transmitted diseases (STDs) as well. Sexual partners who have been exposed in the past 30 days should be examined, and specimens should be obtained.

Interventions
- Drug therapy for uncomplicated gonorrhea may include any of these regimens:
  1. Ceftriaxone (Rocephin): 125 mg IM

2. Cefixime (Suprax), 400 mg in a single dose, *plus* azithromycin (Zithromax), 1 g orally in a single dose
3. Doxycycline (Monodox, Doxy-Caps, Doxycin ✦): 100 mg orally twice daily for 1 week

- Sexual partners also must be treated.
- Advise the patient to return for a follow-up examination if symptoms persist after treatment.
- Treatment of DGI usually requires hospitalization and includes IV or IM ceftriaxone (1 g every 24 hours). If symptoms resolve within 24 to 48 hours, the patient may be discharged to home to continue oral antibiotic therapy for at least a week.
- Teach the patient about:
  1. Transmission and treatment of gonorrhea
  2. Prevention of reinfection
  3. Complications of chronic gonorrhea
     a. Pelvic inflammatory disease (PID)
     b. Ectopic pregnancy
     c. Infertility
     d. Chronic pelvic pain
  4. Avoiding sexual activity until the antibiotic therapy is completed
  5. Condom use if abstinence is not possible
  6. The need to report the disease
  7. The need for all sexual contacts to be examined and treated for gonorrhea and chlamydia infections
- Encourage patients to express their feelings during assessments and teaching sessions.
- Provide privacy for teaching and maintain confidentiality of medical records.

GOUT

OVERVIEW

- Gout, or gouty arthritis, is a systemic disease in which urate crystals deposit in the joints and other body tissues, causing inflammation.
- There are two major types of gout:
  1. *Primary gout* results from one of several inborn errors of purine metabolism that allows the production of uric acid to exceed the excretion capability of the kidneys. Urate is deposited in synovium and other tissues, resulting in inflammation. A number of patients have a family history of gout. It is most common in middle-aged and older men and postmenopausal women.

2. *Secondary gout* results from excessive uric acid crystals that are present in the blood (hyperuricemia) as a result of another disease, condition, or treatment. Causes include renal insufficiency, diuretic therapy, "crash" diets, certain chemotherapeutic agents, and diseases such as multiple myeloma and certain carcinomas. Treatment for secondary gout focuses on management of the underlying disorder.

- There are three clinical stages of primary gout:
  1. *Asymptomatic hyperuricemic stage,* in which these are no symptoms but the serum uric acid level is elevated
  2. *Acute stage,* in which the patient experiences excruciating pain and inflammation in one or more small joints, usually the metatarsophalangeal joint of the great toe, called *podagra*
  3. *Chronic tophaceous stage,* which occurs after repeated episodes of acute gout have caused deposits of urate crystals under the skin and within the major organs, particularly in the renal system. This stage can begin between 3 and 40 years after the initial gout symptoms occur.

PATIENT-CENTERED COLLABORATIVE CARE

Assessment
- Obtain patient information about:
  1. Age
  2. Gender
  3. Family history of gout
  4. Medical history and drug history to determine whether gout has been caused by another problem
- For acute gout, assess for and document joint inflammation and pain.
- For chronic gout, assess for and document:
  1. Presence of tophi (skin deposits of urate crystals)
     a. Outer ear
     b. Arms and fingers near the joints
  2. Infected skin areas
  3. Manifestations of kidney (stones) or kidney dysfunction
     a. Severe pain
     b. Changes in urine output
- Diagnostic assessment may include:
  1. Serum uric acid level
  2. Urinary uric acid levels
  3. Kidney function tests (in chronic gout)
  4. Synovial fluid aspiration (arthrocentesis)

Interventions
- Drug therapy during acute attacks

1. Colchicine (Colsalide, Novocolchicine ❧)
2. NSAID, such as indomethacin (Indocin, Novomethacin ❧) or ibuprofen (Motrin, Amersol ❧)
- Drug therapy for chronic gout
  1. Allopurinol (Zyloprim)
  2. Probenecid (Benemid, Benuryl ❧)
  3. Combination drugs that contain probenecid and colchicine (e.g., ColBenemid)

> 🗲 **Clinical Landmine** ◆ Aspirin should be avoided because it inactivates the effects of the drug therapy.

- Nutritional therapy with a low-purine diet by avoidance of:
  1. Organ meats
  2. Red meats
  3. Shellfish
  4. Oily fish with bones (e.g., sardines)
  5. Teach patients to determine which foods precipitate acute attacks and try to avoid them.
- Other restrictions include:
  1. All forms of aspirin
  2. Diuretics
  3. Excessive physical or emotional stress, which can exacerbate the disease
- Teach the patient to drink plenty of fluids, especially:
  1. Water
  2. Citrus juices
  3. Milk

GUILLAIN-BARRÉ SYNDROME

OVERVIEW

- Guillain-Barré syndrome (GBS) is an acute autoimmune disorder characterized by various degrees of motor weakness and paralysis.
- Three stages make up the acute course:
  1. Acute phase, which begins with the onset of the first definitive symptoms and ends when no further deterioration is noted (usually 1 to 4 weeks)
  2. Plateau phase, which is a time of little change and lasts several days to 2 weeks
  3. Recovery phase, which is thought to coincide with remyelination and axonal regeneration and usually lasts 4 to 6 months (sometimes up to 2 years)

- Chronic inflammatory demyelinating polyneuropathy (CIDP) is an unusual type of GBS that progresses over a longer period; complete recovery rarely occurs.
- The cause of GBS remains obscure, although most evidence implicates a cell-mediated immunologic reaction.
- The patient often relates a history of acute illness, trauma, surgery, or immunization 1 to 8 weeks before the onset of neurologic signs and symptoms.

Cultural Considerations

- GBS has a worldwide distribution and affects people of all races and ages.
- The highest rates have been observed for people 45 years old or older.
- The incidence is higher among whites than blacks.

PATIENT-CENTERED COLLABORATIVE CARE

Assessment

- Record the patient's medical and surgical history, including:
  1. Occurrence of antecedent illness 1 to 8 weeks before the onset of GBS
  2. Description of symptoms (in chronologic order)
- Assessment findings include:
  1. Paresthesia (numbness or tingling) and pain
  2. Cranial nerve dysfunction
     a. Facial weakness
     b. Dysphagia
     c. Diplopia
  3. Difficulty walking
  4. Muscle weakness or flaccid paralysis without muscle wasting in an ascending, distal-to-proximal progression
  5. Respiratory compromise or failure
     a. Dyspnea
     b. Decreased breath sound
     c. Decreased tidal volume or vital capacity
  6. Bowel and bladder incontinence
  7. Autonomic dysfunction evidenced by:
     a. Labile blood pressure
     b. Cardiac dysrhythmias
     c. Tachycardia
  8. Decreased or absent deep tendon reflexes
  9. Ability to cope with illness
  10. Anxiety, fear, and panic
  11. Anger and depression

Planning and Implementation

❖**NDx:** Ineffective Breathing Pattern, Ineffective Airway Clearance, Impaired Gas Exchange

- Perform a respiratory assessment:
  1. Assess every 4 hours; auscultate breath sounds.
  2. Observe for dyspnea, air hunger, adventitious breath sounds, cyanosis, and confusion.
  3. Measure vital capacity every 2 to 4 hours.
  4. Obtain arterial blood gases, as indicated by the patient's clinical status.
  5. Remove secretions by encouraging coughing or suctioning; monitor the color, consistency, and amount of secretions obtained.
  6. Administer humidified air or oxygen, as appropriate.
  7. Administer ultrasonic nebulizer treatments, as appropriate.
  8. Keep equipment for intubation and a ventilator available.
  9. Perform chest physiotherapy; encourage the patient to cough and breathe deeply.

❖**NDx:** Impaired Physical Mobility and Self-Care Deficit Related to Weakness, Paralysis, and Ataxia

- The health care team collaborates with the patient to develop interventions to prevent complications of immobility and address deficits in self-care.
  1. Assess motor function with vital signs.
  2. Assist the patient's hygiene, toileting, and feeding, as needed.
  3. Collaborate with physical therapy and occupational therapy to determine the type and duration of daily exercises or activity, such as transfer to chair, repositioning in bed, ambulation, and ADLs.
  4. Monitor the patient's response to or tolerance of activity.
  5. Provide adequate rest periods between activities.
  6. Collaborate with the nutritionist to develop a nutritional plan, and assist with meals, as needed.
  7. Monitor intake and output, and assess the patient for urinary retention every shift.
  8. Monitor for complications of immobility: atelectasis, pneumonia, pressure ulcers, deep vein thrombosis, and pulmonary emboli.

▼**Nursing Patient Safety Goal**

Assess and periodically reassess each patient's risk for developing a pressure ulcer, and take action to address any identified risks. Prevention of hospital-acquired pressure ulcers is a priority for all patients.

❖**NDx:** Acute Pain Related to Paresthesias
- Assess the severity and nature of the patient's pain, which is typically worse at night.
- Pain is best treated with opiates, which can be administered by a patient-controlled analgesia (PCA) pump or continuous IV drip. Document the patient's response to pain drug.
- Other interventions include frequent positioning, massage, ice, heat, relaxation techniques, guided imagery, and distractions.

❖**NDx:** Impaired Verbal Communication Related to Intubation or Paralysis of the Muscles Required for Speech
- Assist the patient to develop a communication system in collaboration with the speech-language pathologist.
- Develop a communication board that lists common requests.

❖**NDx:** Powerlessness, Anxiety and Fear Related to the Inability to Perform ADLs and Usual Role Responsibilities
- Encourage the patient to verbalize feelings concerning the illness and its effects.
- Provide information regarding the disease process.
- Encourage the patient to participate in his or her care and to make as many choices as possible.
- Provide encouragement and positive reinforcement.
- Identify factors that increase coping abilities by asking the patient and family to describe situations that they have successfully coped with in the past.
- Keep necessary items (call light, radio, or television control) within the patient's reach.
- Use the patient's own personal items, when feasible.
- Other collaborative care includes administering medications and providing plasmapheresis.
- Immunoglobulin therapy may be used.
  1. Monitor for side effects such as chills, mild fever, myalgia, headache, anaphylaxis, aseptic meningitis, retinal necrosis, and acute kidney injury.
- Plasma exchange, also known as plasmapheresis, may be used to remove the circulating antibodies, which are thought to be responsible for the disease. Plasma is selectively separated from whole blood; blood cells are returned to the patient without the plasma.
  1. Provide information and reassurance to the patient.
  2. Weigh the patient before and after treatment.
  3. If a shunt is used, maintain patency of the shunt, check for flow every 2 to 4 hours, and observe the puncture site for bleeding or ecchymosis after a treatment session.
  4. Monitor vital signs during treatment, including cardiac rhythm.

5. Keep double bulldog clamps at the bedside.
6. Monitor intake and output, and weigh the patient daily.
7. Monitor for complications of plasmapheresis: hypovolemia, hypokalemia, hypocalcemia, temporary circumoral and distal extremity paresthesia, muscle twitching, nausea, and vomiting.

Community-Based Care
- Discharge planning includes:
  1. Providing a detailed plan of care at the time of discharge for patients to be transferred to a long-term care or rehabilitation facility (rehabilitation may be lengthy)
  2. Assessing the patient and family's knowledge and understanding of the disease
  3. Providing oral and written information on therapeutic positioning and mobility
  4. Ensuring that patient and family members understand how to use assistive or adaptive devices
  5. Referring the patient to local or community agencies for assistance in the home setting
  6. Referring the patient to the Guillain-Barré Foundation for information about local resources and educational materials

HEADACHE, CLUSTER

- Cluster headaches manifest as unilateral, oculotemporal, or oculofrontal pain described as excruciating, boring, and nonthrobbing.
- They occur every 8 to 12 (and up to 24) hours daily at the same time for a period of 6 to 8 weeks (hence the term cluster), followed by a period of remission for 9 months to a year.
- Cluster headaches occur more often in adult men between 20 and 50 years of age than in women.
- The headache, which lasts typically 30 to 90 minutes, is accompanied by ipsilateral (same side) tearing of the eye, rhinorrhea or congestion, ptosis, miosis, bradycardia, flushing or pallor of the skin, increased intraocular pressure, and increased skin temperature.
- Management includes:
  1. Administering drugs to treat pain, similar to migraine therapy: triptans, ergotamine preparations, and anti-epileptic drug. Additional drugs include calcium channel blockers, especially verapamil (Calan), lithium, and corticosteroids.
  2. In addition to drugs, 100% oxygen by mask with the patient in a sitting position may be administered for 15 to 30 minutes and is discontinued when the headache is relieved.

3. Oxygen reduces cerebral blood flow and inhibits the activity of the carotid bodies.
4. Instructing the patient to wear sunglasses and sit away from windows while the headache is occurring
5. Helping the patient identify precipitating factors such as bursts of anger, excessive physical activity, and excitement
6. Teaching the patient the importance of a consistent sleep-wake cycle
7. Surgical interventions for drug-resistant cluster headaches include percutaneous stereotactic rhizotomy and electrical stimulation of the posterior hypothalamus.

HEADACHE, MIGRAINE

- A migraine headache is an episodic disorder manifested by unilateral, frontotemporal, throbbing pain in the head, which is often worse behind one eye or ear.
- This type of headache is often accompanied by a sensitive scalp, anorexia, photophobia, and nausea with or without vomiting.
- Three categories of migraine headache are migraine with aura (*classic migraine*), migraine without aura, and atypical migraines.
- Management focuses on:
  1. Implementing trigger avoidance. Collaborate with the patient to determine factors, if any, that may trigger the development of a headache, such as, the consumption of monosodium glutamate [MSG], aged cheese, chocolate, nitrates, and red wine. Many patients are sensitive to odors from tobacco products, paint or gasoline fumes, perfumes, or aftershave lotion.
  2. Teaching the patients the importance of regularly using preventative drug therapy
     a. NSAIDs
     b. Beta blockers such as propranolol (Inderal, Apo-Propranolol ✹) and timolol (Blocadren, Apo-Timol ✹)
     c. Calcium channel blockers
     d. Tricyclic or selective serotonin reuptake inhibitor antidepressants
     e. Antiepileptics (AEDs): Topiramate (Topamax) is the most common AED used for migraines, but it should be used in low doses because it can unmask mental health disorders, leading to suicide.
     f. Riboflavin (vitamin B_2)

3. Using drug therapy to treat pain after the headache starts, including:
   a. NSAIDs such as acetaminophen (Tylenol, Abenol ❦), ibuprofen (Motrin, others), or naproxen (Naprosyn, others) for mild pain
   b. Triptans such as sumatriptan (Imitrex), but triptans are contraindicated in patients with actual or suspected ischemic heart disease, hypertension, or peripheral vascular disease and in pregnant women
   c. Ergotamine derivatives such as dihydroergotamine (DHE), but DHE should not be given within 24 hours of a triptan preparation
   d. Isometheptene combinations that are used when ergotamine derivatives are not tolerated
   e. Antiemetics if nausea and vomiting occur with the migraine
   f. Complementary and alternative therapies that may be used include yoga, meditation, biofeedback, relaxation techniques, acupuncture, and various herbals. A dark room and rest may mitigate the migraine if used early during onset of the headache pain.

HEADACHE, TENSION

- Tension headaches are the most common type of long-duration headache and are characterized by neck and shoulder muscle tenderness and bilateral pain at the base of the skull and in the forehead.
- Nausea, vomiting, photophobia, phonophobia, and aggravation of the headache with activity may occur.
- Treatment includes non-opioid analgesics, NSAIDs, and muscle relaxants. Alternative treatments such as biofeedback and relaxation techniques can also be helpful.

HEARING LOSS

OVERVIEW

- Hearing loss, one of the most common handicaps in North America, may be conductive, sensorineural, or a combination of the two.
   1. *Conductive hearing loss* occurs when sound waves are blocked from contact with inner ear nerve fibers because of inflammation or obstruction of the external or middle ear by cerumen or foreign objects, otitis media, tumors, scar tissue buildup, or overgrowth of soft or bony tissue on the ossicles.

2. *Sensorineural hearing loss* occurs when hair cells or the inner ear sensory nerve fibers from the auditory nerve (cranial nerve VIII) that lead to the cerebral cortex are damaged. Causes include prolonged exposure to loud noise, ototoxic drugs, deficiencies of vitamin B_{12} or folic acid, atherosclerosis, hypertension, infections, prolonged fever, Ménière's disease, diabetes mellitus, and ear surgery. *Presbycusis* is a sensorineural hearing loss that occurs as a result of aging.
3. *Combined or mixed hearing loss* has components of both conductive and sensorineural loss.

- About one third of people between the ages of 65 and 75 years have a hearing loss. As many as one half of people older than 85 years have some degree of hearing loss.
- The type and cause of hearing loss determine the degree to which loss can be corrected and the amount of hearing that can return.

Genetic Considerations

- Some hearing loss in adults can have a genetic origin, such as Usher's syndrome and Alport's syndrome. These syndromes usually occur with other physical problems.
- One type of adult onset hearing loss that does not have any other physical problems is associated with a mutation in the *GJB2* gene on chromosome 13. This form of hearing loss has an autosomal dominant pattern of inheritance.

PATIENT-CENTERED COLLABORATIVE CARE

Assessment

- Obtain patient information about:
  1. Any differences in his or her ears or hearing and whether the changes occurred suddenly or gradually, including:
     a. Feeling of ear fullness or congestion
     b. Dizziness or vertigo
     c. Tinnitus
     d. Difficulty understanding conversations, especially in a noisy room
     e. Difficulty hearing sounds
     f. The need to strain to hear
     g. The need to turn the head to favor one ear or the need to lean forward to hear
     h. Pain
  2. Age
  3. Occupational exposure to loud or continuous noises
  4. Current or previous use of ototoxic drugs

5. History of external ear or middle ear infection and whether eardrum perforation occurred with the infection
6. History of ear trauma
7. Whether any family members are hearing impaired
8. Recent upper respiratory infection and allergies affecting the nose and sinuses
9. Functional hearing
   a. Frequency of asking people to repeat statements
   b. Withdrawal from social interactions or large groups
   c. Shouting in conversation
   d. Failing to respond when not looking in the direction of the sound
   e. Answering questions incorrectly

- Assess for and document:
  1. External ear features (pinna)
     a. Size
     b. Position
  2. Otoscopic examination findings
     a. Patency of the external canal; presence of cerumen or foreign bodies, edema, or inflammation
     b. Condition of the tympanic membrane: intact, scars, edema, fluid, inflammation
  3. Abnormal Rinne test findings
     a. Air conduction greater than bone conduction in *conductive* hearing loss
     b. Bone conduction greater than air conduction in *sensorineural* hearing loss
  4. Abnormal Weber test findings
     a. Lateralization to the affected ear in *conductive* hearing loss
     b. Lateralization to the unaffected ear in *sensorineural* hearing loss
  5. Psychosocial issues
     a. Social isolation
     b. Depression, fear, and despair

- Diagnostic studies include audiometry to determine type and extent of hearing loss and imaging to determine possible causes.

Planning and Implementation

❖**NDx:** Disturbed Sensory Perception (Auditory)

Nonsurgical Management

- Early detection helps correct the problem causing the hearing loss.
- Drug therapy is used to correct an underlying pathologic change or to reduce side effects of problems occurring with hearing loss.
  1. Antibiotic therapy
  2. Analgesics

3. Antiemetics
4. Antivertiginous drugs
- Hearing-assistive devices
  1. Telephone amplifiers
  2. Therapy dogs
  3. Portable audio amplifiers
  4. Hearing aids
     a. Teach the patient to start using the hearing aid slowly, at first wearing it only at home and only during part of the day.
     b. Remind him or her that background noise will be amplified along with voices.
     c. Teach him or her to care for the hearing aid by:
        (1) Keeping the hearing aid dry
        (2) Cleaning the ear mold with mild soap and water while avoiding excessive wetting
        (3) Cleaning debris from the hole in the middle of the part that goes into the ear with a toothpick or a pipe cleaner
        (4) Turning off the hearing aid and removing the battery when not in use
        (5) Checking and replacing the battery frequently
        (6) Keeping extra batteries on hand
        (7) Keeping the hearing aid in a safe place
        (8) Avoiding dropping the hearing aid or exposing it to temperature extremes
        (9) Adjusting the volume to the lowest setting that allows hearing to prevent feedback squeaking
        (10) Avoiding using hair spray, cosmetics, oils, or other hair and face products that may come into contact with the receiver
  5. Cochlear implantation

Surgical Management
- The type of operative procedure selected depends on the cause of the hearing loss.
  1. *Tympanoplasty reconstruction* of the middle ear can improve conductive hearing loss. The procedures vary from simple reconstruction of the eardrum (myringoplasty or type I tympanoplasty) to replacement of the ossicles within the middle ear (type II tympanoplasty).
  2. *Stapedectomy* is the removal of the head and neck of the stapes and, less often, the footplate. After removal of the bone, a small hole is drilled or made with a laser in the footplate, and a prosthesis in the shape of a piston is connected between the incus and the footplate.

- Provide preoperative care, including:
  1. Routine preoperative instructions as described in Part One
  2. Using systemic antibiotics
  3. Irrigating the ear with a solution of equal parts of vinegar and sterile water to restore normal ear pH
  4. Instructing the patient to avoid people with upper respiratory infections, get adequate rest, eat a balanced diet, and drink adequate amounts of fluid
  5. Assuring the patient that hearing loss immediately after surgery is normal because of canal packing
  6. Explaining the importance of deep breathing after surgery
  7. Reinforcing the information provided by the surgeon
- Provide postoperative care, including:
  1. Routine postoperative care as described in Part One
  2. Keeping the dressing clean and dry, using sterile technique for changes
  3. Keeping the patient flat, with the head turned to the side and the operative ear facing up for at least 12 hours after surgery
  4. Using communication techniques for the hearing impaired
  5. Giving prescribed antibiotics to prevent infection
  6. Giving prescribed analgesics
  7. Giving prescribed antivertiginous drugs
  8. Assessing for and reporting complications (stapedectomy)
     a. Asymmetric appearance or drooping of features on the affected side of the face
     b. Patient reports changes in facial perception of touch and in taste.
  9. Assisting the patient with ambulating
  10. Reminding the patient to move his or her head slowly when changing position to avoid vertigo
  11. Teaching the patient about care and activity restrictions:
      a. Not using small objects, such as cotton-tipped applicators, matches, toothpicks, or hairpins, to clean the external ear canal
      b. Washing the external ear and canal daily in the shower or while washing the hair
      c. Blowing the nose gently
      d. Not occluding one nostril while blowing the nose
      e. Sneezing with the mouth open
      f. Wearing sound protection around loud or continuous noises
      g. Avoiding activities with high risk for head or ear trauma, such as wrestling, boxing, motorcycle riding, and skate-

H

boarding; wearing head and ear protection when engaging in these activities

h. Keeping the volume on head receivers at the lowest setting that allows hearing

i. Frequently cleaning objects that come into contact with the ear (e.g., headphones, telephone receivers)

j. Avoiding environmental conditions with rapid changes in air pressure

❖**NDx:** Impaired Verbal Communication

- Use best practices for communicating with a hearing-impaired patient, including:
    1. Positioning yourself directly in front of the patient
    2. Making sure that the room is well lighted
    3. Getting the patient's attention before you begin to speak
    4. Moving closer to the better-hearing ear
    5. Speaking clearly and slowly
    6. Keeping hands and other objects away from your mouth when talking to the patient
    7. Attempting to have conversations in a quiet room with minimal distractions
    8. Having the patient repeat your statements rather than just indicating assent
    9. Rephrasing sentences and repeat information to aid in understanding
    10. Using appropriate hand motions
    11. Writing messages on paper if the patient is able to read

> 🦴 Clinical Landmine ◆ Do not shout to the patient, because the sound may be projected at a higher frequency, making him or her less able to understand.

- Having the patient use hearing-assistive devices described earlier
- Encouraging the patient to use lip-reading
- Having the patient and family learn a sign language, such as American Sign Language (ASL)
- Managing anxiety and promoting social interaction by:
    1. Enhancing communication as described earlier
    2. Working with the patient to identify his or her most satisfying activities and social interactions and determine the amount of effort necessary to continue them
    3. Suggesting the use of closed-captioning for television programming

Community-Based Care

- Teach patients who have persistent vertigo and their families to determine the best ways to maintain adequate self-care abilities, maintain a safe environment, decide about assistance needs, and provide needed care.

- Give patients written instructions about how to take drugs and when to return for follow-up care.
- Teach patients how to instill eardrops and irrigate the ears, and obtain a return demonstration.
- Refer patients and families to a home care agency if needed for help with meal preparation, cleaning, and personal hygiene.
- Support patients by listening to their concerns and giving additional information when needed.
- Provide information about public and private agencies that offer hearing evaluations and that supply information and counseling for patients with hearing disorders.

HEART FAILURE

OVERVIEW

- Heart failure (HF), also called pump failure, is the inadequacy of the heart to pump blood throughout the body.
- HF causes insufficient perfusion of body tissue with vital nutrients and oxygen.
- Basic cardiac physiologic mechanisms such as stroke volume, heart rate, cardiac output, and contractility are altered in HF.
- The American College of Cardiology (ACC) and American Heart Association (AHA) have evidence-based guidelines for staging and managing HF as a chronic, progressive disease. These guidelines are combined with the New York Heart Association (NYHA) functional classification system that is used to describe symptoms exhibited by the patient to aid in determining response to interventions and prognostication.
- The major types of HF are:
  1. Left HF, which is characterized by pulmonary edema and further subdivided into systolic HF and diastolic HF
     a. Systolic HF (systolic ventricular dysfunction)
        (1) Systolic failure results when the heart is unable to contract forcefully enough during systole to eject adequate amounts of blood into the circulation, resulting in diminished tissue perfusion.
        (2) Preload increases with decreased contractility and afterload increases as a result of increased peripheral resistance.
        (3) The ejection fraction drops from a normal of 50% to 70% to below 40%.
        (4) Tissue perfusion diminishes and blood accumulates in the pulmonary vessels.

    b. Diastolic HF (diastolic ventricular function)

        (1) Diastolic failure occurs when the left ventricle is unable to relax adequately during diastole, which prevents the ventricle from filling with sufficient blood to ensure an adequate cardiac output.

        (2) The ejection fraction may remain near normal.

  2. Right HF occurs when the right ventricle is unable to empty completely. Right HF in the absence of left failure is most often the result of pulmonary problems. Increased volume and pressure develop in the systemic veins, and systemic venous congestion develops with peripheral edema.

  3. High-output failure can occur when cardiac output remains normal or above normal and is caused by increased metabolic needs or hyperkinetic conditions such as septicemia, anemia, and hyperthyroidism.

- When cardiac output is insufficient to meet the demands of the body, compensatory mechanisms operate to improve cardiac output. Although these mechanisms may initially increase cardiac output, they eventually have a damaging effect on pump function. Compensatory mechanisms contribute to increased myocardial oxygen consumption, leading to worsening signs and symptoms of HF. Compensatory mechanisms include:

  1. Sympathetic nervous system stimulation: Increased sympathetic nervous system response causes increased heart rate, increased force of contraction, and arterial vasoconstriction that increases afterload.

  2. Renin-angiotensin aldosterone system (RAAS) activation: Renin, angiotensin, and aldosterone work together to cause sodium and water retention when blood flow to the kidney decreases during HF. Angiotensin also increases arterial constriction or afterload.

  3. Other neurohumoral responses, such as the synthesis and release of B-type natriuretic peptide from the overstretched atrium: This hormone acts on kidneys to promote diuresis and decrease preload. Growth factors are also released.

  4. Myocardial hypertrophy: Growth of existing mycoardial cells in size (not numbers of cells) provides more muscle mass.

Considerations for Older Adults

- Heart failure is caused by systemic hypertension in 75% of cases.
- Long-term nonsteroidal anti-inflammatory drugs and thiazolidinediones used for diabetic patients can cause fluid and sodium retention, leading to hypertension and subsequently to heart failure.
- Prevalence of HF increases with age.

PATIENT-CENTERED COLLABORATIVE CARE

- Assessment findings include:
  1. History of hypertension, acute coronary syndrome, or myocardial disease such as myocarditis
  2. Dyspnea, orthopnea, breathlessness
  3. Decreased oxygen saturation (SpO_2) or PaO_2
  4. Increased respiratory rate and work of breathing including use of accessory muscles
  5. Crackles or rhonchi on auscultation
  6. Cough
  7. Frothy sputum
  8. Dysrhythmias, especially tachycardia
  9. Weak, thready peripheral pulses
  10. Cool, clammy skin
  11. Decreased mentation, restlessness, or anxiety
  12. Increased vascular or interstitial fluid on chest radiograph
  13. S_3 or S_4 heart sounds
  14. Cardiomegaly by palpation, electrocardiograph (ECG), or chest radiograph
  15. Increased serum B-type natriuretic peptide (BNP)
  16. Peripheral edema
  17. Jugular venous distention
  18. Enlarged liver and spleen, especially with right sided HF
  19. Reduced renal function including oliguria and increased blood urea nitrogen (BUN) and serum creatinine
  20. Anxiety and depression or other markers of psychological distress

Planning and Implementation
Nonsurgical Management
❖**NDx:** Impaired Gas Exchange
- Interventions include:
  1. Monitoring for improving or worsening pulmonary edema by assessing respiratory rate, rhythm, and character every 1 to 4 hours and auscultating breath sounds
  2. Titrating the amount of supplemental oxygen delivered to maintain oxygen saturation at 92% or greater
  3. Placing the patient experiencing respiratory difficulty in a high-Fowler position with pillows under each arm to maximize chest expansion and improve oxygenation
  4. Encouraging the patient to deep breathe and reposition self every 2 hours while awake and in bed

❖**NDx:** Decreased Cardiac Output
- Drug therapy is used to improve myocardial function.
  1. Angiotensin-converting enzyme (ACE) inhibitors are used to prevent conversion of angiotensin I to angiotensin II, resulting in reduction of arterial constriction. ACE inhibitors also

block aldosterone, which prevents sodium and water retention, decreasing fluid overload. Monitor blood pressure, especially orthostatic pressure in older adults. Monitor serum potassium level for hyperkalemia, serum creatinine level for renal dysfunction, and the patient for development of a cough. Monitor blood pressure to determine the patient's response to effective doses.

2. Beta blockers reduce the heart rate and interfere with the sympathetic nervous system compensatory mechanisms that promote adverse myocyte remodeling. Monitor for heart rates below 60 beats/min that cause the patient to exhibit symptomatic bradycardia.

3. Diuretics reduce intravascular volume, especially during an episode of exacerbation of HF. Monitor intake, output, and daily weights to determine fluid balance.

4. Oxygen therapy can maintain or increase Spo$_2$ above 92%.

5. Digoxin (Lanoxin) increases contractility, reduces the heart rate, slows conduction through the arteriovenous node, and inhibits sympathetic activity while enhancing parasympathetic activity. Older patients, particularly those who are hypokalemic, are susceptible to digoxin toxicity.

> **Clinical Landmine** ◆ Heart failure is managed with polypharmacy; typically, three or more drugs are used. The potential for drug interactions increases when three or more drugs are used regularly. Advise your patient and assist him or her in identifying potential drug interactions, including the use of NSAIDs, which can further cause significant acute kidney injury in the presence of low cardiac output.

- Diet therapy is used to reduce sodium and promote ideal body weight. Collaborate with the nutritionist and patient to select foods that meet a heart-healthy, sodium-restricted diet and to understand the importance of eliminating table salt and salt used in cooking. Increase the patient's intake of potassium-rich foods if using a loop or thiazide diuretic.
- Fluid restriction and monitoring
  1. Limit the patients in AHA class 3 or 4 to 2 L/day of fluids, including IV fluids; other HF patients may be restricted to 2.5 to 3 L/day. Weigh the patient every morning before breakfast using the same scale; this is the most reliable indicator of fluid gain or loss (1 kg of weight gain or loss equals 1 L of fluid retained or lost).
  2. Monitor and record intake and output.

3. Monitor for and prevent potassium deficiency from diuretic therapy. If the patient's potassium level is below 4.0 m Eq/L, a potassium supplement may be prescribed.
4. Recognize that patients with renal problems may develop hyperkalemia, especially with the use of potassium supplements, ACE inhibitors, or potassium-sparing diuretics. Renal problems are indicated by a creatinine level higher than 1.8 mg/dL.

- Other options to treat HF
  1. Continuous positive airway pressure (CPAP) improves sleep apnea (oxygen desaturation) and supports cardiac output and ejection fraction.
  2. Cardiac resynchronization therapy (CRT) uses a permanent pacemaker alone or in combination with an implantable cardioverter-defibrillator to provide biventricular pacing.
  3. Investigative stem cell and gene therapy replaces damaged myocytes or genes by a series of injections into the left ventricle.

❖**NDx:** Activity Intolerance

- The most common symptom reported by patients with HF is fatigue. The purpose of collaborative care is to regulate energy, prevent fatigue, and optimize function.
  1. Provide periods of uninterrupted rest.
  2. Assess the patient's response to increased activity. Check for changes in blood pressure, pulse, and oxygen saturation before and after an episode of new or increased activity.

> 🔲 Critical Rescue ◆ An increase in the heart rate of more than 20 beats/min, a change (increase or decrease) in systolic blood pressure of more than 20 mm Hg, or a decrease in the Spo_2 of more than 5% indicates activity intolerance. The physician should be informed about these findings in case it is necessary to alter drug therapy or initiate a physical therapy consultation to promote rehabilitation.

Surgical Management

- Heart transplantation is the ultimate choice for end-stage HF.
- Procedures to improve cardiac output in patients who are not candidates for heart transplant or are awaiting transplant include:
  1. Left ventricular assist device (LVAD)
  2. Right ventricular assist device (RVAD)
- Surgical therapies to reshape the left ventricle in patients with HF include:
  1. Partial left ventriculectomy

2. Endoventricular circular patch
3. Acorn cardiac support device
4. Myosplint cardiac support device perioperatively

- Care for the HF patient who is receiving a surgical intervention to improve pump failure is similar to patients receiving coronary revascularization or other open-heart surgery. Specific monitoring and interventions include:

  1. Assessing the patient with HF for acute pulmonary edema. Clinical manifestations include extreme anxiety; tachycardia; air hunger; moist cough productive of frothy, blood-tinged sputum; cold, clammy, cyanotic skin; crackles in lung bases; disorientation; and confusion.
  2. Administering rapid-acting diuretics, as prescribed
  3. Providing oxygen and maintaining the patient in a high Fowler position
  4. Administering morphine sulfate intravenously to reduce venous return (preload), decrease anxiety, and reduce the work of breathing
  5. Administering other drugs such as bronchodilators and vasodilators
  6. Monitoring vital signs closely including pulse oximetry
  7. Monitoring intake and output; weighing daily

Community-Based Care

- Collaborate with the case manager or social worker to assess the patient's needs for health care resources (e.g., home care nurse) and social support (family and friends to help with care if needed), and facilitate appropriate placement.
- Discharge preparation includes:

  1. Encouraging the patient to stay as active as possible and developing a regular exercise program; investigating the possibility of a rehabilitation program referral

     a. If the patient experiences chest pain or pronounced dyspnea while exercising or experiences excessive fatigue, he or she is probably advancing the activity too quickly and should be returned to the previous level for 24 to 48 hours.

  2. Instructing the patient to watch for and report to the physician

     a. Weight gain of more than 3 pounds in 1 week or 1 to 2 pounds overnight
     b. Decrease in exercise tolerance lasting 2 to 3 days
     c. Cold symptoms (cough) lasting more than 3 to 5 days
     d. Frequent urination at night
     e. Development of dyspnea or angina at rest, or worsening angina
     f. Increased swelling in the feet, ankles, and hands

3. Providing oral and written instructions concerning drugs
4. Teaching the patient and caregiver how to take and record the pulse rate and blood pressure to help monitor response to drug and exercise regimens
5. Instructing the patient to weigh himself or herself each day in the morning
6. Reviewing the signs and symptoms of hypokalemia for patients on diuretics and providing information on foods high in potassium
7. Recommending that the patient restrict dietary sodium, providing written instructions on low-salt diets, and identifying food flavorings to use as a substitute for salt, such as lemon, garlic, and herbs
8. Discussing the importance of advance directives with the patient or family. If resuscitation is desired, the family should know how to activate the Emergency Medical System and how to provide cardiopulmonary resuscitation (CPR) until an ambulance arrives. If CPR is not desired, the patient and family should be given resources on what to do and how to respond.
9. Referring the patient to the American Heart Association (AHA) for information and support groups

> **Critical Rescue** ♦ A weight gain of 1 kg (2.2 pounds) is equivalent to an additional liter of fluid in the vascular and tissue compartments. Intravascular fluid overload can decrease myocardial recoil, promoting permanent, adverse changes in the heart.

HEMATOPOIETIC STEM CELL TRANSPLANTATION (BONE MARROW TRANSPLANTATION)

OVERVIEW

- *Hematopoietic stem cell transplantation (HSCT)* is the process of collecting stem cells from one person (the donor) and transplanting them into another person (the recipient) or into the same person at a later time.
- Stem cells are immature and undifferentiated cells that can mature into any blood cell type.
- Sources of stem cells include the bone marrow, circulating peripheral blood, and cord blood from newborns.
- When stem cells are obtained from the bone marrow, the process is called *bone marrow transplantation (BMT)*.

- When stem cells are transplanted into a recipient, the new cells go to the marrow and then begin the process of hematopoiesis, which results in normal, properly functioning WBCs, RBCs, and platelets.
- Disorders that can be cured by HSCT include acute leukemia, lymphoma, multiple myeloma, aplastic anemia, sickle cell disease, and many solid tumors.
- After successful HSCT, the recipient has the blood type and the immune function of the donor.
- The three types of transplantation are:
  1. *Allogeneic transplantation,* in which the stem cells are taken from a sibling or human leukocyte antigen (HLA)–matched, unrelated donor
  2. *Autologous transplantation,* in which the donor receives his or her own stem cells (collected before any cytotoxic treatment)
  3. *Syngeneic transplantation,* in which the stem cells are taken from the patient's own identical sibling

🌐 Cultural Awareness

About 70% of people on the bone marrow donor lists are white. The chance of finding an HLA-matched, unrelated donor is estimated at 30% to 40% for white people, but for African Americans, the chance is less than 20% because there are fewer African Americans among registered donors. Although blood types are common in all racial groups, tissue types can be very different among racial and ethnic groups. Nationally, efforts are made to publicize the need for donors from all cultural backgrounds. Research in this area has identified several potential barriers to stem cell donation among African Americans. These include fear of or not trusting the system, concern about costs to the donor, and concern that the recipient may be a drug abuser or person that would not appreciate the sacrifice of a donation. Targeted education efforts may reduce these barriers.

- The five phases of HSCT are:
  1. *Stem cell obtainment,* which involves taking stem cells either from the patient directly (autologous stem cells) or from an HLA-matched person (allogeneic stem cells)
  2. *Conditioning regimen,* which involves either "wiping out" the patient's own bone marrow, thus preparing the patient for optimal graft take, or giving higher than normal doses of chemotherapy or radiotherapy to rid the person of cancer cells (myeloablation). Usually a period of 5 to 10 days is required.

3. *Transplantation,* which is the actual infusion of the stem cells through the patient's central catheter like an ordinary blood transfusion
4. *Engraftment,* which is the process of the transplanted cells moving into the recipient's bone marrow and beginning to make new, functioning blood cells
5. *Post-transplantation recovery,* which is the time period between when engraftment begins and full recovery of immune function, RBC function, and platelet function occurs

PATIENT-CENTERED COLLABORATIVE CARE

- In addition to the recipient of an HSCT, allogeneic stem cell transplantation using bone marrow cells and plasma pheresis harvesting involves the donor as a patient.
- Patient care for the donor
  1. Bone marrow harvest is a surgical procedure performed under general anesthesia.
  2. About 500 to 1000 mL of bone marrow are aspirated through multiple sites from the donor's iliac crests.
     a. After the procedure, monitor the donor for:
        (1) Pain
        (2) Fluid loss
        (3) Bleeding from harvest sites
     b. Teach the donor about:
        (1) Inspecting the harvest sites for bleeding
        (2) Taking prescribed analgesics for pain
  3. Peripheral blood stem cells (PBSCs) are stem cells that have been released from the bone marrow and circulate within the blood.
  4. PBSC harvesting requires three phases: mobilization, collection by pheresis, and infusion or reinfusion.
     a. Mobilization phase involves giving the donor hematopoietic growth factors for several days before pheresis to increase the numbers of stem cells in the peripheral blood.
     b. Pheresis is the collection of stem cells by withdrawing whole blood, filtering out the cells, and returning the plasma to the patient. One to five pheresis procedures, each lasting 2 to 4 hours, are needed to obtain enough stem cells for transplantation.
     c. Infusion is the placement of collected stem cells into the recipient by infusion through a central venous catheter.
  5. During pheresis, monitor the patient for:
     a. Hypotension
     b. Catheter clotting

    c. Hypocalcemia
- (1) Numbness or tingling in the fingers and toes or around the mouth
- (2) Abdominal or muscle cramping
- (3) Chest pain

- Patient care for the recipient
  1. Conditioning
     a. The day the patient receives the stem cells is day T-0. Before transplantation, the conditioning days are counted in reverse order from T-0, just like a rocket countdown. After transplantation, days are counted in order from the day of transplantation.
     b. The conditioning regimen is individually tailored to each patient and usually includes high-dose chemotherapy and sometimes includes total-body irradiation (TBI).
     c. A typical conditioning regimen is:
        (1) *Days T-5 through T-4*: high-dose chemotherapy to obliterate the patient's own bone marrow cells or to kill off any remaining cancer cells (if part of cancer treatment)
        (2) *Days T-3 through T-1*: delivery of TBI. The total radiation dose for TBI is 1200 rads given as 200 rads twice daily over 3 days.
     d. Immediate side effects from conditioning are intense or severe and include:
        (1) Nausea and vomiting
        (2) Mucositis
        (3) Capillary leak syndrome
        (4) Diarrhea
        (5) Bone marrow suppression
            (i) Neutropenia
            (ii) Anemia
            (iii) Thrombocytopenia

> 🔲 **Critical Rescue** ◆ During conditioning and before engraftment, the patient has no immune function and is at great risk for life-threatening infection. Infection protection is the priority for management at this time.

    e. Late effects from the conditioning regimen are also common 3 to 10 years after transplantation. These problems include veno-occlusive disease (VOD), skin toxicities, cataracts, lung fibrosis, second cancers, cardiomyopathy, endocrine complications, and neurologic complications.

2. Transplantation
   a. Frozen marrow, PBSCs, or umbilical cord blood cells are thawed and then infused.

> **Clinical Landmine** ◆ Do not use blood administration tubing because the cells can get caught in the filter and not enter the patient's body.

   b. Side effects of all types of stem cell transfusions are similar and may include:
      (1) Fever
      (2) Hypertension
      (3) Fluid overload
      (4) Red urine (resulting from RBC breakage in the infused stem cells)
3. Engraftment
   a. The successful "take" of the transplanted cells in the patient's bone marrow is key to the whole transplantation process.
   b. Engraftment takes 8 to 12 days for PBSC transplantation and 12 to 28 days for bone marrow stem cell transplantation.
   c. To aid engraftment, growth factors, such as granulocyte colony-stimulating factor (G-CSF) or granulocyte-macrophage colony-stimulating factor (GM-CSF), may be given. When engraftment occurs, the patient's WBC, RBC, and platelet counts begin to rise.
   d. Nursing care focuses on prevention of complications, which include:
      (1) Infection
      (2) Bleeding
      (3) Failure to engraft (*If the transplanted cells fail to engraft, the patient will die unless another transplantation is successful.*)
      (4) Development of graft-versus-host disease (GVHD), in which the immunocompetent cells of the donated marrow recognize the patient's (recipient) cells, tissues, and organs as foreign and start an immunologic attack against them. GVHD occurs most often in the skin, intestinal tract, and liver, and more than 15% of the patients who develop GVHD die of its complications. Manifestations are:
         (i) Excessive peeling of the skin
         (ii) Profuse, watery diarrhea
         (iii) Liver tenderness, with jaundice

(5) Development of veno-occlusive disease (VOD), which is the blockage of liver blood vessels by clotting and inflammation (phlebitis). Manifestations include:
   (i) Jaundice
   (ii) Pain in the right upper quadrant
   (iii) Ascites
   (iv) Weight gain
   (v) Liver enlargement
(6) Depression (contributing factors include prolonged hospitalization, limited activity, intense therapy side-effects, uncertain treatment outcome)

HEMOPHILIA

OVERVIEW

- Hemophilia is two different hereditary bleeding disorders resulting from clotting factor deficiencies, which impair the formation of stable fibrin clots and lead to excessive bleeding.
  1. *Hemophilia A (classic hemophilia)* is a deficiency of factor VIII and accounts for 80% of cases of hemophilia.
  2. *Hemophilia B (Christmas disease)* is a deficiency of factor IX and accounts for 20% of cases.

Genetic Considerations

- Hemophilia A is an X-linked recessive trait. Women who are *carriers* (able to pass on the gene without actually having the disorder) have a 50% chance of passing the hemophilia gene to their daughters (who then are carriers) and to their sons (who then have hemophilia).
- It affects mostly men, none of whose sons will have the gene for hemophilia and all of whose daughters will be carriers.
- About 30% of hemophilia arises from a new gene mutation and has no family history.
- Abnormal bleeding occurs in response to any trauma because of a deficiency of the specific clotting factor. Bleeding may be mild, moderate, or severe, depending on the degree of factor deficiency.

PATIENT-CENTERED COLLABORATIVE CARE

- Assess for and document:
  1. Excessive bleeding from minor cuts, bruises, or abrasions
  2. Joint and muscle hemorrhages that lead to disabling long-term problems
  3. A tendency to bruise easily
  4. Prolonged and potentially fatal hemorrhage after surgery

5. Prolonged partial thromboplastin time (PTT), a normal bleeding time, and a normal prothrombin time (PT)
- The bleeding problems of hemophilia A are managed by regularly scheduled infusions of factor VIII cryoprecipitate (Bioclate, Helixate, ReFacto) or by intermittent infusions, as needed.

HEMORRHOIDS

- Hemorrhoids are unnaturally swollen or distended veins in the anorectal region that are common and not significant unless they cause pain or bleeding.
- Increased intra-abdominal pressure causes elevated systemic and portal venous pressure, which is transmitted to the anorectal veins.
- Internal hemorrhoids cannot be seen on inspection of the perianal area and lie above the anal sphincter.
- External hemorrhoids can be seen on inspection and lie below the anal sphincter.
- Prolapsed hemorrhoids can become thrombosed or inflamed, or they can bleed.
- Common causes of repeated increased abdominal pressure are straining at stool, pregnancy, and portal hypertension.
- Assessment findings include:
  1. Bleeding, which is characteristically bright red and found on toilet tissue or outside the stool
  2. Pain associated with thrombosis
  3. Itching
  4. Mucous discharge
- Diagnosis is made by inspection, digital examination, and proctoscopy, if needed.

Nonsurgical Management

- Conservative management focuses on reducing symptoms and includes:
  1. Application of cold packs to the anorectal area followed by tepid sitz baths
  2. Witch hazel soaks and topical anesthetics such as lidocaine (Xylocaine)
  3. OTC remedies such as Nupercainal ointment used temporarily, because prolonged use can mask worsening symptoms and delay diagnosis of a severe disorder
  4. High-fiber diet and fluids to promote regular bowel movements without straining
  5. Stool softeners
  6. Teaching the patient to cleanse the anal area with moistened cleaning tissues and to gently dab the area rather than wipe

Surgical Management
- Ultrasound, sclerotherapy, circular stapling, or hemorrhoidectomy may be indicated for recurring symptoms.
- Postoperative care
  1. Monitor for bleeding and pain.
  2. Apply moist heat (e.g., sitz baths) three to four times each day after the first 12 hours postoperatively.
  3. Administer stool softeners such as docusate sodium (Colace).
  4. Administer opioid analgesia postoperatively and before the first defecation.

HEMOTHORAX

- Hemothorax is blood loss into the thoracic cavity and is a common result of blunt chest trauma or penetrating injuries.
  1. A *simple* hemothorax is a blood loss of less than 1500 mL.
  2. A *massive* hemothorax is a blood loss of more than 1500 mL.
- Bleeding is caused by lung contusions or lacerations that can occur with rib and sternal fractures.
- Massive internal chest bleeding in blunt chest trauma may stem from the heart, great vessels, or the intercostal arteries.
- Physical assessment findings depend on the size of the hemothorax.
  1. A smaller hemothorax may cause no symptoms.
  2. Symptoms of a large hemothorax may include:
     a. Respiratory distress
     b. Reduced breath sounds
     c. Blood in the pleural space (seen on a chest x-ray and confirmed by diagnostic thoracentesis)
- Interventions, aimed at removing the blood in the pleural space to normalize pulmonary function and to prevent infection, include front and back chest tube insertion.
- A large hemothorax, greater than an initial blood loss of 1500 to 2000 mL, may require an open thoracotomy.
- Nursing interventions include:
  1. Monitoring vital signs
  2. Carefully monitoring chest tube drainage for excessive blood loss
  3. Measuring intake and output
  4. Assessing the patient's response to the chest tubes
  5. Infusing IV fluids and blood as prescribed
- The blood lost through chest drainage can be autotransfused back into the patient if needed.

HEPATITIS

OVERVIEW

- Hepatitis is the widespread inflammation of liver cells, resulting in enlargement of the liver and congestion with inflammatory cells.
- Viral hepatitis is the most prevalent type and is caused by one of five common viruses.
  1. Hepatitis A virus (HAV)
     a. HAV is a ribonucleic acid (RNA) virus of the enterovirus family. It is a hardy virus and survives on human hands. HAV is spread by the fecal-oral route, consuming contaminated food, or by person-to-person contact (e.g., oral-anal sexual activity). Unsanitary water, shellfish caught in contaminated water, and food contaminated by food handlers infected with the HAV are all potential sources of infection.
     b. It is characterized by a mild course and often goes unrecognized. HAV is the most common type of viral hepatitis.
     c. The incubation period is usually 15 to 50 days.
  2. Hepatitis B virus (HBV)
     a. HBV is a double-shelled particle containing deoxyribonucleic acid (DNA) composed of a core antigen (HBcAg), a surface antigen (HBsAg), and another antigen found within the core (HBeAg) that circulates in the blood.
     b. Formerly known as serum hepatitis, HBV is transmitted through broken skin or mucous membranes by infected blood and serous fluids. Lower concentrations of HBV are also found in semen, vaginal fluid, and saliva.
     c. HBV is spread by sexual contact, shared needles, accidental needle sticks or injuries from sharp instruments, blood transfusion, hemodialysis, acupuncture, tattooing, ear or body piercing, and mother-fetal route.
     d. The clinical course is varied, with an insidious onset and mild symptoms (anorexia, nausea, vomiting, fever, fatigue, dark urine with light stool).
     e. The incubation period is generally between 25 and 180 days.
  3. Hepatitis C virus (HCV)
     a. The causative virus is an enveloped, single-strand RNA virus that is transmitted by exposure of the skin and mucous membrane to infected blood or serum.
     b. HCV is spread by contaminated items such as illicit IV drug needles, blood and blood products and transplanted

H

organs received before 1992, needle stick injury with HCV-contaminated blood, tattoo, and intranasal cocaine use.

   c. It is not transmitted by casual contact or intimate household contacts. However, those infected should not share razors, toothbrushes, or pierced earrings because there may be microscopic blood on these items.

   d. The incubation period is 21 to 140 days, with an average incubation period of 7 weeks.

   e. Chronic liver disease occurs in 85% of those infected. HCV cirrhosis is the leading indicator for liver transplantation.

4. Hepatitis D (delta hepatitis or HDV)

   a. HDV is a defective RNA virus that needs the helper function of HBV for viral replication. HDV co-infects with HBV.

   b. Incubation period is 14 to 56 days.

   c. HDV is transmitted primarily by parenteral routes.

5. Hepatitis E virus (HEV)

   a. HEV was originally identified by its association with epidemics of hepatitis in the Indian subcontinent and has since been found in epidemics in Asia, Africa, Mexico, the Middle East, and Central and South America.

   b. In the U. S. and Canada, HEV has occurred in people who have visited these endemic areas.

   c. HEV is transmitted by the oral-fecal route and most commonly causes infection from contaminated food or water. The incubation period is 15 to 64 days.

- Toxic and drug-induced forms of hepatitis result from exposure to hepatotoxins such as industrial toxins, alcohol, or drugs. Treatment is supportive.
- Hepatitis may occur as a secondary infection during the course of other viral infections, such as cytomegalovirus, Epstein-Barr virus, herpes simplex virus, and varicella-zoster virus.
- Fulminant hepatitis is a failure of the liver cells to regenerate, with progression of the necrotic process that is often fatal.
- Liver inflammation persisting longer than 6 months is considered chronic hepatitis.

PATIENT-CENTERED COLLABORATIVE CARE

Assessment

- Record patient information.
  1. Known exposure to persons with hepatitis infection
  2. Blood transfusions or organ transplantation

3. History of hemodialysis
4. Sexual preferences
5. Injectable drug use
6. Recent ear or body piercing
7. Recent tattooing
8. Living accommodations, including crowded facilities
9. Health care employment history
10. Recent travel to foreign countries
11. Recent ingestion of shellfish
12. HIV infection
13. History of alcohol abuse

- Assessment findings for viral hepatitis include:
  1. Abdominal pain
  2. Changes in skin or sclera (icterus)
  3. Arthralgia (joint pain) or myalgia (muscle pain)
  4. Diarrhea or constipation; clay-colored stools
  5. Dark or amber colored urine
  6. Fever
  7. Lethargy
  8. Malaise
  9. Nausea and vomiting
  10. Pruritus (itching)
  11. Liver tenderness in the right upper quadrant
  12. Elevated serum liver enzymes
  13. Elevated total bilirubin (serum and urine)
  14. Serologic markers for hepatitis A, B, C, or D
- The clinical manifestations of toxic and drug-induced hepatitis depend on the causative agent.
- Patients may be angry about being sick and being fatigued; may feel guilty about having exposed others to the disease; may be embarrassed by the isolation and hygiene precautions that are necessary; and may be worried about the loss of wages, cost of hospitalization, and general financial issues.
- Family members may be afraid of contracting the disease and therefore distance themselves from the patient.

Planning and Implementation
- Promote rest.
  1. Maintain physical rest alternating with periods of activity to promote liver cell regeneration by reducing the liver's metabolic needs.
  2. Individualize the patient's plan of care and change it to reflect the severity of symptoms, fatigue, and results of liver function tests and enzyme determinations.
  3. Promote emotional and psychological rest.

- Provide diet therapy. A special diet is not needed, but diet should be high in carbohydrates and calories with moderate amounts of fat and protein.
  1. Determine food preferences.
  2. Provide small, frequent meals.
  3. Provide high-calorie snacks as needed.
- Drug therapy includes:
  1. Supplemental vitamins
  2. Antiemetics, such as trimethobenzamide hydrochloride (Tigan, Tegamide) or dimenhydrinate (Dramamine, Travamine ✤) to relieve nausea
  3. Antiviral drugs and immunomodulators for HBV and HCV
- Liver transplantation may be performed for patients with end stage liver disease from chronic hepatitis.

Community-Based Care

- Provide health teaching, including:
  1. Modes of transmission of hepatitis
  2. Observation of measures to prevent infection transmission
  3. Avoiding alcohol and checking with the health care provider before taking any OTC drug or any vitamin, supplement, or herbal preparation
  4. Determination of activity tolerance and rest
  5. Eating small, frequent meals of high-carbohydrate and low-fat foods
  6. Avoiding sexual activity until HBV surface antigen (HBsAg) testing results are negative

HERNIA

OVERVIEW

- A hernia is a weakness in the abdominal muscle wall through which a segment of bowel or other abdominal structure protrudes. Increased intra-abdominal pressure can contribute to hernia formation.
- Hernias are labeled by anatomic location, combined with the severity of protrusion:
  1. Indirect inguinal hernia, a sac formed from the peritoneum that contains a portion of the intestine or omentum; in men, indirect hernias can become large and descend into the scrotum
  2. Direct inguinal hernia, which passes through a weak point in the abdominal wall
  3. Femoral hernia, which occurs through the femoral ring as a plug of fat in the femoral canal that enlarges and pulls the peritoneum and the bladder into the sac

4. Umbilical hernia, which is congenital (infancy) or acquired as a result of increased intra-abdominal pressure, most often in obese persons

5. Incisional (ventral) hernia, which occurs at the site of a previous surgical incision as a result of inadequate healing, postoperative wound infection, inadequate nutrition, or obesity

6. A reducible hernia allows the contents of the hernial sac to be reduced or placed back into the abdominal cavity.

7. An irreducible, or incarcerated, hernia cannot be reduced or placed back into the abdominal cavity. It requires immediate surgical evaluation.

8. A strangulated hernia results when the blood supply to the herniated segment of the bowel is cut off by pressure from the hernial ring, causing ischemia and obstruction of the bowel loop; this can lead to bowel necrosis and perforation, which are surgical emergencies.

Considerations for Older Adults

The older adult with a strangulated hernia may not complain of pain but usually has nausea and vomiting. Direct inguinal hernias occur more often in older adults than in younger persons.

PATIENT-CENTERED COLLABORATIVE CARE

- Assess for a hernia when the patient is lying down and again when the patient is standing. If a hernia is reducible, it may disappear when the patient is lying flat.
- Listen for bowel sounds (absence may indicate GI obstruction).

Nonsurgical Management

- A truss (a pad with firm support) may be used for older or debilitated patients who are poor surgical risks.

Surgical Management

- Herniorrhaphy, the surgical treatment of choice, involves replacing the contents of the hernial sac into the abdominal cavity and closing the opening.
- Hernioplasty reinforces the weakened muscular wall with a mesh patch.
- Postoperative instructions
  1. Avoid coughing but encourage deep breathing.
  2. Turn frequently and promote early, progressive mobility.
  3. For inguinal hernia repair, wear a scrotal support and apply an ice bag to the scrotum to prevent swelling. Elevate the scrotum with a soft pillow when in bed.
  4. Avoid bladder and bowel distention.

   a. Using techniques to stimulate voiding, such as assisting a man to stand

   b. Catheterizing the patient every 6 to 8 hours if he or she is unable to void

   c. Avoiding constipation and teaching the patient to avoid straining with stool during healing

Community-Based Care
- Teach the patient:
  1. How to care for the incision if surgery corrects the muscle defect
  2. To limit activity, including avoiding lifting and straining, for 2 weeks after surgery
  3. To report symptoms such as fever and chills, wound drainage, redness or separation of the incision, and increasing incisional pain to the health care provider

HERNIA, HIATAL

OVERVIEW

- Hiatal hernias, also called diaphragmatic hernias, involve the protrusion of the stomach through the esophageal hiatus of the diaphragm into the thorax.
- There are two major types of hiatal hernias:
  1. Sliding hernia, which occurs when the esophagogastric junction and a portion of the fundus of the stomach slide upward through the esophageal hiatus into the thorax, with the hernia moving freely and sliding into and out of the thorax when there are changes in position or intra-abdominal pressure increases
  2. Paraesophageal, or rolling, hernia, which occurs when the gastroesophageal junction stays below the diaphragm but the fundus and portions of the greater curvature of the stomach roll through the esophageal hiatus and into the thorax beside the esophagus; risk for volvulus, obstruction, and strangulation are high

PATIENT-CENTERED COLLABORATIVE CARE

- Assessment findings include:
  1. Heartburn
  2. Regurgitation (esophageal reflux)
  3. Pain
  4. Dysphagia
  5. Belching
  6. Symptoms of sliding hernia are associated with reflux

7. Symptoms of rolling hernia include a feeling of fullness after eating or a feeling of breathlessness or suffocation
8. Increased symptoms when in a recumbent position
9. Confirmation via a barium swallow study with fluoroscopy as the most specific diagnostic test.

Interventions

Nonsurgical Management

- Drug therapy includes the use of antacids and histamine receptor antagonists to control esophageal reflux and its symptoms.
- Teach the patient to avoid fatty foods, coffee, tea, cola, chocolate, alcohol, spicy foods, and acidic foods such as orange juice.
- Encourage the patient to eat four to six small meals each day and consume liquids between meals to avoid abdominal distension.
- Teach the patient to avoid nighttime snacking to ensure that the stomach is empty before bedtime.
- Encourage weight reduction because obesity increases intra-abdominal pressure.
- Elevate the head of the bed 6 inches to reduce the incidence of esophageal reflux.
- Instruct the patient to avoid lying down several hours after eating, straining or excessively vigorous exercise, or wearing tight or constrictive clothing.

Surgical Management

- Elective surgery is indicated when the risk of complications such as aspiration are high and damage from chronic reflux is severe.
- Provide routine preoperative care.
- Inform the patient that he or she will have an nasogastric (NG) tube after surgery.
- Determine whether the patient will have a chest tube after surgery and include this information in preoperative teaching.
- Surgical approaches for sliding hernias involve reinforcement of the lower esophageal sphincter (LES) to restore sphincter competence and prevent reflux through some degree of fundoplication, or the wrapping of a portion of the stomach fundus around the distal esophagus to anchor it and reinforce the LES.
- Provide postoperative care similar to that for any patient with esophageal surgery with a focus on:
  1. Assessing for complications of surgery, such as temporary dysphagia after oral feeding begins, gas bloat syndrome, atelectasis or pneumonia, and obstruction of the NG tube
  2. Providing adequate pain relief

3. Elevating the head of the bed at least 30 degrees
4. Teaching the patient to support the incisional area during coughing and deep breathing
5. Ensuring correct placement and patency of the NG tube
6. Teaching the patient to avoid drinking carbonated beverages, eating gas-producing foods (especially high-fat foods), chewing gum, and drinking with a straw
7. Encouraging frequent position changes and early ambulation

Community-Based Care

- Advise the patient:
   1. To avoid straining and lifting and restrict stair climbing for 2-6 weeks following surgical repair
   2. To inspect the surgical wound daily and report the incidence of swelling, redness, tenderness, or discharge to the physician
   3. About the importance of reporting fever to the physician
   4. To avoid prolonged coughing episodes to prevent dehiscence of the fundoplication
   5. To stop smoking
   6. About diet modifications, including weight loss goals if needed, eating small portions, avoiding irritating foods and liquids, and reporting recurrence of reflux symptoms to the physician
   7. To avoid straining and prevent constipation while having a bowel movement; stool softeners or bulk laxatives may be needed.

HERPES, GENITAL

OVERVIEW

- Genital herpes (GH) is an acute, recurring, incurable viral disease.
- The two types of herpes simplex virus (HSV) are:
   1. Type 1 (HSV-1), which causes most nongenital lesions such as cold sores
   2. Type 2 (HSV-2), which causes most of the genital lesions

> **Clinical Landmine** ◆ Either type of virus can produce oral or genital lesions through oral-genital contact with an infected person.

- The incubation period is 2 to 20 days, with the average period being 1 week, and many people do not have symptoms during this time.
- Recurrences are not caused by re-infection, and outbreaks are usually less severe and of shorter duration than the primary

infection. *However, there is viral shedding, and the patient is infectious.*

- Long-term complications of GH include the risk of neonatal transmission and an increased risk for acquiring HIV infection.

PATIENT-CENTERED COLLABORATIVE CARE

Assessment

- Obtain patient information about:
  1. The sensation of itching or tingling felt in the skin 1 to 2 days before the outbreak
  2. Whether he or she has had headaches or general malaise
  3. Presence of painful urination or urinary retention
  4. Factors that can trigger a recurrence, such as stress, fever, sunburn, poor nutrition, menses, and sexual activity
- Assess for and document:
  1. The presence of *vesicles* (blisters) in a typical cluster on the penis, scrotum, vulva, vagina, cervix, or perianal region
  2. The presence of painful erosions
  3. Swelling of inguinal lymph nodes
- Diagnostic tests for GH include:
  1. Viral culture
  2. Serology testing to identify the HSV type
  3. Type-specific rapid assays
     a. POCkit HSV-2 Rapid Test
     b. HerpeSelect 1 and 2 Immunoblot IgG test

Interventions

- Interventions to decrease the discomfort from painful ulcerations, promote healing without secondary infection, decrease viral shedding, and prevent infection transmission include:
  1. Drug therapy with antiviral agents
     a. Acyclovir (Zovirax, Avirax ✦)
     b. Famciclovir (Famvir)
     c. Valacyclovir (Valtrex)
  2. Intermittent or continuous suppressive antiviral therapy offered to patients to lessen or prevent outbreaks
  3. Therapy for severe recurrent outbreaks is most beneficial if it is started within 1 day of the appearance of lesions or during the pre-lesion period.
- Emphasize the risk for neonatal infection to all patients, both male and female.
- Teach patients to avoid transmission by:
  1. Adhering to suppressive therapy
  2. Abstaining from sexual activity while lesions are present
  3. Using condoms during all sexual exposures
  4. Keeping the skin in the genital region clean and dry

5. Washing hands thoroughly after contact with lesions and laundering towels that have had direct contact with lesions
6. Wearing gloves when applying ointments
- Help patients and their partner's cope with the diagnosis by:
  1. Assessing the patient's and partner's emotional responses to the diagnosis of genital herpes
  2. Being sensitive and supportive during assessments and interventions
  3. Encouraging social support
  4. Referring them to support groups such as HELP (local support groups of the National Herpes Resource Center [*www.healthywomen.org*])

HIV DISEASE (HIV/AIDS)

OVERVIEW

- HIV disease is a continuum of immune deficiency problems that occur as a result of infection with the human immunodeficiency virus (HIV).
- From the onset of HIV infection through progression to acquired immunodeficiency syndrome (AIDS), the late and final stage, HIV disease represents a continuing battle between the virus and the patient's immune system.
- The HIV is a retrovirus, which carries special enzymes and has RNA as its genetic material. These features give HIV major advantages for infecting living human cells and replicating within them.
- HIV is transmitted in three ways:
  1. *Sexual:* genital, anal, or oral sexual contact with exposure of mucous membranes to infected semen or vaginal secretions
  2. *Parenteral:* sharing of needles or equipment contaminated with infected blood or receiving contaminated blood products
  3. *Perinatal:* from the placenta, from contact with maternal blood and body fluids during birth, or from breast milk from an infected mother to child
- Needle stick or "sharps" injuries are the main means of occupation-related HIV infection for health care workers. Health care workers also can be infected through exposure of nonintact skin and mucous membranes to blood and body fluids.
- Everyone who has AIDS has HIV infection; however, not everyone who has HIV infection has AIDS.
- A diagnosis of AIDS requires that the person is HIV positive and has one of the following:
  1. A CD4$^+$ T-cell count of less than 200 cells/mm^3
  2. An opportunistic infection

- Immune system abnormalities resulting from HIV disease include:
  1. Lymphocytopenia (decreased numbers of lymphocytes, especially CD4⁺ T-cell levels)
  2. Increased production of incomplete and nonfunctional antibodies
  3. Abnormally functioning macrophages
- *The person with HIV infection can transmit the virus to others at all stages of disease.*
- As a result of these abnormalities, the patient is at risk for bacterial, fungal, and viral infections, as well as for some opportunistic cancers.
- *Opportunistic infections* are those caused by organisms that are present as part of the normal environment and are kept in check by normal immune function.
- Once AIDS is diagnosed, even if the patient's cell count goes higher than 200 cells/mm³ or if the infection is successfully treated, the AIDS diagnosis remains and the patient never reverts to being just HIV positive.
- The time from the beginning of HIV infection to development of AIDS ranges from months to years, depending on:
  1. How HIV was acquired
  2. Personal factors, such as frequency of re-exposure to HIV, presence of other sexually transmitted diseases (STDs), nutritional status, and stress
  3. Interventions used

Genetic Considerations

- About 1% of people with HIV infection are *long-term nonprogressors* (LTNPs). These people have been infected with HIV for at least 10 years, have remained asymptomatic, and have CD4⁺ T-cell counts within the normal range.
- A genetic difference for this population is that their CCR5/CXCR4 co-receptors on the CD4⁺ T-cells are abnormal and nonfunctional. This mutation creates a defective receptor that does not bind to the HIV docking proteins.
- Cells with this defective receptor successfully resist the entrance of the HIV.

Cultural Awareness

- More than 72% of new HIV infections reported in the U. S. occur in racial and ethnic minority groups, particularly among African Americans and Hispanics.

- Factors that may increase the incidence of HIV infection and progression to AIDS among minority groups include:
  1. Fear of or lack of faith in the U. S. health care system
  2. Poverty and limited access to high-cost drugs
  3. Health beliefs about HIV treatment

Considerations for Older Adults

- Infection with HIV can occur at any age and older patients should be assessed for risk behaviors, including a sexual and drug use history.
- Age-related decline in immune function increases the likelihood that the older adult will develop the infection after an HIV exposure.
- In the older woman, thinning of vaginal tissue as a result of decreased estrogen may increase susceptibility to all sexually transmitted diseases (STDs), including HIV infection.

Women's Health Considerations

- Women are the fastest growing group with HIV infection and AIDS in North America.
- In less affluent countries, 50% of cases occur among women.
- Risk factors are sexual exposure (75%) and injection drug use (25%).
- Women with HIV infection have a poorer outcome with a shorter mean survival time than men. This outcome may be the result of late diagnosis and social or economic factors that reduce access to medical care.
- Gynecologic problems, especially persistent or recurrent vaginal candidiasis, may be the first signs of HIV infection in women. Other common problems include genital herpes, pelvic inflammatory disease, and cervical dysplasia or cancer.
- The effect of HIV on pregnancy outcomes includes a higher incidence of premature delivery, low-birth-weight infants, and transmission of the disease to the infant.

PATIENT-CENTERED COLLABORATIVE CARE

Assessment
- Obtain patient information about:
  1. Age and gender
  2. Occupation
  3. Current illness
     a. Nature of
     b. When it started
     c. Severity of symptoms

  d. Associated problems
  e. Interventions to date
 4. When HIV infection was diagnosed
 5. Chronologic history of infections and clinical problems since the diagnosis
 6. Health history, including transfusion history
 7. Sexual practices, STDs, and any major infectious diseases, including tuberculosis and hepatitis
 8. Injection drug use, including needle exposure and needle sharing
 9. Level of knowledge regarding the diagnosis, symptom management, diagnostic tests, treatments, community resources, and modes of HIV transmission
 10. Understanding and use of safer sex practices
- Assess for and document:
 1. Immune system changes
  a. Low WBC count
  b. Hypergammaglobulinemia
  c. Opportunistic infections
  d. Lymphadenopathy
  e. Fatigue
 2. Skin changes
  a. Dry, itchy, irritated skin
  b. Rashes
  c. Folliculitis
  d. Eczema
  e. Psoriasis
  f. Poor wound healing
  g. Purple lesions
 3. Respiratory changes
  a. Shortness of breath
  b. Cough
 4. Central nervous system (CNS) changes
  a. Confusion
  b. AIDS dementia complex
  c. Fever
  d. Headache
  e. Visual changes
  f. Memory loss
  g. Personality changes
  h. Pain
  i. Peripheral neuropathies
  j. Gait changes, ataxia
  k. Seizures

H

5. GI changes
    a. Diarrhea
    b. Nausea
    c. Weight loss
6. Opportunistic infections
    a. Protozoal infections
        (1) *Pneumocystis jirovecii* pneumonia (PCP)
        (2) *Toxoplasma gondii*
        (3) *Cryptosporidium*
    b. Fungal infections
        (1) *Candida albicans*
        (2) *Cryptococcus neoformans*
        (3) *Histoplasma capsulatum*
    c. Bacterial infections
        (1) *Mycobacterium avium*
        (2) *Mycobacterium intracellulare*
        (3) *Mycobacterium tuberculosis*
    d. Viral infection
        (1) Cytomegalovirus (CMV)
        (2) Herpes simplex virus (HSV)
        (3) Varicella-zoster virus (VZV)
7. Malignancies
    a. Kaposi's sarcoma
    b. Hodgkin's lymphoma
    c. Non-Hodgkin's lymphoma
    d. Invasive cervical cancer
8. Endocrine changes
    a. Gonadal dysfunction
    b. Adrenal insufficiency
    c. Diabetes mellitus
    d. Hyperlipidemia
9. Abnormal laboratory findings
    a. WBC count of less than 3500 cells/mm^3
    b. CD4$^+$ T-cell numbers decreased
    c. Low ratio of CD4+ to CD8+ T-cells
- Assess psychosocial issues, such as:
    1. Availability of a support system, such as family and significant others
        a. Learn who in this support system is aware of the patient's diagnosis.
        b. Identify whether a health care proxy or durable power-of-attorney document has been signed.
    2. Employment status and occupation
    3. Changes in performance of ADLs
    4. Living arrangements

5. Financial resources, including health insurance
6. Alcohol or recreational drug use
7. Anxiety level, mood, cognitive ability, and level of energy
8. Self-esteem and changes in body image
9. Suicidal ideation, depression
10. Use of support groups or other community resources
11. Energy level

- Diagnostic testing includes:
  1. Antibody tests
     a. Enzyme-linked immunosorbent assay (ELISA)
     b. Western blot analysis
  2. Viral load testing (also called viral burden testing) by Quantitative RNA assays
     a. Reverse transcriptase-polymerase chain reaction (RT-PCR)
     b. Branched deoxyribonucleic acid method (bDNA)
     c. Nucleic acid sequence–based assay (NASBA)
  3. Other laboratory tests to monitor the overall health of the patient
     a. Blood chemistries
     b. CBC with differential and platelets
     c. Toxoplasmosis antibody titer
     d. Liver function tests
     e. Serologic test for syphilis (STS)
     f. Antigens to hepatitis A, hepatitis B, and hepatitis C

Planning and Implementation

❖**NDx:** Risk for Infection

- The patient with AIDS is at high risk for opportunistic infections.
- Drug therapy for HIV/AIDS prolongs immune function and prevents opportunistic infections.
- *Antiretroviral therapy only inhibits viral replication and does not kill the virus.*
- Multiple drugs are used together in regimens popularly called "cocktails" consisting of combinations of different types of antiretroviral agents, an approach called *highly active antiretroviral therapy (HAART).*

> 🔃 Critical Rescue ◆ Ensure that HAART drugs are not missed, delayed, or administered in lower than prescribed doses in the in-patient setting to prevent the development of drug resistance in the virus.

1. *Nucleoside analogue reverse transcriptase inhibitors* (NARTI) suppress production of reverse transcriptase (RT) and inhibit viral DNA synthesis and replication. Drugs in this class

include zidovudine (Retrovir), didanosine (ddI, Videx), zalcitabine (ddC, HIVID), lamivudine (Epivir, 3TC ♣), stavudine (d4T, Zerit), tenofovir (Viread), emtricitabine (Emtriva), and abacavir (Ziagen).

2. *Non-nucleoside reverse transcriptase inhibitors* (NNRTI) inhibit synthesis of reverse transcriptase and suppress viral replication. These drugs include nevirapine (Viramune), delavirdine (Rescriptor), efavirenz (Sustiva), and etravirine.

3. *Protease inhibitors* block the HIV protease enzyme, preventing viral replication and release of viral particles. These drugs include ritonavir (Norvir), indinavir (Crixivan), saquinavir (Invirase), nelfinavir (Viracept), lopinavir (Kaletra), atazanavir (Reyataz), fosamprenavir (Lexiva), and darunavir (Prezista).

4. *Fusion inhibitors* work by blocking the fusion of HIV with a host cell by blocking the ability of gp41 to fuse with the host cell. The major drug in this category is enfuvirtide (Fuzeon).

5. *Entry inhibitors* work to *prevent* infection by blocking the CCR5 receptor on $CD4^+$ T-cells. The major drug in this category is maraviroc (Selzentry).

6. *Integrase inhibitors* work to *prevent* infection by inhibiting the enzyme, integrase, which is needed to insert the viral DNA into the host cell's human DNA. The major drug in this category is raltegravir (Isentress).

- Nursing measures to prevent infection in the patient with HIV/AIDS include:
  1. Placing the patient in a private room whenever possible
  2. Using good handwashing technique or use alcohol-based hand rubs before touching the patient or any of his or her belongings
  3. Ensuring that the patient's room and bathroom are cleaned at least once daily
  4. Not using supplies from common areas. For example, keeping a sleeve or box of paper cups in the patient's room and not sharing this box with any other patient. Other articles include drinking straws, plastic knives and forks, dressing materials, gloves, and bandages.
  5. Limiting the number of health care personnel entering the patient's room
  6. Monitoring vital signs and temperature every 4 hours
  7. Inspecting the patient's mouth at least every 8 hours for open lesions or white patches
  8. Inspecting the patient's skin and mucous membranes (especially the anal area) for the presence of fissures and abscesses at least every 8 hours

9. Inspecting open areas, such as IV sites, every 4 hours for manifestations of infection
10. Changing wound dressings daily
11. Obtaining specimens of all suspicious areas for culture (as specified by the agency), and promptly notify the physician
12. Assisting the patient in performing coughing and deep-breathing exercises
13. Encouraging activity at a level appropriate for the patient's current health status
14. Changing IV tubing daily
15. Keeping frequently used equipment in the room for use with this patient only (e.g., blood pressure cuff, stethoscope, thermometer)
16. Limiting visitors to healthy adults
17. Using strict aseptic technique for all invasive procedures
18. Avoiding the use of indwelling urinary catheters
19. Keeping fresh flowers and potted plants out of the patient's room
20. Teaching the patient to eat a low-bacteria diet (e.g., avoiding raw fruits or vegetables; undercooked meat, eggs, or fish; and pepper and paprika as seasonings sprinkled on food right before eating)

❖**NDx:** Impaired Gas Exchange

- Drug therapy is a mainstay for gas exchange problems resulting from *Pneumocystis* pneumonia (PCP).
  1. Trimethoprim/sulfamethoxazole (Apo-Sulfatrim ❉, Bactrim, Cotrim, Septra)
  2. Pentamidine isethionate (Pentacarinat ❉, Pentam), given IV, IM, or by aerosol
  3. Dapsone (Avlosulfon)
  4. Atovaquone (Mepron)
- Nursing interventions include:
  1. Respiratory support and maintenance:
     a. Assessing the respiratory rate, rhythm, and depth; breath sounds; and vital signs and monitoring for cyanosis at least every 8 hours
     b. Applying oxygen and humidifying the room as prescribed
     c. Monitoring mechanical ventilation
     d. Performing suctioning, as needed
     e. Performing chest physical therapy, as needed
     f. Evaluating blood gas results
  2. Comfort
     a. Assessing the patient's comfort

b. Elevating the head of the bed

c. Pacing activities to reduce shortness of breath and fatigue

3. Rest and activity changes

a. Pacing activities to conserve energy

b. Guiding the patient in active and passive ROM exercises

c. Scheduling non–time-critical activities, such as bathing, so that he or she is not fatigued at mealtime

❖**NDx:** Pain

- Pain with HIV/AIDS has many origins, including enlarged organs stretching the viscera or compressing nerves, tumor invasion of bone and other tissues, peripheral neuropathy, and generalized joint and muscle pain.

- Drug therapy with different classes of drugs is used to manage pain from different causes.

1. Arthralgia and myalgia respond to NSAIDs.

2. Neuropathic pain of peripheral neuropathy

a. Tricyclic antidepressants, such as amitriptyline (Elavil)

b. Anticonvulsant drugs, such as phenytoin (Dilantin) or carbamazepine (Tegretol)

3. General pain managed opioids

a. Weaker opioids: oxycodone or codeine

b. Stronger opioids: morphine, hydromorphone (Dilaudid), or fentanyl transdermal (Duragesic)

- Comfort measures

1. Pressure-relieving mattress pads

2. Warm baths or other forms of hydrotherapy

3. Massage

4. Application of heat or cold to painful areas

5. Use of lift sheets to avoid pulling or grasping the patient with joint pain

6. Frequent position changes

- Complementary and alternative therapies

1. Guided imagery

2. Distraction

3. Progressive relaxation

4. Body-talk

5. Biofeedback

❖**NDx:** Imbalanced Nutrition Less Than Body Requirements

- Poor nutrition has many causes and requires an interdisciplinary team to determine the exact cause or causes.

1. Drug therapy

a. Administering antifungal agents for esophagitis, such as ketoconazole (Nizoral) or fluconazole (Diflucan)

b. Administering antiemetics for nausea and vomiting

2. Comfort measures
   a. Providing frequent mouth care
   b. Keeping the environment pleasant and free from offensive odors
3. Nutritional therapy
   a. Assessing food preferences and any dietary cultural or religious practices
   b. Monitoring weight, intake and output, and calorie count
   c. Teaching the patient about a high-calorie, high-protein, nutritionally sound diet
   d. Encouraging him or her to avoid dietary fat
   e. Collaborating with the nutritionist
   f. Providing small, frequent meals
   g. Administering prescribed supplemental vitamins
   h. Providing prescribed tube feedings or total parenteral nutrition

❖**NDx:** Diarrhea
- Nursing interventions include:
  1. Administering antidiarrheals, such as diphenoxylate hydro-chloride (Diarsed ♣, Lomotil) or loperamide (Imodium), as prescribed
  2. Consulting with the nutritionist to offer less roughage; less fatty, spicy, and sweet food; and no alcohol or caffeine
  3. Assessing the perineal skin every 8 to 12 hours
  4. Providing a bedside commode or a bedpan if needed

❖**NDx:** Impaired Skin Integrity
- Kaposi's sarcoma (KS) is the most common skin lesion.
  1. Lesions may be localized or widespread; monitor for progression.
  2. Lesions are managed with local radiation, intralesional chemotherapy, or cryotherapy.
  3. For rapidly progressive disease or with major involvement of the intestinal tract, lungs, or other organs, therapy may include:
     a. Chemotherapy
     b. Interferon-alpha
     c. Zidovudine
  4. Clean and dress open, weeping KS lesions.
  5. To disguise the lesions, teach patients to:
     a. Use makeup over intact lesions.
     b. Wear long-sleeved shirts.
     c. Wear hats.
- Herpes simplex viral (HSV) lesions, or shingles, may occur and form abscesses.
  1. Provide good skin care to keep the area clean and dry.

   2. Clean abscesses at least once per shift with normal saline and allow them to air-dry.
   3. Provide Burrow's solution (Domeboro) soaks.
   4. Administer prescribed antiviral drugs, including acyclovir (Zovirax) or valacyclovir (Valtrex).

❖**NDx:** Disturbed Thought Processes
   ● Nursing interventions include:
      1. Assessing baseline neurologic and mental status
      2. Evaluating the patient for subtle changes in memory, ability to concentrate, affect, and behavior
      3. Reorienting the confused patient to person, time, and place
      4. Reminding the patient of your identity and explain what is to be done at any given time
      5. Giving simple directions
         a. Using short, uncomplicated sentences
         b. Explaining activities in simple language
         c. Involving the patient in planning the daily schedule
      6. Asking relatives or significant others to bring in familiar items from home
      7. Arranging all items in the patient's environment in the same location as at home
      8. Making the environment safe and comfortable
      9. Administering prescribed psychotropic drugs, antidepressants, or anxiolytics
     10. Assessing the patient with neurologic manifestations for increased intracranial pressure

   > 🔲 **Critical Rescue** ◆ Report immediately any changes in level of consciousness (one of the earliest signs of increased intracranial pressure), vital signs, pupil size or reactivity, or limb strength to the physician for appropriate intervention.

❖**NDx:** Chronic Low Self-Esteem
   ● Self esteem is affected by dramatic changes in appearance that alter the person's body image; abrupt, significant changes in their relationships with others; and changes in day-to-day activities, employment, or other productive activities.
   ● Nursing interventions include:
      1. Providing a climate of acceptance
      2. Promoting a trusting relationship
      3. Helping patients identify positive aspects of themselves
      4. Allowing for privacy but not avoiding or isolating the patient

5. Encouraging self-care, independence, control, and decision making
6. Helping the patient set short-term, attainable goals
7. Offering praise when goals are achieved

❖**NDx:** Social Isolation
- Nursing interventions include:
  1. Explaining the rationale for the use of Standard Precautions
  2. Establishing a therapeutic nurse-patient relationship
  3. Spending time and being present with the patient
  4. Reducing barriers to social contact
  5. Assessing the patient's social support resources
  6. Teaching family and significant others about HIV transmission and the use of Standard Precautions to reduce anxiety and increase contact with the patient
  7. Encouraging the patient to state feelings about self, coping skills, and a sense of control over the situation
  8. Helping the patient identify support systems
  9. Teaching the patient, family, and significant other about prevention of HIV transmission

Community-Based Care
- Collaborate with the health care team members, patient, and family to plan what will be needed and how they will manage at home with self-care and ADLs.
  1. Assess the patient's status, ability to perform self-care activities, and identify the potential need for care, such as:
     a. Assistance with ADLs
     b. Around-the-clock nursing care
     c. Drug administration
     d. Nutritional support
  2. Assess available resources, including family members and significant others willing and able to be caregivers.
  3. Help the family make arrangements for outside caregivers or respite care, if needed.
  4. Refer the patient to support groups, financial counselor, social worker, legal services, and spiritual counselor.
  5. Determine the need for assistance with funeral arrangements.
- Teach the patient, family, and significant others about:
  1. Modes of HIV transmission and preventive behaviors
  2. Guidelines for safer sex
  3. Not sharing toothbrushes, razors, and other potentially blood-contaminated articles

H

4. Manifestations of infection
   a. Temperature higher than 100° F (38° C)
   b. Persistent cough (with or without sputum)
   c. Pus or foul-smelling drainage from any open skin area or normal body opening
   d. Presence of a boil or abscess
   e. Urine that is cloudy or foul smelling or that causes burning on urination
5. Good infection control practices, such as:
   a. Avoiding crowds and other large gatherings of people who may be ill
   b. Not sharing personal toilet articles, such as toothbrushes, toothpaste, washcloths, or deodorant sticks, with others
   c. Bathing daily, using an antimicrobial soap. If total bathing is not possible, washing the armpits, groin, genitals, and anal area twice daily with an antimicrobial soap
   d. Cleaning the toothbrush daily by running it through the dishwasher or rinsing it in liquid laundry bleach
   e. Washing hands thoroughly with an antimicrobial soap before eating or drinking, after touching a pet, after shaking hands with anyone, returning home from any outing, and after using the toilet
   f. Washing dishes between uses with hot, sudsy water or using a dishwasher
   g. Not drinking water, milk, juice, or other cold liquids that have been standing for longer than an hour
   h. Not reusing cups and glasses without washing
   i. Not changing pet litter boxes; if unavoidable, using gloves and washing hands immediately
   j. Avoiding turtles and reptiles as pets
   k. Not feeding pets raw or undercooked meat
6. Teaching good dietary habits, including:
   a. Proper nutrition
   b. Eating a low-bacteria diet
   c. Avoiding salads; raw fruit and vegetables; undercooked meat, fish, or eggs; pepper; and paprika
   d. Thoroughly washing fruit and vegetables
   e. Refrigerating perishable foods
7. Psychosocial preparation
   a. Helping identify ways to avoid problems with social stigma and rejection
   b. Identifying coping strategies for difficult situations
   c. Supporting family members and friends in efforts to help the patient and provide protection from discrimination

d. Encouraging patients to continue as many usual activities as possible
e. Supporting patients in their selection of friends and relatives with whom to discuss the diagnosis
f. Reminding the patient that sexual partners and care providers should be informed of the diagnosis
g. Making referrals to community resources, mental health or behavioral health professionals, and support groups

HUNTINGTON'S DISEASE

- Huntington's disease is a hereditary disorder transmitted as an autosomal dominant trait at the time of conception.
- It is most prevalent in people of western European ancestry.
- The two main symptoms of the disease are progressive mental status changes leading to dementia and choreiform movements.
- Other clinical manifestations of Huntington's disease include poor balance, hesitant or explosive speech, dysphagia, impaired respirations, and bowel and bladder incontinence. Mental status changes include decreased attention span, poor judgment, memory loss, personality changes, and later, dementia.
- There is no known cure or treatment of the disease.
- The only way to prevent transmission of the gene is for those affected to refrain from having children.
- Genetic testing is an option for people at risk for Huntington's disease to determine whether they have the gene on chromosome 4; however, results of the test are subject to error.
- Management of the disease is symptomatic: Physical and occupational therapy and social support can promote function and engagement.

HYDROCELE

- A hydrocele usually is a painless cystic mass filled with a straw-colored fluid that forms around the testis.
- It is caused by impaired lymphatic drainage of the scrotum, leading to swelling of the tissue surrounding the testes.
- Unless the swelling becomes large and uncomfortable or begins to impair blood flow to the testis, no treatment is necessary.
- When a hydrocele is large, uncomfortable, or cosmetically unacceptable, intervention is done by one of two methods:
  1. Drainage through a needle and syringe
  2. Surgical removal

- Provide postoperative care, including:
  1. Explaining the importance of wearing a scrotal support (jock strap) for the first 24 to 48 hours after surgery to keep the dressing in place and to prevent edema
  2. Assessing for pain and wound complications (infection or bleeding)
  3. Instructing the patient to schedule a follow-up visit with the surgeon
  4. Instructing the patient to stay off his feet for several days and to limit physical activity for a week
  5. Reassuring him that this swelling is normal and eventually subsides

HYDRONEPHROSIS, HYDROURETER, AND URETHRAL STRICTURE

- Several disorders are associated with obstruction of the outflow of urine.
- In hydronephrosis, the kidney becomes enlarged as urine accumulates in the renal pelvis and the calyces. Obstruction within the pelvis or ureteropelvic junction results in renal pelvic distention, and extensive damage to the vasculature and renal tubules can result.
- Hydroureter is the obstruction of the ureter at the point of the iliac vessel crossing or the ureterovesical entry. Dilation of the ureter occurs at the point proximal to the obstruction as urine accumulates.
- A urethral stricture is the most distal point of obstruction, with bladder distention occurring before hydroureter and hydronephrosis.
- Urinary tract obstruction results in direct pressure buildup on the tissue, causing structural damage.
- Within the nephron, the tubular filtrate pressure increases as drainage through the collecting system is impaired, resulting in altered glomerular filtration and renal failure.
- Causes of hydronephrosis and hydroureter include tumors, stones, trauma, congenital structural defects, and retroperitoneal fibrosis; pregnancy may cause ureteral dilation.
- Urethral stricture occurs from chronic inflammation.
- Management includes:
  1. Recording history of renal or urologic disorders
  2. Documenting pattern of urination, including amount and frequency
  3. Describing urine, including color, clarity, and odor

4. Reporting new symptoms, including flank or abdominal pain, chills, fever, and malaise
5. Assessing for flank asymmetry and pain
6. Assessing for abdominal tenderness or pain
7. Determining the presence of urinary retention by assessing for bladder distention and urine leakage with abdominal pressure
8. Monitoring urinalysis for bacteria or WBCs to determine if infection is present
9. Anticipating an enlarged ureter or kidney on x-ray and IV pyelography
10. Treating the cause of urinary obstruction to prevent in renal failure

HYPERALDOSTERONISM

OVERVIEW

- Hyperaldosteronism is increased secretion of aldosterone by the adrenal glands that results in mineralocorticoid excess.
- *Primary hyperaldosteronism* (Conn's syndrome), which results from excessive secretion of aldosterone from one or both adrenal glands, is most often caused by a benign adrenal tumor (adrenal adenoma).
- *Secondary hyperaldosteronism* is excessive secretion of aldosterone because of high levels of angiotensin II that are stimulated by high plasma renin levels. Causes include kidney hypoxemia and the use of thiazide diuretics.
- Regardless of the cause, hyperaldosteronism is manifested by hypernatremia, hypokalemia, metabolic alkalosis, and hypertension.

PATIENT-CENTERED COLLABORATIVE CARE

Assessment

- Obtain patient information about:
  1. Headache
  2. Fatigue
  3. Muscle weakness
  4. Nocturia (excessive urination at night)
  5. Polydipsia (excessive fluid intake)
  6. Polyuria (excessive urine output)
  7. Paresthesias (sensations of numbness and tingling)
- Assess for and document:
  1. Hypertension
  2. Elevated serum levels of sodium
  3. Low serum levels of potassium

- Diagnostic assessment includes:
  1. Serum electrolyte levels
  2. Serum renin levels (low)
  3. Serum aldosterone levels (high)
  4. X-rays
  5. Imaging with CT scans or MRI

Interventions

- Adrenalectomy of one or both adrenal glands is the most common treatment for early-stage hyperaldosteronism.
- Provide preoperative care, including:
  1. Implementing routine preoperative care, as described in Part One
  2. Correcting the serum potassium levels by administering prescribed potassium supplements, potassium-sparing diuretics, or aldosterone antagonists
  3. Providing a low-sodium diet
- Provide postoperative care, including:
  1. Implementing routine postoperative care as described in Part One
  2. Teaching the patient about glucocorticoid replacement (replacement is lifelong if both adrenal glands are removed)
  3. Instructing him or her to wear a medical alert bracelet while taking glucocorticoids
- For patients who do not have surgery and must remain on spironolactone therapy to control hypokalemia and hypertension, teach them about:
  1. Avoiding potassium supplements and foods rich in potassium
  2. Increasing dietary sodium
  3. Reporting symptoms of hyponatremia
     a. Mouth dryness
     b. Thirst
     c. Lethargy or drowsiness
  4. Side effects of spironolactone therapy
     a. Gynecomastia
     b. Diarrhea
     c. Drowsiness
     d. Headache
     e. Rash, urticaria (hives)
     f. Confusion
     g. Erectile dysfunction
     h. Hirsutism
     i. Amenorrhea

HYPERCALCEMIA

OVERVIEW

- Hypercalcemia is a total serum calcium level above 10.5 mg/dL or 2.75 mmol/L.
- Because the normal range for serum calcium is so narrow, even small increases have severe effects.
- The effects of hypercalcemia occur first in excitable tissues.
- Common causes of hypercalcemia include:
  1. Increased absorption of calcium
     a. Excessive oral intake of calcium
     b. Excessive oral intake of vitamin D
  2. Decreased excretion of calcium
     a. Kidney failure
     b. Use of thiazide diuretics
  3. Increased bone resorption of calcium
     a. Hyperparathyroidism
     b. Malignancy
     c. Hyperthyroidism
     d. Immobility
     e. Use of glucocorticoids
  4. Dehydration

PATIENT-CENTERED COLLABORATIVE CARE

Assessment

- Assess for and document:
  1. Cardiovascular changes, which are the most serious and life threatening
     a. Increased heart rate and blood pressure (early)
     b. Slow heart rate (late or severe)
     c. Cyanosis and pallor
     d. Dysrhythmias on electrocardiograph (ECG), especially a shortened QT interval
     e. Slowed or impaired blood flow
        (1) Measure calf circumferences.
        (2) Assess foot temperature, color, and capillary refill.
  2. Neuromuscular changes, which include:
     a. Severe muscle weakness
     b. Decreased deep tendon reflexes without paresthesia
     c. Altered level of consciousness (confusion, lethargy, coma)
  3. Intestinal changes, which include:
     a. Constipation, anorexia, nausea, vomiting, and abdominal pain

b. Hypoactive or absent bowel sounds
c. Increased abdominal size

Interventions

- Measures to prevent increases in calcium
  1. Discontinuing IV solutions containing calcium (lactated Ringer's solution)
  2. Discontinuing oral drugs containing calcium or vitamin D (e.g., calcium-based antacids, OTC vitamin supplements)
  3. Discontinuing thiazide diuretics that increase kidney calcium reabsorption
- Drug therapy
  1. Fluid volume replacement with IV normal saline (0.9% sodium chloride)
  2. Diuretics that enhance calcium excretion, such as furosemide (Lasix, Furoside ♦)
  3. Calcium chelators (calcium binders)
     a. Plicamycin (Mithracin)
     b. Penicillamine (Cuprimine, Pendramine ♦).
  4. Drugs that inhibit calcium resorption from bone
     a. Calcitonin (Calcimar)
     b. Bisphosphonates (etidronate)
     c. Prostaglandin synthesis inhibitors (aspirin, NSAIDs)
- Dialysis by hemodialysis or blood ultrafiltration may be needed for rapid calcium reduction when levels are life threatening.
- Continuous cardiac monitoring may be requested.
  1. Compare recent electrocardiographic (ECG) tracings with the patient's baseline tracings (when calcium was normal).
  2. Examine for changes in the T waves, QT interval, and heart rate and rhythm.
- Additional nursing actions include:
  1. Monitoring intake and output
  2. Assessing for fluid overload
  3. Encouraging mobilization to prevent bone resorption

HYPERCORTISOLISM (CUSHING'S SYNDROME)

OVERVIEW

- Excessive secretion of cortisol from the adrenal cortex results in hypercortisolism, also known as Cushing's disease.
- Excess cortisol secretion can be a result of a problem in the adrenal cortex, the anterior pituitary gland, or the hypothalamus. Glucocorticoid therapy also can lead to hypercortisolism.
- Regardless of cause, the excess glucocorticoid affects metabolism and all body systems to some degree.

- Causes of hypercortisolism include oversecretion of adrenocorticotropic hormone (ACTH) from the anterior pituitary gland as a result of a pituitary adenoma, an adrenal adenoma, or drug therapy with corticosteroids for another health problem.

PATIENT-CENTERED COLLABORATIVE CARE

Assessment

- Obtain patient information about:
  1. History of other health problems and drug therapies
  2. Age, gender, and usual weight
  3. Weight gain
  4. Increased appetite
  5. Change in activity or sleep patterns, fatigue, and muscle weakness
  6. Bone pain or a history of fractures
  7. Frequent infections
  8. Easy bruising
  9. Cessation of menses
  10. GI ulcers
- Assess for and document:
  1. General appearance
     a. Buffalo hump on shoulder
     b. Enlarged trunk
     c. Moon face
     d. Thin arms and legs
     e. Generalized muscle wasting and weakness
  2. Skin changes
     a. Bruises
     b. Thin, translucent skin
     c. Wounds that have not healed
     d. Reddish purple striae ("stretch marks") on the abdomen, thighs, and upper arms
     e. Acne
     f. Fine coating of hair over the face and body
  3. Cardiac changes
     a. Elevated heart rate
     b. Hypertension
     c. Edema formation
  4. Emotional lability, mood swings, irritability, confusion, depression
  5. Hyperglycemia
  6. Hypernatremia
- Diagnostic assessment includes:
  1. Elevated blood, salivary, and urine cortisol levels
  2. Dexamethasone suppression testing

3. Abnormal serum electrolyte values (increased sodium, decreased calcium, decreased potassium)
4. X-rays
5. CT scans
6. MRI
7. Arteriography

Planning and Implementation

❖**NDx:** Excess Fluid Volume

Nonsurgical Management

- Patient safety includes preventing fluid overload from becoming worse, leading to pulmonary edema and heart failure.
  1. Monitor for indicators of increased fluid overload (increased pulse quality, increasing neck vein distention, presence of crackles in lungs, increasing peripheral edema, reduced urine output) at least every 2 hours.

> 🚑 Critical Rescue ◆ Notify the health care provider of any change that indicates the fluid overload is not responding to therapy or is becoming worse.

  2. Prevent skin breakdown by:
     a. Using a pressure-reducing or pressure-relieving overlay on the mattress
     b. Assessing skin pressure areas daily for signs of redness or open areas
     c. Assisting the patient to change positions every 2 hours
- Drug therapy
  1. Administer prescribed drugs to interfere with adrenocorticotropic hormone (ACTH) production or adrenal hormone synthesis:
     a. Aminoglutethimide (Elipten, Cytadren)
     b. Metyrapone (Metopirone)
     c. Cyproheptadine (Periactin)
     d. Mitotane (Lysodren)
  2. Monitor the patient for response to drug therapy:
     a. Weight loss
     b. Increased urine output
  3. Assess laboratory findings, especially sodium and potassium values.
- Nutrition therapy
  1. Restriction of sodium
  2. Restriction of fluids
- Radiation therapy for hypercortisolism caused by pituitary adenomas

1. Observe for any changes in the patient's neurologic status, such as headache, elevated blood pressure or pulse, disorientation, or changes in pupil size or reaction.
2. Assess for skin dryness, redness, flushing, or alopecia at the radiation site.

Surgical Management

- The surgical treatment of adrenocortical hypersecretion depends on the cause of the disease.
- When adrenal hyperfunction results from increased pituitary secretion of ACTH, removal of a pituitary adenoma may be attempted.
- When hypercortisolism is caused by adrenal tumors, a partial or complete adrenalectomy (removal of the adrenal gland) may be performed by open abdominal procedures or laparoscopic procedures.
- Provide preoperative care, including:
  1. Implementing routine preoperative care as described in Part One
  2. Implementing prescribed drug and diet therapy to correct electrolyte imbalances
  3. Monitoring blood potassium, sodium, and chloride levels
  4. Monitoring ECG for dysrhythmias
  5. Monitoring blood glucose levels
  6. Preventing infection with handwashing and aseptic technique
  7. Decreasing the risk for falls by raising bed siderails and encouraging the patient to ask for assistance when getting out of bed
  8. Teaching the patient about the care needs for after surgery and the need for long-term drug therapy
- Provide postoperative care, including:
  1. Implementing routine postoperative care as described in Part One
  2. Assessing the patient every 15 minutes for shock (e.g., hypotension, a rapid and weak pulse, decreasing urine output) during the first 6 hours
  3. Monitoring vital signs and other hemodynamic variables
     a. Central venous pressure
     b. Pulmonary wedge pressure
     c. Intake and output
     d. Daily weights
     e. Serum electrolyte levels
  4. Teaching about the need (after bilateral adrenalectomy) for lifelong glucocorticoid replacement

❖**NDx:** Risk for Injury

- Prevent skin injury by:
    1. Assessing the patient's skin for reddened areas, excoriation, breakdown, and edema.
    2. Turning or assisting him or her to turn every 2 hours
    3. Padding bony prominences
    4. Teaching the patient activities to avoid trauma:
        a. Use a soft toothbrush.
        b. Use an electric shaver.
        c. Keep the skin clean and dry it thoroughly after washing.
        d. Use a moisturizing lotion.
    5. Using tape sparingly and taking care when removing it
    6. Exerting pressure over an injection or venipuncture site
- Prevent pathologic fractures by:
    1. Using a lift sheet to move the patient instead of grasping him or her
    2. Reminding the patient to call for help when ambulating
    3. Reviewing the use of ambulatory aids (walkers or canes), if needed
    4. Keeping rooms free of extraneous objects that may cause a fall
    5. Teaching unlicensed assistive personnel (UAPs) to use a gait belt when ambulating the patient
    6. Teaching the patient about safety issues and dietary needs
- Prevent gastrointestinal (GI) bleeding by:
    1. Implementing prescribed drug therapy
        a. Antacids
        b. H_2 histamine receptor blockers
            (1) Cimetidine (Tagamet, Peptol ✤, Novo-Cimetine ✤)
            (2) Ranitidine (Zantac, Apo-Ranitidine ✤)
            (3) Famotidine (Pepcid)
            (4) Nizatidine (Axid)
        c. Proton pump inhibitors
            (1) Omeprazole (Losec ✤, Prilosec)
            (2) Esomeprazole (Nexium)
    2. Encouraging the patient to reduce or eliminate habits that contribute to gastric irritation, such as:
        a. Consuming alcohol or caffeine
        b. Smoking
        c. Fasting
        d. Taking NSAIDs and drugs that contain aspirin or other salicylates

❖**NDx:** Risk for Infection
- Protect the patient from infection by:
  1. Using aseptic technique when performing any invasive procedure
  2. Performing frequent, thorough handwashing
  3. Ensuring that anyone with an upper respiratory tract infection who must enter the patient's room wears a mask
  4. Continually assessing the patient for the presence of infection
     a. Monitoring the daily CBC with differential WBC count and absolute neutrophil count (ANC)
     b. Inspecting the mouth during every shift for lesions and mucosa breakdown
     c. Assessing the lungs every 8 hours for crackles, wheezes, or reduced breath sounds
     d. Assessing all urine for odor and cloudiness
     e. Asking the patient about any urgency, burning, or pain present on urination
     f. Taking vital signs at least every 4 hours to assess for fever
  5. Providing skin care and daily hygiene
  6. Turning the immobile patient every 2 hours and applying skin lubricants
  7. Performing pulmonary hygiene every 2 to 4 hours
  8. Assessing the lungs for crackles, wheezes, or reduced breath sounds
  9. Urging the patient to cough and deep breathe or to perform sustained maximal inhalations every hour while awake

❖**Collaborative Problem:** Potential for Acute Adrenal Insufficiency
- Teach the patient who must take glucocorticoids to:
  1. Take the drug in divided doses, with the first dose in the morning and the second dose between 4 and 6 PM.
  2. Take the drug with meals or snacks.
  3. Weigh himself or herself daily, record it, and compare it with previous weights.
  4. Increase the dosage as directed for increased physical stress or severe emotional stress, including surgery, dental work, influenza, fever, pregnancy, and family problems.
  5. *Never skip a dose of drug.* If the patient has persistent vomiting or severe diarrhea and cannot take the drug by mouth for 24 to 36 hours, he or she must call the physician. If the patient cannot reach the physician, he or she must go to the nearest emergency department because an injection may be needed in place of the usual oral drug.

6. Always wear his or her medical alert bracelet or necklace.
7. Make regular visits for health care follow-up.
8. Learn how to give himself or herself an IM injection of hydrocortisone.

Community-Based Care

- Instruct the patient taking exogenous glucocorticoids to call his or her health care provider if more than 3 pounds are gained in a week or more than 1 to 2 pounds is gained in a 24-hour period.
- Urge him or her to use proper hygiene and to avoid crowds or others with infections.
- Encourage the patient and all people living in the same home with him or her to have yearly influenza vaccinations.

HYPERKALEMIA

OVERVIEW

- Hyperkalemia is a serum potassium level greater than 5.0 mEq/L (5.0 mmol/L).
- The normal range for serum potassium values is narrow, so even slight increases above normal values can affect excitable tissues, especially the heart.
- The consequences of hyperkalemia can be life threatening, and the imbalance usually is not seen in people with normally functioning kidneys.
- Causes include:
  1. Overingestion of potassium-containing foods or drugs
     a. Salt substitutes
     b. Potassium chloride
     c. Potassium-sparing diuretics
  2. Rapid infusion of potassium-containing IV solution
  3. Bolus IV potassium injections
  4. Transfusions of whole blood or packed cells
  5. Adrenal insufficiency (Addison's disease, adrenalectomy)
  6. Kidney failure
  7. Tissue damage (crushing injuries, burns)
  8. Acidosis
  9. Hyperuricemia
  10. Uncontrolled diabetes mellitus
- The problems that occur with hyperkalemia are related to how rapidly extracellular fluid (ECF) potassium levels increase. Sudden rises in serum potassium cause severe problems at potassium levels between 6 and 7 mEq/L. When serum potassium rises slowly, problems may not occur until potassium levels reach 8 mEq/L or higher.

PATIENT-CENTERED COLLABORATIVE CARE

Assessment

- Obtain patient information about:
  1. Age
  2. Chronic illnesses (particularly kidney disease and diabetes mellitus)
  3. Recent medical or surgical treatment
  4. Urine output, including frequency and amount of voidings
  5. Drug use, particularly potassium-sparing diuretics and angiotensin-converting enzyme (ACE) inhibitors
  6. Diet history to determine the intake of potassium-rich foods or the use of salt substitutes (which contain potassium)
  7. Palpitations, skipped heartbeats, and other cardiac irregularities
  8. Muscle twitching and weakness in the leg muscles
  9. Unusual tingling or numbness in the hands, feet, or face
  10. Recent changes in bowel habits, especially diarrhea
- Assess for and document:
  1. Cardiovascular changes
     a. Bradycardia
     b. Hypotension
     c. Electrocardiographic (ECG) changes
        (1) Tall, peaked T waves
        (2) Prolonged PR intervals
        (3) Flat or absent P waves
        (4) Wide QRS complexes
  2. Neuromuscular changes, early
     a. Skeletal muscle twitches
     b. Tingling and burning sensations followed by numbness in the hands and feet and around the mouth
  3. Neuromuscular changes, late
     a. Muscle weakness
     b. Flaccid paralysis first in hands and feet, then moving higher
  4. Intestinal changes
     a. Increased motility
     b. Hyperactive bowel sounds
     c. Frequent watery bowel movements
  5. Laboratory data: serum potassium level greater than 5.0 mEq/L

Interventions

- Interventions for hyperkalemia are aimed at rapidly reducing the serum potassium level, preventing recurrences, and ensuring patient safety during the electrolyte imbalance.

- Drug therapy
  1. IV therapy
     a. Discontinuing potassium-containing infusions
     b. Keeping the IV catheter open
     c. Administering IV preparation of 100 mL of 10% to 20% glucose with 10 to 20 units of regular insulin
  2. Withholding oral potassium supplements
  3. Potassium-excreting diuretics, such as furosemide
  4. Sodium polystyrene sulfonate (Kayexalate) exchange resins
- Hemodialysis or ultrafiltration
- Nursing care priorities include:
  1. Cardiac monitoring for early recognition of dysrhythmias and other manifestations of hyperkalemia on cardiac function

> ▓ **Critical Rescue** ◆ Notify the health care provider or Rapid Response Team if the patient's heart rate falls below 60 beats/min or if the T waves become spiked.

  2. Teaching the patient to avoid:
     a. Meats, especially organ meat and preserved meat
     b. Dairy products
     c. Dried fruit
     d. Fruits high in potassium (bananas, cantaloupe, kiwi, oranges)
     e. Vegetables high in potassium (avocados, broccoli, dried beans or peas, lima beans, mushrooms, potatoes, soybeans, spinach)

HYPERNATREMIA

OVERVIEW

- Hypernatremia is a serum sodium level greater than 145 mEq/L and is often accompanied by changes in fluid volumes.
- It makes excitable tissues more easily excited, a condition known as irritability, and leads to cellular dehydration.
- Common causes include:
  1. NPO status
  2. Dehydration
  3. Watery diarrhea
  4. Excessive diaphoresis
  5. Excessive oral sodium ingestion
  6. Excessive administration of sodium-containing IV fluids
  7. Fever
  8. Increased rate of metabolism
  9. Hyperventilation
  10. Infection

11. Hyperaldosteronism
12. Kidney failure
13. Corticosteroids
14. Cushing's syndrome or disease

PATIENT-CENTERED COLLABORATIVE CARE

Assessment

- Assess for and document:
  1. Nervous system changes
     a. Decreased attention span and recall of recent events
     b. Agitation or confusion
     c. Lethargy, drowsiness, stupor, or coma (when accompanied by fluid overload)
  2. Skeletal muscles changes
     a. Muscle twitching and irregular muscle contractions (mild hypernatremia)
     b. Muscle weakness
     c. Reduced or absent deep tendon reflexes
  3. Cardiovascular changes differ with fluid status.
     a. Hypovolemia leads to increased pulse rate, hypotension, and reduced quality of peripheral pulses.
     b. Hypervolemia leads to slow to normal bounding pulses, full peripheral pulses, neck veins distention, and elevated diastolic blood pressure.
  4. Respiratory changes occur with hypervolemia.
     a. Pulmonary edema
     b. Decreased oxygen saturation

Interventions

- Restore fluid balance when hypernatremia caused by fluid loss with hypotonic IV infusions, usually 0.225% or 0.45% sodium chloride.
- Restore fluid balance when hypernatremia is caused by fluid and sodium losses requires fluid replacement with IV infusions of isotonic sodium chloride (NaCl) solutions.
- Drug therapy includes diuretics that promote sodium loss, such as furosemide (Lasix, Furoside ♣) or bumetanide (Bumex).
- Assess the patient hourly for symptoms of excessive fluid and sodium or potassium losses.
- Dietary sodium restriction may be needed to prevent sodium excess when renal problems are present.
- Fluid restriction may also be needed.
- Priorities for nursing care of the patient with hypernatremia include monitoring the patient's response to therapy and preventing hyponatremia and dehydration.
  1. Patient safety to prevent fluid overload from becoming worse, leading to pulmonary edema and heart failure.

a. Monitor for indicators of increased fluid overload at least every 2 hours.

> **Critical Rescue** ♦ Pulmonary edema can occur very quickly and can lead to death. Notify the health care provider about any change that indicates the fluid overload is not responding to therapy or is becoming worse.

b. Use a pressure-reducing or pressure-relieving overlay on the mattress.
c. Assess skin pressure areas, especially the coccyx, elbows, hips, and heels, daily for signs of redness or open areas.
d. Assist the patient to change positions every 2 hours.

2. Monitor for patient response to drug therapy:
   a. Weight loss
   b. Increased urine output
3. Observe for manifestations of electrolyte imbalance:
   a. Changes in electrocardiographic (ECG) patterns
   b. Changes in sodium and potassium values
4. Nutrition therapy, teach patients and families about:
   a. Sodium restriction
   b. Fluid restriction

HYPERPARATHYROIDISM

OVERVIEW

- Hyperparathyroidism results from increased levels of parathyroid hormone (PTH) that act directly on the kidney, causing increased kidney reabsorption of calcium and increased phosphate excretion. These processes cause hypercalcemia (excessive calcium) and hypophosphatemia (inadequate phosphate).
- Primary hyperparathyroidism results when one or more parathyroid glands do not respond to the normal feedback mechanisms for serum calcium levels. The most common cause is a benign tumor in one parathyroid gland.
- Secondary hyperparathyroidism is a response to the hypocalcemia associated with chronic kidney disease and vitamin D deficiency, which leads to hyperplasia of the parathyroid glands.

PATIENT-CENTERED COLLABORATIVE CARE

Assessment

- Obtain patient information about:
  1. Bone fractures
  2. Recent weight loss
  3. Arthritis

4. Psychological distress
5. History of radiation treatment to the head or neck
6. History of kidney stones
- Assess for and document:
1. Waxy pallor of the skin
2. Bone deformities in the extremities and back
3. GI manifestations
   a. Anorexia, nausea, vomiting
   b. Epigastric pain
   c. Constipation
4. Fatigue and lethargy
5. Confusion, coma (severe hyperparathyroidism)
6. Laboratory values
   a. High serum calcium levels
   b. High serum PTH levels
   c. Low serum phosphorus levels
- Diagnostic studies include:
1. Serum electrolyte levels
2. Serum PTH and urine cyclic adenosine monophosphate (cAMP) levels
3. X-rays
4. Arteriography
5. CT
6. Venous catheterization of the thyroid veins

Interventions

Nonsurgical Management

- Diuretic and hydration therapies are used most often for reducing serum calcium levels in patients who are not candidates for surgery.
- Nursing management includes:
1. Monitoring cardiac function (continuous electrocardiographic [ECG] monitoring)
   a. Compare current ECG tracings with baseline tracings.
   b. Examine for changes in the T waves and the QT interval.
   c. Assess heart rate and rhythm.
2. Measuring intake and output 2 to 4 hours
3. Closely monitoring serum calcium levels

> **Critical Rescue** ◆ Immediately report any sudden drop in the calcium level to the health care provider.

4. Assessing for tingling and numbness in the hands, feet, and around the mouth
5. Preventing injury by:
   a. Teaching all members of the health care team to handle the patient carefully

    b. Using a lift sheet to reposition the patient rather than pulling him or her

    c. Ensuring that the patient is accompanied when ambulating to prevent falls

- Drug therapy when hydration and furosemide do not correct hypercalcemia
  1. Oral phosphates
  2. Calcium chelators
     - a. Plicamycin (Mithracin)
     - b. Penicillamine (Cuprimine, Pendramine ♦)
  3. Drugs that inhibit calcium resorption from bone
     - a. Calcitonin (Calcimar)
     - b. Bisphosphonates (etidronate)
     - c. Prostaglandin synthesis inhibitors (aspirin, NSAIDs)

Surgical Management

- Surgical management of hyperparathyroidism is parathyroidectomy. It involves a transverse incision in the lower neck. All four parathyroid glands are examined for enlargement. If a tumor is present on one side but the other side is normal, the surgeon removes the glands containing tumor and leaves the remaining glands on the opposite side intact. If all four glands are diseased, they are all removed.
- Provide preoperative care, including:
  1. Implementing routine preoperative care as described in Part One
  2. Teaching the patient how to perform coughing and deep-breathing exercises and instructing him or her to perform them hourly after surgery
  3. Reminding the patient that talking may be painful for the first day or two
  4. Teaching about neck support by having the patient place both hands behind the neck to assist in elevating the head
- Provide postoperative care, including:
  1. Implementing routine postoperative care as described in Part One
  2. Closely observing the patient for respiratory distress, which may occur from calcium gluconate, compression of the trachea by hemorrhage or swelling of neck tissues
  3. Ensuring that emergency equipment, including suction, oxygen, and tracheostomy equipment, is at the bedside

> **Critical Rescue** ◆ If severe swelling occurs and the airway begins to be obstructed, notify the Rapid Response Team to remove the clips from the incision to preserve the airway.

4. Monitoring vital signs and identifying any change in status
5. Checking the neck dressing for abnormal amounts of drainage or bleeding
6. Checking serum calcium levels immediately after surgery and every 4 hours thereafter until calcium levels stabilize
7. Monitoring for manifestations of hypocalcemia
   a. Tingling and twitching in the extremities and face
   b. Positive Trousseau's sign
   c. Positive Chvostek's sign (see Hypocalcemia)
8. Assess for damage to the recurrent laryngeal nerve.
   a. Changes in voice patterns
   b. Hoarseness

- If all four parathyroid glands are removed, the patient will need lifelong treatment with calcium and vitamin D because the resulting hypoparathyroidism is permanent.

HYPERPITUITARISM

OVERVIEW

- Hyperpituitarism is a condition of hormone oversecretion that occurs with pituitary tumors or hyperplasia.
- Tumors occur most often in the anterior pituitary cells that produce growth hormone (GH), prolactin (PRL), and adrenocorticotropic hormone (ACTH).
- Overproduction of growth hormone results in gigantism or acromegaly.
  1. *Gigantism* occurs with excessive growth hormone (GH) levels before or during puberty and results in rapid proportional growth in the length of all bones.
  2. *Acromegaly* occurs when excessive growth hormone (GH) levels are produced after puberty and results in increased skeletal thickness, hypertrophy of the skin, and enlargement of all visceral organs.
- Excess ACTH overstimulates the adrenal cortex, resulting in excessive production of glucocorticoids, mineralocorticoids, and androgens, which leads to the development of Cushing's disease.

Genetic Considerations

- An uncommon cause of hyperpituitarism is type 1 multiple endocrine neoplasia (MEN1), in which there is inactivation of a suppressor gene. This problem has an autosomal dominant inheritance pattern and is usually expressed as a benign tumor that affects the pituitary, parathyroid glands, and pancreas.

- In pituitary function, MEN1 leads to excessive production of growth hormone (GH) and acromegaly.

PATIENT-CENTERED COLLABORATIVE CARE

Assessment

- Obtain patient information about:
  1. Age and gender
  2. Family history of endocrine problems
  3. Any change in hat, glove, ring, or shoe size
  4. Fatigue and lethargy
  5. Backache
  6. Arthralgias (joint pain)
  7. Headaches and changes in vision
  8. Menstrual changes (e.g., amenorrhea, irregular menses, difficulty in becoming pregnant)
  9. Changes in sexual functioning (e.g., decreased libido, painful intercourse, impotence)
  10. Loss of or change in secondary sexual characteristics
  11. Weight gain or loss (unplanned)
- Assess for and document:
  1. Changes in the facial features (e.g., increases in lip and nose sizes; prominent brow ridge; increases in head, hand, and foot sizes)
  2. Moon face
  3. Extremity muscle wasting
  4. Acne
  5. Hirsutism
  6. Striae
  7. Hypertension
  8. Areas of uneven pigmentation or hyperpigmentation
  9. Tachycardia or bradycardia
  10. Dysrhythmias
- Diagnostic testing may include:
  1. Blood test for hormone levels (any or all may be elevated)
  2. Skull x-rays
  3. CT
  4. MRI
  5. Angiography (brain)
  6. Hormone suppression tests

Interventions

Surgical Management

- Surgical removal of the pituitary gland and tumor (hypophysectomy) is the most common treatment for hyperpituitarism.
- A transsphenoidal hypophysectomy is the most commonly used surgical approach and is microscopic surgery performed with

the patient under general anesthesia. The surgeon makes an incision just above the upper lip and reaches the pituitary gland through the sphenoid sinus.

- A craniotomy may be needed if the tumor cannot be reached by a transsphenoidal approach.
- Provide preoperative care, including:
  1. Implementing routine preoperative care as described in Part One
  2. Explaining that hypophysectomy decreases hormone levels, relieves headaches, and may reverse changes in sexual functioning.
  3. Reminding the patient that body changes, organ enlargement, and visual changes are not usually reversible.
  4. Explaining that because nasal packing is present for 2 to 3 days after surgery, it will be necessary to breathe through the mouth, and a "mustache dressing" ("drip pad") will be placed under the nose.
  5. Instructing the patient not to brush teeth, cough, sneeze, blow the nose, or bend forward after surgery.
- Provide postoperative care, including:
  1. Implementing routine postoperative care as described in Part One
  2. Monitoring neurologic responses hourly for the first 24 hours and then every 4 hours and documenting any changes in vision, mental status, altered level of consciousness, or decreased strength of the extremities
  3. Observing for complications such as transient diabetes insipidus, CSF leakage, infection, and increased intracranial pressure (ICP)
  4. Measuring intake and output, especially for output greater than intake
  5. Instructing the patient to report any postnasal drip, which may indicate leakage of CSF
  6. Keeping the head of the bed elevated
  7. Assessing nasal drainage for quantity, quality, and the presence of glucose (which indicates that the fluid is CSF)
  8. Instructing the patient to avoid coughing early after surgery and reminding him or her to perform deep breathing exercises hourly while awake
  9. Instructing the patient to avoid bending at the waist for any reason, because this position increases intracranial pressure (ICP)
  10. Performing frequent oral rinses and applying water soluble jelly to dry lips

11. Assessing for manifestations of meningitis
    a. Headache
    b. Fever
    c. Nuchal (neck) rigidity
12. Teaching the patient self-administration of the prescribed hormones

Nonsurgical Management

- The goals of therapy for the patient who has hyperpituitarism are to return hormone levels to normal or near normal, reduce or eliminate headache and visual disturbances, prevent complications, and reverse as many of the body changes as possible.
- Encourage the patient to express concerns and fears about his or her altered physical appearance.
- Help him or her identify personal strengths and positive characteristics.
- Drug therapy (may be used alone or in combination with surgery or radiation)
    1. Dopamine agonists to stimulate dopamine receptors in the brain and inhibit the release of many pituitary hormones, especially prolactin and growth hormone (GH)
        a. Bromocriptine mesylate (Parlodel)
        b. Cabergoline (Dostinex)
        c. Pergolide (Permax)
    2. Somatostatin analogs and growth hormone (GH) receptor blockers (for growth hormone (GH) secreting tumors)
        a. Octreotide (Sandostatin)
        b. Pegvisomant (Somavert)
- Radiation therapy regimens take a long time to complete, and several years may pass before a therapeutic effect can be seen. Side effects of radiation therapy include hypopituitarism, optic nerve damage, and other eye and vision problems.

HYPERTENSION

OVERVIEW

- Hypertension is defined as systolic blood pressure (SBP) greater than or equal to 140 mm Hg or diastolic blood pressure (DBP) greater than or equal to 90 mm Hg, or both, occurring in a patient on at least two separate occasions. In patients with diabetes, hypertension is defined as an SBP greater than 130 mm Hg.
- Prehypertension is defined as an SBP of 120 to 139 mm Hg or a DBP of 80 to 89 mm Hg.
- Hypertension is the major risk factor for coronary, cerebral, renal, retinal (vision), and peripheral vascular disease.

- There are two major classifications of hypertension:
  1. Primary, with no known cause and associated with risk factors such as a family history of hypertension, age older than 60 years, hyperlipidemia, stress, and smoking
  2. Secondary hypertension results from specific diseases, such as renal vascular and renal parenchymal disease, primary aldosteronism, Cushing's disease, coarctation of the aorta, brain tumors and encephalitis, psychiatric disorders, and some drugs, such as estrogen-containing oral contraceptives, glucocorticoids, mineralocorticoids, cyclosporine, and erythropoietin
- Malignant hypertension is a severe type of hypertension that progresses rapidly and leads to renal failure, left ventricular failure, and stroke unless intervention occurs promptly.

Cultural Considerations

The prevalence of hypertension in African Americans is among the highest in the world and continues to increase. When compared with Euro-Americans, they develop high blood pressure earlier in life, making them much more likely to die of strokes, heart disease, and kidney disease. The reason for these differences is not known, but genetics and environmental factors may play a role.

PATIENT-CENTERED COLLABORATIVE CARE

Assessment

- Record patient information:
  1. Age
  2. Race or ethnic origin
  3. Family history of hypertension
  4. Average daily intake of calories, sodium, and potassium-containing foods
  5. Alcohol intake
  6. Smoking history
  7. Exercise habits
  8. Past and present history of renal or cardiovascular disease
  9. Drug use (prescribed and OTC)
  10. Blood pressure readings in both arms
  11. Blood pressure readings in supine and erect positions
  12. Peripheral pulse rate, rhythm, and force
  13. Psychosocial stressors

National Patient Safety Goal

Accurately and completely reconcile medications from home used to treat hypertension so that those drugs can be continued in the hospital.

- Assessment findings include:
  1. No obvious symptoms
  2. Headache, dizziness, or fainting
  3. Edema
  4. Nocturia
  5. Lethargy
  6. Nosebleeds
  7. Vision changes or retinal changes on funduscopic examination
  8. Signs of kidney injury, such as elevated blood urea nitrogen (BUN) or creatinine levels or low urine output
  9. Physical findings related to vascular damage, including atherosclerosis, acute coronary syndrome, and heart failure
     a. Abdominal, carotid, or femoral bruits
     b. Tachycardia, sweating, and pallor
     c. Decreased or absent femoral pulses
     d. Cardiomegaly or left ventricular hypertrophy

Planning and Implementation
❖**NDx:** Deficient Knowledge
  1. In collaboration with the nutritionist:
     a. Advising the patient to decrease sodium intake by not adding table salt to food, not cooking with salt, and not adding seasonings that contain sodium and to limit eating canned, frozen, and other processed foods
     b. Suggesting that the patient use spices, herbs, fruits, and other non–salt-containing substances such as powdered garlic and onion or a salt substitute to enhance the flavor of food
     c. Advising the patient to consider strategies to promote ideal body weight
     d. Developing a plan to reduce saturated fat and cholesterol in the diet
  2. Advising the patient to restrict alcohol intake and smoking
  3. Collaborating with the physician and physical therapist to assist the patient in developing a regular exercise program
  4. Teaching or referring the patient to stress management programs including yoga, massage, biofeedback, and hypnosis programs
  5. Encouraging lifestyle choices that promote a heart healthy diet, regular exercise, and adherence to prescribed drugs
  6. Providing drug therapy as prescribed. Most patients require two drugs from different classes to control hypertension
     a. Thiazide diuretics prevent sodium and water reabsorption in the distal tubules of the kidneys while promoting potassium excretion.

b. Loop diuretics depress sodium reabsorption in the ascending loop of Henle and promote potassium excretion.

c. Potassium-sparing diuretics act on the distal tubules of the kidneys to inhibit reabsorption of sodium in exchange for potassium ions, retaining potassium. Aldosterone inhibitors also interfere with the renin-angiotensin-aldosterone system, promoting vascular health.

d. Angiotensin-converting enzyme (ACE) inhibitors convert angiotensin I to angiotensin II, resulting in vasorelaxation and diuresis.

e. Angiotensin receptor blockers (ARBs) selectively block the binding of angiotensin II in the vascular and adrenal tissue.

f. Beta-adrenergic blockers lower blood pressure by blocking beta receptors in the heart and peripheral vessels, reducing the cardiac rate and blocking renin release.

g. Central alpha agonists act on the central nervous system, preventing reuptake of norepinephrine, resulting in lower peripheral vascular resistance and blood pressure.

h. Calcium channel blockers lower blood pressure by interfering with transmembrane influx of calcium ions, resulting in vasoconstriction.

▼ National Patient Safety Goal

Improve the safety of using drugs to treat hypertension by standardizing the drug concentrations used within the organization and identifying look-alike and sound-alike drugs to determine how to prevent errors involving the interchange of these drugs.

> **⊠ Critical Rescue ◆** Monitor the patient's serum potassium level when administering a diuretic, ACE inhibitor, or ARB.

- Additional nursing diagnoses that guide interventions
  1. Risk for Ineffective Therapeutic Regimen Management related to nonadherence to treatment
  2. Ineffective Tissue Perfusion (Renal, Cerebral, Cardiopulmonary, and Peripheral) related to decreased perfusion
  3. Risk for Imbalanced Nutrition More than Body Requirements related to learned eating behaviors, ethnic and cultural values, lack of social support for weight loss, or imbalance between activity level and caloric intake
  4. Fatigue related to altered body chemistry (drug, electrolyte interactions) and disease state
  5. Sexual Dysfunction related to altered body function from drug therapy

6. Ineffective Coping related to inadequate level of perception of control
7. Excessive Fluid Volume related to compromised regulatory mechanism
8. Risk for Noncompliance related to knowledge and skill relevant to the regimen behavior

Community-Based Care

- Provide educational information for hypertension control, especially:
  1. Salt restriction
  2. Weight maintenance or reduction
  3. Consider diet intake record to increase self-awareness of food selections.
  4. Stress reduction
  5. Alcohol restriction
  6. Exercise program
  7. Taking prescribed antihypertensive drugs even in the absence of symptoms
  8. Regular, ongoing follow-up with healthcare provider
- Give oral and written information on drug therapy, including:
  1. Rationale for use, dose, and time of administration
  2. Side effects and vigilance for drug interactions
  3. The importance of taking the drugs even when there are no symptoms
- Instruct the patient and family members in the technique of blood pressure monitoring at home.
- Teach the patient or family member to obtain heart rate and record blood pressure readings in a logbook or diary.
- Refer the patient to home care agency, if necessary.
- Refer the patient to the American Heart Association (AHA) for information and support.

HYPERTHYROIDISM

OVERVIEW

- Hyperthyroidism is excessive thyroid hormone secretion from the thyroid gland. It is one of the most common endocrine disorders and affects women 5 to 10 times more often than men.
- The manifestations of hyperthyroidism are called *thyrotoxicosis*, regardless of the origin of the thyroid hormones.
- Thyroid hormones affect metabolism in all body organs, and excesses produce many different manifestations.
- The most common cause is Graves' disease, an autoimmune disorder in which antibodies are made and attach to the thyroid-

stimulating hormone (TSH) receptor sites on the thyroid tissue. The thyroid-stimulating immunoglobulins (TSIs) bind to the thyroid gland, increasing its size and overproducing thyroid hormones.

Genetic Considerations

- Graves' disease appears to have a strong association with other autoimmune disorders, such as diabetes mellitus, vitiligo, and rheumatoid arthritis.
- It often occurs in both members of identical twins, with an inheritance pattern of familial clustering or complex polygenic inheritance.

- Other causes include benign or malignant tumors and excessive use of thyroid replacement drugs.
- *Thyroid storm*, or *thyroid crisis*, is a life-threatening condition of an extreme state of hyperthyroidism that can occur when the condition is untreated or poorly controlled or when the patient is severely stressed.

PATIENT-CENTERED COLLABORATIVE CARE

Assessment

- Obtain patient information about:
  1. Age and gender
  2. Usual weight and any unplanned weight loss
  3. Increased appetite
  4. Increased number of daily bowel movements
  5. Heat intolerance
  6. Diaphoresis (increased sweating) even when environmental temperatures are comfortable for others
  7. Palpitations or chest pain
  8. Dyspnea (with or without exertion)
  9. Visual changes, especially exophthalmos (specific to Graves' disease)
  10. Fatigue, weakness
  11. Insomnia (common)
  12. Irritability, depression
  13. Amenorrhea or a decreased menstrual flow (common)
  14. Changes in libido
  15. Previous thyroid surgery or radiation therapy to the neck
  16. Past and current drugs, especially the use of thyroid hormone replacement or antithyroid drugs
- Assess for and document:
  1. Exophthalmos (Graves' disease)
  2. Photophobia

3. General appearance
   a. Eyelid retraction (Grave's disease)
   b. Eyeball lag (upper eyelid pulls back faster than the eyeball when the patient gazes upward) (Grave's disease)
4. Presence or absence of a goiter (enlarged thyroid gland)
5. Hypertension
6. Tachycardia
7. Dysrhythmias
8. Fine, soft, silky hair
9. Warm, moist skin
10. Tremors
11. Hyperactive deep tendon reflexes

- Psychosocial issues or changes may include:
  1. Wide mood swings
  2. Irritability
  3. Decreased attention span
  4. Mild to severe hyperactivity

- Diagnostic assessment may include:
  1. Blood tests for:
     a. Triiodothyronine (T_3)
     b. Thyroxine (T_4)
     c. T_3 resin uptake (T_3RU)
     d. Thyroid-stimulating hormone (TSH)
     e. Antibodies to TSH (TSH-RAb) (Graves' disease)
  2. Thyroid scan
  3. Ultrasonography of the thyroid gland
  4. Electrocardiograph (ECG)
     a. Tachycardia
     b. Atrial fibrillation
     c. Dysrhythmias
     d. Changes in P and T waveforms

Interventions

- Interventions are described for Graves' disease because it is the most common form of hyperthyroidism. The goals of management are to decrease the effect of thyroid hormone on cardiac function and to reduce thyroid hormone secretion.

Nonsurgical Management

- Monitoring, including:
  1. Measuring the apical pulse and blood pressure at least every 4 hours
  2. Checking temperature at least every 4 hours

> 🔲 **Critical Rescue** ◆ Immediately report a temperature increase of even 1° F because it may indicate impending thyroid crisis.

   3. Instructing the patient to immediately report:
      a. Palpitations
      b. Dyspnea
      c. Vertigo
      d. Chest pain
- Reducing stimulation
   1. Keeping the environment as quiet as possible
   2. Closing the door to the patient's room
   3. Limiting visitors
   4. Eliminating or postponing nonessential care or treatments
- Promoting comfort
   1. Reducing the room temperature
   2. Ensuring that the patient always has a fresh pitcher of ice water
   3. Changing bed linen when it becomes damp from diaphoresis
   4. Assisting the patient to take a cool shower several times each day
- Drug therapy
   1. Antithyroid drugs
      a. Propylthiouracil (PTU)
      b. Methimazole (Tapazole)
   2. Iodine preparations
   3. Lithium
   4. Supportive drug therapy with propranolol (Inderal, Detensol ♣) to relieve diaphoresis, anxiety, tachycardia, and palpitations
- Radioactive iodine (RAI) therapy
   1. Is not used in pregnant women because ^{131}I crosses the placenta and can damage the fetal thyroid gland
   2. Can be delivered as an oral drug or by IV
   3. Dosage depends on the thyroid gland's size and sensitivity to radiation
   4. Destroys some of the cells that produce thyroid hormone
   5. Performed on an outpatient basis
   6. One dose may be sufficient, although a second or third dose may be needed.
   7. Radiation dose is low enough that radiation precautions are not needed.
   8. Results may take 4 to 8 weeks.
   9. Some patients become hypothyroid as a result of this treatment.

Surgical Management
- Surgery to remove all (total thyroidectomy) or part of the thyroid gland (subtotal thyroidectomy) may be needed for patients who have a large goiter causing tracheal or esophageal

compression or who do not have a good response to antithyroid drugs.

- A thyroidectomy is performed with the patient under general anesthesia. The surgeon makes a "collar incision" just above the clavicle.
- After a total thyroidectomy, patients must take lifelong thyroid hormone replacement.
- Provide preoperative care, including:
  1. Implementing routine preoperative care as described in Part One
  2. Administering antithyroid drugs and iodine preparations to decrease the secretion of thyroid hormones and reduce thyroid size and vascularity
  3. Ensuring that hypertension, dysrhythmias, and tachycardia are controlled before surgery
  4. Teaching the patient to support the neck when coughing or moving by placing both hands behind the neck when moving
  5. Explaining that hoarseness may be present for a few days as a result of endotracheal tube placement during surgery
  6. Reassuring the patient by calmly explaining the surgery and the care after surgery
  7. Reminding him or her that a drain and dressing may be in place after surgery
  8. Answering any questions the patient and family have
- Providing postoperative care, including:
  1. Implementing routine postoperative care as described in Part One
  2. Monitoring vital signs every 15 minutes until the patient is stable and then every 30 minutes
  3. Assessing the patient's level of discomfort
  4. Using sandbags or pillows to support the head and neck
  5. Placing the patient, while he or she is awake, in a semi-Fowler position
  6. Decreasing tension on the suture line by avoiding neck extension
  7. Humidifying the air
  8. Assisting the patient to cough and deep-breathe every 30 minutes to 1 hour
  9. Suctioning oral and tracheal secretions when necessary
  10. Preventing complications
      a. Respiratory distress
         (1) Listening for laryngeal stridor (harsh, high-pitched respiratory sounds)

(2) Keeping emergency tracheostomy equipment in the patient's room

(3) Ensuring that oxygen and suctioning equipment are nearby and in working order

> 🛟 **Critical Rescue** ◆ If symptoms of obstruction occur, notify the Rapid Response Team. In some agencies, the nurse can remove clips or sutures when medical assistance is not immediately available and swelling at the surgical site is obstructing the airway.

b. Hemorrhage
(1) Inspecting the neck dressing and behind the patient's neck for blood at least every 2 hours for the first 24 hours
(2) Assessing drainage for amount, color, and character
c. Hypocalcemia and tetany
(1) Asking the patient hourly about any tingling around the mouth or of the toes and fingers
(2) Assessing for muscle twitching
(3) Ensuring calcium gluconate or calcium chloride is available
d. Laryngeal nerve damage
(1) Assessing the patient's voice at 2-hour intervals
(2) Reassuring the patient that hoarseness is usually temporary
- Emergency management of thyroid storm or thyroid crisis
1. Thyroid storm or crisis is a life-threatening event that occurs in patients with uncontrolled hyperthyroidism and occurs most often with Graves' disease.
2. Manifestations develop quickly and are often triggered by stressors such as trauma, infection, diabetic ketoacidosis, and pregnancy.
3. Other conditions that can lead to thyroid storm include vigorous palpation of the goiter, exposure to iodine, and radioactive iodine (RAI) therapy.
4. Key manifestations include fever, tachycardia, and systolic hypertension.
5. Even with treatment, thyroid storm may lead to death.
a. Maintain a patent airway and adequate ventilation.
b. Give antithyroid drugs as prescribed: propylthiouracil (PTU, Propyl-Thyracil 🍁), 300 to 900 mg daily, and methimazole (Tapazole), up to 60 mg daily.
c. Administer sodium iodide solution, 2 g IV daily, as prescribed.

   d. Give propranolol (Inderal, Detensol ✿), 1 to 3 mg IV, as prescribed. Give slowly over 3 minutes; the patient should be connected to a cardiac monitor, and a central venous pressure catheter should be in place.

   e. Give glucocorticoids, as prescribed: hydrocortisone, 100 to 500 mg IV daily; prednisone, 4 to 60 mg orally daily; or dexamethasone 2 mg IM or IV every 6 hours.

   f. Monitor continually for cardiac dysrhythmias.

   g. Monitor vital signs every 30 minutes.

   h. Provide comfort measures, including a cooling blanket.

   i. Give nonsalicylate antipyretics, as prescribed.

   j. Correct dehydration with normal saline infusions.

   k. Apply cooling blanket or ice packs to reduce fever.

Community-Based Care

- Teach the patient and family about:
  1. The manifestations of hyperthyroidism and instructing them to report an increase or recurrence of symptoms
  2. The manifestations of hypothyroidism and the need for thyroid hormone replacement
  3. The need for regular follow-up because hypothyroidism can occur several years after radioactive iodine (RAI) therapy
  4. Pertinent information about any prescribed drugs, including side effects
  5. Inspecting the incision area and reporting redness, tenderness, drainage, or swelling to the surgeon
  6. Possible continued mood changes, reassuring the patient and family that these effects will decrease with continued treatment

HYPOCALCEMIA

OVERVIEW

- Hypocalcemia is a total serum calcium ($Ca^{2}+$) level less than 9.0 mg/dL or 2.25 mmol/L.
- Because the normal blood level of calcium is so low, any change in calcium levels has major effects on function.
- Common causes of hypocalcemia include:
  1. Decreased calcium absorption
     a. Inadequate oral intake of calcium
     b. Lactose intolerance
     c. Malabsorption syndromes (celiac disease [sprue], Crohn's disease)
     d. Inadequate intake of vitamin D
  2. Increased calcium excretion
     a. End-stage kidney disease

b. Kidney failure (polyuric phase)
c. Diarrhea
d. Steatorrhea
e. Wound drainage (especially GI)
3. Conditions that keep calcium out of the blood
  a. Hyperproteinemia
  b. Alkalosis
  c. Calcium chelators or binders (citrate, mithramycin, penicillamine, sodium cellulose phosphate [Calcibind], Aredia)
  d. Acute pancreatitis
  e. Hyperphosphatemia
  f. Immobility
  g. Removal or destruction of parathyroid glands
- Low serum calcium levels increase sodium movement across excitable membranes, allowing depolarization to occur more easily and at inappropriate times.
- The more rapidly hypocalcemia occurs and the more severe it is, the more likely life-threatening manifestations will occur.

Cultural Considerations

- Lactose intolerance caused by a deficiency of the enzyme lactase occurs in 75% to 90% of all Asians, blacks, and American Indians.
- People with lactose intolerance cannot use the nutrients in milk and have cramping, diarrhea, and abdominal pain after ingesting dairy products. Dairy products, especially milk, are common and rich sources of calcium and vitamin D.
- People with lactose intolerance may have difficulty obtaining enough calcium and vitamin D from other sources to maintain normal calcium levels in the blood and bones.

Women's Health Considerations

- Postmenopausal women are at risk for chronic calcium loss as a result of reduced weight-bearing activities and a decrease in estrogen levels.
- Many older women decrease weight-bearing activities, such as running and walking.

PATIENT-CENTERED COLLABORATIVE CARE
Assessment
- Assess for and document:
  1. Neuromuscular changes (most common)
    a. Paresthesias with sensations of tingling and numbness

    b. Muscle twitches, painful cramps, and spasms

    c. Anxiety, irritability

    d. Hyperactive deep tendon reflexes

    e. Positive Trousseau's sign: Place a blood pressure cuff around the upper arm, inflate the cuff to greater than the patient's systolic pressure, and keep the cuff inflated for 1 to 4 minutes. Under these hypoxic conditions, a positive Trousseau's sign occurs when the hand and fingers go into spasm in palmar flexion.

    f. Positive Chvostek's sign: Tap the face just below and in front of the ear (over the facial nerve) to trigger facial twitching of one side of the mouth, nose, and cheek.

2. Cardiovascular changes
   a. Bradycardia
   b. Weak, thready pulse
   c. Hypotension
   d. Electrocardiographic (ECG) changes (prolonged ST interval, prolonged QT interval)

3. GI changes
   a. Hyperactive bowel sounds
   b. Abdominal cramping
   c. Diarrhea

4. Skeletal changes (thin, brittle, and fragile bones)
   a. Overall loss of height
   b. Presence of spinal curvatures
   c. Unexplained bone pain

Interventions

- Drug therapy with:
  1. Direct calcium replacement (oral and IV)
  2. Drugs that enhance the absorption of calcium, such as aluminum hydroxide and vitamin D
  3. Drugs that decrease nerve and muscle responses (magnesium sulfate and various muscle relaxants)
- Nutrition therapy with a high-calcium diet (collaborate with a nutritionist to teach patients about foods high in calcium)
- Additional interventions include:
  1. Environmental management to reduce stimulation
     a. Keeping the room quiet
     b. Limiting visitors
     c. Adjusting the lighting
     d. Using a soft but reassuring voice
  2. Keeping emergency equipment (e.g., oxygen, suction, emergency drugs, endotracheal tray) readily available
  3. Injury prevention strategies
     a. Using a lift sheet when lifting or moving a patient with fragile bones

b. Observing for normal range of joint motion and for any unusual surface bumps or depressions over bony areas

HYPOFUNCTION, ADRENAL (ADRENAL INSUFFICIENCY)

OVERVIEW

- Decreased production of adrenocortical steroids may occur as a result of inadequate secretion of adrenocorticotropic hormone (ACTH), dysfunction of the hypothalamic-pituitary control mechanism, or direct dysfunction of adrenal gland tissue.
- Primary hypofunction, or Addison's disease, develops gradually as adrenal function is reduced and can no longer supply normal levels of glucocorticoids or mineralocorticoids. Causes include tuberculosis, autoimmune factors, HIV/AIDS, adrenal tumors, hemorrhage, sepsis, irradiation of the adrenal glands, and adrenalectomy.
- The most common cause of secondary adrenal insufficiency is the sudden cessation of long-term, high-dose glucocorticoid therapy.
- Manifestations of adrenal hypofunction include:
  1. Hyperkalemia
  2. Hyponatremia
  3. Hypotension
  4. Hypoglycemia
  5. Shock
- *Acute adrenal insufficiency, or Addisonian crisis, is a life-threatening event in which the need for cortisol and aldosterone is greater than the available supply. Manifestations may appear suddenly, without warning. Death from hypoglycemia, shock, and hyperkalemic-associated cardiac problems can occur unless interventions are implemented rapidly.*

PATIENT-CENTERED COLLABORATIVE CARE

Assessment

- Obtain patient information about:
  1. Change in activity level
  2. Increased salt craving or intake
  3. GI problems, such as anorexia, nausea, vomiting, diarrhea, and abdominal pain
  4. Unplanned weight loss
  5. History of irradiation to the abdomen or head
  6. Past or current medical problems (e.g., tuberculosis or previous intracranial surgery)

7. Past and current drugs, especially steroids, anticoagulants, opioids, or cytotoxic drugs
- Assess for and document:
  1. Manifestations of hypoglycemia (low blood glucose level, sweating, headaches, tachycardia, and tremors)
  2. Manifestations of hypovolemia (postural hypotension and dehydration)
  3. Cardiac problems from hyperkalemia (dysrhythmias, bradycardia, irregular heart rate, cardiac arrest)
  4. Skeletal muscle weakness
  5. Electrolyte abnormalities (elevated serum potassium and low serum sodium levels)
  6. Areas of increased pigmentation, decreased pigmentation, or patchy pigmentation
  7. Decreased alertness, forgetfulness, confusion
- Diagnosis is based on clinical manifestations and:
  1. Laboratory findings of low serum cortisol, low fasting blood glucose, low sodium, and elevated potassium levels
  2. Low urinary 17-hydroxycorticosteroid and 17-ketosteroid levels
  3. Skull x-rays, CT, MRI, and arteriography
  4. CT scans of the adrenal gland
  5. ACTH stimulation testing

Interventions
- Cortisol and aldosterone deficiencies are corrected by replacement therapy with hydrocortisone (corrects glucocorticoid deficiency) and fludrocortisone (corrects aldosterone deficiency).
  1. For hydrocortisone therapy, divided doses are usually given, with two thirds given in the morning and one third in the late afternoon (or as prescribed).
  2. Dosage adjustment of fludrocortisone may be needed, especially in hot weather, when more sodium is lost because of excessive perspiration.
- Nursing interventions to promote fluid balance, monitor for fluid deficit, and prevent hypoglycemia include:
  1. Weighing the patient daily and recording intake and output
  2. Assessing vital signs every 1 to 4 hours
  3. Checking for dysrhythmias or postural hypotension
  4. Monitoring laboratory values to identify hemoconcentration (e.g., increased hematocrit or blood urea nitrogen [BUN])

> **Clinical Landmine** ◆ Do not implement salt restriction or diuretic therapy for anyone with severe adrenal hypofunction because it may lead to an adrenal crisis.

HYPOKALEMIA

OVERVIEW

- Hypokalemia is a serum potassium level less than 3.5 mEq/L (3.5 mmol/L).
- It can be life threatening because every body system is affected.
- With hypokalemia, the cell membranes of all excitable tissues, such as nerve and muscle, are *less* responsive to normal stimuli.
- Rapid reduction of serum potassium levels causes dramatic changes in function, whereas gradual reductions may not show changes in function until the level is very low.
- Common causes include:
  1. Inappropriate or excessive use of drugs
     a. Diuretics
     b. Digitalis
     c. Corticosteroids
  2. Increased secretion of aldosterone
  3. Cushing's syndrome/disease
  4. Diarrhea
  5. Vomiting
  6. Wound drainage (especially GI)
  7. Prolonged nasogastric suction
  8. Excessive diaphoresis
  9. Kidney disease impairing reabsorption of potassium
  10. NPO status
  11. Alkalosis
  12. Hyperinsulinism
  13. Hyperalimentation
  14. Total parenteral nutrition
  15. Water intoxication
  16. IV therapy with potassium-poor solutions

PATIENT-CENTERED COLLABORATIVE CARE

Assessment

- Obtain patient information about:
  1. Age
  2. Drugs, especially diuretics, corticosteroids, digoxin, beta-adrenergic agonists or antagonists, and potassium supplements
  3. Presence of any acute or chronic disease
  4. Diet history
- Assess for and document:
  1. Respiratory changes

> 🔲 **Critical Rescue** ◆ Skeletal muscle weakness results in shallow respirations. Respiratory status should be assessed first in any patient who may have hypokalemia.

    a. Breath sounds
    b. Ease of respiratory effort
    c. Color of nail beds and mucous membranes
    d. Rate and depth of respiration
    e. Oxygen saturation
  2. Musculoskeletal changes for weakness
    a. Weak hand grasps
    b. Decreased deep tendon reflexes
    c. Flaccid paralysis
  3. Cardiovascular changes
    a. Rapid, thready pulse
    b. Peripheral pulses difficult to palpate
    c. Dysrhythmias and electrocardiographic (ECG) changes
      (1) ST-segment depression
      (2) Flat or inverted T waves
      (3) Increased U waves

> 🔲 **Critical Rescue** ◆ Dysrhythmias can lead to death, particularly in older adults who are taking digoxin. Report ECG changes consistent with hypokalemia to the physician or Rapid Response Team.

    d. Orthostatic hypotension
  4. Neurologic changes
    a. Altered mental status
    b. Irritability and anxiety
    c. Lethargy, acute confusion, coma
  5. GI changes
    a. Hypoactive bowel sound
    b. Nausea, vomiting
    c. Constipation
    d. Abdominal distention
    e. Paralytic ileus
  6. Serum potassium value below 3.5 mEq/L (3.5 mmol/L)

Interventions
- Interventions for hypokalemia aim to prevent potassium loss, increase serum potassium levels, and provide a safe environment for the patient.

- Medical interventions include:
  1. Drug therapy
     a. Oral potassium supplements
     b. IV potassium for severe hypokalemia

▼ **National Patient Safety Goal**

Potassium is available in different concentrations, and this drug carries a high alert warning as a concentrated electrolyte solution. Although the drug is usually added to the IV solution in the pharmacy, it may be added on the nursing unit. Check and re-check the concentration of the drug in the vial with another registered nurse, a pharmacist, or a physician, and carefully calculate the required dilution before adding it to the IV solution. A dilution of no more than 1 mEq/10 mL of solution is recommended. The maximum recommended infusion rate is 5 to 10 mEq/hr; this rate is never to exceed 20 mEq/hr under any circumstances. Because rapid infusion of potassium can cause cardiac arrest, potassium is not given by IV push.

> 🔪 **Clinical Landmine** ◆ Potassium is a severe tissue irritant and is never given by IM or subcutaneous injection.

     c. Potassium-sparing diuretics
        (1) Spironolactone (Aldactone, Novospiroton 🍁)
        (2) Triamterene (Dyrenium)
        (3) Amiloride (Midamor)
  2. Nutrition therapy to increase dietary potassium intake
- The priorities for nursing care of the patient with hypokalemia are ensuring adequate oxygenation, patient falls prevention, prevention of injury from potassium administration, and monitoring the patient's response to therapy.
  1. Implementing safety measures
     a. Instituting falls precautions
     b. Eliminating hazards in the ambulation path
     c. Assisting with ambulation
  2. Performing respiratory monitoring at least hourly for severe hypokalemia
     a. Rate and depth (checking for increasing rate and decreasing depth)
     b. Oxygen saturation by pulse oximetry
     c. Patient's ability to cough
     d. Evaluation of arterial blood gas values (when available)

HYPONATREMIA

OVERVIEW

- Hyponatremia is a serum sodium (Na+) level less than 136 mEq/L (136 mmol/L), and it often occurs with fluid volume imbalances.
- The problems caused by hyponatremia involve reduced excitable depolarization and cellular swelling.
- Common causes of hyponatremia include:
  1. Poor intake of sodium or excessive sodium loss
     a. Excessive diaphoresis
     b. Diuretics (high-ceiling diuretics)
     c. Wound drainage (especially GI)
     d. Decreased secretion of aldosterone
     e. Hyperlipidemia
     f. Kidney disease (scarred distal convoluted tubule)
     g. NPO status
     h. Low-salt diet
  2. Dilution of serum sodium
     a. Excessive ingestion of hypotonic fluids
     b. Freshwater submersion accident
     c. Kidney failure (nephrotic syndrome)
     d. Irrigation with hypotonic fluids
     e. Syndrome of inappropriate antidiuretic hormone (SIADH)
     f. Hyperglycemia
     g. Heart failure

PATIENT-CENTERED COLLABORATIVE CARE

Assessment

- Assess for and document:
  1. Cerebral changes
     a. Acute confusion
     b. Reduced level of cognition
     c. Seizure activity
  2. Neuromuscular changes
     a. General muscle weakness, especially in arms and legs
     b. Diminished deep tendon reflexes

> 🛟 Critical Rescue ◆ If the patient has muscle weakness, immediately check respiratory effectiveness, because ventilation depends on adequate strength of respiratory muscles.

  3. GI changes
     a. Increased motility

b. Diarrhea
c. Abdominal cramping
d. Hyperactive bowel sounds
4. Cardiovascular changes
    a. Hyponatremia with hypovolemia
        (1) Rapid, weak, thready pulse
        (2) Reduced peripheral pulses
        (3) Hypotension
    b. Hyponatremia with hypervolemia
        (1) Full bounding pulse
        (2) Normal or high blood pressure
        (3) Edema

Interventions

- Drug therapy
    1. Discontinuing or reducing drugs that increase sodium loss, such as loop diuretics and thiazide diuretics
    2. Hyponatremia with a fluid deficit: IV saline infusions are prescribed to restore both sodium and fluid volume. Severe hyponatremia may be treated with small-volume infusions of hypertonic (2% to 3%) saline.
    3. Hyponatremia with fluid excess: Osmotic diuretics that promote the excretion of water rather than sodium, such as mannitol (Osmitrol), or conivaptan (Vaprisol)
    4. Hyponatremia caused by inappropriate secretion of antidiuretic hormone (ADH): Therapy includes agents that antagonize ADH, such as lithium and demeclocycline (Declomycin).
- Nutrition therapy
    1. Increased oral sodium intake
    2. Fluid restriction when hyponatremia occurs with fluid excess
- Priorities for nursing care of the patient with hyponatremia include monitoring the patient's response to therapy and preventing hypernatremia and fluid overload.
    1. Patient safety to prevent fluid overload from becoming worse, leading to pulmonary edema and heart failure
        a. Monitor for indicators of increased fluid overload at least every 2 hours.

> 🛟 Critical Rescue ◆ Pulmonary edema can occur very quickly and can lead to death. Notify the health care provider or Rapid Response Team about any change that indicates the fluid overload is not responding to therapy or is becoming worse.

    b. Use a pressure-reducing or pressure-relieving overlay on the mattress.

    c. Assess skin pressure areas, especially the coccyx, elbows, hips, and heels, daily for signs of redness or open areas.

    d. Assist the patient to change positions every 2 hours.

2. Monitor for patient response to drug therapy:
   a. Weight loss
   b. Increased urine output
3. Observe for manifestations of electrolyte imbalance:
   a. Changes in ECG patterns
   b. Changes in sodium and potassium values
4. Nutritional therapy, teach patients and families about:
   a. Increased sodium intake
   b. Fluid restriction

HYPOPARATHYROIDISM

OVERVIEW

- Hypoparathyroidism is a rare endocrine disorder in which parathyroid function is decreased, resulting in a deficiency of circulating parathyroid hormone (PTH) levels.
- The main result is hypocalcemia.
- There are two forms:
  1. *Iatrogenic hypoparathyroidism,* the most common form, is caused by the removal of all parathyroid tissue during total thyroidectomy or by deliberate surgical removal of the parathyroid glands.
  2. *Idiopathic hypoparathyroidism,* which is rare and probably caused by an autoimmune problem

PATIENT-CENTERED COLLABORATIVE CARE

Assessment

- Obtain patient information about:
  1. Any head or neck surgery
  2. History of head or neck radiation therapy
  3. History of serious neck injury by car crash or strangulation
  4. Presence of mild tingling and numbness around the mouth or in the hands and feet
  5. Presence of severe muscle cramps and spasms of the hands and feet
- Assess for and document:
  1. Irritability
  2. Psychosis
  3. Excessive or inappropriate muscle contractions that cause finger, hand, and elbow flexion

4. Positive Chvostek's sign (see Hypocalcemia)
5. Positive Trousseau's sign (see Hypocalcemia)
6. Bands or pits encircling the crowns of the teeth
- Diagnostic tests for hypoparathyroidism include:
  1. Electroencephalography (EEG)
  2. Serum electrolyte tests and parathyroid hormone (PTH) levels
  3. CT
  4. Urine cyclic adenosine monophosphate (cAMP) levels

Interventions

- Medical management focuses on correcting hypocalcemia, vitamin D deficiency, and hypomagnesemia.
  1. IV calcium is given as a 10% solution of calcium chloride or calcium gluconate over 10 to 15 minutes.
  2. Calcitriol (Rocaltrol), 0.5 to 2 mg daily for vitamin D deficiency
  3. Magnesium sulfate 50%, 2-mL doses (up to 4 g daily) either IM or IV for hypomagnesemia
  4. Long-term oral therapy of calcium, 0.5 to 2 g daily, in divided doses
  5. Long-term therapy with 50,000 to 400,000 units of ergocalciferol daily
- Nursing management includes:
  1. Teaching about the drug regimen and interventions to reduce anxiety
  2. Teaching the patient to eat foods high in calcium but low in phosphorus (milk, yogurt, and processed cheeses are avoided because of their high phosphorus content)
  3. Stressing that therapy for hypocalcemia is lifelong
  4. Advising the patient to wear a medical alert bracelet

HYPOPITUITARISM

OVERVIEW

- Hypopituitarism is a deficiency of one or more anterior pituitary hormones, resulting in metabolic problems and sexual dysfunction.
- Decreased production of *all* anterior pituitary hormones is a rare condition known as *panhypopituitarism*.
- Usually, there is a decrease in the secretion of one hormone and a lesser decrease in the other hormones.
- Clinical features depend on which hormone is undersecreted.
- Deficiencies of adrenocorticotropic hormone (ACTH) and thyroid-stimulating hormone (TSH) are the *most* life threatening because they result in a corresponding decrease in the secretion of vital hormones from the adrenal and thyroid glands.

- Causes of hypopituitarism include pituitary tumors, severe malnutrition or rapid loss of body fat, shock or severe hypotension, head trauma, brain tumors or infection, radiation or surgery of the head and brain, and AIDS.

PATIENT-CENTERED COLLABORATIVE CARE

Assessment

- Assess for and document:
  1. Loss of secondary sexual characteristics (men)
     a. Facial and body hair loss
     b. Impotence
     c. Decreased libido
  2. Loss of secondary sexual characteristics (women)
     a. Absence of menstrual periods
     b. Painful intercourse
     c. Infertility
     d. Decreased libido
     e. Breast atrophy
     f. Decreased amount or absence of auxiliary and pubic hair
  3. Changes in vision
     a. Loss of visual acuity, especially peripheral vision
     b. Temporal headaches
     c. Diplopia (double vision)
     d. Ocular muscle paralysis, limiting eye movement
- Diagnostic assessment may include:
  1. Blood levels of pituitary hormones
  2. Hormone stimulation testing
  3. Skull x-rays
  4. CT scans
  5. MRI
  6. Angiography (brain)

Interventions

- Management of the patient with hypopituitarism focuses on replacement of deficient hormones.
- Instruct the patient about the hormone replacement method and regimen.
  1. Men with gonadotropin deficiency receive sex steroid replacement therapy with androgens (testosterone) by IM injections or transdermal testosterone patches.
     a. High doses are used until virilization (presence of male secondary sex characteristics) occurs, and then maintenance doses are used.
     b. Side effects may include gynecomastia (development of breast tissue in men), acne, baldness, and prostate enlargement.
     c. Fertility is difficult and requires additional therapy.

2. Women who have gonadotropin deficiency receive hormone replacement with a combination of estrogen and progesterone.
   a. Drugs are taken orally or by transdermal patch.
   b. Complications include hypertension and deep vein thrombosis.
   c. Additional therapy is needed for fertility.
3. Adult patients with growth hormone (GH) deficiency may be treated with injections of GH.

HYPOTHYROIDISM

OVERVIEW

- Hypothyroidism is the underproduction of thyroid hormones by the thyroid gland, resulting in decreased whole-body metabolism.
- Most cases of hypothyroidism in the U. S. occur as a result of thyroid surgery and radioactive iodine (RAI) treatment of hyperthyroidism.
- Worldwide, hypothyroidism is common in areas where the soil and water have little natural iodide, causing endemic goiter.
- Other causes of hypothyroidism include autoimmune thyroid destruction; infection of thyroid tissue; congenital absence or hypoplasia of thyroid tissues; neck surgery, irradiation, or trauma; and a wide variety of drugs.
- Women are affected much more frequently than men.
- Myxedema coma is a rare, serious complication of untreated or poorly treated hypothyroidism.

PATIENT-CENTERED COLLABORATIVE CARE

Assessment
- Obtain patient information about:
  1. Activity levels now compared with those a year earlier
  2. Amount of time spent sleeping
  3. Generalized weakness, anorexia, muscle aches, and paresthesias
  4. Constipation
  5. Cold intolerance (use of more blankets at night or sweaters and extra clothing, even in warm weather)
  6. Change in libido
  7. Heavy, prolonged menses or amenorrhea
  8. Impotence and infertility
  9. Current or previous use of drugs, such as lithium, amiodarone, aminoglutethimide, sodium or potassium perchlorate, thiocyanates, or cobalt

10. Medical history, including whether the patient has ever been treated for hyperthyroidism and what specific treatment was used
11. Recent weight gain

- Assessment for and document:
  1. Overall appearance
     a. Coarse features
     b. Edema around the eyes and face
     c. Blank expression
     d. Thick tongue
  2. Slow muscle movement
  3. Slurred or unclear speech
  4. Slow response to questions
  5. Bradycardia
  6. Hypotension
  7. Slow respiratory rate
  8. Low core body temperature
  9. Presence or absence of a goiter

> 🐾 **Clinical Landmine** ◆ A goiter may or may not be present with hypothyroidism and can be present with some types of hyperthyroidism. Therefore, do not use the presence of a goiter to determine whether the thyroid problem is excessive hormone secretion or too little hormone secretion.

- Psychosocial assessment and issues may include:
  1. Depression
  2. Lethargy, apathy, drowsiness
  3. Reduced attention span and memory
- Diagnostic assessment may include:
  1. Blood tests for:
     a. Triiodothyronine (T_3)
     b. Thyroxine (T_4)
     c. Thyroid stimulating hormone (TSH) levels

Interventions

- Drug therapy is the mainstay of management for hypothyroidism.
- The patient requires lifelong thyroid hormone replacement; the most commonly used drug is levothyroxine sodium (Synthroid, T_4, Eltroxin ♦).
  1. Therapy is started with a low dose that is gradually increased over a period of weeks.
  2. The patient with more severe symptoms of hypothyroidism is started on the lowest dose of thyroid hormone replacement, because starting at too high a dose or increasing the

dose too rapidly can cause severe hypertension, heart failure, and myocardial infarction.

   a. Teach patients and the families of patients who are beginning thyroid replacement hormone therapy to take the drug exactly as prescribed and not to change the dose or schedule without consulting the health care provider.

   b. Assess the patient for chest pain and dyspnea during initiation of therapy.

3. The final dosage is determined by blood levels of TSH and the patient's physical responses.

4. Monitor for and teach the patient and family about the manifestations of hyperthyroidism, including:

   a. Tachycardia

   b. Intolerance to heat

   c. Difficulty sleeping

   d. Diarrhea

   e. Excessive weight loss

   f. Fine tremors of the hands

- Management of myxedema coma

   1. Myxedema coma is a severe and life-threatening form of hypothyroidism in which the patient's overall metabolism slows to the point that cardiac and respiratory arrest can occur.

   2. Factors leading to myxedema coma include acute illness, surgery, chemotherapy, discontinuing thyroid replacement therapy, and the use of sedatives or opioids.

   3. Manifestations include:

      a. Coma

      b. Respiratory failure

      c. Hypotension

      d. Hyponatremia

      e. Hypothermia

      f. Hypoglycemia

   4. Untreated myxedema coma leads to shock, organ damage, and death.

   5. Treatment is instituted quickly according to the patient's manifestations and without waiting for laboratory confirmation.

   6. Best practices for emergency care of the patient with myxedema coma are:

      a. Maintaining a patent airway

      b. Replacing fluids with IV normal or hypertonic saline

      c. Giving levothyroxine sodium IV, as prescribed

      d. Giving glucose IV, as prescribed

    e. Giving corticosteroids, as prescribed

    f. Checking the patient's temperature hourly

    g. Monitoring blood pressure hourly

    h. Covering the patient with warm blankets

    i. Monitoring for changes in mental status

    j. Turning every 2 hours

    k. Instituting aspiration precautions

Community-Based Care

- Hypothyroidism is usually a chronic condition, and the patient may live in any type of environment. Ensure that whoever is responsible for overseeing the patient's daily care is aware of the condition and understands its treatment.
- Discuss the need for extra heat or clothing because of cold intolerance.
- The patient who has a decreased attention span may need help from family, friends, or a home care aide with the drug regimen.
- Develop a plan for drug therapy, and be sure that one person is clearly designated as responsible for drug preparation and delivery so that doses are neither missed nor duplicated.
- Teach the patient and family about hormone replacement therapy and it side effects:
  1. Emphasize the need for lifelong drugs.
  2. Review the manifestations of both hyperthyroidism and hypothyroidism.
  3. Teach the patient to wear a medical alert bracelet.
  4. Instruct the patient not to take any OTC drugs because thyroid hormone preparations interact with many other drugs.
  5. Advise the patient to eat a well-balanced diet with adequate fiber and fluid intake to prevent constipation.
  6. Caution patients that the use of fiber supplements may interfere with the absorption of thyroid hormone and to not take these supplements within 4 hours of taking the hormone.
- Teach the family to orient the patient often and to explain everything clearly, simply, and as often as needed.
- Teach the patient to monitor himself or herself for therapy effectiveness by assessing the need for sleep and the frequency of bowel elimination.
  1. When the patient requires more sleep and is constipated, the dose of replacement hormone may need to be increased.
  2. When the patient has difficulty getting to sleep and has more bowel movements than normal for him or her, the dose may need to be decreased.

IMMUNODEFICIENCIES

OVERVIEW

- Immunodeficiency is a failure of the immune system to recognize infectious agents or foreign proteins as a result of a missing or damaged immune component.
- A *primary (congenital) immunodeficiency* is a condition in which one or more parts of the system are not functioning properly from birth.
- A *secondary immunodeficiency* is acquired after birth as the result of viral infection, contact with a toxin, or medical therapy.
- The immunodeficient patient is at increased risk for infection, cancer, and other diseases.
- Types of congenital or primary antibody-mediated immunodeficiencies that adults may have include:
  1. Bruton's Agammaglobulinemia
     a. A classic congenital antibody-mediated immune deficiency that has an X-linked pattern of inheritance.
     b. Boys born with this disease usually start to have problems at about age 6 months with manifestations of recurrent otitis, sinusitis, pneumonia, furunculosis, meningitis, and septicemia.
     c. Laboratory assessment shows an absence of circulating immunoglobulin (antibodies).
     d. The overall prognosis is good if antibody replacement is started early.
     e. Antibiotics are used for specific infections, and long-term prophylactic antibiotic therapy may also be used.
  2. Common variable immune deficiency
     a. Affects men and women
     b. Patients have low levels of circulating antibodies (immunoglobulins) of all classes.
     c. It usually first appears later (in adolescence or young adulthood), and the infections are less severe than those seen in patients with Bruton's agammaglobulinemia.
     d. Common problems include giardiasis (intestinal infection with *Giardia lamblia*), pneumonia, sinusitis, gastric cancer, bronchiectasis, and gallstones.
     e. Management requires regular infusions of immune serum globulin and regular or intermittent use of antibiotics to protect the affected person against infection.
  3. Selective immunoglobulin A (IgA) deficiency
     a. Is the most common congenital immunodeficiency seen in adults

b. May be asymptomatic or have chronic or recurrent upper respiratory tract infections, skin infections, urinary tract infections, vaginal infections, and diarrhea
c. It does not reduce the life span.
d. Management is limited to vigorous treatment of infections.

> **Clinical Landmine ◆** Unlike other immunoglobulin deficiencies, IgA deficiency should never be treated with exogenous immune globulin. Because patients with IgA deficiency make normal amounts of all other antibodies, they are at high risk for severe allergic reactions to exogenous immune globulin.

- Types of iatrogenic or therapy-induced immunodeficiencies include:
  1. Drug-induced immune deficiencies caused by:
     a. Cytotoxic drugs used in the treatment of cancer and autoimmune disorders
     b. Corticosteroids used to treat many autoimmune diseases, neoplasms, and endocrine disorders
     c. Cyclosporine (Sandimmune, Neoral), a specific immunosuppressant that is used to prevent organ transplant rejection and graft-versus-host disease and is occasionally used for other disorders, such as uveitis, rheumatoid arthritis, and other autoimmune disorders
  2. Radiation-induced immunodeficiency when the iliac and femur in adults are exposed to high doses of radiation (these are the blood cell–producing sites of adults)
- Management of treatment-induced immune deficiency aims to improve immune function and protect the patient from infection.
- Usually, treatment-related immunodeficiencies resolve after the suppressive drug or radiation therapy is stopped and the hematopoietic cells recover.
- Teach the patient how to protect himself or herself from infection by:
  1. Avoiding crowds and other large gatherings of people who might be ill
  2. Not sharing personal toilet articles, such as toothbrushes, toothpaste, washcloths, or deodorant sticks, with others
  3. Bathing daily, using an antimicrobial soap, and, if total bathing is not possible, washing the armpits, groin, genitals, and anal area twice daily with an antimicrobial soap

4. Cleaning the toothbrush daily by running it through the dishwasher or rinsing it in liquid laundry bleach
5. Washing hands thoroughly with an antimicrobial soap before eating or drinking, after touching a pet, after shaking hands with anyone, returning home from any outing, and after using the toilet
6. Washing dishes between uses with hot, sudsy water, or using a dishwasher
7. Not drinking water, milk, juice, or other cold liquids that have been standing for longer than an hour
8. Not reusing cups and glasses without washing
9. Not changing pet litter boxes or, if unavoidable, using gloves and washing hands immediately
10. Avoiding turtles and reptiles as pets
11. Not feeding pets raw or undercooked meat
12. Avoiding salads; raw fruit and vegetables; undercooked meat, fish, or eggs; pepper; and paprika
13. Thoroughly washing fruit and vegetables
14. Refrigerating perishable foods

INCONTINENCE, URINARY

OVERVIEW

- Urinary incontinence (UI) is the involuntary loss of urine that is severe enough to cause social or hygienic problems. It may be transient or permanent. It is *not* a normal change associated with aging.
- Common forms of urinary incontinence (UI)
  1. Stress incontinence is the loss of small amounts of urine during coughing, sneezing, jogging, or lifting. Patients are unable to tighten the urethra sufficiently to overcome the increased detrusor pressure, and leakage of urine results.
  2. Urge urinary incontinence (UI) is the involuntary loss of urine associated with a sudden, strong desire to urinate. Patients are unable to suppress the signal for bladder contractions. It is also known as *overactive bladder*.
  3. Mixed incontinence is a combination of stress and urge incontinence.
  4. Reflex incontinence occurs when the bladder has reached a specific bladder volume. There is a decreased or absent ability to sense a full bladder, usually from neurologic impairment or bladder damage.
  5. Functional incontinence is leakage of urine caused by factors other than pathology of the lower urinary tract, such as impaired cognition, impaired vision, or inability to reach a toilet.

- In adult patients younger than 65 years, incontinence occurs twice as often in women than in men.

PATIENT-CENTERED COLLABORATIVE CARE

Assessment

- Obtain patient information:
  1. Presence and severity of incontinence with effective screening questions. Ask the patient to respond with *always*, *sometimes*, or *never* to the following questions:
     a. Do you ever leak urine when you do not want to?
     b. Do you ever leak urine or water when you cough, laugh, or exercise?
     c. Do you ever leak urine on the way to the bathroom?
     d. Do you ever use pads, tissue, or cloth in your underwear to catch urine?
  2. Risk factors for urinary incontinence (UI)
     a. Age
     b. Menopausal status
     c. Disease that may affect the autonomic nervous system or cognition, such as:
        (1) Parkinson disease
        (2) Dementia
        (3) Multiple sclerosis
        (4) Stroke
        (5) Neurogenic complications from diabetes mellitus
     d. Childbirth
     e. Urologic procedures
     f. Spinal cord injuries
     g. Drugs, especially drugs that affect the autonomic nervous system
     h. Bowel pattern
     i. Stress or anxiety level
  3. Limited mobility, reduced ability to ambulate and to transfer to a chair or toilet
  4. Reduced cognitive awareness
  5. Communication pattern
  6. Barriers to toileting
     a. Privacy
     b. Restrictive clothing
     c. Access to toilet
  7. Presence of urinary tract infection (cystitis)
     a. Assess for and document the findings:
        (1) Palpate the abdominal area for evidence of bladder fullness.

(2) Percuss the abdomen, and listen for the dull sound of a distended bladder.

(3) Observe for urine leakage while the patient strains by coughing or bearing down in the standing position.

(4) With a physician's order, determine the amount of residual urine by portable ultrasound or by catheterizing the patient immediately after voiding.

(5) Inspect the external genitalia of women to determine urethral or uterine prolapse, cystocele, or rectocele.

(6) Describe any secretions from the genitourinary openings.

(7) Inspect the urinary meatus of men for the presence of discharge or other characteristics.

(8) Query the patient regarding the effects of incontinence on socialization, family relationships, and emotional status.

(9) Monitor the urine for color, odor, and presence of sediment or cloudiness, and monitor the results of a urinalysis.

(10) Review the results of the voiding cystourethrogram, which detects the anatomic structure and function of the bladder, as well as the postvoiding residual.

Planning and Implementation

❖**NDx:** Stress Urinary Incontinence (UI)

Nonsurgical Management

- Nonsurgical management of incontinence may include:
  1. Drug therapy to reduce urgency and frequency
     a. Phenylpropanolamine, an alpha-adrenergic agonist
     b. Tricyclic antidepressants: imipramine (Tofranil, Novo-Pramine)
     c. Estrogen for postmenopausal women
     d. Tolterodine, an anticholinergic
  2. Dietary counseling to assist the obese patient with weight loss and to encourage all patients to avoid alcohol and caffeine (bladder stimulants)
     a. Collaborate with the nutritionist.
  3. Exercise therapy
     a. Teach women how to do Kegel exercises to strengthen the muscles of the pelvic floor; biofeedback devices may be used to help the patient detect the effectiveness of the exercises.
     b. Instruct the patient in the correct use of vaginal cones.
        (1) The lightest cone is inserted into the vagina with the string to the outside for a 1-minute test period.

(2) If the patient is able to hold the first cone in place without its slipping out while she walks around, she proceeds to the second cone and repeats the procedure.

(3) Treatment is begun with the heaviest cone that the patient can hold in her vagina for the 1-minute test period.

(4) The treatment is for 15 minutes twice daily; when the patient can hold the cone comfortably in her vagina for 15 minutes, proceed to the next heaviest weight.

4. Other treatments include behavior modification, psychotherapy, and electrical devices for the inhibition of bladder contraction.

   a. The Reliance insert is a tampon-like device inserted into the urethra. The patient inflates the attached balloon, which prevents urine flow.

Surgical Management

- Provide preoperative care as described earlier.
- Operative procedures for women are used to elevate the bladder and urethra into a normal intra-abdominal position, increase the length of the urethra, and decrease hypermobility of the bladder neck.

   1. Anterior vaginal repair (colporrhaphy) to elevate the urethra and repair any cystocele

   2. Retropubic suspension to elevate the urethra and provide longer-lasting results

   3. Needle bladder neck suspension (Pereyra or Stamey procedure) to elevate the urethra and provide a longer-lasting result without a long operative time

   4. Pubovaginal sling procedure, in which a sling made of synthetic material is placed under the urethrovesical junction to elevate the bladder neck

   5. An artificial sphincter, a mechanical device that opens and closes the urethra, placed around the anatomic urethra; the procedure is used for men more often than for women.

- Provide postoperative care as described earlier, and take the following steps:

   1. Secure the urethral catheter to prevent unnecessary movement or traction on the bladder neck.

   2. Monitor the suprapubic catheter, if present, for leakage of urine and serosanguineous drainage.

❖**NDx:** Urge Urinary Incontinence (UI)

- Interventions for urge urinary incontinence (UI) include drug and behavioral interventions such as bladder and habit training. Surgery is not recommended.

1. Drug therapy includes:
   a. Anticholinergic agents and anticholinergics with smooth muscle relaxant properties
   b. Tricyclic antidepressants
2. Diet therapy includes:
   a. Instructing the patient to avoid foods that have a bladder-stimulating effect, such as caffeine and alcohol
   b. Instructing the patient to space fluids throughout the day and to limit fluids after dinner
3. Bladder training is an educational program to help patients gain control of their bladder.
   a. A regular schedule of voiding is established.
   b. The patient is instructed to void during the established time frame and to ignore any urge to urinate that occurs between the mandated interval.
   c. After the patient is comfortable with the initial interval, the interval time is increased by 15 to 30 minutes.
4. Habit training is a variation of bladder training that is useful for cognitively impaired patients. The caregiver assists the patient to void every 2 hours.
5. Exercise therapies, such as Kegel exercises and vaginal cone therapy, are also useful.
6. Electrical stimulation with a variety of intravaginal and intra-rectal devices has been used to treat both stress and urge urinary incontinence (UI).

❖**NDx and Collaborative Problem:** Reflex Urinary Incontinence (UI)

- Interventions for reflex incontinence include surgery, drugs, and teaching the patient interventions to empty the bladder.
  1. Surgery, which includes removal of the prostate and repair of genital prolapse to relieve the obstruction of the bladder outlet.
  2. Drug therapy includes bethanechol chloride for the short-term management of urinary retention.
  3. Interventions can assist with bladder emptying:
     a. Using or teaching the Credé maneuver, Valsalva maneuver, or double-voiding technique to assist in promoting bladder contraction
     b. Teaching intermittent self-catheterization to patients with long-term problems of incomplete bladder emptying

❖**NDx:** Functional Urinary Incontinence (UI)

- The primary focus of the intervention is to treat reversible causes of incontinence. When that is not possible, the goal is to contain the urine and protect the patient's skin. Interventions include:

1. Altering the environment so the patient can reach the toilet easily
2. Implementing habit training for the cognitively impaired patient
3. Using absorbent pads and briefs to collect urine and keep the patient's skin and clothing dry
4. Using an external catheter for men or any patient, inserting a Foley catheter, or implementing intermittent catheterization, especially when perineal skin impairment is present

> **Critical Rescue** ♦ Assessing the patient's risk for incontinence while he or she is hospitalized is an essential step in preventing iatrogenic skin damage and preventing pressure ulcer formation.

Community-Based Care
- Discharge planning includes:
    1. Assessing the home environment for barriers that impede access to the toileting facilities
    2. Considering the personal, physical, emotional, and social resources of the patient
    3. Considering who the primary caretaker will be and what circumstances or factors exist in the environment that will influence the effectiveness of the plan
    4. Assisting the patient to control or manage fears and anxieties related to incontinence while in public
    5. Referring the patient to home care agencies
- Teach the patient and family about:
    1. The causes of incontinence and treatment options available
    2. Prescribed drugs (purpose, dosage, method, route of administration, and expected and potential side effects)
    3. The importance of weight reduction and dietary modification
    4. Options available for external devices or incontinence pads, considering the patient's lifestyle and resources
    5. The technique of self-catheterization, ensuring that a return demonstration is correct

IRRITABLE BOWEL SYNDROME

OVERVIEW

- Irritable bowel syndrome (IBS) is a functional GI disorder characterized by chronic or recurrent diarrhea, constipation, and abdominal pain and bloating.

- No pathologic changes in the GI mucosa occur.
- The disease is thought to result from impairment in the motor or sensory function of the GI tract.
- The disease exacerbates ("flares up") whenever the patient is exposed to causative agents. Factors such as diet, stress, and anxiety may precipitate exacerbations.
- Twice as many women as men are affected by IBS.

PATIENT-CENTERED COLLABORATIVE CARE

Assessment

- Obtain patient information about symptoms collectively known as the Manning criteria:
  1. Abdominal pain relieved by defecation or falling asleep
  2. Abdominal pain associated with changes in stool frequency or consistency
  3. Abdominal distention
  4. The sensation of incomplete evacuation of stool
  5. The presence of mucus with stool passage
- Assess for and document:
  1. Pain in the lower left quadrant of the abdomen that increases after eating and is relieved by a bowel movement
  2. Nausea associated with mealtime and defecation
  3. Diarrhea or constipation
  4. Belching, gas, anorexia, and bloating
  5. Bowel sounds
  6. Weight
  7. Nutritional status

Interventions

- Diet therapy includes:
  1. Suggesting a symptom diary to help identify triggers and bowel habits
  2. Helping the patient identify and eliminate foods associated with exacerbations
  3. Advising the patient to limit caffeine and avoid alcohol and beverages that contain sorbitol or fructose and advising avoidance of milk and milk products if lactose intolerance is suspected
  4. Consulting with the nutritionist
  5. Teaching the patient to ingest 30 to 40 g of fiber daily
  6. Teaching the patient to drink 8 to 10 cups of liquid per day
- Drug therapy includes:
  1. Bulk-forming laxatives, such as psyllium hydrophilic mucilloid (Metamucil), taken at mealtimes with a glass of water to prevent dry, hard, or liquid stools

2. Antidiarrheal agents to decrease cramping and frequency of stools
3. Muscarinic-3 blocking agents (anticholinergic drugs specific to GI receptors)
4. Serotonin (5-HT4) drugs for women with constipation-predominant IBS
5. Tricyclic antidepressants for pain associated with IBS (These drugs have anticholinergic properties and pain relief effects.)
- Stress management includes:
  1. Assisting the patient to learn relaxation techniques
  2. Encouraging the patient to implement a regular exercise program to promote bowel elimination and reduce stress
  3. Personal counseling
- Complementary and alternative therapies include peppermint oil, ginger, aloe, yoga, and acupuncture.

KIDNEY DISEASE, POLYCYSTIC

OVERVIEW

- Polycystic kidney disease (PKD) is an inherited kidney disorder in which fluid-filled cysts develop in nephrons.
- Growing cysts damage the glomerular and tubular membranes, reducing nephron and kidney function.
- The kidney tissue is eventually replaced by nonfunctioning cysts; each cystic kidney may enlarge to two to three times its normal size, causing discomfort and abdominal organ displacement. The fluid-filled cysts are at increased risk for infection, rupture, and bleeding.
- Most patients with PKD have high blood pressure and heart problems.
- Cysts may occur in other tissues, such as the liver or blood vessels.

PATIENT-CENTERED COLLABORATIVE CARE

Assessment

- Obtain patient information about:
  1. Genetic status, because PKD can be autosomal dominant (most common form of PKD with several different subtypes) or autosomal recessive (which is more severe, with death typically occurring in early childhood)
  2. Current health status
  3. Family history of PKD

4. Age of parent at diagnosis of PKD and any related complications
5. Family history of sudden death from a stroke
6. History of constipation
7. Changes in urine or frequency of urination
8. High blood pressure
9. History of headaches

- Assess for and document:
  1. Pain (flank or abdominal)
  2. Distended abdomen
  3. Enlarged, tender kidney on palpation
  4. Hematuria or cloudy urine
  5. Dysuria
  6. Nocturia
  7. Hypertension
  8. Edema
  9. Uremic symptoms: nausea, vomiting, pruritus, and fatigue
  10. Anger, resentment, futility, sadness, or anxiety related to chronicity or inheritable condition

- Diagnostic studies may include:
  1. Urinalysis with proteinuria and hematuria
  2. Urine culture and sensitivity if infection is suspected
  3. Serum creatinine and blood urea nitrogen (BUN) to assess kidney function
  4. Renal sonography, CT scan, or MRI to assess presence and size of cysts

Interventions

- Control pain.
  1. Provide drug therapy:
     a. Administer analgesics for comfort; use NSAIDs cautiously, and avoid aspirin-containing products.
     b. Administer antibiotics such as trimethoprim/sulfamethoxazole (Bactrim, Septra, Trimpex) or ciprofloxacin (Cipro) if a cyst infection is causing discomfort.
  2. Provide other interventions:
     a. Apply dry heat to the abdomen or flank.
     b. Teach relaxation or distraction techniques to self-manage pain and discomfort.

- Prevent constipation:
  1. Nutrition management
  2. Regular exercise
  3. Fluid management
  4. Appropriate use of stool softeners and bulk agents and careful use of laxatives

- Provide hypertension and kidney failure management:
  1. Administer antihypertensive agents, including angiotensin-converting enzyme (ACE) inhibitors, vasodilators, beta blockers, and calcium channel blockers, as ordered.
  2. Administer diuretics, as ordered, for patients with renal insufficiency.
  3. Monitor daily weight.
  4. Provide a low-sodium diet unless the patient has a salt-wasting condition.
  5. Maintain protein restriction if kidney injury progresses.
  6. Provide counseling, support, and teaching about health maintenance to promote self-management (see Hypertension Chronic Kidney Failure).
  7. Encourage the patient to verbalize feelings or frustrations and identify successful coping strategies.
- Teach the patient and family:
  1. How to measure and monitor blood pressure and weight
  2. Diet considerations to promote health; salt, protein, and fiber intake may need special attention or nutritionist consultation
  3. Self-administration of drugs and potential adverse effects of prescribed drugs, including antihypertensive drugs and diuretics
  4. Measures and their rationale for preventing constipation
  5. Resources that are available for research and education, such as the Polycystic Kidney Research Foundation and the National Kidney and Urologic Disease division of the National Institutes of Health

KIDNEY INJURY, ACUTE (ACUTE KIDNEY FAILURE)

OVERVIEW

- Acute kidney injury (AKI), formerly known as acute renal failure, is a rapid decrease in kidney function leading to the accumulation of metabolic wastes in the body.
- AKI can result from conditions that reduce blood flow to the kidneys (prerenal failure); damage to the glomeruli, interstitial tissue, or tubules (intrarenal or intrinsic renal failure); or obstruction of urine flow (postrenal failure).
- AKI is characterized by oliguria. A diuretic phase may follow oliguria; the diuretic phase may include output of up to 10L/day. Some patients may have a nonoliguric form of AKI.

- AKI is classified by the extent of changes in serum creatinine, decreases in urine output, and persistence of symptoms. There are five classes, ranging from risk to end-stage disease:

Risk, Injury, Failure, Loss, and End-Stage Kidney (RIFLE) Classification

Class	Glomerular Filtration Rate Criteria	Urine Output Criteria
Risk	Serum creatinine × 1.5	<0.5 mL/kg/hr × 6 hr
Injury	Serum creatinine × 2	<0.5 mL/kg/hr × 12 hr
Failure	Serum creatinine × 3 or serum creatinine ≥ 4 mg/dL with an acute rise > 0.5 mg/dL	<0.3 mL/kg/hr × 24 hr or anuria × 12 hr
Loss	Persistent acute renal failure: complete loss of kidney function > 4 wk	
End-stage kidney disease	Loss of kidney function > 3 months	

PATIENT-CENTERED COLLABORATIVE CARE

Assessment

- Obtain patient information about:
  1. Exposure to nephrotoxins, including:
     a. Contrast dye used in imaging procedures
     b. Drugs, especially antibiotics, angiotensin-converting enzyme inhibitors, and NSAIDs
  2. Recent surgery or trauma
  3. Transfusions
  4. History of diseases that impair kidney function such as diabetes mellitus, systemic lupus erythematosus, and hypertension
  5. History of acute illnesses, including influenza, colds, gastroenteritis, and sore throat or pharyngitis
  6. History of intravascular volume depletion
  7. History of urinary obstructive disease, such as prostatic hypertrophy or kidney stones
- Assess for and document:
  1. Hypotension
  2. Tachycardia
  3. Decreased or absent urine output
  4. Decreased cardiac output
  5. Decreased or increased central venous pressure
  6. Lethargy

   7. Peripheral edema
   8. Electrocardiographic (ECG) changes indicating electrolyte abnormalities
   9. Shortness of breath
   10. Rales or crackles
   11. Nausea and vomiting
   12. Anorexia
   13. Flank pain
- Diagnostic studies may include:
   1. Urinalysis
   2. Urine and serum electrolytes, creatinine, and BUN
   3. Abdominal or pelvic x-ray to assess the size of the kidneys and CT without contrast dye to identify obstruction
   4. Renal biopsy to determine uncertain cause of AKI or if immunologic disease is suspected

Interventions
- Monitor fluid and electrolyte status. The patient may move from the oliguric phase (fluids and electrolytes are retained) to the diuretic phase, in which hypovolemia and electrolyte loss are the main problems.
- The patient with AKI receives multiple drugs.
   1. As kidney function changes, drug dosages are modified.
   2. Monitor for drug side effects and interactions.
- Fluid challenges and diuretics are commonly used to promote renal perfusion.
   1. Monitor for fluid overload.
- A low-dose dopamine infusion may be used to promote renal perfusion although the drug is no longer recommended for this purpose.
- Hypercatabolism during illness, surgery, or trauma results in the breakdown of muscle for protein, which leads to increased azotemia. Patients require increased calories. Total parenteral nutrition with intralipid infusion may be required to reduce catabolism if the patient is unable to tolerate oral or enteral feeding.
- Indications for hemodialysis or peritoneal dialysis in patients with AKI are symptomatic of uremia, persistent hyperkalemia, uncompensated metabolic acidosis, excess fluid volume, uremic pericarditis, and uremic encephalopathy (see Kidney Failure, Chronic, for a discussion of dialysis).
- Continuous hemofiltration, an alternative to dialysis, may be used in the intensive care unit (ICU).

Community-Based Care
- The needs of the patient depend on the status of the disease on discharge (see Community-Based Care under Kidney Failure, Chronic).

- Follow-up care may include medical visits, laboratory tests, consultation with a nutritionist, temporary dialysis, home nursing care, and social work assistance.

KIDNEY DISEASE, CHRONIC

OVERVIEW

- Chronic kidney failure (CKD) is a progressive, irreversible kidney injury; kidney function does not recover.
- The progression toward CKD occurs in three stages:
  1. Stage 1: reduced renal reserve
     a. There is a 30% to 50% reduction in renal functioning without accumulation of metabolic wastes.
     b. The unaffected nephrons may compensate for the diseased nephrons.
  2. Stage 2: renal insufficiency
     a. Metabolic wastes begin to accumulate in the blood because the unaffected nephrons no longer compensate.
     b. Levels of blood urea nitrogen (BUN), serum creatinine, uric acid, and phosphorus are elevated in proportion to the amount of nephrons lost.
  3. Stage 3: end-stage kidney disease (ESKD)
     a. ESKD occurs when excessive amounts of urea and creatinine accumulate in the blood.
     b. The kidneys are unable to maintain homeostasis and require dialysis.
- Pathologic alterations include disruptions in the glomerular filtration rate (GFR), abnormal urine production, poor water excretion, electrolyte imbalance, and metabolic anomalies.
- When less than 20% of nephrons are functional, hyposthenuria (loss of urine concentrating ability) and polyuria occur; left untreated, severe dehydration occurs.
- Urea is the primary product of protein metabolism and is normally excreted by the kidney; BUN varies with dietary intake of protein.
- Creatinine is derived from creatine and phosphocreatine; the normal rate of excretion depends on muscle mass, physical activity, and diet.
- Azotemia is increased accumulation of nitrogenous waste (BUN) in the blood and is a classic indicator of kidney failure.
- Variations in sodium excretion occur and depend on the stage of CKD.
  1. There is increased risk for hyponatremia, or sodium depletion, in early CKD.

2. Hyponatremia occurs because the reduced number of functional nephrons is insufficient to reabsorb sodium, and sodium is lost in the urine.
- Hyperkalemia results from an increase in potassium load, including ingestion of potassium in drugs, failure to restrict potassium in the diet, blood transfusions, and excess bleeding.
- Other metabolic derangements in CKD include changes in pH (metabolic acidosis), calcium (hypocalcemia) and phosphorus (hyperphosphatemia) imbalances, and vitamin D insufficiency.
  1. Renal osteodystrophy caused by hypocalcemia and phosphorus retention results in skeletal demineralization manifested by bone pain, pseudofractures, sclerosis of the spine, skull demineralization, osteomalacia, reabsorption of bone, and loss of tooth lamina.
- Cardiovascular alterations include anemia, hypertension, hyperlipidemia, heart failure, and pericarditis.
- GI alterations include uremic stomatitis, anorexia, peptic ulcer disease, nausea, and vomiting.

PATIENT-CENTERED COLLABORATIVE CARE

Assessment

- Obtain patient information about:
  1. Age and gender
  2. Height and weight, including recent weight gain or loss
  3. Current and past medical conditions
  4. Drugs, prescription and nonprescription
  5. Family history of kidney disease
  6. Dietary and nutritional habits, including food preferences
  7. History of GI problems, such as nausea, vomiting, anorexia, diarrhea, or constipation
  8. Current energy level
  9. Recent injuries and abnormal bruising or bleeding
  10. Weakness and fatigue and related changes in daily routine
  11. Shortness of breath
  12. Detailed urinary elimination history
- Assess for and document:
  1. Neurologic manifestations of CKD
     a. Changes in mentation or new lethargy
     b. Changes in sensation or weakness in extremities indicating uremic neuropathy
  2. Cardiovascular manifestations of CKD from fluid overload, hypertension, or cardiac disease

    a. Systolic blood pressure (SBP) higher than 130 mm Hg or diastolic blood pressure (DBP) higher than 80 mm Hg (lower tolerance for elevations in blood pressure with CKD)

    b. Cardiomyopathy

    c. Uremic pericarditis

    d. Peripheral edema

    e. Heart failure

    f. Pericardial friction rub or effusion

3. Respiratory manifestations

    a. Breath that smells like urine (uremic fetor or halitosis)

    b. Deep sighing or yawning

    c. Tachypnea or shortness of breath

    d. Pulmonary edema or pleural effusion

    e. Kussmaul's respiration with acidemia

    f. Uremic lung or hilar pneumonitis

4. Hematologic manifestations of CKD

    a. Anemia

    b. Abnormal bleeding: bruising petechiae, abnormal vaginal bleeding, GI bleeding

5. GI disruptions

    a. Mouth ulceration

    b. Abdominal pain or cramping

    c. Nausea or vomiting

6. Urinary findings

    a. Change in urinary amount, frequency, and appearance of urine

    b. Proteinuria or hematuria

7. Integumentary or dermatologic manifestations

    a. Yellow coloration from pigment deposition; darkening of skin for some African Americans

    b. Severe itching (pruritus)

    c. Uremic frost: layer of uremic crystals from evaporated sweat on the face, eyebrows, axilla, and groin (rare)

    d. Bruises or purple patches and rashes

8. Immunologic considerations: increased susceptibility to infections

- Diagnostic testing may include:
  1. Serum creatinine, BUN, sodium, potassium, calcium, phosphorus, bicarbonate, hemoglobin, and hematocrit
  2. Urinalysis
  3. A 24-hour urinanalysis for creatinine and creatine clearance
  4. Ultrasound, CT scan, or x-ray to observe progression, which manifests as small and fibrotic kidneys

K

Planning and Implementation

❖**NDx:** Imbalanced Nutrition, Less Than Body Requirements

- The goal is to provide food and fluids to prevent malnutrition.
- The nutritional need and diet restrictions for the patient with CKD vary according to the degree of remaining renal function and the type of renal replacement therapy used.
- Common changes include control of protein intake; fluid intake limitation; restriction of potassium, sodium, and phosphorus intake; taking vitamin and mineral supplements; and eating enough calories to meet metabolic demand.
- Consult with the nutritionist to provide nutritional teaching and planning and to assist the patient in adapting the diet to food preferences, ethnic background, and budget.

❖**NDx:** Excess Fluid Volume

- The goal is to achieve and maintain acceptable fluid balance. Indicators include:
  1. Blood pressure
  2. Heart rate
  3. Body weight
  4. Central venous pressure
  5. Serum electrolyte
- Diuretic drugs may be used in patients with stage 1 or 2 CKD.

❖**NDx:** Decreased Cardiac Output

- The goal is to attain and maintain adequate cardiac output. Indicators include:
  1. Systolic and diastolic blood pressures
  2. Ejection fraction
  3. Peripheral pulses
  4. Cognitive status
- Interventions include:
  1. Administering calcium channel blockers, angiotensin-converting enzyme (ACE) inhibitors, alpha- and beta-adrenergic blockers, and vasodilators
  2. Teaching the family to measure the patient's blood pressure and weight daily and to bring these records when visiting the physician, nurse, or nutritionist
  3. Monitoring the patient for decreased cardiac output, heart failure, congestive heart failure, and dysrhythmias

❖**NDx:** Risk for Infection

- The goals are to prevent infection and detect infection early by monitoring for:
  1. Fever
  2. Lymph node enlargement

3. Positive urine or other culture
4. Tenderness, redness or drainage at dialysis access site
5. WBC count

❖**NDx:** Risk for Injury

- The goals are to prevent the following problems: falls, pathologic fractures, bleeding, and toxic effects of prescribed drugs. Interventions include:

1. Monitoring the patient closely for drug-related complications
2. Teaching the patient to avoid certain drugs that can increase kidney damage, such as NSAIDs, antibiotics, antihypertensives, and diuretics in the presence of hypovolemia
3. Anticipating dosage adjustment as kidney function decreases
4. Administering agents to control phosphorus excess, such as calcium acetate, calcium carbonate, and aluminum hydroxide
5. Instructing the patient to avoid compounds containing magnesium
6. Administering opioid analgesics cautiously because the effects may last longer and uremic patients are sensitive to the respiratory depressant effects

❖**NDx:** Fatigue

- The goal is to conserve energy and ability to perform self-care, retain interest in surroundings, and sustain mental concentration. Interventions include:

1. Providing vitamin and mineral supplementation
2. Administering erythropoietin and iron supplements to maintain a hematocrit of 28%
3. Monitoring dietary intake; improved appetite challenges patients in their attempts to maintain protein, potassium, and fluid restriction

❖**NDx:** Anxiety

- The goal is to reduce feelings of apprehension and tension. Interventions include:

1. Observing the patient's behavior for signs of anxiety
2. Evaluating the patient's support system
3. Explaining all procedures, tests, and treatments
4. Providing instruction on kidney function and kidney failure
5. Encouraging the patient to discuss current problems, fears, or concerns and to ask questions
6. Facilitating discussion with family members concerning the patient's prognosis and potential impacts on the patient's lifestyle

❖**NDx:** Potential for Pulmonary Edema
- The goal is to remain free of pulmonary edema and maintain optimal fluid balance.
- Interventions include:
  1. Assessing for early signs of pulmonary edema such as restlessness, dyspnea, and crackles
  2. If dyspneic, placing the patient in a high Fowler position and giving oxygen to maximize lung expansion and improve gas exchange
  3. Measuring and recording intake and output
  4. Assessing cardiovascular system for fluid overload: S_3, peripheral edema, jugular venous distention, tachycardia, hypotension, or hypertension
  5. Monitoring serum chemistry results for electrolyte imbalance
  6. Monitoring peripheral oxygenation (Spo_2)
  7. Providing drug therapy
     a. Loop diuretics for stage 1 or 2 CKD; monitor for ototoxicity
     b. Morphine sulfate to reduce myocardial oxygen demands; monitor for respiratory depression
     c. Vasodilators such as nitroglycerin

❖**Collaborative Problem:** Renal Replacement Therapy
- Renal replacement therapy is required when the clinical and laboratory manifestations of kidney failure present complications that are potentially life threatening or that pose continuing discomfort to the patient.
- Hemodialysis removes excess fluid and waste products and restores chemical and electrolyte balance. It is based on the principle of diffusion, in which the patient's blood is circulated through a semipermeable membrane that acts as an artificial kidney.
  1. Dialysis settings include the acute care facility, freestanding centers, and the home.
  2. Total dialysis time is usually 12 hours per week, which usually is divided into three 4-hour treatments.
  3. Vascular access route is needed to perform hemodialysis.
  4. Long-term vascular access for hemodialysis is accomplished by:
     a. Arteriovenous (AV) fistula
     b. AV graft
  5. Complications of vascular access include:
     a. Thrombosis or stenosis
     b. Infection
     c. Ischemia
     d. Aneurysm formation

- Temporary vascular access for hemodialysis is accomplished by a specially designed catheter inserted into the subclavian, internal jugular, or femoral vein.
- Nurses are specially trained to perform hemodialysis.
- Postdialysis care includes:
  1. Closely monitoring for side effects: hypotension, headache, nausea, malaise, vomiting, dizziness, and muscle cramps
  2. Obtaining the patient's weight and vital signs
  3. Avoiding invasive procedures for 4 to 6 hours because of heparinization of the dialysate
  4. Monitoring for signs of bleeding
  5. Monitoring laboratory results
- Complications of hemodialysis include:
  1. Dialysis disequilibrium
  2. Infectious disease
  3. Hepatitis infection
  4. Human immunodeficiency virus (HIV) infection

Considerations for Older Adults

- ESKD occurs most often in people between 65 and 69 years old.
- Patients older than 65 years who are receiving dialysis are more at risk than younger patients for dialysis-induced hypotension. Older adults require more frequent monitoring during and after dialysis.
- Peritoneal dialysis (PD), an alternative and slower dialysis method, is accomplished by the surgical insertion of a silicone rubber catheter (Tenckhoff catheter) into the abdominal cavity to instill dialysis solution into the abdominal cavity.
- Candidates for PD include:
  1. Patients who are unable to tolerate anticoagulation
  2. Patients who lack vascular access
  3. Patients without peritoneal adhesions and without extensive abdominal surgery
- The PD process occurs by means of a transfer of fluid and solutes from the bloodstream through the peritoneum.
- The types of PD include intermittent, continuous ambulatory (CAPD), automated, and others; the type is selected based on patient ability and lifestyle.
- Complications of PD include:
  1. Peritonitis
  2. Pain
  3. Poor dialysate flow
  4. Leakage of the dialysate
  5. Exit site and tunnel infection

- Nursing interventions include:
  1. Implementing and monitoring PD therapy and instilling, dwelling, and draining the solution, as ordered
  2. Maintaining PD flow data and monitoring for negative or positive fluid balances
  3. Obtaining baseline and daily weights
  4. Monitoring laboratory results to measure the effectiveness of the treatment
  5. Maintaining accurate intake and output records
  6. Taking vital signs every 15 to 30 minutes during initiation of PD
  7. Performing an ongoing assessment for signs of respiratory distress or pain
- Kidney transplantation is appropriate for selected patients with ESKD (see Transplantation).

Community-Based Care

- The case manager helps in planning, coordination, and evaluation of care.
  1. The physical and occupational therapist collaborates with the patient and family to evaluate the home environment and to obtain needed equipment before discharge.
  2. Refer the patient to home health nursing as needed.
- Provide in-depth health teaching about diet and pathophysiology of kidney disease and drug therapy.
  1. Provide information and emotional support to assist the patient with decisions about treatment course, personal lifestyle, support systems, and coping.
  2. Teach the patient about the hemodialysis treatment.
  3. Teach the patient about care of the vascular access.
  4. Provide patients with home based renal replacement therapy with extensive teaching and assist the patient to obtain the needed equipment and supplies. Emphasize the importance of strict sterile technique and of reporting manifestations of infection at any dialysis access site.
  5. Assist the patient and family to identify coping strategies to adjust to the diagnosis and treatment regimen.
  6. Instruct patients and family members in all aspects of diet therapy, drug therapy, and complications. Assist patient to schedule drugs so that drugs will not be unintentionally eliminated by dialysis.
  7. Teach patients and family members to report complications, such as fluid overload, bleeding, and infection.
  8. Stress that although uremic symptoms are reduced as a result of dialysis procedures, the patient will not return completely to his or her previous state of well-being.

9. Instruct the family to monitor the patient for any behaviors that may contribute to nonadherence to the treatment plan and to report such to the health care provider.
10. Refer the patient to a home health nurse and to local and state support groups and agencies such as the National Kidney Foundation.

LABYRINTHITIS

- Labyrinthitis is an infection of the labyrinth of the inner ear.
- Causes include complications of acute or chronic otitis media, cholesteatoma, complication of middle ear or inner ear surgery, and aftermath of an upper respiratory infection or mononucleosis.
- Manifestations include hearing loss, tinnitus, nystagmus on the affected side, and vertigo with nausea and vomiting.
- The most common complication is meningitis.
- Management includes:
  1. Systemic antibiotic therapy
  2. Bedrest in a darkened room
  3. Antiemetics
  4. Antivertiginous drugs
  5. Psychosocial support for persistent balance problems and possible hearing loss
  6. Gait training and physical therapy for persistent balance problems

LACERATIONS, EYE

- Lacerations are wounds caused by sharp objects and projectiles.
- The most commonly injured areas involved in eye lacerations are the eyelids and the cornea.
  1. Eyelid lacerations
     a. Bleed heavily and look more severe than they are
     b. Are managed by closing the eye and applying a small icepack, checking visual acuity, and cleaning and suturing the eyelid
     c. Lacerations that involve the eyelid margin, affect the lacrimal system, involve a large area, or have jagged edges should be managed by an ophthalmologist.
  2. Corneal lacerations
     a. Are an emergency because eye contents may prolapse through the laceration

b. Manifestations include severe eye pain, photophobia, tearing, decreased visual acuity, and inability to open the eyelid.

> 🔖 Clinical Landmine ◆ If an object is seen protruding from the eye, do not remove it. The object should be removed only by the ophthalmologist, because it may be holding eye structures in place.

c. Management includes surgical repair and antibiotic therapy.
d. If scarring alters vision, a corneal transplant may be needed.
e. If the eye contents have prolapsed through the laceration or if the injury is severe, *enucleation* (surgical eye removal) may be needed.

LEIOMYOMAS (UTERINE FIBROIDS)

OVERVIEW

- Uterine *leiomyomas*, also called *myomas* and *fibroids* (fibroid tumors) are the most commonly occurring benign pelvic tumors.
- Leiomyomas develop from the uterine myometrium. They may grow within the myometrium or become attached to it by a pedicle or stalk.
- These tumors are classified according to their position in the layers of the uterus and anatomic position.
- The most common types are:
  1. *Intramural tumors*, contained in the uterine wall in the myometrium
  2. *Submucosal tumors*, protrude into the cavity of the uterus
  3. *Subserosal tumors*, protrude through the outer uterine surface and may extend into the broad ligament

PATIENT-CENTERED COLLABORATIVE CARE

Assessment

- Assessment findings include:
  1. Abnormal uterine bleeding
  2. Reports of a feeling of pelvic pressure
  3. Constipation
  4. Urinary frequency or retention
  5. Increased abdominal size
  6. Dyspareunia (painful intercourse)

7. Infertility
8. Abdominal pain occurring with torsion of the fibroid or pedicle
9. Uterine enlargement on abdominal, vaginal, or rectal examination

Planning and Implementation

❖**Collaborative Problem:** Potential for Hemorrhage

Nonsurgical Management

- The patient who has no symptoms or who desires childbearing is observed and examined for changes in the size of the leiomyoma every 4 to 6 months.
- Many fibroids spontaneously shrink after menopause and require no treatment.
- Mild leiomyoma symptoms can be managed with NSAIDs, hormonal contraceptives, or a levonorgestrel IUD.
- Artificial menopause and fibroid shrinkage can be induced with agonists to gonadotropin-releasing hormone (GnRH).
- MRI focused ultrasound pulsed into the uterus can destroy the fibroid.
- Uterine artery embolization or uterine fibroid embolization (UFE) involves the injection of embolic particles into the blood supply of the tumors, occluding the blood supply to the tumor and thereby causing its shrinkage and resorption.

Surgical Management

- Surgical management depends on whether future childbearing is desired, the age of the woman, the size of the fibroid, and the degree of symptoms.
- A *myomectomy* (removal of the leiomyomas with preservation of the uterus) is performed to preserve childbearing capabilities and relieve the symptoms. This procedure can be done as minimally invasive surgery by a laparoscopic approach or by more traditional open abdominal and vaginal approaches.
- A *transcervical endometrial resection* (TCER) involves destroying the endometrium with a diathermy rectoscope or with radioablation.
  1. This procedure manages submucosal fibroids and menorrhagia.
  2. Complications include:
     a. Fluid overload (fluid used to distend the abdomen can be reabsorbed)
     b. Embolism
     c. Perforation of the uterus, bowel, bladder, or ureter
     d. Persistent increased menstrual bleeding
     e. Incomplete suppression of menstruation

- *Hysterectomy*, surgical removal of the uterine body, is the usual surgical management in the older woman who has multiple leiomyomas and unacceptable symptoms.
    1. A *total hysterectomy* involves removal of the uterus by a vaginal approach (total vaginal hysterectomy [TVH]), an open abdominal approach, or minimally invasive surgery by laparoscopy.
    2. *Panhysterectomy*, or *total abdominal hysterectomy* (TAH), includes the removal of the uterus, ovaries, and fallopian tubes.
    3. A *radical hysterectomy* involves removal of the uterus, lymph nodes, upper one third of the vagina, and the surrounding tissues.
- Provide preoperative nursing care, including:
    1. Routine preoperative care as described in Part One
    2. Exploring the patient's feelings about the loss of the uterus and childbearing capability, self-image, femininity, and sexual functioning
    3. Identifying the patient's support system
    4. Discussing any concerns the patient may have regarding possible rejection by her sexual partner
- Provide postoperative care for the patient after abdominal hysterectomy, including:
    1. Routine postoperative care as described in Part One
    2. Assessing for vaginal bleeding (there should be less than one pad saturated every 4 hours)
    3. Assessing the incision for intactness, bruising, or bleeding
    4. Maintaining the Foley catheter for the first 24 hours (or as prescribed)
    5. Monitoring for complications
        a. Paralytic ileus
        b. Thromboembolism
        c. Atelectasis
        d. Pneumonia
        e. Wound dehiscence
        f. Pulmonary embolism
        g. Depression
        h. Decreased libido
- Provide postoperative care for the patient after vaginal hysterectomy, including:
    1. Routine postoperative care as described in Part One
    2. Assessing for vaginal bleeding (there should be less that one pad saturated every 4 hours)
    3. Performing perineal care
        a. Sitz baths
        b. Ice packs

4. Maintaining the Foley catheter for the first 24 hours (or as prescribed)
5. Monitoring for complications
   a. Hemorrhage
   b. Urinary tract problems (retention, infection)
   c. Pulmonary embolism
   d. Depression
   e. Decreased libido

Considerations for Older Adults

- Older women are more at risk for all complications, especially pulmonary complications, than are younger women.
- Obese women are more at risk for all complications than are nonobese women.

Community-Based Care

- Plan health teaching based on the specific management method and the patient's needs.
- Teach the patient who has had an abdominal hysterectomy or a vaginal hysterectomy to:
  1. Avoid or limit stair climbing for 1 month.
  2. Shower rather than bathe in the tub.
  3. Avoid sitting for long periods.
  4. Avoid strenuous activity or lifting more than 5 pounds (2.2 kg).
  5. Expect cessation of menstruation and the inability to become pregnant.
  6. Participate in low-impact exercise, such as walking.
  7. Include foods in the diet that aid in healing, such as those containing protein, iron, and vitamin C.
  8. Avoid sexual intercourse for 3 to 6 weeks.
  9. Check for manifestations of complications, such as infection.
  10. Expect some changes in emotions and responses.

LEUKEMIA

OVERVIEW

- The leukemias are a type of cancer with uncontrolled production of immature WBCs in the bone marrow. This results in bone marrow overcrowding with immature, nonfunctional cells and in decreased production of normal blood cells.
- Leukemia may be *acute*, with a sudden onset and short duration, or *chronic*, with a slow onset and symptoms that persist for a period of years.

- The two major types of leukemia are:
  1. *Lymphocytic* (lymphoblastic), in which the abnormal cells are lymphoid in origin and which can be acute or chronic
  2. *Myelocytic* (myelogenous), in which the abnormal cells are myeloid in origin and which can be acute or chronic
- Acute myelogenous leukemia (AML) is the most common form of adult-onset leukemia.
- Other less common forms in adults are chronic myelogenous leukemia (CML) (20%), acute promyelocytic leukemia (APL) (10%), acute lymphocytic leukemia (ALL) (10%), and chronic lymphocytic leukemia (CLL) (less than 5%).
- Possible causes of leukemia include exposure to ionizing radiation, exposure to chemicals and drugs, bone marrow *hypoplasia* (reduced production of blood cells), genetic factors, immunologic factors, environmental factors, and the interaction of these factors.
- The basic pathologic defect is damage to the genes of early precursor leukocyte cells, causing excessive growth of a specific type of immature leukocyte. These cells are abnormal, and their excessive production in the bone marrow stops normal bone marrow production of RBCs, platelets, and mature leukocytes. Anemia, thrombocytopenia, and leukopenia result. Without treatment, the patient will die of infection or hemorrhage. In acute leukemia, these changes occur rapidly and, without intervention, progress to death. Chronic leukemia may be present for years before changes appear.
- Leukemic cells can invade all tissues and organs.

PATIENT-CENTERED COLLABORATIVE CARE
Assessment
- Obtain patient information about:
  1. Age
  2. Environmental exposure to agents that increase the risk for leukemia
  3. Previous illnesses and exposure to ionizing radiation or drugs
  4. History of infections, such as colds, influenza, pneumonia, bronchitis, or unexplained fevers
  5. Any excessive bleeding episodes, including:
     a. Tendency to bruise easily
     b. Nosebleeds
     c. Increased menstrual flow
     d. Bleeding from the gums
     e. Rectal bleeding

      f. Hematuria
      g. Prolonged bleeding after minor abrasions or cuts
  6. Weakness and fatigue
  7. Associated symptoms (headaches, behavior changes, increased somnolence, decreased attention span, lethargy, muscle weakness, loss of appetite, or weight loss)
- Assess for and document:
  1. Cardiovascular changes
      a. Anemia
      b. Tachycardia
      c. Hypotension
      d. Murmurs and bruits
      e. Slow capillary refill
      f. Bleeding from the gums
  2. Respiratory changes
      a. Increased respiratory rate
      b. Coughing and shortness of breath
      c. Abnormal breath sounds
  3. Skin changes
      a. Pallor on the face, around the mouth, and in the nail beds
      b. Coolness to the touch
      c. Pale conjunctiva and palmar creases
      d. Petechiae
      e. Ecchymosis
      f. Mouth sores that do not heal
  4. GI changes
      a. Nausea and anorexia
      b. Weight loss
      c. Rectal fissures
      d. Bloody stools
      e. Reduced bowel sounds
      f. Constipation
      g. Enlarged liver and spleen
      h. Abdominal tenderness
  5. Central nervous system (CNS) changes (in advanced disease)
      a. Papilledema
      b. Seizures
      c. Coma
  6. Miscellaneous changes
      a. Bone and joint tenderness
      b. Lymph node enlargement
  7. Psychosocial issues and concerns, especially anxiety and fear about the diagnosis, treatment, and outcome

8. Laboratory abnormalities
   a. Decreased hemoglobin and hematocrit levels
   b. Low platelet count
   c. WBC count (low, normal, or elevated)
- Diagnosis of leukemia is based on findings from bone marrow aspiration and biopsy. The bone marrow is full of leukemic *blast phase cells* (immature cells that are dividing). The leukemia type is diagnosed by cell surface antigens and chromosomal or gene markers.

Planning and Implementation
❖**NDx:** Risk for Infection

- Infection is a major cause of death in the patient with leukemia because the WBCs are immature and unable to function, and sepsis is a common complication.
- Infection occurs through *autocontamination* (normal flora overgrows and penetrates the internal environment) and *cross-contamination* (organisms from another person or the environment are transmitted to the patient).
- The three most common sites of infection are the skin, respiratory tract, and intestinal tract.
- Implement infection control and patient protection measures:
  1. Frequent, thorough handwashing before any patient contact
  2. If you have an upper respiratory tract infection, wear a mask when entering the patient's room.
  3. Observe strict aseptic procedures when performing dressing changes or accessing a central venous catheter.
  4. Place the patient in a private room, if possible.
  5. Reduce environmental sources of contamination.
     a. No standing collections of water in vases, denture cups, or humidifiers in the patient's room
     b. Use of a *minimal bacteria diet* (no raw fruits and vegetables, undercooked meat, pepper, or paprika)
     c. Use of high-efficiency particulate air (HEPA) filtration or laminar airflow systems
  6. Monitor for infection:
     a. Monitor the daily CBC with differential WBC count and absolute neutrophil count (ANC).
     b. Inspect the mouth during every shift for lesions and mucosa breakdown.
     c. Assess the lungs every 8 hours for crackles, wheezes, or reduced breath sounds.
     d. Assess all urine for odor and cloudiness.
     e. Ask the patient about any urgency, burning, or pain present on urination.

    f. Take vital signs, including temperature, at least every 4 hours.

  7. Provide meticulous skin care to maintain skin integrity.

  8. Implement pulmonary hygiene to prevent pulmonary infection.

> **Critical Rescues ◆** A temperature elevation of even 1° F (or 0.5° C) above baseline is significant for a patient with leukopenia and indicates infection until it has been proved otherwise.

  9. Implement agency neutropenia protocols for cultures, infection identification, and initiation of anti-infective therapy when infection is suspected.

- Drug therapy for acute leukemia (for patients with AML) is divided into three distinctive phases:
  1. Induction therapy is intense and consists of combination chemotherapy started at the time of diagnosis. The goal of this therapy is to achieve a rapid, complete remission of all manifestations of disease. These agents cause extreme side effects and toxicities. Care issues for chemotherapy are described under Cancer Treatment, General, in Part One.
  2. Consolidation therapy often consists of another course of the same drugs used for induction at a different dosage or a different combination of chemotherapy drugs. This treatment occurs early in remission, and its intent is to cure.
  3. Maintenance therapy may be used after successful induction and consolidation therapies for patients with acute lymphoblastic leukemia (ALL) and acute promyelocytic leukemia (APL). The purpose is to maintain the remission achieved through induction and consolidation. Drugs are milder and are often given orally for 2 to 5 years.

- Targeted therapy with imatinib mesylate (Gleevec) may be used for chronic myelocytic leukemia (CML) that is Philadelphia chromosome positive. Rituximab (Rituxin) may be used as targeted therapy for chronic lymphocytic leukemia (CLL). Care issues for targeted therapies are listed under Cancer Treatment, General, in Part One.

- Drug therapy for infection may include:
  1. Antibiotic and antibacterial drugs
     a. Aminoglycoside antibiotics
     b. Penicillin or a third-generation cephalosporin
  2. Systemic antifungal drugs
     a. Amphotericin B
     b. Ketoconazole (Nizoral)

    c. Voriconazole (Vfend)

    d. Fluconazole (Diflucan)

    e. Nystatin (Mycostatin, Nadostine ♣, Nilstat)

  3. Antiviral drugs, most commonly, acyclovir

- The definitive treatment for cure of leukemia after remission is achieved is a hematopoietic stem cell transplantation (HSCT). Care issues for this procedure are discussed under Hematopoietic Stem Cell Transplantation (Bone Marrow Transplantation).

❖**NDx:** Risk for Injury

- Normal bone marrow production of platelets is severely limited as a result of the disease or its treatment, leading to thrombocytopenia and increasing the risk for excessive bleeding in response to minimal trauma.
- Nursing interventions
  1. Institute bleeding precautions:
     a. Handle the patient gently.
     b. Use and teach unlicensed assistive personnel (UAPs) to use a lift sheet when moving and positioning the patient in bed.
     c. Avoid IM injections and venipunctures.
     d. When injections or venipunctures are necessary, use the smallest-gauge needle for the task.
     e. Apply firm pressure to the needle stick site for 10 minutes or until the site no longer oozes blood.
     f. Apply ice to areas of trauma.
     g. Test all urine and stool for the presence of occult blood.
     h. Observe IV sites every 4 hours for bleeding.
     i. Instruct alert patients to notify nursing personnel immediately if any trauma occurs or if bleeding or bruising is noticed.
     j. Avoid trauma to rectal tissues.
     k. Instruct the patient to use an electric shaver rather than a razor.
     l. Provide mouth care using a soft-bristle toothbrush or tooth sponges, and do not floss.
     m. Instruct the patient not to blow the nose or insert objects into the nose.
     n. Ensure that the patient wears shoes with firm soles when ambulating.
  2. Monitoring laboratory values daily, especially platelets
  3. Assessing the patient for bleeding
  4. Administering prescribed erythropoietic growth factors

❖**NDx:** Fatigue

- Normal production of RBCs is limited in leukemia, causing anemia, which results in fatigue.
- Interventions aim to reduce fatigue through energy management and improving RBC counts.
  1. Nutrition therapy
     a. Collaborate with a nutritionist.
     b. Provide small, frequent meals high in protein and carbohydrates.
  2. Transfusion therapy
  3. Drug therapy with colony-stimulating factors
     a. Epoetin alfa (Epogen or Procrit)
     b. Darbepoetin alfa (Aranesp)
  4. Energy management by eliminating or postponing activities that do not have a direct positive effect on the patient's condition

Community-Based Care

- Teach the patient and family about:
  1. Measures to prevent infection
  2. The importance of continuing therapy and medical follow-up
  3. The need to report manifestations of infection or bleeding immediately to the health care provider
  4. Assessing for petechiae, avoiding trauma and sharp objects, applying pressure to wounds for 10 minutes, and reporting blood in the stool or urine or headache that does not respond to acetaminophen
  5. The importance of eating a healthy diet
  6. Resources for psychological and financial support and for role and self-esteem adjustment
  7. Care of the central catheter if in place at discharge
- Assess the need for a home care nurse, aide, or equipment.

LIVER, FATTY

- Fatty liver is caused by the accumulation of triglycerides and other fats in the hepatic cells.
- The most common cause is chronic alcoholism.
- Other causes include malnutrition, diabetes mellitus, obesity, pregnancy, prolonged parenteral nutrition, and exposure to toxic drugs.
- The patient usually has no symptoms; the typical finding is hepatomegaly (an enlarged liver).
- Assess for:
  1. Right upper abdominal pain

2. Ascites
3. Edema
4. Jaundice
5. Fever
6. Signs of cirrhosis (see Cirrhosis)

- Liver biopsy confirms the diagnosis.
- Interventions are aimed at removing the underlying cause of the infiltration and dietary restrictions.

LUPUS ERYTHEMATOSUS

OVERVIEW

- *Systemic lupus erythematosus* (SLE) is a chronic, progressive, inflammatory connective tissue disease that can cause major body organs and systems to fail.
- The main mechanism of organ damage is the formation of immune complexes that form in organ tissues and in blood vessels, which deprive the organ of essential oxygen.
- It is classified as an autoimmune disease and has periods of spontaneous remissions and exacerbations (flares).
- *Discoid lupus erythematosus* (DLE) affects only the skin and is not as common as SLE.
- Lupus mainly affects women between 15 and 40 years of age and has wide variations in symptoms.
- The cause is unknown, although like many autoimmune disorders, a genetic predisposition is likely.

PATIENT-CENTERED COLLABORATIVE CARE

Assessment

- Assess for and document:
  1. Dry, scaly, raised rash on the face (butterfly rash) or upper body
  2. Individual round lesions (scarring lesions of discoid lupus)
  3. Joint involvement
     a. Initial changes are similar to rheumatoid arthritis.
     b. Later changes may include joint deformity.
  4. Muscle atrophy
  5. Muscle aches
  6. Fever
  7. Various degrees of weakness, fatigue, anorexia, and weight loss
  8. Renal involvement, such as reduced urine output, proteinuria, hematuria, and fluid retention

9. Pulmonary effusions or pneumonia
10. Pericarditis (the most common cardiovascular change)
    a. Tachycardia
    b. Chest pain
    c. Myocardial ischemia
11. Neurologic changes
    a. Psychoses
    b. Seizures
    c. Paresis
    d. Migraine headaches
    e. Cranial nerve palsies
12. Raynaud's phenomenon
13. Abdominal pain
14. Liver enlargement
15. Osteonecrosis
16. Body image changes
17. Social isolation
18. Fear, anxiety
- Diagnostic tests include:
  1. Skin biopsy
  2. Positive blood tests for:
     a. Rheumatoid factor
     b. Antinuclear antibodies
     c. Erythrocyte sedimentation rate
     d. Anti-SS-A (Ro), anti-SS-B (La), anti-Smith (anti-SM), anti-DNA, extractable nuclear antigens (ENA)
  3. Serum protein electrophoresis
  4. CBC
  5. Electrolyte levels
  6. Renal function tests, cardiac and liver enzymes

Interventions

- Drug therapy may include:
  1. Topical steroid preparations
  2. Hydroxychloroquine (Plaquenil) to reduce inflammatory responses
  3. Chronic oral steroid therapy
  4. Immunosuppressive agents, such as methotrexate (Rheumatrex) or azathioprine (Imuran) for renal or central nervous system (CNS) lupus
  5. Antineoplastic drugs, such as cyclophosphamide (Cytoxan, Procytox ✦)
- Teach the patient how to protect the skin by:
  1. Minimizing exposure to sunlight and other forms of ultraviolet light
     a. Wearing long sleeves and wide-brimmed hats

    b. Using sun blocking agents with a sun protective factor of at least 30

  2. Cleaning the skin with a mild soap and avoiding harsh, perfumed products

  3. Using cosmetics with moisturizers and sun protectants

  4. Using mild protein shampoo and avoiding hair bleaching agents, permanents, and dyes

- Reinforce measures for joint protection and energy conservation (see Arthritis, Rheumatoid).
- Help the patient identify coping strategies and support systems that can help him or her deal with the unpredictable nature of the exacerbations.
- Teach the patient about:
  1. The importance of monitoring for fever (the first sign of exacerbation)
  2. The importance of joint protection and energy conservation
  3. Sexual counseling for risk of pregnancy and for contraception options
  4. Resources such as the Lupus Foundation and the Arthritis Foundation
  5. Drug therapy information for scheduling, side effects, and any precautions

LYME DISEASE

- Lyme disease is transmitted by infected deer ticks.
- The disease can be prevented by avoiding heavily wooded areas or areas with thick underbrush; by wearing long-sleeved tops, long pants, and socks; and by using an insect repellent on skin and clothing when in an area where infected ticks are likely to be found.
- Symptoms appear in three stages.
  1. Stage I symptoms appear in 3 to 32 days after the tick bite:
     a. Fever and chills
     b. Swollen glands
     c. Headache
     d. Joint and muscle aches
     e. Spreading, oval or circular rash (erythema migrans)
     f. Drug therapy includes doxycycline, amoxicillin, or cefuroxime.
  2. Stage II symptoms appear 2 to 12 weeks after the tick bite:
     a. Cardiac symptoms (dysrhythmia, dizziness, palpitations, dyspnea)

    b. Neurologic symptoms (meningitis, cranial neuropathy, peripheral neuritis)

    c. Drug therapy includes ceftriaxone or cefotaxime.

3. Stage III, chronic persistent Lyme disease, occurs weeks to years after the tick bite and may lead to chronic complications:

    a. Arthralgia and arthritis (may be the only symptom of Lyme disease)

    b. Memory and thinking problems

    c. Fatigue

    d. Enlarged lymph nodes

    e. Drug therapy includes oral tetracycline or IV cephalosporins (for severe disease).

- Testing for Lyme disease is not accurate until 4 to 6 weeks after the initial tick bite.
- Vaccination against Lyme disease is available and should be encouraged for adults living in high-risk areas.
- Refer patients to the Lyme Disease Foundation.

L

LYMPHOMA, HODGKIN'S AND NON-HODGKIN'S

OVERVIEW

- *Hodgkin's lymphoma* (HL) is a cancer of the lymphoid tissues with abnormal overgrowth of one type of leukocyte, the lymphocyte. It usually starts in a single lymph node or a single chain of nodes and contains a specific cancer cell type, the Reed-Sternberg cell. HL usually spreads from one group of lymph nodes to the next in an orderly fashion.
- *Non-Hodgkin's lymphoma* (NHL) includes all lymphoid cancers that do not have the Reed-Sternberg cell. There are more than 12 subtypes of NHL, and they usually spread through the lymphatic system in a less orderly way than HL.
- The exact cause of either type of lymphoma is unknown.
- HL affects any age-group, but it is most common among teens and young adults and among adults in their 50s and 60s. NHL is more common in white, older men.
- The most common manifestation of either lymphoma type is a large but painless lymph node or nodes.
- Other manifestations of either type may include fever, drenching night sweats, and unexplained weight loss.
- Diagnosis is made on the basis of findings from lymph node biopsy. After diagnosis, lymphoma is classified by subtype and staged to determine extent of disease (which determines exact therapy).

PATIENT-CENTERED COLLABORATIVE CARE

- HL is one of the most treatable types of cancer. Generally, for stage I and stage II disease, the treatment is external irradiation of involved lymph node regions. With more extensive disease, irradiation and combination chemotherapy are used to achieve remission.
- Treatment options for patients with NHL vary based the subtype of the tumor, international prognostic index (IPI) score, stage of the disease, performance status, and overall tumor burden. Options include combinations of chemotherapy drugs, targeted therapies, localized radiation therapy, radiolabeled antibodies, hematopoietic stem cell transplantation, and newer investigational agents.
- Nursing management of the patient undergoing chemotherapy treatment for HL or NHL focuses on the side effects of therapy, especially:
  1. Drug-induced pancytopenia, which increases the risk for infection, anemia, and bleeding
  2. Severe nausea and vomiting
  3. Constipation or diarrhea
  4. Impaired hepatic function
  5. Specific interventions are listed under Cancer Treatment, General, in Part One.
- Nursing management of the patient undergoing radiation therapy for HL or NHL focuses on side effects of therapy, especially:
  1. Skin problems at the site of radiation
  2. Fatigue and taste changes
  3. Permanent sterility for men receiving radiation to the abdominopelvic region in the pattern of an inverted Y in combination with specific chemotherapy drugs
  4. Specific interventions are listed under Cancer Treatment, General, in Part One.

MACULAR DEGENERATION

OVERVIEW

- Macular degeneration is the deterioration of the macula (the area of central vision), and it can be *atrophic* (age-related) or *exudative*.
- Age-related macular degeneration (AMD) has two types.
  1. Dry AMD, caused by gradual blockage of retinal capillaries, allowing retinal cells in the macula to become ischemic and necrotic. Central vision declines first, but eventually, the

person loses all central vision. It is more common and progresses at a faster rate among smokers.

2. Wet AMD, caused by the growth of new blood vessels in the macula, which have thin walls and leak blood and fluid (*wet* AMD)

- Exudative macular degeneration is also *wet*, but it can occur at any age. The condition may occur only in one eye or in both eyes. Patients have a sudden decrease in vision after a serous detachment of pigment epithelium in the macula.

PATIENT-CENTERED COLLABORATIVE CARE

- Management of dry AMD aims to maximize remaining vision.
- The loss of central vision reduces the ability to read, write, recognize safety hazards, and drive.
- Suggest alternative strategies (e.g., large-print books, public transportation) and referrals to community organizations that provide a wide range of adaptive equipment.
- See Visual Impairment (Reduced Vision) for more discussion of patients' care needs.
- Management of wet macular degeneration focuses on slowing the process and identifying further changes in visual perception.
- Laser therapy to seal the leaking blood vessels in or near the macula can limit the extent of the damage.
- Photodynamic therapy (PDT) can also seal leaking retinal blood vessels. The patient is given an IV agent to increase photosensitivity. After the agent is absorbed, a special laser light is applied in the specific area to activate the agent, occluding the leaking vessels and preventing excessive formation of new vessels.
- The photosensitizer used in PDT increases the sensitivity of the eye and the skin to sunlight and other bright lights for weeks. During this time, the patient is at high risk for skin and retinal burns and must take steps to stay out of the sun and avoid bright lights.

MALABSORPTION SYNDROME

- Malabsorption syndrome is associated with a variety of disorders and intestinal surgical procedures and interferes with the ability to absorb nutrients as a result of altered mucosa of the small intestine.
- Physiologic mechanisms limit absorption because of one or more abnormalities, including:
  1. Bile salt deficiencies
  2. Enzyme deficiencies

3. Presence of bacteria
4. Disruption of the mucosal lining of the small intestine
5. Alteration in lymphatic or vascular circulation
6. Decreased gastric or intestinal surface area

- Clinical manifestations of malabsorption include diarrhea, steatorrhea, weight loss, fatigue, bloating and flatus, decreased libido, easy bruising, anemia, bone pain, and edema.
- Interventions focus on avoiding dietary substances that aggravate malabsorption, supplementing nutrients, and surgical or nonsurgical management of the primary causative disease.

MALNUTRITION

OVERVIEW

- Malnutrition, also known as undernutrition, results from inadequate nutrient intake, increased nutrient loss, and increased nutrient requirements.
- Protein-calorie malnutrition (PCM) affects all aspects of immune function; it causes reduced energy and protein synthesis and increases the risk for infection.
- There are three forms of PCM:
  1. Marasmus, a calorie malnutrition in which body fat and protein are wasted. Serum proteins are often preserved.
  2. Kwashiorkor, a lack of protein quantity and quality in the presence of adequate calories. Body weight is normal, and serum levels of proteins are low.
  3. Marasmic-kwashiorkor is a combined protein and energy malnutrition.
- Unrecognized dysphagia is a common problem in elderly patients and can cause malnutrition.
- Anorexia nervosa (self-induced starvation) and bulimia nervosa (binge eating followed by purging behavior such as self-induced vomiting) also lead to malnutrition.
- Clinical manifestations include:
  1. Leanness and cachexia
  2. Decreased effort tolerance and lethargy
  3. Intolerance to cold
  4. Ankle edema
  5. Dry, flaking skin, dermatitis, or other skin impairment
  6. Poor wound healing
  7. A higher than usual incidence of postoperative infection

≋ Consideration for Older Adults

Body weight and the body mass index (BMI) usually increase throughout adulthood until about 60 years of age. As people get older, they become less hungry and eat less, even if they are healthy. Older adults should have a BMI between 23 and 27.

PATIENT-CENTERED COLLABORATIVE CARE

- Treatment
  1. Identify and treat the precipitating cause.
  2. Examine and treat oral conditions (e.g., caries, pain, ill fitting dentures) that may contribute to impaired oral intake.
  3. Determine the patient's height and weight, and calculate a BMI.
  4. Provide high-calorie, high-protein diet.
  5. Monitor the patient's ability to eat the ordered diet and the amount eaten.
  6. Obtain a dietary consultation.
  7. Provide an environment conducive to eating.
  8. Drugs such as megestrol acetate (Megace) may be given to stimulate appetite.
  9. Provide nutritional supplements or partial enteral nutrition; total parenteral nutrition or peripheral parenteral nutrition.
  10. Maintain a daily calorie count, and weigh the patient daily. Evaluate whether nutrients consumed are sufficient to meet basal and stress-related energy needs.
  11. Assess and monitor laboratory values for electrolytes, serum albumin, prealbumin, and leukocyte count.
- Promote adequate nutrition with enteral feeding:
  1. Prevent tube clogging by rinsing with at least 60 mL of water whenever feeding is interrupted (when giving a drug or stopping feeding).
  2. Mark the tube at the nares or lip, and evaluate tube placement by noting migration of the mark every 4 hours.
  3. Monitor intake and output to determine fluid excess or dehydration.
  4. Prevent aspiration by maintaining backrest elevation greater than 35 degrees unless contraindicated by the patient's condition.
  5. Prevent contamination of the enteral solution and equipment; replace every 24 hours.

> Clinical Landmine ◆ Undernutrition is a risk factor for development of iatrogenic pressure ulcers. Implement nutritional consultation and skin pressure–relieving interventions for patients with a BMI less than 18.

MASTOIDITIS

- Mastoiditis is an infection of the mastoid air cells that are embedded in the temporal bone.
- It is caused by untreated or inadequately treated otitis media and can be acute or chronic.
- Manifestations include swelling behind the ear and pain with minimal movement of the tragus, the pinna, or the head. Cellulitis develops on the skin or external scalp over the mastoid process, and the ear is pushed sideways and down.
- Otoscopic examination shows a red, dull, thick, immobile eardrum with or without perforation.
- Other manifestations include low-grade fever, malaise, ear drainage, loss of appetite, and enlarged lymph nodes.
- Hearing loss is common.
- Management involves IV antibiotics and surgical removal of the infected tissue if the infection does not respond to antibiotic therapy. A simple or modified radical mastoidectomy with tympanoplasty is the most common treatment.
- Complications of surgery include damage to cranial nerves VI and VII, decreasing the patient's ability to look sideways (cranial nerve VI), and causing a drooping of the mouth on the affected side (cranial nerve VII). Other complications include vertigo, meningitis, brain abscess, chronic purulent otitis media, and wound infection.

MELANOMA

OVERVIEW

- Melanomas are pigmented cancers arising in the melanin-producing epidermal cells.
- Melanoma is highly metastatic, and a person's survival depends on early diagnosis and treatment.
- Risk factors include genetic predisposition, excessive exposure to UV light, and the presence of one or more precursor lesions that resemble unusual moles.
- It occurs most often among light-skinned races and people older than 60 years.

PATIENT-CENTERED COLLABORATIVE CARE

Assessment

- Obtain patient information about:
  1. Age and race
  2. Family history of skin cancer
  3. Any past surgery for removal of skin growths

4. Recent changes in the size, color, or sensation of any mole, birthmark, wart, or scar
5. Geographic regions where the patient has lived or currently lives
6. Sun exposure
7. Exposure to arsenic, coal tar, pitch, radioactive waste, or radium

- Assess for and document all lesions for:
  1. Location, size, color
  2. Surface features
     a. *A*symmetry of shape
     b. *B*order irregularity
     c. *C*olor variation within one lesion
     d. *D*iameter greater than 6 mm
- Diagnosis is made on the bases of biopsy findings.

Interventions

Surgical Management

- Surgical intervention is the management of choice for melanoma.
  1. *Excision* is used for biopsy of small lesions, and a sentinel node biopsy can determine whether tumor spread has started.
  2. *Wide excision* for deeper melanoma often involves removing full-thickness skin in the area of the lesion. Subcutaneous tissues and lymph nodes may also be removed, and grafting may be needed for wound closure.

Nonsurgical Management

- Drug therapy may involve systemic chemotherapy, biotherapy, or targeted therapy.
  1. Systemic chemotherapy with a combination of agents. General management issues for care of patients undergoing chemotherapy are presented in Part One under Cancer Therapy.
  2. Biotherapy with interferon
  3. Targeted therapy with experimental drugs such as a CTLA4 receptor blocker
- Radiation therapy for melanoma may be helpful for patients with metastatic disease when used in combination with systemic corticosteroids. General management issues for care of patients undergoing radiation therapy are presented in Part One under Cancer Therapy.

MELANOMA, OCULAR

- Melanoma is the most common malignant eye tumor in adults and is associated with exposure to UV light. Because of its rich blood supply, a melanoma can spread easily into nearby tissue and the brain.

- Manifestations may not be readily apparent, and the tumor may be discovered during a routine examination.
- Manifestations vary with the exact location and may include blurred vision, reduced visual acuity, increased intraocular pressure (IOP), change in iris color, and visual field loss.
- Diagnostic tests usually include ultrasonography or MRI.
- Management depends on the tumor's size and growth rate and on the condition of the other eye.
  1. *Enucleation* (surgical removal of the entire eyeball) with insertion of a ball implant to provide a base for fitting the socket prosthesis (in about 1 month)
  2. *Radiation therapy* using an implanted radioactive disk to reduce the size and thickness of melanoma
     a. Complications include vascular changes, retinopathy, glaucoma, necrosis of the sclera, cataract formation, and vitreous hemorrhage.
     b. Cycloplegic eyedrops and an antibiotic-steroid combination are used during the therapy period.

MÉNIÈRE'S DISEASE

OVERVIEW

- Ménière's disease is an excess of endolymphatic fluid that distorts the entire inner canal system.
- This fluid excess leads to tinnitus, one-sided sensorineural hearing loss, and vertigo, occurring in intermittent attacks that can last for several days.
- At first, hearing loss is reversible, but repeated damage to the cochlea from increased fluid pressure leads to permanent hearing loss.
- The disease usually begins in people between the ages of 20 and 50 years and is more common in men and in white people.

PATIENT-CENTERED COLLABORATIVE CARE

Assessment

- Assess patients for:
  1. Sensation of a feeling of fullness in one ear before an attack
  2. *Tinnitus*, a continuous, low-pitched roar or a humming sound, which worsens just before and during a severe attack
  3. Hearing loss that occurs first with the low-frequency tones but worsens to include all levels after repeated episodes

4. *Vertigo*, periods of a whirling sensation that may cause patients to fall. The vertigo is severe and usually lasts 3 to 4 hours.
5. Nausea and vomiting
6. Rapid eye movements (*nystagmus*)
7. Severe headaches

Interventions

Nonsurgical Management

- Teach patients about attack prevention strategies, including:
  1. Making slow head movements to prevent worsening of the vertigo
  2. Stopping smoking
  3. Participating in the hydrops diet, which includes:
     a. Distributing food and fluid intake evenly throughout the day and from day to day
     b. Avoiding foods or fluids that have a high salt content
     c. Drinking adequate amounts of fluids (low in sugar) daily
     d. Avoiding caffeine-containing fluids and foods
     e. Limiting alcohol intake to one glass of beer or wine each day
     f. Avoiding foods containing monosodium glutamate (MSG)
- Drug therapy to control the vertigo and vomiting and restore normal balance
  1. Mild diuretics
  2. Nicotinic acid
  3. Antihistamines (just before and during an acute attack)
     a. Diphenhydramine hydrochloride (Benadryl, Allerdryl ♣)
     b. Dimenhydrinate (Dramamine, Gravol ♣)
  4. Antiemetics
  5. Intratympanic therapy with gentamycin and steroids
- Use of the Meniett device, which applies low-pressure micro-pulses to the inner ear for 5 minutes three times daily

Surgical Management

- Surgical treatment of Ménière's disease is a last resort, because the hearing in the affected ear is often lost from the procedure.
- The specific surgical procedure depends on the degree of serviceable hearing, the severity of the spells, and the condition of the opposite ear.
- A *labyrinthectomy* is performed through the ear canal.
- Endolymphatic decompression is performed with drainage and a shunt.

MENINGITIS

OVERVIEW

- Meningitis is inflammation of the meninges that surround the brain and spinal cord.
- The infecting organism produces an inflammatory response in the pia mater, the arachnoid, the cerebral spinal fluid (CSF), and the ventricles.
- Bacterial meningitis is potentially life threatening; viral meningitis is usually self-limiting; and cryptococcal meningitis is the most common fungal meningitis.

PATIENT CENTERED COLLABORATIVE CARE

Assessment

- Obtain patient information about:
  1. Recent viral or respiratory diseases and exposure to communicable disease
  2. Head trauma or ear, nose, or sinus infection
  3. Heart disease, diabetes mellitus, cancer, immunosuppressive therapy, and neurologic surgery or procedures that increase risk for infection or invading organisms
- Assess for and document:
  1. Fever, neck stiffness, headache, and altered mental status
  2. Photophobia
  3. Nuchal rigidity and Kernig's and Brudzinski's signs, which are present in only a small percentage of patients with definite meningitis
  4. Seizure and focal neurologic deficits, especially with bacterial meningitis
  5. Change in level of consciousness
  6. Possible syndrome of inappropriate antidiuretic hormone (SIADH) (see Syndrome of Inappropriate Antidiuretic Hormone)
  7. Complications of meningitis, including coagulopathy resulting in emboli that compromise peripheral circulation
- Diagnostic studies may include:
  1. Lumbar puncture to obtain cerebrospinal fluid for cell count, differential, protein, and culture
  2. Serum levels of WBCs and electrolytes, especially to detect low sodium levels associated with diuresis
  3. CT scan to detect inflamed meninges, abscess, and intracranial hypertension

Interventions

- Assess and record the patient's neurologic status with vital signs and peripheral circulation at least every 4 hours. Level of consciousness is the most sensitive indicator of change in patient status.

- Assess and record with particular attention to cranial nerves III, IV, VI, VII, and VIII (pupillary response to light and ability to move eyes through four quadrants promotes early detection, concerning deterioration of patient condition).
- Administer drugs such as antibiotics and analgesics, as ordered.
- Maintain isolation precautions according to hospital policy.
- Implement seizure precautions, when indicated.
- Monitor for complications such as vascular compromise from emboli, shock, coagulation disorders, prolonged fever, and septic complications.

METABOLIC SYNDROME

- Metabolic syndrome, also called *syndrome X*, is classified as the simultaneous presence of metabolic factors known to increase risk for developing type 2 diabetes and cardiovascular disease.
- Features of the syndrome include:
  1. *Abdominal obesity*, with waist circumference of at least 40 inches (100 cm) for men and 35 inches (88 cm) for women
  2. *Hyperglycemia*, with an elevated fasting blood glucose level of 100 mg/dL or more or on drug treatment for elevated glucose
  3. *Hypertension*, with a systolic blood pressure of 130 mm Hg or more, diastolic blood pressure of 85 mg Hg or more, or on drug treatment for hypertension
  4. *Dyslipidemia*, with a triglyceride level 150 mg/dL or more or on drug treatment for elevated triglycerides; high-density lipoprotein (HDL) cholesterol less than 40 mg/dL for men or less than 50 mg/dL for women
- Any one of these health problems increases the rate of atherosclerosis and the risk for stroke, coronary heart disease, and early death.
- Teach patients about the lifestyle changes that can improve health, including:
  1. Reducing weight to within 20% of ideal or body mass index (BMI) to less than 25 kg/m^2 by modifying diet
  2. Increasing physical activity (moderate-intensity exercise for at least 30 minutes three times per week; low-intensity exercise for at least 30 minutes five times per week)
  3. Adhering to drug therapy to achieve desired lipid and blood pressure goals

M

METHICILLIN-RESISTANT *STAPHYLOCOCCUS AUREUS* (MRSA)

OVERVIEW

- Methicillin-resistance *Staphylococcus aureus* (MRSA) is an increasingly common skin infection that can range from mild folliculitis to extensive furuncles.
- It is easily spread to other body areas and to other people through direct contact with infected skin and by contact with articles of clothing, bed linens, athletic equipment, towels, and other objects used by a person with MRSA.
- The infection does not respond to cleansing with antibacterial soaps or to most types of topical and many oral antibiotic therapies.
- If MRSA infects a wound or gains access into the blood, deep wound infection, sepsis, organ damage, and death can occur.
- The incidence of the problem is highest among adults living in communal environments, such as dormitories or prisons, and among patients in hospitals or other health care residential settings.

PATIENT-CENTERED COLLABORATIVE CARE

- Drug therapy for patients infected with MRSA may include IV vancomycin, oral linezolide, or oral clindamycin.
- Nursing care focuses on teaching the patient and family techniques to prevent the spread of MRSA, including:
  1. Avoiding close contact with others, including participation in contact sports, until the infection has cleared
  2. Taking all prescribed antibiotics exactly as prescribed for the entire time prescribed
  3. Keeping the infected skin area covered with clean, dry bandages
  4. Changing the bandage whenever drainage seeps through it
  5. Placing soiled bandages in a plastic bag and sealing it closed before placing it in the regular trash
  6. Washing hands with soap and warm water before and after touching the infected area or handling the bandages
  7. Showering (rather than bathing) daily using an antibacterial soap
  8. Washing all uninfected skin areas before washing the infected area or using a fresh washcloth to wash the uninfected areas
  9. Using each washcloth only once before laundering and avoiding using bath sponges or puffs

10. Sleeping in a separate bed from others until the infection is cleared
11. Avoiding sitting on or using upholstered furniture
12. Not sharing clothing, washcloths, towels, athletic equipment, shavers or razors, or any other personal items
13. Cleaning surfaces that may have come into contact with infected skin, drainage, or used bandages (e.g., bathroom counters, shower or bath stalls, toilet seats) with household disinfectant or bleach water mixed daily (1 tablespoon of liquid bleach to 1 quart water)
14. Washing all soiled clothing and linens with hot water and laundry detergent; drying clothing in a hot dryer or outside on a clothesline in the sun
15. Urging family members and close friends to shower daily with an antibacterial soap
16. Ensuring that anyone who assists changing the bandages uses disposable gloves, pulls them off inside out when finished, places them with the soiled bandages in a sealed bag, and washes his or her hands thoroughly

MYASTHENIA GRAVIS

M

OVERVIEW

- Myasthenia gravis (MG) is a chronic autoimmune disease characterized by fatigue and weakness primarily in muscles innervated by the cranial nerves, as well as in skeletal and respiratory muscles.
- MG is caused by an autoantibody attack on the acetylcholine receptors (AChR) in the muscle end plate membranes. As a result, nerve impulses are not transmitted to the skeletal muscle at the neuromuscular junction.
- Women are affected three times more often than are men, with a peak onset between 20 and 30 years of age.
- In *Eaton-Lambert syndrome*, a form of myasthenia often observed in combination with small cell carcinoma of the lung, the muscles of the trunk and the pelvic and shoulder girdles are most commonly affected.

PATIENT-CENTERED COLLABORATIVE CARE

Assessment

- Obtain patient information about:
    1. Muscular weakness that increases on exertion or as the day wears on and improves with rest (with a temporary increase in weakness sometimes noted after vaccination, menstruation, and exposure to extremes in environmental temperature)

2. Rapid, temporary onset of fatigue or weakness associated with infection, emotional upset, pregnancy, or anesthesia and after vaccination, menstruation, and exposure to extremes in environmental temperature
3. Inability to perform ADLs
4. Ptosis, diplopia or weakness in facial muscles
5. Difficulty swallowing (dysphagia), choking
6. Respiratory distress
7. Family history of MG or thymic disorder
8. Weakness of voice
9. Decreased sensation (paresthesia) or aching in weakened muscles

- Assess for and document:
  1. Progressive paresis of affected muscle groups that is resolved by rest, at least in part
  2. Symptoms related to involvement of the levator palpebrae or extraocular muscles:
     a. Ocular palsies
     b. Ptosis
     c. Diplopia
     d. Weak or incomplete eye closure
  3. Involvement of muscles for facial expression, chewing, and speech
     a. The patient's smile may turn into a snarl.
     b. The jaw hangs.
     c. Difficulty chewing and swallowing may lead to severe nutritional deficits.
  4. Because of proximal limb weakness, the patient has difficulty climbing stairs, lifting heavy objects, or raising arms overhead.
  5. Mild or severe neck weakness
  6. Difficulty sustaining a sitting or walking posture
  7. Respiratory distress
  8. Bowel and bladder incontinence
  9. Weakness of the pelvic and shoulder girdles (seen in Eaton-Lambert syndrome, a special form of MG often observed in combination with small cell carcinoma of the lung)
  10. Disturbed body image
  11. Feelings of loss, fear, helplessness, and grief
  12. Usual coping methods
  13. Positive ACh receptor antibodies
  14. Significant improvement after Tensilon testing
- Diagnostic studies may include:
  1. Serum thyroid function tests

2. Serum protein electrophoresis tests to evaluate presence of autoantibodies
3. Serum acetylcholine receptor antibodies
4. Chest x-ray and CT scan to evaluate the thymus gland in the mediastinum
5. Pharmacologic tests with the cholinesterase inhibitors edrophonium chloride (Tensilon) and neostigmine bromide (Prostigmin); anticipate a marked improvement of muscle tone that lasts 4 to 5 minutes.
6. Electromyography to test muscle contraction after electrical stimulation

Interventions

Nonsurgical Management

- Promote balance between activity and rest including:
  1. Assessing respiratory function before and after periods of activity to prevent compromise from overexertion
  2. Providing assistance with mobilization as necessary and assessing motor strength before and after activity
  3. Teaching the patient to plan activities early in the day or during the energy peaks that follow the administration of drugs
  4. Planning rest periods for the patient to avoid excessive fatigue
  5. Providing pressure-relieving interventions such as heel protectors or air mattress to prevent pressure ulcer formation with reduced mobility
- Administer drugs for MG on time to avoid respiratory compromise and muscular weakness:
  1. Cholinesterase inhibitor drugs, also referred to as anticholinesterase drugs, typically pyridostigmine (Mestinon, Regonol) to prevent the breakdown of acetylcholine by enzymes in the neuromuscular junction, thereby increasing the response of muscles to nerve impulses and improving strength
     a. The drug is given with a small amount of food to minimize GI side effects; meals are provided 45 minutes to 1 hour after taking drug.
     b. Drugs containing magnesium, morphine or its derivatives, curare, quinine, quinidine, procainamide, hypnotics, or sedatives are avoided because they may increase weakness.
     c. Antibiotics such as neomycin, kanamycin, streptomycin, polymyxin B, and certain tetracyclines increase myasthenic symptoms by impairing transmitter release.
  2. Immunosuppression may be accomplished with the use of corticosteroids or with chemotherapeutic agents.

M

- Observe for myasthenic crisis, an exacerbation of the myasthenic symptoms caused by underdosing with anticholinergic drugs or by infection.
  1. Maintain adequate respiratory functioning (ABCs of emergency care); intubation and mechanical ventilation may be needed.
  2. Withhold cholinesterase-inhibiting drugs because they increase respiratory secretion and are usually ineffective for the first few days after the crisis begins.
  3. Anticipate restarting drugs gradually at lower doses.
- Observe for cholinergic crisis, an acute exacerbation of muscle weakness caused by overdosing with cholinergic (anticholinesterase) drugs.
  1. Withhold cholinesterase-inhibiting drugs until symptoms resolve.
  2. Anticipate administration of atropine to treat excess acetylcholine. Atropine may thicken secretions, causing more difficulty with airway clearance and possible development of mucous plugs.
- Monitor the patient's responses and vascular access for plasmapheresis. Plasmapheresis is a method by which autoantibodies are removed from the plasma.
- Implement frequent respiratory monitoring and anticipate respiratory support including:
  1. Performing a respiratory assessment at least every 8 hours
  2. Reporting respiratory distress: dyspnea, shortness of breath, air hunger, and confusion
  3. Encouraging the patient to turn, cough, and deep breathe every 2 hours
  4. Performing chest physiotherapy, including postural drainage, percussion, and vibration to aid in removal of secretions
  5. Keeping an Ambu bag, equipment for oxygen administration, and endotracheal intubation equipment at the bedside in case of respiratory distress
  6. Monitoring the patient's response to drugs
- Enhance self-care, including:
  1. Assessing the patient's ability to perform ADLs to establish his or her abilities and limitations
  2. Encouraging the patient to perform activities as independently as possible
  3. Planning activities to follow the administration of drug to maximize independence and successful attempts at self-care
  4. Collaborating with physical and occupational therapists to identify the need for assistive devices

- Assist with communication:
  1. Collaborate with the speech-language pathologist to develop communication strategies as needed.
  2. Instruct the patient to speak slowly and repeat information to verify that it is correct.
  3. Develop alternative communication systems such as flash cards.
- Ensure adequate nutritional support:
  1. Provide small, frequent meals and high-calorie snacks. Record calorie counts.
  2. Measure intake and output, serum albumin levels, and daily weight.
  3. Assess the patient's gag reflex and ability to chew and swallow. Observe the patient for choking, nasal regurgitation, and aspiration.
  4. Promote or provide oral hygiene.
  5. Obtain a dietary consultation to optimize nutritional strategies.
- Maintain eye protection:
  1. Apply artificial tears to keep corneas moist and free from abrasion.
  2. Consider a lubricant gel and eye shield at bedtime.
  3. To help relieve diplopia, cover alternate eyes with a patch for 2 to 3 hours at a time.

Surgical Management

- Thymectomy may be performed early in the disease. Remission may not occur even with a thymectomy or may take up to 2 years to show effect.
- Provide routine preoperative care as outlined in Part One, including:
  1. Administering pyridostigmine (Mestinon), as ordered, to keep the patient stable throughout surgery
  2. If steroids have been used, administering before surgery but tapering postoperatively
  3. Giving antibiotics before and after surgery
- Provide routine postoperative care as outlined in Part One, including:
  1. Observing for signs of pneumothorax or hemothorax such as chest pain, sudden shortness of breath, diminished or absent breath sounds, and restlessness or a change in vital signs
  2. Focusing on respiratory health, including using spirometry, coughing, deep breathing, and frequent monitoring for respiratory distress
  3. Observing for signs and symptoms of wound infection
  4. Providing chest tube care if indicated

Community-Based Care

- Emphasize specific points concerning the disease process:
  1. MG is characterized by episodic exacerbations (worsening of symptoms). If rest does not relieve symptoms or respiratory distress occurs, contacting your health care provider is indicated.
  2. Avoid factors that predispose the patient to exacerbation, such as infection, stress, surgery, and hard physical exercise.
  3. Recognition of symptoms of myasthenic crisis and cholinergic crisis
  4. Promote lifestyle adaptations, such as avoiding heat (sauna, sunbathing), crowds, overeating, and erratic changes in sleep habits.
- Provide information concerning the drug regimen, and include the name, effects, side effects, and the importance of taking drugs on time and not missing doses.
- Encourage the patient's family to become certified in cardiopulmonary resuscitation (CPR).
- Refer the patient to community agencies and support groups such as the Myasthenia Gravis Foundation.

NEPHROSCLEROSIS

- Nephrosclerosis is a problem of thickening in the nephron blood vessel, resulting in narrowing of the lumen, decreased renal blood flow, and chronically hypoxic kidney tissue.
- Ischemia and fibrosis develop over time.
- Nephrosclerosis is associated with hypertension, atherosclerosis, and diabetes mellitus.
- Prevention of renal damage includes control of lipidemia, glycemia, and hypertension.

NEPHROTIC SYNDROME

- Nephrotic syndrome is a condition of increased glomerular permeability that allows larger molecules to pass through the membrane into the urine and be removed from the blood.
- Nephrotic syndrome is commonly caused by changes in an immune or inflammatory process.
- The main features are severe proteinuria, hypoalbuminemia, hyperlipidemia, lipiduria, edema, and derangements in blood pressure.
- Treatment depends on what is causing the disorder (identified by renal biopsy) and may include:
  1. Angiotensin-converting enzyme inhibitors

2. Cholesterol-lowering drugs
3. Immunosuppressive agents, steroids
4. Heparin
5. Mild diuretics
6. Diet changes, including sodium restriction
- Assess the patient's hydration status, and monitor for dehydration. If the plasma volume is depleted, renal problems worsen.

NEUROMA, ACOUSTIC

- An acoustic neuroma is a benign tumor of cranial nerve VIII (vestibulocochlear nerve, also known as the auditory or acoustic nerve). Damage to hearing, facial movements, and sensation can occur as the tumor grows.
- Manifestations begin with tinnitus and progress to gradual sensorineural hearing loss in most patients. Constant, mild vertigo occurs later.
- Diagnosis is made by CT scanning, MRI, audiograms, and cerebrospinal fluid assays.
- Surgical removal is achieved by a craniotomy, and the remaining hearing is lost. Extreme care is taken to preserve the function of the facial nerve (cranial nerve VII). For care of the patient having a craniotomy, see Surgical Management under Tumors, Brain. See Hearing Loss for a review of care needs for the patient whose hearing is reduced.

OBESITY

OVERVIEW

- Obesity refers to an excess amount of body fat compared with lean body mass.
- An obese person weighs at least 20% above the upper limit of the normal range for ideal body weight (IBW) and has a body mass index (BMI) of 30 cm/kg^2 or more.
- Morbid obesity, also called extreme obesity, refers to a weight that has a severely negative effect on health—usually more than 100% above IBW or a BMI of 40 cm/kg^2 or more.
- More than one third of the U. S. population is obese, and another third is overweight. At least 10% of adults are morbidly obese. This problem is the second leading cause of preventable deaths in the U. S.
- Obesity involves complex interrelationships among genetic, environmental, psychological, social, cultural, pathologic, behavioral, and physiologic factors.

- Causes of obesity include high-fat and high-cholesterol diets, physical inactivity, drug treatment (corticosteroids, NSAIDs), and familial and genetic factors.
- Complications include diabetes mellitus, hypertension, hyperlipidemia, cardiac disease, sleep apnea, cholelithiasis, chronic back pain, early degenerative arthritis, susceptibility to infections, and certain cancers.

⬛ National Patient Safety Goal

The Joint Commission Patient Care Standards require that a nutritional screening occur within 24 hours after the patient's hospital admission. If indicated, an in-depth nutritional assessment should be performed. When patients are in the hospital for more than a week, nutritional assessment should be part of the daily plan of care.

PATIENT-CENTERED COLLABORATIVE CARE

- Obtain patient information about:
  1. Economic status
  2. Usual food intake
  3. Eating behaviors
  4. Cultural background
  5. Attitude toward food and current weight
  6. Appetite
  7. Drugs
  8. Physical activity
  9. Height and weight
  10. Chronic diseases
  11. Family history of obesity
  12. 24-hour diet history recall
- Management includes:
  1. Diet programs managed through close interaction among the patient, nutritionist, and health care provider
  2. Exercise program
  3. Drug therapy
     a. Anorectic drugs suppress appetite, which reduces food intake and over time may result in weight loss.
     b. Orlistat (Xenical) inhibits lipase and leads to partial hydrolysis of triglycerides. Because fats are only partially digested and absorbed, calorie intake is decreased.
  4. Behavioral treatment including reinforcement techniques and cognitive restructuring
- Surgery is indicated for the patient who is morbidly obese or who has a BMI greater than 35 with comorbidities that contribute to poor health.

1. Surgical procedures include three types: gastric restrictive, malabsorption, or both. *Restrictive* surgeries decrease the volume capacity of the stomach to limit the amount of food that can be eaten at one time. As the name implies, *malabsorption* procedures interfere with the absorption of food and nutrients from the GI tract.
2. Bariatrics is a branch of medicine that manages obesity and its related diseases.

- Provide routine postoperative care after bariatric surgery:
  1. Attention to airway management, as a thick neck may lead to a compromised airway.
  2. Focus on patient and staff safety, using specialized bariatric equipment to promote mobility and reduce skin complications.
  3. Monitor the patency of the nasogastric (NG) tube and record the amount of drainage.
  4. Monitor for manifestations of anastomotic leak, the most common and life-threatening complication after gastric bypass surgery. Manifestations of leak are increasing back, shoulder, or abdominal pain; restlessness; unexplained tachycardia; and oliguria (scant urine). Report any of these findings to the surgeon immediately.
  5. Apply an abdominal binder to prevent wound dehiscence.
  6. Place the patient in a semi-Fowler position or use continuous positive airway pressure (CPAP) ventilation at night to improve ventilation and decrease risk for sleep apnea.
  7. Observe skin areas and folds for redness, excoriation, or breakdown, and treat these problems early.
  8. Use absorbent padding between skin folds to prevent pressure ulcers, particularly from tubes and catheters.
  9. Remove the NG tube on the third postoperative day if bowel sounds are present and the patient is passing flatus; then begin clear fluids.
  10. Give 1 oz of water in a small cup and instruct the patient to slowly sip the water over a 1-hour period when oral intake is initially prescribed. Additional liquids, puréed foods, juices, and soups thinned with broth, water, or milk are added to the diet 24 to 48 hours after water is tolerated.
  11. Observe for dumping syndrome, manifested by frequent liquid stools.

Community-Based Care

- Give the patient a list of community resources, such as Weight Watchers, Overeaters Anonymous, and Take Off Pounds Sensibly (TOPS).

- In collaboration with the nutritionist, provide health teaching regarding the diet and the importance of maintaining a healthy eating pattern.
- Encourage the patient to increase physical activity, decrease fat intake and reliance on drug use, establish a normal eating pattern in response to physiologic hunger, and address medical and psychological problems.

OBSTRUCTION, INTESTINAL

OVERVIEW

- Intestinal obstruction can be partial or complete; intestinal contents accumulate at or above the obstruction.
- Intestinal obstruction can occur in the small intestine or large intestine (bowel). It can be either mechanical or nonmechanical (paralytic).
  1. Mechanical obstruction occurs when the bowel is physically obstructed by disorders outside the intestine (adhesions or hernias) or blockages in the lumen of the intestine (tumors, fecal impactions, and strictures).
  2. Nonmechanical obstruction (paralytic or adynamic ileus) occurs when peristalsis is decreased or absent, resulting in a slowing of the movement or a backup of intestinal content caused by physiologic, neurogenic, or chemical imbalances.
     a. Paralytic ileus is associated with trauma, abdominal surgery, hypokalemia, myocardial infarction, or vascular insufficiency.
- Distention results from the inability of the intestine to absorb and mobilize intestinal contents. Increased peristalsis occurs, leading to additional distention, edema of the bowel, and increased capillary permeability. Absorption of fluid and electrolytes into the vascular space is decreased, and reduced circulatory blood volume and electrolyte imbalances occur. Hypovolemia ranges from mild to extreme.
- Strangulated obstruction results when there is obstruction with compromised blood flow. This is a surgical emergency.

PATIENT-CENTERED COLLABORATIVE CARE

Assessment

- Obtain patient information about:
  1. Medical history, including abdominal surgical procedures, radiation therapy, and bowel diseases such as Crohn's disease, ulcerative colitis, diverticular disease, gallstones, hernias, trauma, and peritonitis
  2. Diet history

3. Bowel elimination patterns, including the presence of blood in the stool
4. Familial history of colorectal cancer
5. Nausea and vomiting, including color of emesis

- Assess for and document:
  1. Quality of abdominal pain, onset, and aggravating and alleviating factors associated with pain
  2. Bowel sounds: High pitched bowel sounds (borborygmi) may be heard early in an obstructive process and absent bowel sounds in later stages.
  3. Abdominal distention (hallmark sign)
  4. Nausea, vomiting, and character of emesis
     a. Obstruction above the ileum causes early and profuse vomiting of partially digested food and chyme, changing to watery contents containing bile and mucus.
     b. Obstruction in the large intestine produces vomitus with an orange-brown color and a foul odor caused by bacterial overgrowth, which may be fecal contamination.
  5. No passage of stool (obstipation), which is characteristic of total small- and large-bowel mechanical obstruction
  6. Hiccups (singultus), which is common with all types of intestinal obstruction

- Diagnostic studies may include:
  1. Flat-plate and upright abdominal x-rays
  2. Abdominal ultrasound or CT scan is used to further pinpoint the location and cause of the obstruction.

> **Critical Rescue** ◆ The sudden change in abdominal pain from dull to sharp or local to generalized may indicate a perforation after obstruction. Inform the physician immediately of this change in patient pain, along with current vital signs and oxygen status. A perforation is a surgical emergency.

Interventions
Interventions are aimed at uncovering the cause and relieving the obstruction.

Nonsurgical Management
- Decompress the GI tract by inserting or maintaining a gastric or intestinal tube, which can be inserted nasally or orally.
  1. Ensure that the patient receives nothing by mouth or decompressive tube.
  2. Maintain patency of decompressive tube:
     a. The Salem sump or Anderson suction tube sits distally in the stomach and is connected to low continuous suction.
     b. Levine tubes are connected to low intermittent suction.

3. Monitor and record quantity and character of NG or nasointestinal tube output every 4 hours.
4. Assess the nares for integrity at the site of tube insertion.
5. Mark the tube at the nares to provide ongoing confirmation of placement.
6. Record the passage of flatus and the amount and character of bowel movements.
7. Measure the patient's abdominal girth daily.
8. Inform the health care provider if gastric or intestinal outflow stops or becomes bloody.

- Obstruction caused by fecal impaction resolves after disimpaction and enema.
- Intussusception (telescoping of bowel) may resolve with hydrostatic pressure changes during a barium enema or with manipulation under fluoroscopy.
- Administer fluid and electrolyte replacement:
  1. Administer IV fluid because of vascular fluid losses from lack of normal reabsorption in the intestine, increased intestinal secretions, nasogastric (NG) suction, and NPO status (normal saline solutions with potassium replacement are used according to electrolyte results).
  2. Provide blood products in case of strangulated obstruction because of blood loss into the bowel or peritoneal cavity.
  3. Provide oral care, which may include ice chips.
  4. Monitor vital signs and other measures of fluid status (urinary output, skin turgor, and mucous membranes).
  5. Measure intake and output.
  6. Assess the patient for edema and ascites.
  7. Weigh the patient daily.
  8. Administer total parenteral nutrition, as ordered.
- Provide pain management:
  1. Report changes in pain to the physician, including pain that significantly increases or changes from a colicky, intermittent type to constant discomfort (changes could indicate perforation or peritonitis).
  2. Opioid analgesics can be given in the diagnostic period while waiting for a surgical consult.
  3. Provide a position of comfort, including semi-Fowler's, that helps to relieve the pressure of abdominal distention and facilitates thoracic excursion and normal breathing patterns.
- Broad-spectrum antibiotics are given if strangulation is suspected.

Surgical Management
- Surgical management is required for complete mechanical obstruction and for many cases of incomplete mechanical obstruction.

- An exploratory laparotomy is performed to locate the obstruction and determine the nature of the problem.
- The specific surgical procedure performed depends on the cause and location of the obstruction. Examples of procedures include lysis of adhesions, colon resection with anastomosis for obstruction resulting from tumor or diverticulitis, and embolectomy or thrombectomy for intestinal infarction. A colon resection and colostomy may be necessary.
- Nursing care for abdominal surgery is similar to that described under Cancer, Colorectal.

Community-Based Care

- Patient and family education depends on the specific cause and treatment of the obstruction.
  1. Report signs that may indicate recurrent obstruction, including abdominal pain or distention, nausea, vomiting, or constipation (for nonmechanical obstruction after surgery or trauma).
  2. Develop a structured bowel regimen, including a high-fiber diet, daily exercise, and psyllium hydrophilic mucilloid (e.g., Metamucil) with copious amounts of water for prevention of recurrences of fecal impaction.
- Information about incision care (if surgery was performed), drug therapy, and activity restriction is given to the patient and family.

O

OBSTRUCTION, UPPER AIRWAY

OVERVIEW

- Upper airway obstruction, a life-threatening emergency, is an interruption in airflow through the nose, mouth, pharynx, or larynx.
- Causes include:
  1. Foreign-body aspiration
  2. Edema of the tongue or larynx
  3. Occlusion by the tongue
  4. Peritonsillar or pharyngeal abscess
  5. Head and neck cancer
  6. Thick secretions
  7. Stroke and cerebral edema
  8. Smoke inhalation edema
  9. Facial, tracheal, or laryngeal trauma
  10. Burns of the head or neck area
  11. Anaphylaxis
- Partial obstruction may have only subtle or general manifestations such as diaphoresis, tachycardia, and elevated blood

pressure. To rule out a tumor, foreign body, or infection, diagnostic procedures, such as a chest x-ray, neck films, laryngoscopic examination, and CT scan, are performed.

- Observe for hypoxia and hypercarbia, restlessness, increasing anxiety, sternal retractions, a "seesawing" chest, abdominal movements, or a feeling of impending doom related to actual air hunger.
- Use pulse oximetry for ongoing monitoring of oxygen saturation. Continually assess for stridor, cyanosis, and changes in level of consciousness.

> 📷 **Critical Rescue** ♦ Early recognition is essential to prevent further complications, including respiratory arrest. Unexplained or persistent recurrent symptoms warrant evaluation even if the symptoms are vague.

PATIENT-CENTERED COLLABORATIVE CARE

- Management depends on the cause of the obstruction:
  1. For tongue occlusion, slightly extend the patient's head and neck and insert a nasal or oral airway.
  2. For secretions, suction to remove obstructing secretions.
  3. For foreign body, perform abdominal thrusts.
  4. For complete obstruction from edema, cancer, or abscesses:
     a. Direct laryngoscopy
     b. Cricoidectomy
     c. Endotracheal intubation
     d. Tracheotomy

OSTEOARTHRITIS

OVERVIEW

- Osteoarthritis (OA), formerly called degenerative joint disease (DJD), is the most common arthritis, with joint pain and loss of function leading to disability.
- The disease course includes progressive deterioration and loss of cartilage in one or more joints (articular cartilage), especially the hips and knees, the vertebral column, and the hands.
- The major pathologic problems are thinning and deteriorating joint cartilage, narrowing of the joint space, bone spur formation, inflammation, and joint deformity leading to immobility, pain, muscle spasm, and muscle atrophy.
- Known risk factors for OA include obesity, joint trauma, and smoking.

Considerations for Older Adults

- Age is the biggest risk factor for OA, because the proteoglycans in the joint cartilage decrease with age, reducing cartilage strength.

Genetic Considerations

- Some patients report a family history of OA, which supports a possible genetic cause, especially for women who have hand involvement.
- Interleukin-1 (IL-1) is a cytokine that increases the rate of cartilage degradation. Variations in the IL-1 gene family have been shown to increase the risk of other bone diseases.
- Another possible genetic predisposition for OA is an increase in discoid domain receptor 2 (DDR-2) expression in diseased joint cartilage.

PATIENT-CENTERED COLLABORATIVE CARE

Assessment

- Obtain patient information about:
  1. The course of the disease
     a. Nature and location of joint pain
     b. Location and duration of joint stiffness
     c. When and where any joint swelling has occurred
     d. What relieves or controls pain or stiffness
     e. Any loss of function or difficulty in performing ADLs
  2. Age and gender
  3. Occupation and nature of work
  4. History of trauma
  5. Weight history
  6. Smoking history
  7. Current or previous involvement in sports
  8. Family history of arthritis
  9. Any medical condition that may cause joint manifestations
- Assess for and document:
  1. Chronic joint pain and stiffness that diminishes after rest and intensifies after activity or that occurs with slight motion or even when at rest
  2. Joint pain or tenderness by palpation or by putting the joint through its ROM
  3. Crepitus (a continuous grating sensation felt or heard as the joint goes through its ROM)
  4. Joint enlarged from bony hypertrophy
  5. Any joint warmth or inflammation (indicates a secondary synovitis)

6. Hand changes with Heberden's nodes (at the distal interphalangeal [DIP] joints) and Bouchard's nodes (at the proximal interphalangeal [PIP] joints)
7. Joint effusions (excess joint fluid), especially in the knee
8. Atrophy of skeletal muscle from disuse
9. Loss of range of joint motion, loss of function
10. Compression of spinal nerve roots that produces radiating pain, stiffness, and muscle spasms in one or both extremities
11. Reduced level of mobility and function
12. Changes in ability to perform self-care

- Assess for psychosocial issues:
  1. Change in role and self-esteem
  2. Depression, anger, stress
- Laboratory changes may include:
  1. Elevated erythrocyte sedimentation rate (ESR)
  2. Elevated high-sensitivity C-reactive protein (hsCRP)
- Imaging assessment may include x-rays or MRI.

Planning and Implementation

❖**NDx:** Chronic Pain

Nonsurgical Management

- Drug therapy
  1. Analgesic drugs
     a. Acetaminophen (Tylenol, Exdol, Datril)
     b. Propoxyphene (Darvon, Novapropoxyn)
  2. Topical drug applications
     a. Lidocaine 5% patches
     b. Topical salicylates (Aspercreme, 1% diclofenac sodium [Voltaren])
  3. NSAIDs
     a. Celecoxib (Celebrex)
     b. Ibuprofen (Advil)
  4. Joint injection
     a. Cortisone
     b. Hyaluronate (Hyalgan)
     c. Hylan GF 20 (Synvisc)
  5. Muscle relaxants (cyclobenzaprine hydrochloride [Flexeril])
- Nonpharmacologic measures
  1. Joint rest
     a. Local joint rest with an immobilizer
     b. Systemic rest with napping and 8 to 10 hours of nighttime sleep
     c. Balancing rest and activity

2. Joint positioning
   a. Avoid excessive flexion of involved joint.
   b. Maintain normal extension.
3. Heat or cold applications (hot showers and baths, hot packs or compresses, moist heating pads)
4. Weight control
5. Complementary and alternative therapies (topical capsaicin products, acupuncture, acupressure, tai chi, music therapy)
6. Cognitive-behavioral therapies (imagery, prayer, meditation)
7. Dietary supplements (gamma-linolenic acid [GLA, Efamol], glucosamine, and chondroitin)

Surgical Management

- Surgery may be indicated when conservative measures no longer provide pain control, when mobility becomes so restricted that the patient cannot participate in enjoyable activities, or when he or she is unable to maintain the desired quality of life.
  1. Total joint arthroplasty (TJA) (surgical creation of a joint), also known as total joint replacement (TJR), is the most common type of surgery for OA. Almost any synovial joint of the body can be replaced with a prosthetic system that consists of at least two parts, one for each joint surface.
  2. An *osteotomy* (bone resection) may be performed to correct joint deformity, but this procedure is less common because of the success rate of TJR.
- Total hip arthroplasty (THA) with a replacement prosthesis can be done by a traditional open hip incision or, for select patients, by *minimally invasive surgery* (MIS) using one or two smaller 2- to 4-inch incisions with special instruments to reduce muscle cutting. The replacement joint consists of two parts, the acetabular component and the femoral component.
  1. Provide preoperative care:
     a. Performing routine preoperative care as described in Part One
     b. Assessing the patient's level of understanding about the surgery
     c. Reinforcing the surgeon's explanations about the procedure and postoperative expectations
     d. Explaining about transfers, positioning, ambulation, and postoperative exercises
     e. Demonstrating assistive/adaptive devices for ADLs
     f. Teaching patients having MIS how to perform muscle-strengthening exercises at home before the procedure
     g. Explaining the importance of having any necessary dental procedures done *before* the surgery

h. Assessing the patient's risk factors for clotting problems and administering any prescribed anticoagulants

i. Determining whether the patient has made an autologous blood donation and ensuring that the blood is ready before surgery

j. Administering or teaching the patient to administer any prescribed synthetic erythropoietin (epoetin alfa [Epogen, Procrit, Eprex ✦])

k. Administering any prescribed IV therapy before the initial surgical incision is made

2. Provide postoperative care:

a. Performing routine postoperative care as described in Part One

b. Preventing dislocation by:

(1) Maintaining correct positioning (supine position with the head slightly elevated)

(2) Placing a trapezoid-shaped abduction pillow, wedge, sling, or splint (with or without straps) between the legs to prevent adduction beyond the midline of the body

(3) Placing and supporting the affected leg in neutral rotation

(4) Keeping the patient's heels off the bed to prevent skin breakdown, particularly for older adults

(5) Following agency policy or surgeon preference for postoperative turning

(6) Observing for signs of possible hip dislocation (increased hip pain, shortening of the affected leg, and leg rotation)

> 🔲 **Critical Rescue** ✦ If manifestations of hip dislocation occur, keep the patient in bed and notify the surgeon immediately.

c. Preventing thromboembolic complications by:

(1) Administering prescribed anticoagulants, such as warfarin (Coumadin, Warfilone ✦), subcutaneous low-molecular-weight (LMW) heparin, or factor Xa inhibitors

(2) Assessing for manifestations of deep vein thrombosis (swelling, pain)

(3) Teaching leg exercises (plantar flexion and dorsiflexion, circles of the feet, gluteal and quadriceps muscle setting, straight-leg raises)

(4) Applying prescribed antiembolic stockings or devices

d. Preventing infection:
   (1) Monitoring the surgical incision and vital signs carefully—every 4 hours for the first 24 hours and every 8 hours thereafter
   (2) Observing for signs of infection (elevated temperature and excessive or foul-smelling drainage from the incision)

> ⬛ **Critical Rescue** ◆ An older patient may not have a fever with infection but instead may experience an altered mental state. Consider infection in any older patient with new-onset confusion or inability to rouse.

e. Preventing anemia:
   (1) Observing the surgical hip dressing for bleeding or other type of drainage at least every 4 hours or when vital signs are taken
   (2) Emptying and measuring the bloody fluid in the surgical drains every shift
   (3) Checking the results of the periodic hemoglobin and hematocrit (H&H) tests
f. Preventing neurovascular complications:
   (1) Checking and documenting color, temperature, distal pulses, capillary refill, movement, and sensation
   (2) Comparing these parameters with those of the nonoperative leg
   (3) Reporting any changes to the surgeon
g. Managing pain by:
   (1) Assessing the patient's pain level
   (2) Ensuring proper use of pain control devices such as epidural analgesia, intraspinal analgesia, patient-controlled analgesia (PCA), and IV opioid analgesia
   (3) Administering prescribed analgesics as needed
h. Progressing activity by assisting the patient with getting out of bed by:
   (1) Standing on the same side of the bed as the affected leg
   (2) Teaching the patient to stand on the unaffected leg and pivot to the chair
   (3) Assisting the patient to a sitting position
   (4) Ensuring that the patient does not flex the hips beyond 90 degrees
   (5) Preventing hyperflexion of the replaced joint with the use of raised toilet seats, straight-back chairs, and reclining wheelchairs

3. Weight bearing on the affected leg depends on the surgeon, type of prosthesis, and surgical procedure.

4. Work with the physical therapist (PT) to teach the patient how to follow weight-bearing restrictions and progress to full-weight-bearing (FWB) status.

5. The occupational therapist (OT) may recommend assistive-adaptive devices to help with ADLs, especially for those patients having traditional surgery.

6. For patients who have *traditional surgery*, the length of stay in the acute care hospital for patients after traditional surgery is typically 3 days; those who have *MIS procedures* may be discharged on the second postoperative day or, in a few cases, on the day of surgery.

7. The interdisciplinary team provides written instructions for posthospital care and reviews them with patients and their family members.

8. Complete recovery may take 6 weeks or more.

- Total knee arthroplasty (TKA) can be performed by traditional open surgery or by MIS procedures for some patients.

  1. Provide preoperative care:
     a. Routine preoperative care described in Part One
     b. Care as described for THA
     c. Explanation and demonstration of a continuous passive motion (CPM) machine (if prescribed)

  2. Provide postoperative care:
     a. Routine postoperative care as described in Part One
     b. Care to prevent complications as described for THA
     c. Implementing the CPM machine as prescribed for ROM and cycles per minute
        (1) Checking the cycle and ROM settings at least once every 8 hours
        (2) Ensuring that the joint being moved is properly positioned on the machine
        (3) Placing the controls to the machine out the reach of a confused patient
        (4) Assessing the patient's response to the machine
        (5) Turning off the machine while the patient is having a meal
        (6) Storing the machine off the floor when it is not in use
     d. Applying ice packs or a Hot/Ice device to decrease surgical site swelling
     e. Ensuring safe use of continuous peripheral nerve blockade (CPNB) for pain control:
        (1) Performing neurovascular assessments every 2 to 4 hours or according to hospital protocol

  (2) Assessing that the patient can plantar flex and dorsiflex the affected foot but does not feel pain in the extremity

  (3) Checking for movement, sensation, warmth, color, pulses, and capillary refill

  (4) Monitoring for symptoms of systemic infusion of the nerve-blocking drug (a metallic taste, tinnitus, restlessness, nervousness, slurred speech, bradycardia, hypotension, decreased respirations)

 f. Maintaining the knee in a neutral position and not rotated internally or externally

 g. Ensuring that the surgical knee is not hyperextended

 h. Monitoring neurovascular status frequently to check for compromise to the distal operative leg every time vital signs are taken

- Total shoulder arthroplasty (TSA) can be performed either as a total joint replacement or as a *hemiarthroplasty* (replacement of part of the joint, typically the humeral component). These surgeries are most commonly performed using traditional open incisions, but minimally invasive shoulder arthroplasty can be used instead for some patients.
  1. Preoperative care and postoperative care are similar to those for other joint replacement surgeries.
  2. A sling is applied to immobilize the joint and prevent dislocation until therapy begins.
  3. The hospital stay for TSA is usually 1 to 2 days until pain is controlled.
  4. Rehabilitation with an occupational therapist (OT) usually takes 2 to 3 months.
- Other joints that can be replaced include:
  1. Elbow (total elbow arthroplasty [TEA])
  2. Hand or foot joints (phalangeal joint, metacarpal or metatarsal arthroplasties)
  3. Any bone of the wrist
  4. Ankle (total ankle arthroplasty [TAA]), which has more postoperative complications than other arthroplasties

❖**NDx:** Impaired Physical Mobility

- Reinforce the techniques and principles of exercise, ambulation, promotion of ADLs, and use of assistive devices developed by the physical therapist (PT) and occupational therapist (OT) to meet the goal of independent function.
- The ideal time for exercise is immediately after the application of heat.
- Teach the patient to follow these instructions:
  1. Follow the exercise instructions that have been specifically prescribed for you. There are no universal exercises;

your exercises have been specifically tailored to your needs.

2. Do your exercises on both "good" and "bad" days. Consistency is important.

3. Respect pain. If pain increases as you exercise, stop and report this to your health care provider.

4. Use active rather than active-assist or passive exercise whenever possible.

5. Reduce the number of repetitions if the inflammation is severe and you have more pain.

6. Do not substitute your normal activities or household tasks for the prescribed exercises.

7. Avoid resistive exercises if your joints are severely inflamed.

Community-Based Care

- Collaborate with the discharge planner and the health care provider to determine the best placement for the patient with OA at discharge.
- Provide health teaching:
  1. Explaining the general principles of joint protection
     a. Use large joints instead of small ones; for example, place your purse strap over your shoulder instead of grasping the purse with your hand.
     b. Turn doorknobs toward your thumb (rather than toward your little finger) to avoid twisting your arm and promoting ulnar deviation.
     c. Use two hands instead of one to hold objects.
     d. Sit in a chair that has a high, straight back.
     e. When getting out of bed, do not push off with your fingers; use the entire palm of both hands.
     f. Do not bend at your waist; instead, bend your knees while keeping your back straight.
     g. Use long-handled devices, such as a hairbrush with an extended handle.
     h. Use assistive-adaptive devices, such as Velcro closures and built-up utensil handles, to protect your joints.
     i. Do not use pillows in bed, except a small one under your head.
     j. Avoid twisting or wringing your hands.
  2. Explaining the drug protocol, desired and potential side effects, and toxic effects
  3. Emphasizing the importance of reducing weight and eating a well-balanced diet to promote tissue healing
  4. Referring the patient to the Arthritis Foundation for up-to-date information about new treatments and helpful complementary and alternative practices

5. Providing written instructions about the required care, regardless of whether the patient goes home or to another inpatient facility

6. Referring the patient to the nutritionist, counselor, home health nurse, rehabilitation therapist, financial counselor, and local and state support groups as needed

OSTEOMALACIA

OVERVIEW

- Osteomalacia is a softening of the bone tissue that occurs when there are inadequate deposits of calcium and phosphorus in the bone matrix.
- Vitamin D deficiency is the most important factor in its development. This can occur as a result of inadequate exposure to sunlight, poor dietary intake, abnormal metabolism, chronic use of many drugs, or the presence of chronic disease.
- Older adults are most at risk for osteomalacia.

PATIENT-CENTERED COLLABORATIVE CARE

- Obtain patient information about:
  1. Age
  2. Exposure to sunlight and skin pigmentation (darker skin reduces vitamin D activation)
  3. Dietary habits
  4. Current prescribed and OTC drug use
  5. Chronic disease processes of the GI tract
     a. Inflammatory bowel disease
     b. Gastric or intestinal bypass surgery
  6. Renal or liver dysfunction
  7. History of bone fracture
- Assess for and document:
  1. Muscle weakness (causing a waddling and unsteady gait) and cramping
  2. Bone pain (aggravated by activity and worse at night)
  3. Bone tenderness to palpation (especially tibia or rib cage)
  4. Skeletal malalignment (long-bone bowing or spinal deformity)
  5. Hypocalcemia or hypophosphatemia
  6. Presence of radiolucent bands (Looser's lines or zones) on x-ray
- The major intervention for osteomalacia is vitamin D.
  1. Teach patients to take the amount of vitamin D supplementation prescribed by their health care provider.

2. Remind patients, especially those who are homebound, about the importance of daily sun exposure (at least 5 minutes each day) to activate the vitamin.
3. Teach patients to choose foods that are fortified with vitamin D (milk and dairy products) or are rich in vitamin D (eggs, swordfish, chicken, and liver), as well as enriched cereals and bread products.

OSTEOMYELITIS

OVERVIEW

- Osteomyelitis is an infection in bony tissue caused by bacteria, viruses, or fungi and is often severe and difficult to treat.
- It can result in chronic recurrence of infection, loss of function, amputation, and even death.
- The pathologic processes that occur in infected bone tissue include inflammation, blood vessel thromboses, and necrosis.
- Categories of osteomyelitis include:
  1. *Exogenous,* in which infectious organisms enter from outside the body, as in an open fracture
  2. *Endogenous,* also called hematogenous, in which organisms are carried by the bloodstream from other areas of infection in the body
  3. *Contiguous,* in which bone infection results from skin infection of adjacent tissues
- The two major types of osteomyelitis are acute and chronic.
- Common causes include bacteremia, underlying disease, penetrating and nonpenetrating trauma, long-term IV therapy, hemodialysis, *Salmonella* infection of the GI tract, sickle cell disease, poor dental hygiene and periodontal (gum) infection, and skin infection with methicillin-resistant *Staphylococcus aureus* (MRSA).

Considerations for Older Adults

- The most common cause of contiguous spread in older adults is slow-healing foot ulcers in patients with diabetes or peripheral vascular disease.
- Multiple organisms tend to be responsible for osteomyelitis in these patients.

PATIENT-CENTERED COLLABORATIVE CARE

Assessment

- Assess for and document:
  1. Bone pain described as a constant, localized, pulsating sensation that worsens with movement

2. Fever, usually greater than 101° F (38° C) (in acute disease)
3. Swelling, tenderness, erythema, and heat around the site of infection
4. Ulcerations on the feet or hands (if circulation is poor)
5. Sinus tract formation and drainage (with chronic infection)
6. Elevated WBC count and erythrocyte sedimentation rate (ESR)
7. Positive blood cultures

Interventions

Nonsurgical Management

- Nonsurgical interventions include:
  1. Administering IV antibiotic therapy for several weeks, followed by oral antibiotic therapy for weeks or months

> 🔲 **Critical Rescue** ◆ Even if symptoms of the disease appear to be improved, the full course of IV and oral antibiotics must be completed. Teach patients the importance of completing the full course of therapy.

  2. Irrigating the wound either continuously or intermittently, with one or more antibiotic solutions
  3. Using sterile technique at all times
  4. Packing the wound with beads made of bone cement that have been impregnated with an antibiotic
  5. Administering drugs for pain control
  6. Covering the wound to prevent infection spread
  7. Implementing Contact Precautions for severe infections, particularly if the purulent material cannot be adequately contained by a dressing
  8. Administering hyperbaric oxygen (HBO) therapy for patients with chronic, unremitting osteomyelitis

Surgical Management

- Surgery is reserved for patients with chronic osteomyelitis and may include:
  1. Sequestrectomy with excision of dead and infected bone to allow revascularization of tissue
  2. Application of bone *grafts* to repair bone defects
  3. Reconstruction with *microvascular bone transfers* if excision is extensive
  4. Closure of the defect with muscle flaps and skin grafts
  5. Amputation of the affected limb if the infection cannot be controlled or revascularization is not successful
- Provide postoperative care:
  1. Implementing routine postoperative care described in Part One

2. Performing frequent neurovascular (NV) assessments:
   a. Pain
   b. Movement
   c. Sensation
   d. Warmth
   e. Temperature
   f. Distal pulses
   g. Capillary refill

> 🔳 **Critical Rescue** ◆ Immediately report to the surgeon any of these signs of neurovascular compromise: **p**ain that cannot be controlled, **p**aresis or **p**aralysis (weakness or inability to move), **p**aresthesias (abnormal, tingling sensation), **p**allor, and **p**ulselessness.

3. Elevating the affected extremity to increase venous return and control swelling

OSTEOPOROSIS

OVERVIEW

- *Osteoporosis* is a chronic metabolic disease in which bone loss causes decreased density and possible fracture, most often of the wrist, hip, and vertebral column.
- The main mechanism of osteoporosis is an imbalance in the continuous bone remodeling processes such that osteoclastic (bone resorption) activity is greater than osteoblastic (bone building) activity.
- *Generalized* osteoporosis involves many structures in the skeleton and is further divided into two categories:
  1. *Primary* osteoporosis, which is more common and occurs in postmenopausal women and in men in their sixth or seventh decade of life
  2. *Secondary* osteoporosis, which results from other medical conditions, such as hyperparathyroidism; long-term drug therapy, such as with corticosteroids; or prolonged immobility
- *Regional* osteoporosis occurs when a limb is immobilized related to a fracture, injury, or paralysis for longer than 8 to 12 weeks.
- Risk factors include menopause; lean and thin body build, Euro-American or Asian ancestry; sedentary lifestyle; diet deficient in calcium and vitamin D; malabsorption syndromes; high intake of caffeine and carbonated beverages; excessive alcohol

and tobacco use; family history; and long-term use of certain drugs, especially corticosteroids.

🌐 Cultural Awareness

- Although there is some advantage of increased bone density in dark-skinned women, lifestyle and health beliefs about prevention may put all women at equal risk for osteoporosis.
- Many African Americans and Asians have lactose intolerance and cannot drink milk or eat other dairy-based foods, which are good sources of protein and calcium.

PATIENT-CENTERED COLLABORATIVE CARE

Assessment

- Obtain patient information about:
  1. Age, gender, race, body build, weight
  2. Change in height
  3. Back pain after bending, lifting, or stooping (worse with activity, relieved with rest)
  4. Mobility
  5. Muscular weakness
  6. History of falls
  7. Current drugs
- Assess for and document:
  1. Features of the spinal column (presence of classic "dowager's hump," or kyphosis of the dorsal spine)
  2. Location of all painful areas
  3. Manifestations of fractures (swelling and malalignment)
  4. Constipation, abdominal distention
  5. Respiratory compromise
  6. Fear of falling
  7. Body image disturbance
  8. Changes in quality of life and sexuality
- Diagnostic tests may include:
  1. Biochemical markers of spinal changes
     a. Bone-specific alkaline phosphatase (BSAP)
     b. Osteocalcin
     c. Pyridinium (PYD)
     d. N-telopeptide (NTX)
     e. C-telopeptide (CTX)
     f. Levels of serum calcium, vitamin D, phosphorus, and protein
     g. X-rays
     h. Dual x-ray absorptiometry (DXA)
     i. Quantitative computed tomography (QCT)
     j. Quantitative ultrasound (QUS)

Interventions
Nonsurgical Management

- Nutrition therapy
  1. Coordinate health teaching and nutrition planning with the nutritionist.
  2. Teach patients to eat a diet that includes:
     a. Fruits and vegetables
     b. Low-fat dairy and protein sources
     c. Increased fiber
     d. Moderation in alcohol and caffeine intake
     e. Adequate amounts of protein, magnesium, vitamin K, and trace minerals
     f. Increased calcium and vitamin D intake
  3. Work with patients who are lactose intolerant to choose from a variety of soy and rice products, fruit juices, bread, and cereal products that are fortified with or have additional calcium and vitamin D.
- Exercise, which is important in both prevention and management of osteoporosis
  1. Coordinate health teaching with the physical therapist (PT) for exercises to improve posture, support, and pulmonary capacity; strengthen extremity muscles; and improve ROM:
     a. Abdominal muscle tightening
     b. Deep breathing
     c. Pectoral stretching
     d. Extremity muscle tightening, resistive, and ROM exercises
     e. Swimming
     f. Walking for 30 minutes three to five times a week
  2. Teach patients to avoid high-impact recreational activities, such as running, bowling, and horseback riding.
- Teach about other lifestyle changes:
  1. Avoiding tobacco in any form, especially cigarette smoking
  2. Preventing falls
  3. Maintaining a hazard-free environment by avoiding scatter rugs, cluttered rooms, and wet floor areas
- Drug therapy for prevention and management:
  1. Estrogen and hormone therapy in low doses for short durations
  2. Parathyroid hormone (teriparatide [Fortéo])
     a. Teach patients to self-administer Fortéo as a daily subcutaneous injection.
     b. Teach patients to lie down if dizziness or leg cramping occurs and to notify the health care provider as soon as possible.

3. Calcium and vitamin D supplementation
4. Bisphosphonates
   a. Alendronate (Fosamax) (oral drug)
   b. Ibandronate (Boniva) (oral and IV)
   c. Risedronate (Actonel) (oral drug)
   d. Pamidronate (Aredia) (IV drug)
   e. Zoledronic acid (Reclast) (IV drug)

> **Critical Rescue** ◆ Osteonecrosis of the jaw is a rare but serious complication of bisphosphonate therapy. Teach the patient to have an oral assessment and preventive dentistry before beginning therapy and to inform any dentist who is planning invasive treatment, such as a tooth extraction or implant, that he or she is taking a bisphosphonate.

5. Selective estrogen receptor modulators (SERMs) (raloxifene [Evista])
6. Other drugs:
   a. Calcitonin
   b. Androgens (testosterone propionate [Testex, Malogen ♣])

Surgical Management
- *Vertebroplasty* is the injection of bone cement into the vertebral body to reduce a fracture or fill the space created by osteoporosis.
- *Kyphoplasty* includes the use of a balloon in the vertebral body to contain the bone cement.

Community-Based Care
- Ensure that the patient and family understand drug and exercise regimens.
- Help the patient and family identify and correct hazards in the home before discharge.
- Refer the patient to a home health agency.
- Refer the patient and family to community resources, such as the National Osteoporosis Foundation and local osteoporosis specialty clinics.

OTITIS MEDIA

OVERVIEW
- Otitis media is an infection of the middle ear that causes an inflammatory process within the mucosa. Most infections of the middle ear are bacterial.
- The inflammation leads to swelling and irritation of the small bones (ossicles) within the middle ear, a purulent exudate, pain, and temporary hearing loss.

- If otitis progresses or remains untreated, permanent conductive hearing loss may occur.
- Otitis media can be acute, chronic, or serous.

PATIENT-CENTERED COLLABORATIVE CARE

Assessment

- Assess for manifestations of acute or chronic otitis media:
  1. Ear pain with or without movement of the external ear (which is relieved when the ear drum ruptures)
  2. Sensation of fullness in the ear
  3. Reduced or distorted hearing
  4. Tinnitus
  5. Headaches
  6. Dizziness or vertigo
  7. Systemic symptoms
     a. Malaise
     b. Fever
     c. Nausea and vomiting
  8. Otoscopic examination findings
     a. Dilated and red eardrum blood vessels
     b. Red, thickened, or bulging eardrum
     c. Decreased eardrum mobility
     d. Eardrum perforation with pus present in the canal

Interventions

- Nonsurgical management
  1. Bedrest to limit head movements that intensify the pain
  2. Application of heat or cold
  3. Systemic antibiotic therapy
  4. Analgesics
     a. Mild, such as aspirin, ibuprofen (Advil), and acetaminophen (Tylenol, Abenol ♣)
     b. Opioids such as codeine and meperidine hydrochloride (Demerol) for severe pain
  5. Antihistamines and decongestants
- Surgical management with a *myringotomy* (surgical opening of the pars tensa of the eardrum) may be needed.
  1. Preoperative care
     a. Providing reassurance
     b. Administering systemic antibiotic therapy
     c. Cleaning the external canal
  2. Postoperative care
     a. Teach the patient to keep the external ear and canal free of other substances.
     b. Instruct him or her to avoid washing the hair or showering for 48 hours.

OVARIAN CYSTS

OVERVIEW

- There are several types of ovarian cysts:
  1. Follicular cysts, which usually occur in young, menstruating women, are not malignant and do not grow without hormonal influences.
     a. It can develop when a mature follicle fails to rupture or an immature follicle fails to reabsorb follicular fluid during the second half of the menstrual cycle.
     b. The cyst is usually small (2.4 to 3.2 inches [6 to 8 cm]) and may be asymptomatic unless it ruptures.
     c. Rupture of a follicular cyst or torsion (twisting) may cause acute, severe pelvic pain that usually resolves after several days of bedrest and use of mild analgesics.
     d. If the cyst does not rupture, it usually disappears within two or three menstrual cycles without intervention.
     e. For cysts that persist, oral contraceptives may be prescribed for one or two menstrual cycles to suppress ovulation.
     f. Surgery is recommended only after menopause or for cysts that are larger than 3.2 inches.
  2. Corpus luteum cysts
     a. These cysts occur after ovulation and often occur with increased secretion of progesterone.
     b. The cysts are usually small, averaging 1.5 inches (4 cm), and are purplish red as a result of hemorrhage within the corpus luteum.
     c. They are associated with a delay in the onset of menses, irregular or prolonged flow, and low abdominal or pelvic pain on one side.
     d. Cyst rupture can cause intraperitoneal hemorrhage.
     e. Cysts may disappear in one or two menstrual cycles or with suppression of ovulation.
     f. Management is the same as for follicular cysts.
  3. Theca-lutein cysts
     a. These cysts are uncommon and are associated with hydatidiform mole pregnancies. They develop as a result of prolonged stimulation of the ovaries by excessive amounts of human chorionic gonadotropin (hCG).
     b. These cysts regress spontaneously within 3 months after removal of the molar pregnancy or the source of excessive hCG.
- Polycystic ovary syndrome (PCOS) (Stein-Leventhal syndrome) results when high levels of luteinizing hormone (LH) over-stimulate the ovaries, producing multiple cysts on one or both

O

ovaries. High levels of estrogen are produced by these cysts and are unopposed by postovulatory progesterone, resulting in endometrial hyperplasia (tissue overgrowth) or even carcinoma. Patients are usually obese, are hirsute, have irregular menses, and may be infertile because of lack of ovulation.

PATIENT-CENTERED COLLABORATIVE CARE

- Management of the patient with PCOS depends on which problem is of greatest concern to the woman:
  1. Conservative management includes the use of oral contraceptives to inhibit LH production and prevent excessive ovarian stimulation.
  2. For a woman who is older than 35 years and no longer desires childbearing, management may involve a bilateral salpingo-oophorectomy (BSO) (removal of both tubes and ovaries) and hysterectomy (removal of the uterus and cervix).
  3. In women who desire fertility, PCOS can be managed with drugs such as clomiphene citrate (Clomid) to stimulate ovulation.

PAGET'S DISEASE OF THE BONE

OVERVIEW

- Paget's disease, or osteitis deformans, is a chronic metabolic disorder in which bone is excessively broken down (osteoclastic activity) and reformed (osteoblastic activity). The result is structurally disorganized bone that is weak with increased risk of bowing of long bones and fractures.
- There are three phases of the disorder:
  1. *Active*, in which there is a rapid increase in osteoclasts (cells that break down bone), causing massive bone destruction and deformity
  2. *Mixed*, in which the osteoblasts (bone-forming cells) react to compensate in forming new but structurally weak bone
  3. *Inactive*, in which the osteoblastic activity exceeds the osteoclastic activity, resulting in hard, sclerotic bone
- The most common areas of disease involvement are the vertebrae, femur, skull, clavicle, humerus, and pelvis.
- The risk for developing Paget's disease increases as a person ages and is particularly high for those 80 years old or older.
- Most patients with Paget's disease are asymptomatic and have disease confined to one bone. In more severe disease, the manifestations are diverse and potentially fatal.

Genetic Considerations

- Two types of Paget's disease can occur: familial and sporadic. Possible mutation areas for the familial form include the *RANKL/RANK/OPG* gene system, the gene for the valosin-containing protein *(VCP)* that controls complement, and the gene for sequestosome 1 *(SQSTM1)*.
- Teach patients the importance of genetics in familial Paget's disease, and refer them to the appropriate genetic counseling resource.
- Ask the patient whether genetic testing is desired.

PATIENT-CENTERED COLLABORATIVE CARE

Assessment

- Obtain patient information about:
  1. History of fracture
  2. Bone pain (mild to moderate aching, deep, worsened by pressure and weight bearing), especially of the hip and pelvis
  3. Redness and warmth at affected sites
  4. Arthritis at the joints (cartilage) of the affected bones
  5. Nerve impingement in the lumbosacral area of the vertebral column (back pain that radiates along one or both legs)
  6. Any changes in hearing, vision, swallowing, balance, or speech
  7. Loose teeth or difficulty chewing
- Assess for and document:
  1. Posture, stance, and gait for gross bony deformities
  2. Loss of normal spinal curvature, lower extremity malalignment, and decreased height
  3. Kyphosis or scoliosis of the spinal column
  4. Long-bone bowing in the legs or arms
  5. Flexion contracture in the hip joint
  6. Soft, thick, and enlarged skull
  7. Deafness and vertigo
  8. Problems with vision, swallowing, or speech
  9. Hydrocephalus
  10. Bone fractures, especially of the femur or tibia, after minimal trauma
  11. Apathy, lethargy, and fatigue
  12. Hyperparathyroidism and gout (along with an increase in serum and urinary calcium levels and serum uric acid levels)
  13. Kidney stones (renal calculi)
  14. Cardiac complications (heart failure)

P

- Diagnosis is made on the basis of physical findings, increases in serum alkaline phosphatase (ALP) and urinary hydroxyproline levels, x-ray findings, and radionuclide bone scanning.

Interventions

Nonsurgical Management

- Drug therapy for pain management includes:
  1. Aspirin or NSAIDs such as ibuprofen (Motrin, Apo-Ibuprofen ✤) for mild to moderate pain
  2. More potent analgesics for severe pain
- Drug therapy to decrease bone resorption includes:
  1. Bisphosphonates
     a. Alendronate (Fosamax) (oral drug)
     b. Risedronate (Actonel) (oral drug)
     c. Etidronate (Didronel) (oral drug)
     d. Tiludronate (Skelid) (oral drug)
     e. Pamidronate (Aredia) (IV drug)
     f. Zoledronic acid (Reclast) (IV drug)
  2. Calcium: 1500 mg daily
  3. Vitamin D: 800 international units (IU) daily
  4. Calcitonin (subcutaneous injection or nasal spray)
  5. Plicamycin (Mithracin) (potent antineoplastic agent with many side effects)
- Non-impact exercises
- Use of orthotic device to immobilize and provide support for the vertebrae or long bones
- Nutrition therapy with a diet rich in calcium

Surgical Management

- If a patient with Paget's disease has secondary arthritis and pain relief is not achieved, a tibial osteotomy or partial or total joint replacement may be performed.
- Surgical decompression and stabilization of the spine may be used to retain function, decrease pain, and reduce potential cardiac and respiratory complications.

PAIN, BACK

OVERVIEW

- The areas of the back most commonly affected by back pain are the cervical and lumbar vertebrae.
- Acute lumbosacral (low back) pain (LBP) is typically caused by a muscle strain, spasm, ligament sprain, disk degeneration, or herniated nucleus pulposus (usually between the fourth and fifth lumbar vertebrae).
- If back pain continues for 3 months or if repeated episodes occur, back pain is classified as chronic.

- Risk factors for acute back pain include:
  1. Trauma (twisting or hyperflexion during lifting)
  2. Obesity
  3. Congenital spinal problems, such as scoliosis
  4. Smoking (causes premature disk degeneration)

Considerations for Older Adults

- In older adult patients, osteoarthritis and osteoporosis contribute to back pain.
- Cervical pain is also common in patients with advanced rheumatoid arthritis who experience cervical disk subluxation, most often at the C1-2 level (first and second cervical vertebrae).
- Physiologic changes associated with aging, such as spinal stenosis, vertebral malalignment, and vascular changes, contribute to back pain in the older adult.

PATIENT-CENTERED COLLABORATIVE CARE

Assessment

- Assess and document:
  1. Pain location, quality, radiation, severity, alleviating and aggravating factors
  2. Posture and gait
  3. Vertebral alignment and swelling
  4. Muscle spasm
  5. Tenderness of the back and involved extremity
  6. Sensory changes: paresthesia and numbness
  7. Muscle tone and strength
  8. Limitations in movement
  9. Psychosocial reaction to illness
  10. Vertebral changes seen on an x-ray, CT scan, or MRI scan
  11. Abnormal electromyography and nerve conduction studies

Interventions

Nonsurgical Management

- To treat acute LBP:
  1. Have the patient use the Williams position when in bed (semi-Fowler's bed position with the knees flexed). A bed board or firm mattress may be useful for patients with a muscle injury. For patients with a herniated disk, a flat position may aggravate the pain.
  2. Collaborate with the physical therapist to develop an individualized exercise program.
  3. Drug therapy includes muscle relaxants and NSAIDs.
  4. Epidural or local steroid injection may be helpful in some cases.

5. Apply ice and heat therapy.
   a. Apply moist heat in the form of heat packs or hot towels for 20 to 30 minutes four times daily; hot showers or baths also are beneficial for some patients.
   b. Apply ice therapy using ice packs or ice massage over the affected area for 10 to 15 minutes every 1 to 2 hours.
   c. Some patients prefer alternating ice and heat therapy.
   d. Deep heat therapy such as ultrasound treatments and diathermy may be administered by the physical therapist (PT).

- Approaches for treating chronic back pain:
  1. Collaborate with the nutritionist to implement a weight loss program if appropriate.
  2. Have the patient use a custom-fitted lumbosacral brace or corset for LBP.
  3. Have the patient use ergonomic office furniture.
  4. Have the patient use shoe inserts or insoles.
  5. Have the patient use distraction, imagery, and music therapy.

Surgical Management

- Conventional open operative procedures include:
  1. Percutaneous laser disk decompression, which relieves the pain of a herniated disk by drawing the herniated portion away from the nerve root
  2. Diskectomy, in which a portion of the disk is removed
  3. Laminectomy, which is the removal of one or more vertebral laminae, plus osteophytes, and the herniated nucleus pulposus through a 3-inch (7.5-cm) incision
  4. Spinal fusion, which stabilizes the spine if repeated laminectomies are performed
- Minimally invasive operative procedures include:
  1. Percutaneous lumbar diskectomy
     a. A metal cannula is inserted adjacent to the affected disk under fluoroscopy, and a special cutting tool is threaded through the cannula for removal of pieces of the disk that are compressing the nerve root (laser surgery may be used). Inpatient hospitalization is not necessary.
     b. Possible complications: infection and nerve root injury
  2. Microdiskectomy
     a. Microscopic surgery is performed through a 1-inch (2.5-cm) incision.
     b. Possible complications: infection, dural tears, and missed disk fragments
  3. Laser-assisted laparoscopic lumbar diskectomy
     a. A laser with modified standard disk instruments is inserted periumbilically through the laparoscope.

  b. Possible complications: infection and nerve root injury
 4. Disk prosthesis: Insertion of a hard plastic prosthesis that replaces the patient's natural disk and is shaped to allow full spinal movement
- Provide preoperative care as described in Part One and additional care:
  1. Explain to the patient that various sensations may be experienced in the affected leg or both legs (for lumbar surgery) because of manipulation of nerves and muscles during surgery.
  2. Addressing the need for a postoperative brace and bone grafting if the patient is having a spinal fusion
- Provide routine postoperative care as described in Part One and additional care:
  1. Perform neurologic assessment with vital signs every 4 hours during the first 24 hours.
  2. Check the patient's ability to void. An inability to void may indicate damage to sacral spinal nerves. Opioid analgesics have been associated with difficulty voiding.
  3. Log roll the patient if bedrest is prescribed immediately after surgery.
  4. Ensure that a brace or other type of thoracolumbar support is worn when the patient is out of bed (for spinal fusion).

Community-Based Care
- Health teaching includes:
  1. The prescribed exercise program, including daily walking (and patient mastery is ensured by observing correct performance on return demonstration, in collaboration with physical therapy)
  2. Restrictions on climbing stairs, lifting, bending, and activities such as driving
  3. Principles of body mechanics
  4. The use of a firm mattress or bed board, if appropriate
  5. Drug information
  6. A weight-reduction diet, if needed
  7. The use of moist heat
  8. The importance of smoking cessation
  9. For unresolved pain, referral to a pain specialist or clinic

P

PAIN, CERVICAL SPINE

OVERVIEW
- Cervical spine or neck pain is usually related to herniation of the nucleus pulposus in an intervertebral disk (ruptured disk)

between the fifth and sixth vertebrae or to nerve compression caused by osteophyte formation.

- Pain also may result from muscle strain or ligament sprain.

PATIENT-CENTERED COLLABORATIVE CARE

Assessment

- Assess for:
  1. Pain that radiates to the scapula and down the arm when the patient moves his or her neck
  2. Sleep disturbances caused by pain
  3. Headache
  4. Numbness and tingling in the affected arm
  5. Vertebral changes seen on CT or MRI

Interventions

Nonsurgical Management

- Nonsurgical management of cervical spine pain is the same as for back pain, except that the exercises focus on the neck and shoulder.
- A soft collar may be prescribed for the patient; it should not be worn for more than 10 days, because doing so can lead to increased pain and decreased muscle strength and ROM.
- Cervical traction can be done intermittently at home, guided by a physical therapist (PT) initially.

Surgical Management

- Depending on the causative factors, an anterior or a posterior approach may be used.
- Provide routine postoperative care as described in Part One.
  1. Anticipate that the patient will wear some type of cervical collar for several weeks.
  2. Assess the patient's ability to void.
  3. Assist the patient with ambulation, usually on the evening of surgery unless a multilevel fusion was performed.
  4. Monitor for complications:
     a. Hoarseness due to laryngeal injury
     b. Dysphagia
     c. Esophageal, tracheal, or vertebral artery injury
     d. Graft extrusion and screw loosening if a fusion was performed

PANCREATITIS, ACUTE

OVERVIEW

- Acute pancreatitis is a serious and, at times, life-threatening inflammatory process of the pancreas caused by premature activation of pancreatic enzymes and resulting in autodigestion and fibrosis of the pancreas.

- The extent of the inflammation and tissue destruction ranges from mild involvement, characterized by edema and inflammation, to severe, necrotizing hemorrhagic damage leading to diffusely bleeding pancreatic tissue with fibrosis and tissue death.
- Many factors can cause injury to the pancreas:
  1. Biliary tract disease with gallstones
  2. Excessive alcohol ingestion
  3. Postoperative trauma from surgical manipulation after biliary tract, pancreatic, gastric, and duodenal procedures
  4. External blunt trauma
  5. Metabolic disturbances
  6. Renal failure or renal transplant
  7. Drug toxicities, including opiates, sulfonamides, thiazides, steroids, and oral contraceptives
  8. Other medical diseases
- Complications include transient hyperglycemia, pleural effusions, atelectasis, pneumonia, multisystem organ failure, acute lung injury progressing to acute respiratory distress syndrome (ARDS), shock, and coagulation defects.

PATIENT-CENTERED COLLABORATIVE CARE

Assessment

- Obtain patient information about:
  1. History of abdominal pain, especially if related to alcohol ingestion or high intake of fat
  2. Individual and family history of alcoholism, pancreatitis, or biliary tract disease
  3. Previous abdominal surgeries or diagnostic procedures
  4. Medical history, including peptic ulcer disease, renal failure, vascular disorders, hyperparathyroidism, and hyperlipidemia
  5. Recent viral infection
  6. Use of prescription and OTC drugs
- Assess for and document:
  1. Abdominal pain (the most frequent symptom), including sudden-onset pain in a midepigastric or left upper quadrant location with radiation to the back, aggravated by a fatty meal, ingestion of a large amount of alcohol, or lying in the recumbent position
  2. Weight loss, with nausea and vomiting
  3. Jaundice
  4. Gray-blue discoloration of the abdomen and periumbilical area (Cullen's sign)

5. Gray-blue discoloration of the flanks (Turner's sign)
6. Absent or decreased bowel sounds
7. Abdominal tenderness, rigidity, and guarding
8. Dull sound on abdominal percussion, indicating ascites
9. Elevated temperature with tachycardia and decreased blood pressure
10. Adventitious breath sounds, dyspnea, or orthopnea
11. Elevated serum amylase and lipase levels
- Diagnostic studies may include:
   1. Serum lipase, amylase, alkaline phosphatase, alanine aminotransferase (ALT), bilirubin, WBC, hemoglobin, hematocrit, coagulation factors, sodium, potassium, calcium, magnesium, triglycerides, and albumin
   2. Imaging of the pancreas and gallbladder with ultrasound or CT scan

Planning and Implementation

❖**NDx:** Acute Pain

Nonsurgical Management
- Fasting includes:
   1. Withholding food and fluids in the acute period; hydration is maintained with IV fluids
   2. Maintaining nasogastric (NG) intubation to decrease gastric distention and suppress pancreatic secretion
   3. Assessing frequently for the presence of bowel sounds
- Drug therapy may include:
   1. Opioids such as morphine or hydromorphone, often with a patient-controlled analgesia (PCA) device
   2. H_2 histamine receptor blockers or proton pump inhibitors to decrease gastric hydrochloric acid production during fasting
   3. Spasmolytics such a papaverine or nitroglycerin and secretogogue inhibitors such as octreotide or somatostatin to reduce pancreatic activity
   4. Anticholinergics to decrease vagal stimulation and decrease GI motility
   5. Antibiotics for patients with acute necrotizing pancreatitis
- Comfort measures include:
   1. Helping the patient assume a side-lying position to decrease abdominal pain
   2. Avoiding oral stimulation while providing measures to keep mucus membranes from drying
   3. Encouraging the patient to express the emotions and responses he or she is feeling
   4. Providing reassurance and diversional activities to reduce anxiety

Surgical Management

- Surgical management usually is not indicated for acute pancreatitis.
- Patients with complications such as pancreatic pseudocyst or abscess may require surgical drainage.
- Routine postoperative care is provided as described in Part One.
  1. Monitor drainage tubes for patency and recording output.
  2. Protect skin, because pancreatic drainage is particularly excoriating to the skin.
  3. Collaborate with the enterostomal therapist to promote skin integrity; possibilities include the use of ostomy appliances and the application of topical ointments.

❖**NDx:** Imbalanced Nutrition: Less than Body Requirements

- Interventions include:
  1. Withholding oral food and fluids in the early stages of the disease
  2. Providing jejunal enteral or parenteral nutrition (TPN) if fasting is required for more than 48 to 72 hours
  3. When food is tolerated, providing small, frequent, high-carbohydrate and high-protein feedings with limited fats
  4. Providing supplemental liquid diet preparations and vitamins and minerals to boost caloric intake, if needed

Community-Based Care

- Patient and family health teaching is aimed at preventing future episodes and preventing disease progression to chronic pancreatitis.
  1. Encourage alcohol abstinence to prevent further pain and extension of the inflammation and insufficiency.
  2. Teach the patient to notify the physician if he or she is experiencing acute abdominal pain or symptoms of biliary tract disease such as jaundice, clay-colored stools, and dark urine.
  3. Emphasize the importance of follow-up visits with the health care provider.
  4. Refer the patient with an alcohol abuse problem to support groups such as Alcoholics Anonymous.
  5. Refer the patient to home health nursing, as needed.

PANCREATITIS, CHRONIC

OVERVIEW

- Chronic pancreatitis is a progressive, destructive disease of the pancreas with remissions and exacerbations.
- Inflammation and fibrosis of the tissue contribute to pancreatic insufficiency and diminished organ function.

- The disease usually develops after repeated episodes of alcohol-induced acute pancreatitis, also known as chronic calcifying pancreatitis; it may also be associated with chronic obstruction of the common bile duct.
- Chronic pancreatitis is characterized by protein precipitates that plug the ducts and lead to ductal obstruction, atrophy, and dilation, causing metaplasia and ulceration and resulting in fibrosis of the pancreatic tissue.
- Chronic obstructive pancreatitis develops from sclerotic lesions in the head of the pancreas and around the ducts, which cause backflow of pancreatic secretions and enzymes.
- Pancreatic insufficiency is characterized by the loss of exocrine function, which causes a decreased output of enzymes and bicarbonate; loss of endocrine function results in diabetes mellitus.

PATIENT-CENTERED COLLABORATIVE CARE

Assessment

- Obtain patient information about:
  1. History of abdominal pain related to alcohol ingestion or high fat intake with specific information about alcohol intake, including time, amount, and relationship of alcohol to pain development
- Assess for and document:
  1. Abdominal pain (major clinical manifestation): continuous, burning, or gnawing dullness with intense and relentless exacerbations
  2. Left upper quadrant mass, indicating a pseudocyst or abscess
  3. Dullness on abdominal percussion, indicating pancreatic ascites
  4. Steatorrhea, foul-smelling stools that may increase in volume as pancreatic insufficiency progresses
  5. Weight loss and muscle wasting
  6. Jaundice and dark urine
  7. Signs and symptoms of diabetes mellitus
  8. Elevated serum amylase, bilirubin, and alkaline phosphatase levels
  9. Identification of calcification of pancreatic tissue in biopsy specimen

Interventions

Nonsurgical Management

- Drug therapy includes:
  1. Opioid analgesia. The patient may become dependent on opioids with long-term use.

2. Non-opioid analgesics
3. Pancreatic enzyme replacements given with meals or snacks to aid in digestion and absorption of fat and protein
   a. Record the number and consistency of stools per day to monitor the effectiveness of enzyme therapy.
4. Insulin or oral hypoglycemic agents to control diabetes
5. H_2 histamine receptor antagonist or proton pump inhibitor to decrease gastric acid

- Diet therapy includes:
  1. Fasting to avoid recurrent pain exacerbated by eating
  2. Providing jejunal or parenteral (TPN) nutrition if NPO for 3 or more days and for severe nutritional depletion
  3. Providing small, frequent, high-carbohydrate and high-protein feedings with limited fats when able to eat

Surgical Management

- Surgical management is not the primary intervention for chronic pancreatitis. Surgery may be indicated for intractable pain, incapacitating pain relapses, or complications such as pseudocyst and abscess.
- Surgical procedures include:
  1. Incision and drainage for abscesses or pseudocysts
  2. Laparoscopic cholecystectomy or choledochotomy for underlying biliary tract disease
  3. Sphincterotomy (incision of the sphincter) for fibrosis
  4. Pancreatojejunostomy (the pancreatic duct is opened and anastomosed to the jejunum, relieving obstruction) to relieve pain and preserve pancreatic tissue and function
  5. Partial pancreatectomy, which may be performed for advanced pancreatitis or disabling pain
  6. Vagotomy with gastric antrectomy to alter nerve stimulation and decrease pancreatic secretion
- For preoperative and postoperative care, see care of the patient undergoing a Whipple procedure under Cancer, Pancreatic.

Community-Based Care

- Health teaching is aimed at preventing further exacerbations.
  1. Avoid known precipitating factors, such as alcohol and foods with a high-fat content.
  2. Comply with diet instructions: high protein, high carbohydrate, low or no fat.
  3. Follow written instructions and prescriptions for pancreatic enzyme therapy:
     a. How and when to take enzymes
     b. The importance of maintaining therapy

P

c. The importance of notifying the physician of increased steatorrhea, abdominal distention, cramping, and skin breakdown

4. Comply with elevated glucose management, including oral hypoglycemic drugs or insulin injections and monitoring of blood glucose levels.

5. Keep follow-up visits with the physicians.

- Refer the patient to financial counseling, social services, vocational rehabilitation, home health services, and Alcoholics Anonymous, as needed.

PARALYSIS, FACIAL

- Facial paralysis, or Bell's palsy, is an acute paralysis of cranial nerve VII, with maximal paralysis reached within 2 to 5 days of onset.
- The disorder is characterized by an inability to close the eye, wrinkle the forehead, smile, whistle, or grimace; the face appears masklike and sags.
- This syndrome is thought to be caused by inflammation from herpes simplex virus-1 (HSV-1).
- Treatment includes:
  1. Administering antiviral agents early in the syndrome
  2. Administering mild analgesics for pain
  3. Protecting the eye from corneal abrasion or ulceration by patching and administering artificial tears
  4. Teaching the patient to use warm moist heat, massage, and facial exercises such as whistling, grimacing, and blowing air out of the cheeks three or four times a day

PARKINSON DISEASE

OVERVIEW

- Parkinson disease is a debilitating neurologic disorder involving the basal ganglia and substantia nigra. Loss of dopamine in the affected central nervous system (CNS) structures results in difficulty with initiation and coordination of voluntary movement. Loss of other neurotransmitters can contribute to mood disorders and autonomic dysfunction.
- The disease is characterized by muscle rigidity, akinesia (slow movements), postural instability, and tremors.
- The disease involves five stages:
  1. *Stage 1*: Mild disease with unilateral limb involvement
  2. *Stage 2*: Bilateral limb involvement

3. *Stage 3*: Significant gait disturbances and moderate general-ized disability
4. *Stage 4*: Severe disability, akinesia, and muscle rigidity
5. *Stage 5*: Complete dependency in all aspects of ADLs

PATIENT-CENTERED COLLABORATIVE CARE

Assessment

- Obtain patient information about:
  1. Time and progression of symptoms such as resting tremors, bradykinesia, and difficulty in completing fine motor tasks such as handwriting
  2. Family history related to neurologic disorders
  3. History of head injury, which can damage central nervous system (CNS) structures
  4. Use of drugs to treat serious mental illness; some antipsy-chotic medications can have Parkinson-like adverse effects
- Assess for and document:
  1. Rigidity, which is present early in the disease process and progresses over time
     a. Cogwheel rigidity, manifested by a rhythmic interruption of the muscles of movement
     b. Plastic rigidity: mildly restrictive movements
     c. Lead-pipe rigidity: total resistance to movement
  2. Posture
     a. Stooped posture
     b. Flexed trunk
     c. Fingers adducted and flexed at the metacarpophalangeal joint
     d. Wrists slightly dorsiflexed
  3. Gait
     a. Slow and shuffling
     b. Short, hesitant steps
     c. Propulsive gait
     d. Difficulty stopping quickly
  4. Speech
     a. Soft, low-pitched voice
     b. Dysarthria
     c. Echolalia: automatic repetition of what another person says
     d. Repetition of sentences
     e. Change in voice volume, phonation, or articulation
  5. Motor
     a. Bradykinesia or difficulty completing two tasks simultaneously
     b. Akinesia

P

    c. Tremors, especially at rest
    d. "Pill-rolling" movement
    e. Masklike facies
    f. Difficulty chewing and swallowing
    g. Uncontrolled drooling, especially at night
    h. Difficulty getting into and out of bed
    i. Little arm swinging when walking
    j. Change in handwriting, micrographia
6. Autonomic dysfunction
    a. Orthostatic hypotension
    b. Excessive perspiration and oily skin
    c. Flushing, changes in skin texture
    d. Blepharospasm
7. Psychosocial
    a. Emotional lability
    b. Depression
    c. Paranoia
    d. Easily upset
    e. Rapid mood swings
    f. Cognitive impairments
    g. Delayed reaction time
    h. Sleep disturbances

Interventions

- Provide drug therapy:
  1. Administer drug therapy on time to maintain continuous therapeutic drug levels.
     a. Levodopa combinations
     b. Dopamine agonists
     c. Catechol-O-methyltransferase (COMT) inhibitors to interfere with the breakdown of dopamine in the CNS
     d. Anticholinergic drugs, if the patient's primary symptom is tremor
     e. Monoamine oxidase inhibitors
     f. Variety of investigational drugs
  2. Monitor the patient for drug toxicity and side effects such as delirium, cognitive impairment, decreased effectiveness of the drug, postural hypotension, and hallucination.
  3. Treatment of drug toxicity or tolerance includes:
     a. Reduction in drug dosage
     b. Change in drugs or in the frequency of administration
     c. Drug holiday (particularly with levodopa therapy) for up to 10 days with close surveillance
- Other interventions include:
  1. Physical therapy (PT) and occupational therapy (OT) consultations to plan and maintain a mobility and muscle-

stretching program (e.g., traditional exercise, yoga, tai chi) and exercises for the muscles of the face and tongue to facilitate swallowing and speech

2. Providing assistive devices for participation in ADLs; PT and OT consultation to provide training in ADLs and the use of adaptive devices

3. Teaching the patient and family to monitor the patient's sleeping pattern and to discuss whether it is safe for the patient to operate machinery or perform other potentially dangerous tasks

4. Monitoring the patient's ability to eat and swallow; monitoring food and fluid intake; collaborating with the registered dietitian for caloric calculation and diet planning

5. Assessing the need for a speech-language pathologist consultation for evaluation of swallowing dysfunction and communication problems

6. Teaching the patient to speak slowly and clearly; using alternative communication methods such as a communication board

7. Referring the patient and family to a social worker to help with financial and health insurance agencies and to state and social agencies and support groups

8. Instructing the patient with orthostatic hypotension to wear elastic stockings and to change position slowly, especially when moving from a sitting to a standing position

9. Allowing sufficient time for the patient to complete activities; scheduling appointments and activities for late in the morning to prevent rushing the patient, or scheduling them at the time of the patient's optimal level of functioning

10. Implementing interventions to prevent complications of immobility such as constipation, pressure ulcers, contractures, and atelectasis

- Surgical interventions may be used to treat severe or early onset of Parkinson disease.

1. Stereotactic pallidotomy can be a very effective treatment for Parkinson disease. Through a probe, the target area in the brain receives a mild electrical stimulation to decrease tremor and rigidity. The probe is placed in the ideal location, and a temporary lesion is made. If this is successful, a permanent lesion is made.

2. Unilateral thalamotomy treats the tremor through thermocoagulation of brain cells.

3. Deep brain stimulation involves placing a thin electrode in the thalamus or subthalamus and connecting it to a "pacemaker" that delivers electrical current to interfere with

"tremor cells." The electrodes are connected to an implantable pulse generator that is placed underneath the skin in the patient's chest, something like a cardiac pacemaker.

4. Experimental surgical treatments include brain graft surgery, which consists of transplanting small pieces of the patient's own adrenal gland into the caudate nucleus of the brain; fetal tissue transplantation; and gene therapy, among others.

PELVIC INFLAMMATORY DISEASE

OVERVIEW

- Pelvic inflammatory disease (PID) is a complex infectious process in which organisms from the lower genital tract migrate from the endocervix upward through the uterine cavity into the fallopian tubes.
- It is a major cause of infertility and ectopic pregnancies.
- It is most often caused by sexually transmitted organisms, especially *Chlamydia trachomatis* and *Neisseria gonorrhoeae*. Other organisms may include *Gardnerella vaginalis*, *Haemophilus influenzae*, *Staphylococcus*, *Streptococcus*, and *Escherichia coli*.
- The infection may spread to other organs and tissues, including the uterus, fallopian tubes, and adjacent pelvic structures such as the ovaries, parametrium, and peritoneal cavity.
- Resultant infections include:
  1. Endometritis (infection of the endometrial cavity)
  2. Salpingitis (inflammation of the fallopian tubes)
  3. Oophoritis (ovarian infection)
  4. Parametritis (infection of the parametrium)
  5. Peritonitis (infection of the peritoneal cavity)
  6. Tubal or tubo-ovarian abscess
- Sepsis and death can occur, especially if treatment is delayed or inadequate.
- Although common manifestations include tenderness in the tubes and ovaries (adnexa) and low, dull abdominal pain, some patients have only mild discomfort or menstrual irregularity, and others experience no symptoms at all. These variations can make the diagnosis of PID challenging.

PATIENT-CENTERED COLLABORATIVE CARE

Assessment

- Obtain patient information about:
  1. Medical history
  2. Menstrual history
  3. Obstetric and sexual history

4. Previous episodes of PID or other sexually transmitted diseases
5. Contraceptive use
6. Previous reproductive surgery
7. Abnormal vaginal bleeding
8. Dysuria (painful urination)
9. Increase or change in vaginal discharge
10. Dyspareunia (painful sexual intercourse)
11. Risk factors, including:
    a. Age younger than 26 years
    b. Multiple sexual partners
    c. Intrauterine device (IUD) in place
    d. Smoking
- Assess for and document:
  1. Pain, especially lower abdominal pain
  2. Fever and chills
  3. Discomfort with movement
  4. Hunched-over gait
  5. Abdominal tenderness, rigidity, or rebound tenderness
- Assess for psychosocial issues, such as:
  1. Anxiety and fear
  2. Need for reassurance and support during the physical examination
  3. Embarrassment
  4. Discomfort when discussing symptoms or sexual history
- Diagnosis is made on the basis of manifestations, history, abnormal cervical or vaginal mucopurulent discharge, presence of WBCs on saline microscopy of vaginal secretions, and laboratory documentation of cervical infection with *N. gonorrhoeae* or *Chlamydia*. Other tests that may be helpful include ultrasonography, MRI, and endometrial biopsy.

Planning and Implementation
❖**Collaborative Problem:** Infection
- Uncomplicated PID is usually treated on an ambulatory care basis.
- Hospitalization for PID is recommended if the patient has a more complicated history, does not respond to oral antibiotic therapy, or has severe illness.
- Drug therapy includes:
  1. Oral or parenteral antibiotics, or both, for 14 days
  2. Hospitalization with IV antibiotic therapy and further evaluation if the infection does not respond to earlier antibiotic therapy
- Teaching the patient about the need to:
  1. Obtain adequate rest.

2. Abstain from sexual intercourse.
3. Check her temperature twice a day.
4. Be seen by the health care provider within 72 hours after starting the antibiotics and then at 1 and 2 weeks from the time of the initial diagnosis.

- In a small number of patients, a laparotomy may be needed to remove an abscess.

❖**NDx:** Acute Pain

- Interventions for pain management with PID include:
  1. Administering antibiotic therapy
  2. Administering mild analgesics
  3. Applying heat to the lower abdomen or back
  4. Encouraging the patient to maintain bedrest in a semi-Fowler position

❖**NDx:** Anxiety

- Nursing interventions are aimed at understanding the patient's perspective of the diagnosis and future complications, especially the possibility of infertility.
  1. Provide an atmosphere of comfort for the patient to express feelings and ask questions.
  2. Give accurate information about the diagnosis, treatment, and prognosis.
  3. Help the patient assess the emotional support available from family members or significant others.
  4. Teach about relaxation techniques.

Community-Based Care

- Teach the patient about:
  1. Signs of persistent or recurrent infection (persistent pain, dysmenorrhea, low backache, fever)
  2. Prevention strategies for all sexually transmitted diseases (STDs)
     a. Decrease the number of partners
     b. Consistent condom use
  3. The importance of completing the antibiotic therapy and keeping follow-up appointments
  4. The importance of having sexual partners examined and treated
  5. Contraception methods and the patient's need or desire for it
- Provide nonjudgmental emotional support.
- Allow time for the woman to express her feelings.
- Refer patients with infertility to a clinic specializing in infertility treatment and counseling.
- Collaborate with the case manager or social worker to locate community resources for free or discounted drugs for women who cannot afford the cost.

PERICARDITIS

OVERVIEW

- Acute pericarditis is an inflammation or alteration of the pericardium, the membranous sac enclosing the heart.
- There are two types of pericarditis:
  1. Acute pericarditis, which is most commonly associated with infective organisms (bacteria, viruses, fungi), malignant neoplasms, postmyocardial infarction syndrome, postpericardiotomy syndrome, systemic connective tissue diseases, renal failure, and idiopathic causes
  2. Chronic constrictive pericarditis, which is caused by tuberculosis, radiation therapy, trauma, renal failure, and metastatic cancer, with the pericardium becoming rigid, preventing adequate ventricular filling and resulting in cardiac failure

PATIENT-CENTERED COLLABORATIVE CARE

- Obtain patient information about:
  1. History of cardiac disease, cardiac surgery, chest trauma, or recent systemic infections
  2. History of chest radiation, connective tissue diseases, or cancer
- Assess for and document:
  1. Substernal precordial pain that can radiate to the left neck, shoulder, and back and is aggravated by breathing, coughing, and swallowing
  2. Pericardial friction rub
  3. Acute pericarditis
     a. Elevated WBC count
     b. ST-T wave elevation on electrocardiography (ECG)
     c. Fever (infectious cause)
  4. Chronic constrictive pericarditis
     a. Right-sided heart failure, including dyspnea, exertional fatigue, and orthopnea
     b. Pericardial thickening on echocardiogram and CT scan
     c. Inverted or flat T waves on ECG
     d. Atrial fibrillation
- Treatment depends on the type of pericarditis.
- Acute pericarditis is treated by:
  1. Administering nonsteroidal anti-inflammatory agents
  2. Administering corticosteroid therapy
  3. Administering antibiotics
  4. Encouraging rest
- For chronic constrictive pericarditis, the definitive treatment is surgical excision of the pericardium (pericardiectomy).

- Complications of pericarditis include pericardial effusions and cardiac tamponade, which is manifested by jugular venous distention, paradoxical pulse (systolic blood pressure at least 10 mm Hg higher on expiration than on inspiration), decreased cardiac output, muffled heart sounds, and circulatory collapse.
  1. Treatment of cardiac tamponade includes pericardiocentesis, in which a needle is inserted into the pericardial space. After the needle is properly positioned, a catheter is inserted and the pericardial fluid is withdrawn. IV fluids are administered to improve cardiac output.
  2. For recurrent tamponade or effusions or adhesions resulting from chronic pericarditis, a partial or complete pericardiectomy is done to allow adequate ventricular filling and contraction.

PERITONITIS

OVERVIEW

- Peritonitis is an acute inflammation of the viscera/parietal and endothelial peritoneum (lining of the abdominal cavity).
- Primary peritonitis is an acute bacterial infection that develops as a result of contamination of the peritoneum through the vascular system and is rare.
- Secondary peritonitis is caused by bacterial invasion as a result of perforation or a penetrating wound, such as appendicitis, diverticulitis, peptic ulcer, ascending genital infection, or a gunshot injury to the abdomen. Chemical peritonitis is the result of leakage of bile, pancreatic enzymes, and gastric acid.
- Peritonitis can be life-threatening with accompanying shock, respiratory problems, and paralytic ileus.

PATIENT-CENTERED COLLABORATIVE CARE

Assessment

- Obtain patient information about:
  1. History of abdominal trauma or surgery
  2. Pain that is aggravated by coughing or movement of any type and that is relieved by knee flexion
  3. Abdominal distention
  4. Anorexia, nausea, or vomiting
  5. Hiccups
  6. Low-grade fever or recent spikes in temperature
- Assess for and document:
  1. Character of abdominal pain, onset, duration, location, quality, aggravating and alleviating factors. The cardinal signs of peritonitis are abdominal pain and tenderness.

2. Abdominal rigidity ("boardlike") or distention with rebound tenderness
3. Absent bowel sounds
4. Fever with tachycardia
5. Dehydration as evidenced by dry mucous membranes, poor skin turgor, and decreased urinary output
6. Tachypnea with low peripheral oxygenation (decreased SpO_2)

● Diagnostic tests may include:
1. CBC count if an elevated WBC count is concerning
2. Serum electrolytes, blood urea nitrogen (BUN), and creatinine
3. Abdominal x-rays to determine presence of dilation, edema, and inflammation of the intestines
4. Peritoneal lavage to determine presence of WBCs, pus, bile, or other indicators of perforation and infection

> 🔳 Critical Rescue ◆ A sudden worsening of abdominal pain or a change from localized to generalized abdominal pain may signal a medical emergency. This symptom needs to be communicated, along with vital signs, to the medical provider immediately to avoid patient progression to vascular and respiratory compromise.

Interventions

P

Nonsurgical Management
● Administer IV fluids and broad-spectrum antibiotics.
● Monitor daily weight.
● Record intake and output.
● Keep the patient on NPO status.
● Monitor and record drainage from the nasogastric (NG) tube used for gastric and intestinal decompression.
● Provide pain management with IV analgesics; anticipate use of patient-controlled analgesia (PCA) pump.
● Administer oxygen as prescribed according to the patient's respiratory status.

Surgical Management
● Surgical management may be necessary to identify and repair the underlying cause of the peritonitis.
● Surgery is focused on controlling the contamination, removing foreign material from the peritoneal cavity, and draining fluid collections.
● During surgery, the peritoneum is irrigated with antibiotic solutions, and drainage catheters are inserted.

- Provide routine postoperative care as described in Part One, including:
  1. Close monitoring of the patient's cardiovascular stability for early detection of shock (level of consciousness, heart rate, blood pressure, and urine output should remain within normal limits for the patient)
  2. Providing meticulous wound care; irrigating and packing the wound, as prescribed
  3. Assisting the patient to gradually increase his or her activity level

Considerations for Older Adults

The early signs and symptoms of dehydration in the older adult may consist of a subtle decrease in mental status, such as confusion or lethargy. Do not delay in communicating subtle changes in mentation.

Community-Based Care

- The patient may be discharged home or to a transitional care unit to complete antibiotic therapy and recovery.
- If the patient is discharged home, collaborate with the case manager to determine the need for assistance.
- Provide written and oral postoperative instructions, including:
  1. The necessity to report any redness, swelling, tenderness, or unusual or foul-smelling drainage from the wound
  2. Care of the incision and dressing; ensure that the patient has the necessary equipment to perform wound care (dressings, solutions, catheter-tipped syringe); stress the importance of handwashing.
  3. The need to report fever (typically 101° F [38° C]) or abdominal pain to the physician
  4. Pain drug administration and monitoring
  5. Dietary limitations, if necessary
  6. Activity limitations, including limited lifting until healing has occurred

PHEOCHROMOCYTOMA

OVERVIEW

- Pheochromocytoma is a catecholamine-producing tumor that arises in the adrenal medulla.
- These tumors are most often benign, but at least 10% are malignant.
- They produce, store, and release epinephrine and norepinephrine (NE), which stimulate adrenergic receptors and can have wide-ranging adverse effects mimicking the action of the sympathetic division of the autonomic nervous system.

PATIENT-CENTERED COLLABORATIVE CARE

Assessment

- Obtain patient information about intermittent manifestations, including:
  1. Severe headaches
  2. Palpitations
  3. Profuse diaphoresis
  4. Flushing
  5. Apprehension or sense of impending doom
  6. Pain in the chest or abdomen, with nausea and vomiting
- Assess for and document:
  1. Hypertension
  2. Tremors
  3. Weight loss

> ![] Clinical Landmine ♦ Do not palpate the abdomen, because this action could cause a sudden release of catecholamines and severe hypertension.

- Diagnosis is made on the basis of high urine levels of vanillylmandelic acid (VMA), metanephrine, and catecholamines; the clonidine suppression test; and MRI or CT scans to precisely locate tumors.

Interventions

- Surgery is performed to remove the tumors and the adrenal gland or glands.
- Provide preoperative care:
  1. Implementing routine preoperative care as discussed in Part One
  2. Monitoring blood pressure regularly; placing the cuff consistently on the same arm, with the patient in lying and standing positions
  3. Identifying stressors that may lead to a hypertensive crisis
  4. Teaching the patient to not smoke, drink caffeine-containing beverages, or change position suddenly
  5. Ensuring adequate hydration
  6. Providing a calm, restful environment
  7. Administering prescribed drug therapy to stabilize the patient's blood pressure (usually phenoxybenzamine [Dibenzyline])
- Provide postoperative care:
  1. Implementing routine postoperative care discussed in Part One
  2. Closely monitoring for hypertension, hypotension, and hypovolemia

3. Monitoring for hemorrhage and shock:
   a. Vital signs
   b. Fluid intake and output
4. Checking opioid effects on blood pressure

- If inoperable, tumors are managed with alpha-adrenergic and beta-adrenergic blocking agents and self-measurement of blood pressure with home monitoring equipment.

PHLEBITIS

- Phlebitis is an inflammation of the superficial veins caused by an irritant, commonly IV therapy.
- Phlebitis is manifested as a reddened, warm area radiating up an extremity.
- The patient may experience pain, soreness, and swelling of the extremity.
- Treatment involves application of warm, moist soaks, which dilate the vein and promote circulation. *Do not massage the area.*

PNEUMONIA

OVERVIEW

- *Pneumonia* is an excess of fluid in the lungs resulting from an inflammatory process.
- It can be caused by many infectious organisms and by inhalation of irritating agents or aspiration of stomach contents.
- Infectious pneumonias are categorized as community-acquired (CAP) or hospital-acquired (HAP); HAP is more likely to be resistant to antibiotics than is CAP.
- The inflammation and multiplication of organisms result in local capillary leak, edema, and exudate that reduce gas exchange and lead to hypoxemia, interfering with *oxygenation and tissue perfusion* and possibly leading to death.
- Risk factors for CAP:
  1. Older adult
  2. Never received the pneumococcal vaccination or had received it more than 6 years ago
  3. Not having received the influenza vaccine in the previous year
  4. Presence of a chronic health problem or other coexisting condition
  5. Recent exposure to respiratory viral or influenza infections
  6. Use of tobacco or alcohol

- Risk factors for HAP:
  1. Older adult
  2. Presence of a chronic lung disease
  3. Gram-negative colonization of the mouth, throat, and stomach
  4. Altered level of consciousness
  5. Recent aspiration event
  6. Presence of endotracheal, tracheostomy, or nasogastric (NG) tube
  7. Poor nutritional status
  8. Immunocompromised status (from disease or drug therapy)
  9. Drugs that increase gastric pH
  10. Mechanical ventilation

PATIENT-CENTERED COLLABORATIVE CARE
Assessment
- Obtain patient information about:
  1. Age
  2. Living, work, and school environments
  3. Diet, exercise, and sleep routines
  4. Swallowing problems
  5. Presence of a nasogastrointestinal tube
  6. Tobacco and alcohol use
  7. Past and current use of drugs, including drug addiction or injection drug use
  8. Past respiratory illnesses
  9. Recent exposure to influenza, pneumonia, or other viral infection
  10. Recent skin rashes, insect bites, or exposure to animals
  11. Chronic respiratory problems
  12. Home respiratory equipment use and cleaning
  13. Date of last influenza or pneumococcal vaccine
- Assess for and document:
  1. General appearance
  2. Breathing pattern; use of accessory muscles
  3. Chest or pleuritic pain or discomfort
  4. Chills and fever
  5. Cough
  6. Tachycardia
  7. Dyspnea and tachypnea
  8. Sputum production
  9. Oxygen saturation
  10. Crackles or wheezes
  11. Hypotension

12. Mental status changes (especially in an older adult)
13. Fatigue
14. Anxiety

Considerations for Older Adults

- The older adult with pneumonia often has weakness, fatigue, lethargy, confusion, and poor appetite.
- Fever and cough may be absent, but hypoxemia is usually present.
- The most common manifestation of pneumonia in the older adult patient is confusion from hypoxia rather than fever or cough.

- Diagnosis is based on manifestations, sputum Gram stain or culture, elevated WBC count, chest x-ray, and arterial blood gas (ABG) levels.

Planning and Implementation

❖**NDx:** Impaired Gas Exchange and Ineffective Airway Clearance
- Monitor rate, rhythm, depth, and effort of ventilation.
- Assess pulse oxymetry and administer oxygen by nasal cannula or mask as prescribed.
- Instruct the patient on the correct use of incentive spirometry (sustained maximal inspiration) and encourage him or her to perform 5 to 10 breaths per session every hour while awake.
- Assess the patient's ability to cough effectively.
- Encourage coughing and deep breathing at least every 2 hours.
- Monitor fluid intake and encourage the alert patient to drink at least 3 L of fluid daily unless another health problem requires fluid restriction.
- Administer prescribed bronchodilators and corticosteroids by aerosol nebulizer or by metered-dose inhaler.
- Monitor for complications such as hypoxemia, ventilatory failure, atelectasis, pleural effusion, and pleurisy.

❖**Collaborative Problem:** Potential for Sepsis
- Administer prescribed anti-infective therapy, based on organism sensitivity.
- For pneumonia resulting from aspiration of food or stomach contents, steroids and NSAIDs are used with antibiotics to reduce the inflammatory response.

Community-Based Care

- Teach the patient about:
  1. The importance of completing the full course of antibiotic therapy
  2. Notifying the health care provider if chills, fever, persistent cough, dyspnea, wheezing, hemoptysis, increased sputum

production, chest discomfort, or increasing fatigue recurs or if symptoms fail to resolve

3. The importance of getting plenty of rest and gradually increasing exercise
4. Preventing upper respiratory tract infections and viruses by:
   a. Avoiding crowds
   b. Avoiding people who have a cold or flu
   c. Avoiding exposure to irritants such as smoke
   d. Obtaining an annual influenza vaccination
   e. Obtaining the pneumococcal vaccination
5. The importance of eating a balanced diet with adequate fluid intake

- Encourage the patient to quit smoking, and provide information on smoking-cessation classes through the American Lung Association (ALA) and American Cancer Society.

PNEUMONIA, VENTILATOR-ASSOCIATED

- *Ventilator-associated pneumonia* (VAP) is a hospital-acquired pneumonia that develops in patients who have an endotracheal tube in place for mechanical ventilation.
- Although the presence of a tube providing a direct connection between the environment and the patient's lower respiratory passageways increases the risk for VAP, the risk can be reduced with conscientious assessment and meticulous nursing care.

P

National Patient Safety Goal

Three care actions, known as a *ventilator bundle*, have been shown to reduce the incidence of VAP: hand hygiene, oral care, and elevation of the head of the bed.

- Implement these practices for the ventilator bundle:
  1. If possible, perform oral care with a disinfecting oral rinse immediately *before* the intubation.
  2. Do not wear hand jewelry, especially rings, when providing care to ventilator patients.
  3. Wash hands before and after contact with the patient.
  4. Provide complete oral care at least every 12 hours.
  5. Remove subglottic secretions frequently (at least every 2 hours) or continuously (if the endotracheal tube has a separate lumen that opens directly above the tube cuff).
  6. Keep the head of the bed elevated to at least 30 degrees unless another health problem is a contraindication for this position.

7. Verify that an initial x-ray has been obtained to confirm the placement of any nasogastric (NG) tube before instilling drugs, fluids, or feedings into the tube.
8. Avoid turning the patient or placing him or her in the supine position (even briefly) within 1 hour after a bolus tube feeding.
9. Work with the patient and health care team to assist in the weaning process as soon as possible.

PNEUMOTHORAX

- *Pneumothorax*, also called a *collapsed lung*, is an accumulation of atmospheric air in the pleural space that results in a rise in chest pressure and a reduction in vital capacity.
- It is often caused by blunt chest trauma and may occur with some degree of hemothorax. It also may occur spontaneously.
- Assess for and document:
  1. Reduced breath sounds on auscultation
  2. Hyperresonance on percussion
  3. Prominence of the involved side of the chest, which moves poorly with respirations
  4. Deviation of the trachea away from (closed) or toward (open) the affected side
  5. Pleuritic chest pain
  6. Tachypnea
  7. Subcutaneous emphysema (air under the skin in the subcutaneous tissues)
- An ultrasound examination or a chest x-ray is used for diagnosis.
- Chest tubes may be needed to allow the air to escape and the lung to reinflate.

PNEUMOTHORAX, TENSION

- Tension pneumothorax is a rapidly developing and life-threatening complication of blunt chest trauma that results from an air leak in the lung or chest wall.
- Air forced into the chest cavity causes complete collapse of the affected lung.
- Air that enters the pleural space during inspiration does not exit during expiration, allowing air to continue to collect under pressure, compressing blood vessels, limiting venous return, and reducing cardiac output.
- Causes include blunt chest trauma, mechanical ventilation with positive end-expiratory pressure (PEEP), closed-chest

drainage (chest tubes), and insertion of central venous access catheters.

> 🔳 Critical Rescue ◆ If not promptly detected and treated, tension pneumothorax is quickly fatal.

- Assess for and document:
  1. Asymmetry of the thorax
  2. Tracheal movement *away* from midline to the *unaffected* side
  3. Respiratory distress
  4. Absence of breath sounds on one side
  5. Distended neck veins
  6. Cyanosis
  7. Hypertympanic sound on percussion over the affected side
- Initial management includes insertion of a large-bore needle into the second intercostal space in the midclavicular line of the affected side.
- Chest tube placement into the fourth intercostal space then follows, with water seal drainage until the lung reinflates.

POLIO AND POSTPOLIO SYNDROME

- Poliomyelitis (polio) is an acute viral disease characterized by destruction of the motor cells of the anterior horn of the spinal cord, the brainstem, and the motor strip of the frontal lobe. The disease is rare in North America because immunization during childhood is prevalent. Treatment is symptomatic.
- Postpolio syndrome is a new onset of weakness, pain, and fatigue in people who had poliomyelitis 30 or more years previously. Physical and emotional stressors are contributing factors. Treatment is symptomatic and includes lifestyle modifications and adaptive devices to preserve energy and function.

POLYNEURITIS AND POLYNEUROPATHY

OVERVIEW

- The terms polyneuritis, polyneuropathy, and peripheral neuropathy may be used interchangeably.
- The disorders are characterized by muscle weakness with or without atrophy; pain that is described as stabbing, cutting, or searing; paresthesia or loss of sensation; impaired reflexes; autonomic manifestations; or a combination of these symptoms.
- The most common type is a symmetric polyneuropathy in which the patient experiences decreased sensation along with a

feeling that the extremity is asleep. Tingling, burning, tightness, or aching sensations usually start in the feet and progress to the level of the knee before affecting the hands ("glove and stocking" neuropathy).

- The disorders can result from inflammatory or noninflammatory processes; both can damage cranial and peripheral nerves.
- Factors associated with polyneuropathy include diabetes; renal or hepatic failure; alcoholism; vascular disease; vitamin B_1, B_6, and B_{12} deficiencies; and exposure to heavy metals or industrial solvents.

PATIENT-CENTERED COLLABORATIVE CARE

- Assess for and document:
  1. Light touch sensation and pain in the distal extremities
  2. Position sense and kinesthetic sensation
  3. Any signs of injury
  4. Indications of autonomic dysfunction, such as orthostatic hypotension, abnormal sweating, and miosis
- Treatment consists of elimination or treatment of the underlying cause and symptomatic therapy.
  1. Treat the underlying cause.
  2. Supplement the patient's diet with vitamins.
  3. Provide pain management as needed.
  4. Provide health teaching, including the importance of foot care and of inspecting the extremities for injuries.
  5. Stress the importance of wearing shoes at all times and of purchasing well-fitting shoes.
  6. Teach the patient how to recognize potential hazards, such as exposure to extremes of environmental temperature.
  7. Discourage smoking.
  8. Promote glycemic control.

POLYPS, GASTROINTESTINAL

- GI tract polyps are small growths covered with mucosa that are attached to the intestinal surface; polyps have the potential to become malignant.
- One form of inherited GI polyps is particularly concerning to the health care provider: Familial adenomatous polyposis (FAP) and hereditary nonpolyposis colorectal cancer (HNPCC) are genetic syndromes characterized by the progressive development of colorectal adenomas. If these conditions are left untreated, colorectal cancer will occur.
- Pedunculated polyps are stalklike, with a thin stem attaching them to the intestinal wall.

- Polyps are usually asymptomatic but can cause rectal bleeding, intestinal obstruction, and intussusception.
- Polyps can usually be removed by polypectomy with an electro-cautery snare that fits through a colonoscope, eliminating the need for abdominal surgery.
- After the procedure, monitor for:
  1. Abdominal distention and pain
  2. Rectal bleeding
  3. Mucopurulent rectal drainage
  4. Fever
- Teach the patient about the need for regular, routine monitoring if there is a family history of polyps or a finding of polyps with a screening colonoscopy. Specific follow-up timeframe varies but generally occurs with 3 years.

PRESSURE ULCERS

OVERVIEW

- A *pressure ulcer* is tissue damage that occurs when the skin and underlying soft tissue are compressed between a bony prominence and an external surface for an extended period.
- They form most commonly over the sacrum, hips, and ankles but can occur on any body surface.
- The major pathologic mechanism is tissue compression from pressure that restricts blood flow to the skin, resulting in reduced tissue perfusion and oxygenation and leading to cell death.
- The forces that lead to pressure ulcer formation include:
  1. *Pressure*: A mechanical force occurring as a result of gravity, compressing blood vessels at the point of contact and leading to ischemia, inflammation, and tissue necrosis
  2. *Friction*: A mechanical force occurring when surfaces rub the skin and irritate or directly pull off epithelial tissue (as when the patient is dragged or pulled across bed linen)
  3. *Shear* or *shearing forces*: Mechanical forces occurring when the skin itself is stationary and the tissues below the skin (e.g., fat, muscle) shift or move, reducing the blood supply to the skin and leading to skin hypoxia, anoxia, ischemia, inflammation, and necrosis

Considerations for Older Adults

- Older adults are at particular risk for pressure ulcers because of the presence of age-related skin changes.
- They are exposed to mechanical shearing forces, such as removal of tape or friction from tightly applied restraints.

- Skin moisture and irritation resulting from incontinence and friction over bony prominences can lead to partial-thickness skin destruction and early pressure ulcer formation.
- Once formed, these chronic wounds are slow to heal, resulting in increased morbidity and health care costs.
- Complications include sepsis, kidney failure, infectious arthritis, and osteomyelitis.

- Stages of pressure ulcers:
    1. *Stage I*: The skin is intact, is red, and does not blanch with external pressure.
    2. *Stage II*: The skin is not intact, and there is a partial-thickness skin loss of the epidermis or dermis. It may appear as an abrasion, a blister (open or fluid filled), or a shallow crater, and bruising is *not* present.
    3. *Stage III*: In which skin loss is full thickness and subcutaneous tissues may be damaged or necrotic. Bone, tendon, and muscle are *not* exposed, but the fat may show a deep, crater-like appearance. Undermining and tunneling may or may not be present.
    4. *Stage IV*: In which skin loss is full thickness with exposed or palpable muscle, tendon, or bone. Undermining, tunneling, and sinus tracts may be present. Slough and eschar are often present on at least part of the wound.
    5. *Unstageable*: In which skin loss is full thickness, and the base is completely covered with slough or eschar, obscuring the true depth of the wound.
- Health promotion and maintenance
    1. Pressure ulcers can be prevented if the risk is recognized and intervention begins early.
    2. Identify patients at risk for pressure ulcer formation. Risk factors include:
        a. Mental status changes
        b. Decreased sensory perception
        c. Impaired mobility
        d. Poor nutritional status
        e. Incontinence
- Implement prevention interventions:
    1. Performing proper positioning by:
        a. Padding contact surfaces with foam, silicon gel, air pads, or other pressure-relieving pads
        b. Keeping the head of the bed elevated less than 30 degrees to prevent shearing
        c. Using a lift sheet to move the patient in the bed and not dragging or sliding the patient

  d. Avoiding positioning the patient directly on the trochanter when placing him or her on the side
  e. Repositioning an immobile patient every 2 hours while in bed and every 1 hour while sitting in a chair
  f. Not placing a rubber ring or doughnut under the patient's sacral area
  g. Using a designated slide board or a mechanical lift when moving an immobile patient from a bed to another surface
  h. Keeping the patient's skin directly off plastic surfaces
  i. Keeping the patient's heels off the bed surface with the use of a bed pillow under the ankles
2. Ensuring adequate nutrition by:
  a. Providing a fluid intake of between 2000 and 3000 mL daily
  b. Helping the patient maintain an adequate intake of protein and calories
3. Providing skin care, including:
  a. Performing a daily inspection of the patient's entire skin
  b. Documenting and reporting any manifestations of skin infection
  c. Using moisturizers daily on dry skin, and applying them when skin is damp
  d. Keeping moisture from prolonged contact with skin
  e. Drying areas where two skin surfaces touch, such as the axilla and under the breasts
  f. Placing absorbent pads under areas where perspiration collects
  g. Using moisture barriers on skin areas where wound drainage or incontinence occurs

> **Clinical Landmine** ◆ Do not massage bony prominences.

  h. Humidifying the room
4. Ensuring appropriate skin cleaning by:
  a. Cleaning the skin as soon as possible after soiling occurs and at routine intervals
  b. Using a mild, heavily fatted soap or gentle commercial cleanser for incontinence
  c. Using tepid rather than hot water
  d. Using a disposable cleaning cloth that contains a skin barrier agent when cleaning the perineal area
  e. Using the minimal scrubbing force necessary to remove soil

P

   f. Patting gently rather than rubbing the skin dry

   g. Avoiding the use of powders or talcs directly on the perineum

   h. Applying a commercial skin barrier after cleansing to those areas in frequent contact with urine or feces

5. Using appropriate pressure-relieving and pressure-reducing devices

   a. Pressure-relief devices consistently reduce pressure to less than the capillary closing pressure.

   b. Pressure-reduction devices lower pressure to less than that of a standard hospital mattress or chair surface but do not consistently reduce pressure to less than the capillary closing pressure.

> **Clinical Landmine ♦** These devices are not effective for preventing pressure ulcers when used alone. They must be used together with a turning schedule and other skin care measures.

PATIENT-CENTERED COLLABORATIVE CARE

Assessment

- Obtain patient information about:
  1. The cause and specific circumstances of skin loss
  2. Whether any contributing factors are present, such as prolonged bedrest, immobility, incontinence, diabetes mellitus, inadequate nutrition or hydration, altered mental status (decreased sensory perception), or peripheral vascular disease
- Assess for and document:
  1. The entire body for areas of skin injury or pressure
  2. General appearance for body weight and the proportion of weight to height
  3. Overall cleanliness of the skin, hair, and nails
  4. Any loss of mobility or range of joint motion
- Assess existing wounds daily for:
  1. Location, size, color, extent of tissue involvement, using a clock face approach to the wound, with 12 o'clock in the direction of the patient's head and 6 o'clock in the direction of the patient's feet
     a. Length
     b. Width
     c. Depth
  2. Exudate
  3. Condition of surrounding tissue
  4. Presence of foreign bodies

5. Whether reddened areas blanch with pressure
6. Texture of the wound
7. Presence of undermining and tunneling
8. Comparison of existing wound features with those documented previously, to determine the current state of healing or deterioration
9. Presence of wound infection
   a. Inflammation
   b. Induration
   c. Redness
   d. Foul odor
   e. Moderate to heavy exudate
   f. Cellulitis
   g. Progressive increase in ulcer size or depth
   h. Fever (systemic infection)
   i. Elevated WBC count (systemic infection)
- Assess for psychosocial issues, including:
  1. Altered body image
  2. Coping patterns
  3. Changes in lifestyle and ADL
  4. Financial resources
  5. Patient's and family's willingness and skill in cleaning the wound and applying a dressing
- Assess laboratory data for:
  1. Wound contamination, which is the presence of organisms without any manifestation of infection
  2. Wound infection, which is contamination with pathogenic organisms to the degree that growth and spread cannot be controlled by the body's immune defenses
  3. Systemic infection with bacteremia and sepsis

Planning and Implementation

❖**NDx:** Impaired Skin Integrity

Nonsurgical Management
- Dressing and wound care are the basis for pressure ulcer management. A properly designed dressing can speed healing by removing unwanted debris from the ulcer surface, protecting exposed healthy tissues and creating a barrier between the body and the environment until the ulcer is closed.
  1. *Hydrophobic* (nonabsorbent, waterproof) dressing materials are used when the wound is relatively free of drainage. They protect the ulcer from external contamination.
  2. *Hydrophilic* (absorbent) materials draw excessive drainage away from the ulcer surface, preventing maceration.
- The frequency of dressing changes depends on the amount of necrotic material or exudate.

1. Dry gauze dressings are changed when "strike-through" occurs or when the outer layer of the dressing first becomes saturated with exudate.
2. Gauze dressings used for débridement, such as those that are wetted and placed on a wound, allowed to become damp, and then removed, are changed often enough to take off any loose debris or exudate, usually every 4 to 6 hours.
3. Synthetic dressings are changed when exudate causes the adhesive seal to break and leakage to occur.

- Before reapplying any dressing, gently clean the ulcer surface with saline or a nontoxic wound cleanser as prescribed.
- Drug therapy with topical antibacterial agents is often needed to control bacterial growth.
- Nutrition therapy requires adequate nutritional intake of calories, protein, vitamins, minerals, and water.
  1. Perform a nutritional assessment at least weekly.
  2. Coordinate with the nutritionist to encourage the patient to eat a well-balanced diet, emphasizing protein, vegetables, fruit, whole grain breads and cereals, and vitamins.
- New technologies may be useful for chronic ulcers that remain open for months.
  1. *Electrical stimulation* is the application of a low-voltage current to a wound area to increase blood vessel growth and promote granulation.
  2. *Vacuum-assisted wound closure* (VAC) is the use of a suction tube that is covered by a special sponge and sealed in place for 48 hours. During that time, continuous low-level negative pressure is applied through the suction tube.
  3. *Hyperbaric oxygen* (HBO) therapy is the administration of oxygen under high pressure, which raises the tissue oxygen concentration.
  4. *Topical growth factors* are biologically active substances that stimulate cell movement and growth and are applied to the wound.
  5. *Skin substitutes* are engineered products that aid in the temporary or permanent closure of various types of wounds.

Surgical Management

- Surgical management includes removal of necrotic tissue (surgical débridement) and skin grafting or use of muscle flaps to close wounds that cannot heal by epithelialization and contraction.
- Provide preoperative care:
  1. Implementing routine preoperative care as described in Part One
  2. Monitoring potential donor sites

3. Maintaining the integrity of the donor skin

4. Avoiding minor injuries that may result in infection and graft loss

- Provide postoperative care, including:

   1. Implementing routine postoperative care as described in Part One

   2. Elevating and resting the grafted area to allow revascularization

   3. Maintaining graft site immobilization with bulky cotton pressure dressings for 3 to 5 days

   4. After dressings are removed, monitoring the graft for indications of failure to vascularize, nonadherence to the wound, or graft necrosis:

      a. A pale flap with delayed capillary filling when blanched

      b. A dusky color or sharp line of color change

   5. Caring for donor sites

      a. Protecting the area from injury and infection

      b. Positioning the patient to avoid pressure on the site

      c. Using an overbed cradle to tent the sheets

      d. Trimming the separating gauze (when gauze dressings are used) close to the skin surface reduces the chance of accidentally moving the still adherent gauze before healing is complete

      e. Administering analgesics as prescribed

      f. Using special low-pressure or air-fluidized mattresses when grafts or donor sites are on the posterior body surface

❖Collaborative Problem: Risk for Infection and Wound Extension

- Priority nursing interventions focus on preventing wound infections and on identifying wound infections early to prevent complications.

   1. Monitoring the ulcer's appearance using objective criteria

   2. Re-evaluating the treatment plan if an ulcer shows no progress toward healing within 7 to 10 days or worsens

   3. Checking for manifestations of wound infection:

      a. Increased redness at the wound margins

      b. Edema

      c. Purulent and malodorous drainage

      d. Tenderness of the wound margins

      e. Increase in the size or depth of the lesion

      f. Changes in the color or texture of the granulation tissue

   4. Maintaining a safe environment by:

      a. Performing meticulous wound care

      b. Teaching all personnel to use standard precautions

      c. Disposing properly of soiled dressings and linens

Community-Based Care

- Teach the patient and family how to modify the home and supplies to manage wound care.
- Ensure that the patient or the person who will be performing the wound care demonstrates facility in removing the dressing, cleaning the wound, and applying the dressing.
- Explain the manifestations of wound infection, and remind the patient and family to report these to the health care provider or wound care clinic.
- Stress the need for those with pressure ulcers on the legs to rest frequently, with the leg elevated, to avoid or reduce edema.
- Assist the family of an immobile patient in making arrangements for around-the-clock repositioning, as often as every 2 to 4 hours, to prevent further breakdown.
- Work with the social worker or case manager to obtain special beds or mattress overlays for the home.
- Encourage the patient to eat a balanced diet with frequent high-protein snacks.
- Emphasize the need to keep the skin of an incontinent patient clean and dry.
- Make referrals for home care nursing visits, if needed, to monitor wound progress.

PRIMARY PULMONARY HYPERTENSION

OVERVIEW

- *Primary pulmonary hypertension* (PPH) is a problem of the pulmonary blood vessels in which blood vessel constriction with increasing vascular resistance occurs in the lungs.
- Pulmonary blood pressure rises and blood flow decreases, leading to poor perfusion and hypoxemia. Eventually, the right side of the heart fails (*cor pulmonale*) as a result of the continuous workload of pumping against the high pulmonary pressures.
- PPH can occur as a complication of other lung disorders or for unknown reasons.
- The disorder is rare and occurs mostly in women between the ages of 20 and 40 years.
- Without treatment, death usually occurs within 2 years after diagnosis.

Genetic Considerations

- About 50% of patients with PPH have a genetic mutation in the *BMPR2* gene, which codes for a growth factor receptor. Excessive activation of this receptor allows increased growth of arterial smooth muscle in the lungs, making these arteries thicker.

- Because many more people have mutations in this gene than have PPH, it is thought that the mutations increase susceptibility to PPH when other, often unknown, environmental factors also are present.
- Teach women who have a first-degree relative (parent or sibling) with PPH to have regular health checkups and to consult a health care provider whenever pulmonary problems are present.

PATIENT-CENTERED COLLABORATIVE CARE

Assessment

- Assess for and document:
  1. Dyspnea and fatigue in an otherwise healthy adult
  2. Angina-like chest pain
- Diagnosis is made from the results of right-sided heart catheterization showing elevated pulmonary pressures.

Interventions

- Nonsurgical interventions focus on reducing pulmonary pressures and slowing the development of cor pulmonale.
- Drug therapy involves drugs that dilate pulmonary vessels and prevent clot formation.
  1. Continuous IV infusion of epoprostenol (Flolan) or treprostinil (Remodulin)
  2. Endothelin-receptor antagonists, bosentan (Tracleer)
  3. Warfarin (Coumadin)
  4. Calcium channel blockers, such as nifedipine (Procardia) and diltiazem (Cardizem)

> 🔲 Critical Rescue ◆ Although epoprostenol therapy is very effective, deaths have been reported if drug delivery is interrupted for even a few minutes. Teach the patient to always have backup drug cassettes and battery packs. If these are not available or the line is disrupted, the patient should go to the emergency department immediately.

- Teaching patients about the need to:
  1. Use strict aseptic technique in all aspects of manipulating the drug delivery system.
  2. Notify the pulmonologist at the first sign of any respiratory or systemic infection.
- Surgical management of PPH involves single-lung or whole-lung transplantation.
- If cor pulmonale also is present, the patient may need combined heart-lung transplantation.

PROLAPSE, MITRAL VALVE

- Mitral valve prolapse occurs when the heart valve leaflets prolapse into the left atrium during systole.
- Mitral valve prolapse is usually benign (asymptomatic) but may progress to pronounced mitral regurgitation.
- Assess for and document:
  1. Atypical chest pain; sharp pain localized in the left side of the chest
  2. Dizziness and syncope
  3. Palpitations
  4. Midsystolic click or a late systolic murmur that may be audible at the apex
- Valve replacement surgery is indicated for symptomatic mitral regurgitation.

PROLAPSE, UTERINE

- *Uterine prolapse* is the downward displacement of the uterus. It can be caused by neuromuscular damage of childbirth; increased intra-abdominal pressure related to pregnancy, obesity, or physical exertion; or weakening of pelvic support due to decreased estrogen.
- Whenever the uterus is displaced, other structures such as the bladder, rectum, and small intestine can protrude through the vaginal walls. A *cystocele* is a protrusion of the bladder through the vaginal wall; it can lead to stress incontinence and urinary tract infections. A *rectocele* is a protrusion of the rectum through a weakened vaginal wall.
- Assessment findings include:
  1. Patient's report of feeling as if "something is falling out"
  2. Dyspareunia
  3. Backache
  4. Feeling of heaviness or pressure in the pelvis
  5. Protrusion of the cervix when the woman is asked to bear down
  6. Bowel or bladder problems, such as urinary incontinence, constipation, hemorrhoids, or fecal impaction
- Interventions are based on the degree of prolapse.
  1. Nonsurgical management may include:
     a. Teaching women to improve pelvic support and tone by pelvic floor muscle exercises (PFME, also called Kegel exercises)
     b. Use of space-filling devices such as pessaries or spheres worn intravaginally to elevate the uterine prolapse

   c. Intravaginal estrogen therapy
   d. Bladder training and attention to complete emptying
   e. Promotion of bowel elimination
2. Surgical management, usually with a vaginal approach, may be recommended for severe symptoms.
   a. Anterior colporrhaphy (anterior repair) tightens the pelvic muscles for better *bladder* support.
   b. Posterior colporrhaphy (posterior repair) reduces *rectal* bulging.
   c. If both a cystocele and a rectocele are present, an *anterior and posterior colporrhaphy* (A&P repair) is performed.
3. Nursing care is similar to that for a woman undergoing a vaginal hysterectomy (see Surgical Management under Leiomyomas, Uterine).
   a. Warn the patient to avoid lifting anything heavier than 5 pounds, strenuous exercises, and sexual intercourse for 6 weeks.
   b. Teach her to use heat in the form of a moist heating pad or warm compresses applied to the abdomen.
   c. Instruct her to notify her surgeon if she has signs of infection, such as fever, persistent pain, or purulent, foul-smelling discharge.

PROSTATIC HYPERPLASIA, BENIGN (BPH)

OVERVIEW

- With aging, the glandular units in the prostate undergo tissue hyperplasia (an increase in the number of cells), resulting in prostatic hypertrophy (enlargement).
- The enlarged prostate extends upward into the bladder and inward, causing bladder outlet obstruction.
- The patient has an increased residual urine (stasis) or acute or chronic urinary retention.
- Increased residual urine causes overflow urinary incontinence in which the urine "leaks" around the enlarged prostate, causing dribbling.
- Urinary stasis can result in urinary tract infections and bladder calculi (stones).

PATIENT-CENTERED COLLABORATIVE CARE

Assessment

- Obtain patient information about:
  1. Frequency
  2. Nocturia
  3. Difficulty in starting (hesitancy) and continuing urination

4. Reduced force and size of the urinary stream
5. Sensation of incomplete bladder emptying
6. Postvoid (after voiding) dribbling
7. Hematuria

- Assess for and document:
  1. Bladder distention (by palpation or bedside bladder scan)
  2. Prostate for size and consistency (by the health care provider or advanced practice nurse): uniform, elastic, and nontender enlargement
  3. Laboratory findings:
     a. Evidence of urinary tract infection and hematuria (WBCs and RBCs in the urine)
     b. Prostate-specific antigen (PSA) and a serum acid phosphatase level if prostate cancer is suspected

Interventions
Nonsurgical Management

- "Watchful waiting" observation period with yearly examination
- Drug therapy
  1. Drugs to lower dihydrotestosterone (DHT) levels:
     a. Finasteride (Proscar)
     b. Dutasteride (Avodart)
  2. Alpha-blocking agents that reduce urethral pressure and improve flow:
     a. Tamsulosin (Flomax)
     b. Alfuzosin (Uroxatral)
     c. Doxazosin (Cardura)
     d. Terazosin (Hytrin)
- Complementary and alternative therapies
  1. Palmetto extract
  2. Lycopene
- Prostatic fluid can be released and obstructive symptoms reduced with frequent sexual intercourse.
- Teach the patient about ways to prevent bladder distention, such as:
  1. Avoiding drinking large amounts of fluid in a short period
  2. Avoiding alcohol, diuretics, and caffeine
  3. Voiding as soon as the urge is felt
  4. Avoiding drugs that can cause urinary retention, especially anticholinergics, antihistamines, and decongestants
- Minimally invasive techniques to reduce prostate tissue:
  1. *Transurethral needle ablation* (TUNA), in which low radio frequency energy shrinks the prostate
  2. *Transurethral microwave therapy* (TUMT), in which high temperatures heat and destroy excess tissue

3. *Interstitial laser coagulation* (ILC), in which laser energy coagulates excess tissue
4. *Electrovaporization,* in which high-frequency electrical current cuts and vaporizes excess tissue
5. Placement of prostatic stents into the urethra

Surgical Management

- The most common surgery for BPH is a transurethral resection of the prostate (TURP), in which the enlarged portion of the prostate is cut into pieces and removed through the urethra by an endoscopic instrument. A similar procedure is the transurethral incision of the prostate (TIUP), in which small cuts are made into the prostate to relieve pressure on the urethra.
- Another alternative is an open prostatectomy, although it is rarely performed.
- Newer surgical technologies include holmium laser enucleation of the prostate (HoLEP) and transurethral ultrasound-guided laser incision of the prostate (TULIP).
- Provide preoperative care:
  1. Implementing routine preoperative care as described in Part One
  2. Assessing the patient's anxiety
  3. Correcting any misconceptions about the surgery
  4. Informing the patient that he will have an indwelling bladder catheter for at least 24 hours and may have continuous bladder irrigations (CBI)
  5. Explaining that while the catheter is in place, he will feel the urge to void
  6. Reassuring him that it is normal for the urine to be blood-tinged after surgery
- Provide postoperative care:
  1. Implementing routine postoperative care as described in Part One
  2. Monitoring the patient's urine output every 2 hours and vital signs every 4 hours

> **Critical Rescue** ◆ If arterial bleeding occurs, notify the surgeon immediately, and increase the CBI rate or intermittently irrigate the catheter with normal saline solution according to physician or hospital protocol.

  3. Maintaining traction on the three-way urinary catheter
  4. Monitoring the patient's hemoglobin and hematocrit levels
  5. Reminding the patient not to try to void around the catheter

6. Administering antispasmodic drugs as prescribed
7. Performing CBI with normal saline or other solution as prescribed
8. Keeping the catheter free of obstruction
9. Monitoring the color of the urine output, and adjusting the irrigation fluid rate to maintain a colorless or light pink drainage return
10. Instructing the patient to increase fluid intake to at least 2000 to 2500 mL daily after the catheter is removed to decrease dysuria and keep the urine clear
11. Observing for other possible complications of TURP, such as infection or incontinence
12. Teaching the patient that sexual function should not be affected after TURP, but that retrograde ejaculation is possible

Considerations for Older Adults

- Frequently reorient older men, who may become confused after surgery, and remind them not to pull on the catheter.
- Provide the patient who is restless or "picks" at tubes with a familiar object, such as a family picture, to hold for distraction.
- Do not restrain the patient unless all other alternatives have failed.

Community-Based Care

- Reassure the patient that loss of urine control or dribbling is almost always temporary and will resolve.
- Assist the patient and his family in finding ways to keep his clothing dry until sphincter control returns.
- Instruct him to contract and relax his sphincter frequently to re-establish urinary control (Kegel exercises).

PROSTATITIS

OVERVIEW

- *Prostatitis* is an inflammation of the prostate gland.
- There are four types: acute bacterial prostatitis (ABP), chronic bacterial prostatitis (CBP), nonbacterial prostatitis (NBP) or chronic pelvic pain syndrome (CPPS), and asymptomatic inflammatory prostatitis.
- ABP often occurs with urethritis or an infection of the lower urinary tract.
- Common organisms are *Escherichia coli, Enterobacter, Proteus,* and group D streptococci.

- Manifestations of ABP may include:
  1. Fever and chills
  2. Dysuria (painful urination)
  3. Urethral discharge
  4. Boggy, tender prostate
  5. Urinary tract infections
  6. WBCs in prostatic secretions
- Manifestations of CBP may include:
  1. Hesitancy, urgency, dysuria
  2. Difficulty initiating and terminating the flow of urine
  3. Decreased strength and volume of urine
  4. Discomfort in the perineum, scrotum, and penis
  5. Backache
  6. Hematuria
- Complications include epididymitis and cystitis.

PATIENT-CENTERED COLLABORATIVE CARE

- Treatment includes:
  1. Drug therapy with antimicrobials, which may last from weeks to many months because of poor penetration of antibiotics into prostatic tissue
  2. Comfort measures, such as sitz baths, muscle relaxants, and NSAIDs
  3. Stool softeners to prevent straining and rectal irritation of the prostate during a bowel movement
  4. Drug therapy with alpha blockers such as tamsulosin (Flomax) to promote voiding
- Teach patients about:
  1. Avoiding alcohol, coffee, tea, and spicy foods that irritate symptoms
  2. Avoiding cold preparations containing decongestants or antihistamines that may cause urinary retention
  3. The importance of increasing fluid intake
  4. Activities that drain the prostate:
     a. Sexual intercourse
     b. Masturbation
  5. The fact that prostatitis is not contagious
  6. The importance of adhering to long-term antibiotic therapy for CBP

PSEUDOCYSTS, PANCREATIC

- Pancreatic pseudocysts develop as a complication of acute or chronic pancreatitis or abdominal trauma.

- These "false cysts" do not have an epithelial lining and are encapsulated, saclike structures that form on or surround the pancreas.
- The pancreatic wall is inflamed, vascular, and fibrotic and contains large amounts of straw-colored or dark brown, viscous fluid (enzyme exudate from the pancreas).
- The pseudocyst may be palpated as an epigastric mass.
- The primary symptoms are epigastric pain radiating to the back, abdominal fullness, nausea, vomiting, and jaundice. Serum amylase and lipase may be elevated.
- Complications include rupture; hemorrhage; infection; obstruction of the bowel, biliary tract, or splenic vein; abscess or fistula formation; and pancreatic ascites.
- A pseudocyst may spontaneously resolve.
- Surgical intervention with internal drainage is accomplished by creating an ostomy between the pseudocyst and the stomach, jejunum, or duodenum; external drainage is provided by insertion of a sump drainage tube to remove pancreatic exudate and secretions.

PSORIASIS

OVERVIEW

- Psoriasis is a lifelong scaling skin disorder with underlying dermal inflammation that has exacerbations and remissions.
- It appears to be an autoimmune reaction resulting from over-stimulation of the immune system that leads to increased keratinocyte cell division and plaque formation.

Genetic Considerations

- A strong genetic predisposition has been recognized in at least 30% of cases, and several genes appear to be involved in expression of the disease.
- It is likely that a genetic predisposition exists but environmental factors influence whether the disease ever occurs, its severity, and its response to various treatments.
- Always ask about a family history when assessing the patient with psoriasis.
- Many environmental factors lead to outbreaks and influence the severity of clinical symptoms, including skin trauma, surgery, sunburn, and excoriation.
- Psoriasis seems to improve in warmer climates, where there is more exposure to sunlight.
- Some patients with psoriasis also develop a debilitating arthritis.

PATIENT-CENTERED COLLABORATIVE CARE

Assessment

- Obtain patient information about:
  1. Any family history of psoriasis
     a. Age at onset
     b. Description of the disease progression
     c. Pattern of recurrences
  2. Description of the current flare-up of psoriasis, including:
     a. Whether the onset was gradual or sudden
     b. Where the lesions first appeared
     c. Whether there have been any changes in severity over time
     d. Whether fever and itching are present
  3. Possible precipitating factors, including:
     a. Recent skin trauma
     b. Upper respiratory tract infection
     c. Recent surgeries
     d. Menopause status
     e. Past and current use of drugs
     f. Recent stress
     g. Previous interventions and their effectiveness
- Assess for and document the appearance of psoriasis and its course:
  1. *Psoriasis vulgaris* is the most common type of psoriasis:
     a. Thick, reddened papules or plaques covered by silvery white scales
     b. Sharply defined borders between the lesions and normal skin
     c. Lesions are usually present in the same areas on both sides of the body.
     d. Common lesion sites are the scalp, elbows, trunk, knees, sacrum, and outside surfaces of the limbs.
  2. *Exfoliative psoriasis* (erythrodermic psoriasis) has generalized erythema and scaling that do not form obvious lesions.

Interventions

- Teach the patient about the disease and its treatment, and provide emotional support for the changes in body image often experienced with psoriasis.
- Topical therapy
  1. Corticosteroids applied to skin lesions, followed by warm, moist dressings to increase absorption
  2. Tar preparations applied to the skin lesions as solutions, ointments, lotions, gels, and shampoos
  3. Anthralin (Anthraforte ✥, Drithocreme, Lasan) application alone or in combination with coal tar baths and ultraviolet (UV) light

4. Calcipotriene (Dovonex), a synthetic form of vitamin D that regulates skin cell division
5. Tazarotene (Tazorac), which can cause birth defects even when used topically
- Ultraviolet (UV) radiation therapy decreases dermal growth rates.
  1. Ultraviolet B (UV-B) light
  2. Ultraviolet A (UV-A) light
  3. Psoralen and UV-A (PUVA) treatments involve the ingestion of a photosensitizing agent (psoralen) 2 hours before exposure to UV-A light.
- Systemic therapy
  1. Biologic agents
     a. Alefacept (Amevive)
     b. Efalizumab (Raptiva)
     c. Etanercept (Enbrel)
  2. Low-dose methotrexate (Folex, Mexate)
  3. Immunosuppressive agents
     a. Cyclosporine (Sandimmune)
     b. Azathioprine (Imuran)
- Often patients' self-esteem suffers because of the presence of skin lesions and the unpleasantness of some of the treatments.
  1. Encourage the patient and family members to express their feelings about having an incurable skin problem that can alter appearance.
  2. Urge patients to contact other people with the disorder.
  3. Use touch without gloves during social interactions to communicate acceptance of the person and the skin problem.
- Teach women of childbearing age who are taking tazarotene, biologic agents, methotrexate, or immunosuppressive drugs to use a reliable method of contraception, because these agents can cause birth defects when taken during pregnancy.

PULMONARY CONTUSION

- Pulmonary contusion most often follows injuries caused by rapid deceleration during vehicular accidents. Hemorrhage occurs in and between the alveoli. The resulting edema decreases lung movement and reduces the area for gas exchange.
- Respiratory failure often develops over time rather than immediately after the trauma.
- Manifestations include:
  1. Dyspnea
  2. Hypoxemia
  3. Bloody sputum

4. Decreased breath sounds
5. Crackles and wheezes
6. Hazy opacity on chest x-ray in the lobes or parenchyma
- Management is aimed at maintenance of ventilation and oxygenation:
  1. Monitor central venous pressure (CVP).
  2. Fluid intake is restricted as necessary to reduce edema formation.
  3. Mechanical ventilation with positive end-expiratory pressure (PEEP) may be needed.
  4. Monitor for the complication of acute respiratory distress syndrome (ARDS).

PULMONARY EMBOLISM

OVERVIEW

- Pulmonary embolism (PE) is a collection of particulate matter (solids, liquids, or air), most commonly a blood clot, that enters venous circulation and lodges in the pulmonary vessels.
- Large emboli obstruct pulmonary blood flow, leading to reduced oxygenation of the whole body, pulmonary tissue hypoxia, and, potentially, death.
- The local response includes collection of platelets on the embolus, which triggers the release of substances that cause blood vessel constriction. Widespread pulmonary vessel constriction and pulmonary hypertension impair gas exchange. Deoxygenated blood is moved into the arterial circulation, causing hypoxemia.
- Major risk factors for deep vein thrombosis (DVT) leading to PE:
  1. Prolonged immobility
  2. Central venous catheters
  3. Surgery (especially pelvic or leg surgery)
  4. Obesity
  5. Advancing age
  6. Conditions that increase blood clotting
  7. History of thromboembolism
- Smoking, pregnancy, estrogen therapy, heart failure, stroke, cancer (particularly lung or prostate), and trauma increase the risk for DVT and PE.

PATIENT-CENTERED COLLABORATIVE CARE

Assessment

- Obtain patient information about:
  1. Sudden onset of breathing difficulty
  2. Risk factors for PE

- Assess for manifestations:
  1. Pulmonary manifestations
     a. Dyspnea
     b. Pleuritic chest pain (sharp, stabbing pain on inspiration)
     c. Crackles
     d. Dry cough
     e. Hemoptysis (bloody sputum)
  2. Cardiac manifestations
     a. Rapid heart rate
     b. Distended neck veins
     c. Syncope (fainting or loss of consciousness)
     d. Cyanosis
     e. Hypotension

  > 🔲 Critical Rescue ◆ Assess for the described respiratory and cardiac symptom cluster, and if present, notify the Rapid Response Team.

     f. Abnormal heart sounds, such as an S_3 or S_4
     g. Electrocardiographic (ECG) abnormalities (nonspecific and transient)
  3. Miscellaneous manifestations
     a. Low-grade fever
     b. Petechiae on the skin over the chest and in the axillae
     c. Nausea, vomiting, and general malaise
     d. Low $Paco_2$ (early)
     e. Low Pao_2 (late)
     f. High $Paco_2$ (late)
     g. Low arterial pH (late)
  4. Psychosocial issues
     a. Anxiety and fear
     b. Sense of impending doom
     c. Restlessness
- Diagnosis is most commonly made with spiral CT scans.

  > 🔲 Critical Rescue ◆ If a patient has sudden onset of dyspnea and chest pain, immediately notify the Rapid Response Team. Reassure the patient, and assist him or her to a position of comfort with the head of the bed elevated.

Planning and Implementation
❖NDx: Hypoxemia
- Goals of management for PE are to increase gas exchange, improve lung perfusion, reduce the risk for further clot formation, and prevent complications.

Nonsurgical Management

- Oxygen therapy
  1. Apply oxygen by nasal cannula or by mask in less severe cases.
  2. Institution of mechanical ventilation for the severely hypoxemic patient
  3. Monitor:
     a. Oxygen saturation continually
     b. Vital signs, lung sounds, and cardiac status hourly
  4. Assess for and document increasing or decreasing:
     a. Dyspnea
     b. Dysrhythmias
     c. Distended neck veins
     d. Pedal or sacral edema
     e. Abnormal lung sounds
     f. Cyanosis of the lips, conjunctiva, oral mucosa, and nail beds
- Drug therapy
  1. Anticoagulants keep the embolus from enlarging and prevent the formation of new clots.
     a. Heparin
     b. Fibrinolytic drugs (later to break up the existing clot)
     c. Warfarin (Coumadin, Warfilone 🍁) starting on the third day of heparin use
  2. Review the patient's partial thromboplastin time (PTT) before therapy is started, every 4 hours after therapy begins, and daily thereafter. Therapeutic PTT values usually range between 1.5 and 2.5 times the control value.
  3. Therapy with both heparin and warfarin continues until the patient has an international normalized ratio (INR) of 2.0 to 3.0.

> 🔄 **Critical Rescue** ◆ Keep antidotes to anticoagulant drugs and fibrinolytic therapy on the unit for patients undergoing this therapy. The antidote for heparin is protamine sulfate; the antidote for warfarin is injectable phytonadione (vitamin K_1, AquaMEPHYTON, Mephyton). Antidotes for fibrinolytic therapy include clotting factors, fresh-frozen plasma, and aminocaproic acid (Amicar).

Surgical Management

- *Embolectomy* is the surgical removal of the embolus from pulmonary blood vessels using special thrombectomy catheters that can mechanically break up clots (e.g., AngioJet).

- *Inferior vena cava interruption* with placement of a vena cava filter is a lifesaving measure that prevents further embolus formation for some patients.

❖**NDx:** Decreased Cardiac Output

- IV fluid therapy involves giving crystalloid solutions to restore plasma volume and prevent shock.
    1. Continuously monitor:
        a. ECG
        b. Pulmonary artery pressure
        c. Central venous or right atrial pressure
    2. Assess for signs of right-sided heart failure:
        a. Hypoxemia
        b. Dependent edema
- Drug therapy with agents that increase myocardial contractility:
    1. Milrinone (Primacor)
    2. Dobutamine (Dobutrex)
- Drug therapy with vasodilators, such as nitroprusside (Nipride, Nitropress) to decrease pulmonary artery pressure (if it is impeding cardiac contractility)

❖**NDx:** Anxiety

- The patient with PE is anxious and fearful for many reasons.
- Communication
    1. Acknowledge the anxiety and the patient's perception of a life-threatening situation.
    2. Stay with the patient and speak calmly and clearly, providing reassurance that appropriate measures are being taken.
    3. Explain the rationale and share information with the patient regarding any procedure, assessment, or intervention.
- Drug therapy with an antianxiety drug may be prescribed if the patient's anxiety increases or prevents adequate rest.

❖**NDx:** Risk for Injury (Bleeding)

- Assess at least every 2 hours for evidence of bleeding in the form of oozing, bruises that cluster, petechiae, or purpura.
- Examine all stools, urine, drainage, and vomitus visually for gross blood and test for occult blood.
- Measure any blood loss as accurately as possible.
- Measure the patient's abdominal girth every 8 hours.
- Implement best practices for bleeding prevention:
    1. Handling the patient gently
    2. Using and teaching unlicensed assistive personnel (UAPs) to use a lift sheet when moving and positioning the patient in bed
    3. Avoiding IM injections and venipunctures

4. If injections or venipunctures are necessary, using the smallest-gauge needle for the task
5. Applying firm pressure to the needle stick site for 10 minutes or until the site no longer oozes blood
6. Applying ice to areas of trauma
7. Testing all urine, vomitus, and stool for the presence of occult blood
8. Observing IV sites every 4 hours for bleeding
9. Instructing patients to notify nursing personnel immediately if any trauma occurs or if bleeding or bruising is noticed
10. Avoiding trauma to rectal tissues by:
    a. Instructing UAPs not to take temperatures rectally
    b. Not administering enemas
    c. If suppositories are prescribed, lubricating liberally and administering with caution
11. Instructing the patient and UAPs to use an electric shaver rather than a razor
12. When providing mouth care or supervising others in providing mouth care:
    a. Using a soft-bristled toothbrush or tooth sponges
    b. Not using floss
    c. Checking to make certain that dentures fit and do not rub
13. Instructing the patient to not blow the nose forcefully or insert objects into the nose
14. Instructing UAPs and the patient to wear shoes with firm soles whenever he or she is ambulating
15. Ensuring that antidotes to anticoagulation therapy are on the unit

- Monitor laboratory values daily.
  1. Hematocrit and hemoglobin
  2. Platelet count
  3. PT, aPPT, INR

Community-Based Care

- The patient with PE is discharged after hypoxemia and hemodynamic instability have been resolved and adequate anticoagulation has been achieved.
- Anticoagulation therapy usually continues after discharge.
- Teach the patient and family about:
  1. Bleeding precautions
  2. Activities to reduce the risk for DVT and recurrence of PE
  3. Complications
  4. Need for follow-up care

PULMONARY EMPYEMA

OVERVIEW
- Pulmonary empyema is a collection of pus in the pleural space; the fluid is thick, opaque, exudative, and foul smelling.
- The most common cause is pulmonary infection (pneumonia), lung abscess, or infected pleural effusion that can spread across the pleura, obstructing lymph nodes and leading to a retrograde (backward) flood of infected lymph into the pleural space.
- Other causes include liver or abdominal abscesses that spread infection through the lymphatic system into the lung area, thoracic surgery, and chest trauma.

PATIENT-CENTERED COLLABORATIVE CARE
Assessment
- Obtain patient information about:
  1. Recent febrile illness (including pneumonia)
  2. Chest pain
  3. Dyspnea
  4. Cough
  5. Chest trauma
  6. Fever, chills, night sweats
- Assess for and document:
  1. Character of the sputum
  2. Reduced chest wall motion
  3. Decreased or absent fremitus
  4. Decreased breath sounds
  5. Abnormal breath sounds
  6. Weight loss
  7. Hypotension
  8. Displacement of the cardiac point of maximal impulse (PMI)
- Diagnosis is made by chest x-ray and analysis of pleural fluid obtained by thoracentesis.

Interventions
- Therapy for empyema is focused on emptying the empyema cavity, re-expanding the lung, and controlling the infection.
- Antibiotics appropriate for the identified organism are prescribed.
- Closed-chest drainage is used to promote lung expansion.
- Open thoracotomy and removal of a portion of the pleura may be needed for thick pus or marked pleural thickening.
- Nursing care is the same as for patients with a pleural effusion, pneumothorax, or infection.

PULMONARY SARCOIDOSIS

- *Sarcoidosis* is a granulomatous disorder of unknown cause that can affect any organ, especially the lung.
- It develops over time as an autoimmune disorder in which the normally protective T-lymphocytes increase and cause damaging actions in lung tissue.
- Alveolar inflammation (alveolitis) results from the presence of immune cells in the alveoli, and the chronic inflammation causes fibrosis that reduces lung compliance (elasticity) and the ability to exchange gases.
- Cor pulmonale (right-sided cardiac failure) is often present, because the heart can no longer pump effectively against the stiff, fibrotic lung.
- The disease usually affects young adults.
- Manifestations include enlarged lymph nodes in the hilar area of the lungs, lung infiltrate on chest x-ray, skin lesions, eye lesions, cough, dyspnea, hemoptysis, and chest discomfort.
- The disease may resolve permanently or may lead to progressive pulmonary fibrosis and severe systemic disease.
- The goal of therapy is to lessen symptoms and prevent fibrosis.
- The most common form of management is drug therapy with corticosteroids.

P

PYELONEPHRITIS

OVERVIEW

- Pyelonephritis is an infection of the renal pelvis and refers to the active presence of microorganisms in the kidney or the effects of kidney infections.
- Microorganisms enter the renal pelvis and activate the inflammatory response, which results in mobilization of WBCs and local edema.
- The infection is generally classified as acute or chronic.
- Complications include renal abscess, perinephric abscess, emphysematous pyelonephritis, and septicemia.
- Pregnancy, diabetes mellitus, and chronic renal calculi increase the risk for pyelonephritis.
- Stones, obstruction, and neurogenic impairment involving the voiding mechanism often lead to chronic pyelonephritis.
- Reflux of infected urine from the bladder into the ureters and kidney is responsible for most cases of chronic pyelonephritis.

PATIENT-CENTERED COLLABORATIVE CARE

Assessment

- Obtain patient information about:
  1. History of urinary tract and kidney infections
  2. History of diabetes mellitus, stone disease, or other structural or functional abnormalities of the genitourinary tract
  3. Presence of immunosuppression or immunosuppressive therapy
- Assess for:
  1. Pregnancy, because pyelonephritis is associated with early onset of labor and delivery, and fetal health may be compromised if the mother has pyelonephritis
  2. Flank or abdominal discomfort
  3. Hematuria, cloudy urine
  4. General malaise
  5. Chills and fever
  6. Asymmetry, edema, or erythema at the costovertebral angle
  7. Anxiety, embarrassment, or guilt
  8. Presence of WBCs and bacteria in the urine
- Diagnostic testing may include:
  1. Urinalysis and urine for culture and sensitivity
  2. WBC count with differential
  3. Urography to diagnose stones or obstruction; ensure that the patient is *not* pregnant before any imaging study is performed.

> ▨ Critical Rescue ♦ A decrease in urine output by more than 0.5 mL per kilogram of patient weight per hour or an increase of serum creatinine of more than 1.5 times over baseline indicates worsening kidney function and should be communicated to the physician in a timely manner. Early detection of acute kidney injury can prevent progression to kidney failure.

Interventions

- Administer antibiotics. Drug therapy initially includes broad-spectrum antibiotics. With urine and blood culture sensitivity results, a single antibiotic may be ordered.
- Encourage sufficient calories and protein intake to maintain health; consult with nutritionist.
- Surgical procedures include:
  1. Pyelolithotomy (removal of a stone from the renal pelvis)
  2. Nephrectomy (removal of a kidney)
  3. Ureteral diversion or reimplantation of the ureter to restore the bladder drainage mechanism

- Maintain sufficient perfusion to the kidneys to prevent acute (hypotensive) or chronic (hypertensive) renal injury.
- Maintain sufficient fluid intake to promote urine output greater than 1 mL/kg/hr.
- Assess for signs of acute kidney injury, such as increasing creatinine or decreased urinary output.

Community-Based Care
- Health teaching includes:
  1. Drug administration, including effects, side effects, and importance of following the prescribed duration of therapy
  2. Planning and implementing healthy choices for nutrition and fluid intake
  3. Balancing rest and activity
  4. Limiting activity after surgery
  5. Manifestations of disease reoccurrence, such as functional incontinence, which is leakage of urine caused by factors other than pathology of the lower urinary tract

RAYNAUD'S PHENOMENON AND RAYNAUD'S DISEASE

- Raynaud's *phenomenon* is caused by vasospasm of the arterioles and arteries of the upper and lower extremities, usually unilaterally. It usually occurs in people older than 30 years of age in either gender.
- Raynaud's *disease* occurs bilaterally. It is more common in women and occurs between the ages of 17 and 50 years.
- The pathophysiology is the same for both entities: vasospasm of the arterioles and arteries of the upper and lower extremities.
- Cutaneous vessels are constricted, causing blanching of the extremities, followed by cyanosis.
- When the vasospasm is relieved, the tissue becomes reddened or hyperemic.
- Patients often have an associated systemic connective tissue disease such as systemic lupus erythematosus (SLE) or progressive systemic sclerosis.
- Assess for:
  1. Color changes in the extremity or digits, ranging from blanched to reddened to cyanotic
  2. Numbness of the extremity or digits
  3. Coldness of the extremity or digits
  4. Pain
  5. Swelling
  6. Ulcerations

7. Aggravation of symptoms by cold or stress
8. Gangrene of digits in severe cases
- Interventions include:
  1. Drug therapy to prevent vasoconstriction, including calcium channel blockers
  2. Lumbar sympathectomy to relieve symptoms in the feet
  3. Sympathetic ganglionectomy to relieve symptoms in the upper extremities
- Health teaching emphasizes methods to minimize vasoconstriction.
  1. Smoking cessation
  2. Decreasing the exposure to cold by wearing warm clothes, socks, and gloves and maintaining a warm indoor ambient temperature
  3. Stress management

REGURGITATION, AORTIC

- In aortic regurgitation (insufficiency), the aortic valve leaflets do not close properly during diastole, and the annulus may become dilated, loose, or deformed.
- Regurgitation of blood from the aorta into the left ventricle occurs during diastole; the left ventricle dilates to accommodate the greater blood volume and hypertrophies.
- Nonrheumatic causes include infective endocarditis, congenital anatomic aortic valvular abnormalities, hypertension, and Marfan syndrome (a generalized, systemic connective tissue disease).
- Patients with aortic insufficiency remain asymptomatic for many years because of the compensatory mechanisms of the left ventricle.
- Signs and symptoms include:
  1. Palpitations (severe disease)
  2. Dyspnea on exertion
  3. Orthopnea
  4. Paroxysmal nocturnal dyspnea
  5. Nocturnal angina with diaphoresis
  6. Bounding arterial pulse
  7. Widened pulse pressure
  8. High-pitched, blowing, decrescendo diastolic murmur
- Nonsurgical therapy focuses on drug therapy and rest. Prophylactic antibiotic therapy is recommended for invasive procedures or surgery.
- Surgical treatment is performed after symptoms of left ventricular failure have developed but before irreversible dysfunction occurs.

- Aortic valve repair or replacement surgery is performed to improve cardiac function in symptomatic patients.
- Repair procedures include valvuloplasty, commissurotomy, and annuloplasty (reconstruction).
- Replacement means that the aortic valve is excised during cardiopulmonary bypass surgery and replaced with a prosthetic (synthetic) or biologic (xenographic or tissue) valve.
- The postoperative patient requires lifetime anticoagulation therapy to prevent thrombus formation on the valve.
- For preoperative and postoperative care, see Surgical Management under Coronary Artery Disease.

REGURGITATION, MITRAL

- Mitral regurgitation (insufficiency) results from fibrotic and calcific changes that prevent the mitral valve from closing completely during systole, allowing backflow of blood into the left atrium when the left ventricle contracts.
- During diastole, regurgitant output again flows from the left atrium to the left ventricle along with normal blood flow, increasing the volume of blood to be ejected during the next systole.
- To compensate for the increased volume and pressure, the left atrium and ventricle dilate and hypertrophy.
- Rheumatic heart disease is the predominant factor, usually coexisting with mitral stenosis.
- Signs and symptoms include:
  1. Fatigue and weakness
  2. Dyspnea on exertion
  3. Orthopnea
  4. Anxiety
  5. Atypical chest pains and palpitations
  6. Atrial fibrillation
  7. Neck vein distention
  8. Pitting edema
  9. High-pitched, systolic murmur
- Drug therapy is instituted to maintain normal cardiac output.
- The reparative surgical procedure is mitral annuloplasty, which is performed during cardiopulmonary bypass surgery. Mitral valve leaflets and annuli are reconstructed to narrow the valve orifice.
- The postoperative patient requires lifetime anticoagulation therapy to prevent thrombus formation on the valve.
- For preoperative and postoperative care, see care of the patient undergoing a coronary artery bypass grafting procedure (see Coronary Artery Disease).

R

- Discharge planning includes:
  1. Providing health teaching information
     a. Drug therapy effects, side effects, and monitoring for anticoagulation
     b. The importance of taking antibiotics before any procedure (e.g., dental work, surgery)
  2. Referring the patient to community resources such as the American Heart Association

RESPIRATORY FAILURE, ACUTE

OVERVIEW

- Acute respiratory failure is classified by blood gas abnormalities: pH less than 7.30, Pao_2 less than 60 mm Hg, Sao_2 less than 90%, and $Paco_2$ greater than 50 mm Hg.
- Acute respiratory failure can be defined in three ways, based on the underlying problem.
  1. *Ventilatory failure* is a problem of oxygen intake (ventilation) and blood delivery (perfusion) that causes a ventilation-perfusion $(\dot{V}/\dot{Q})$ mismatch in which perfusion is normal but ventilation is inadequate. It is often the result of a physical problem of the lungs or chest wall, a defect in the respiratory control center in the brain, or poor function of the respiratory muscles, especially the diaphragm. The $Paco_2$ level is greater than 45 mm Hg in patients who have otherwise healthy lungs.
  2. *Oxygenation failure* is a problem in which chest pressure changes are normal and air moves in and out without difficulty but does not oxygenate the pulmonary blood sufficiently. It occurs in the type of $\dot{V}/\dot{Q}$ mismatch in which air movement and oxygen intake (ventilation) are normal but lung blood flow (perfusion) is decreased. Problems leading to this type of failure include impaired diffusion of oxygen at the alveolar level, right-to-left shunting of blood in the pulmonary vessels, $\dot{V}/\dot{Q}$ mismatch, breathing air with a low partial pressure of oxygen (a rare problem), and abnormal hemoglobin that fails to bind oxygen.
  3. *Combined ventilatory and oxygenation failure* involves hypoventilation and impairment of oxygenation at the alveolar-capillary membrane. This type of respiratory failure leads to a more profound hypoxemia than either ventilatory failure or oxygenation failure alone. It is seen in patients who have abnormal lungs (chronic bronchitis, emphysema, or during asthma attacks) and in patients who have cardiac failure along with respiratory failure.

- *Regardless of the underlying cause, the patient in acute respiratory failure is always hypoxemic.*

PATIENT-CENTERED COLLABORATIVE CARE

Assessment
- Assess for and document:
  1. Dyspnea (the hallmark of respiratory failure)
  2. Orthopnea
  3. Changes in the respiratory rate or pattern
  4. Changes in lung sounds
  5. Manifestations of hypoxemia
     a. Pallor
     b. Cyanosis
     c. Increased heart rate
     d. Restlessness
     e. Confusion
  6. Hypercarbia (high arterial blood levels of carbon dioxide)

Interventions
- Management of acute respiratory failure of any origin includes:
  1. Applying oxygen therapy to keep the partial pressure of arterial oxygen (Pao_2) greater than 60 mm Hg
  2. Implementing mechanical ventilation, if needed
  3. Assisting the patient to find a position of comfort that allows easier breathing, usually a more upright position
  4. Assisting the patient to use relaxation, diversion, and guided imagery to reduce anxiety
  5. Instituting energy-conserving measures of minimal self-care and no unnecessary procedures
  6. Administering drug therapy given systemically or by metered dose inhaler (MDI)
  7. Encouraging deep breathing and other breathing exercises

RETINAL HOLES, TEARS, AND DETACHMENTS

OVERVIEW
- A *retinal hole* is a break in the retina, usually caused by trauma or aging.
- A *retinal tear* is a more jagged and irregularly shaped break, often caused by traction on the retina.
- A *retinal detachment* is the separation of the retina from the epithelium. Detachments are classified by the nature of their development.

1. *Rhegmatogenous* detachments occur after a hole or tear in the retina is caused by mechanical force, creating an opening for the vitreous to move under the retina, pushing the retina away from its attachment.
2. *Traction* detachments occur when the retina is pulled away from the support tissue by bands of fibrous tissue in the vitreous.
3. *Exudative* detachments are caused by fluid collecting under the retina.

PATIENT-CENTERED COLLABORATIVE CARE

Assessment

- Subjective manifestations
  1. Bright flashes of light (*photopsia*) or floating dark spots in the affected eye
  2. The sensation of a curtain being pulled over part of the visual field
  3. No pain
- Ophthalmoscopic manifestations
  1. Gray bulges or folds in the retina that quiver
  2. Possibly a hole or tear at the edge of the detachment

Interventions

- For an actual detachment, surgical repair is needed to place the retina in contact with the underlying structures. A common repair procedure is scleral buckling.
- Preoperative care
  1. Reassuring the patient to allay fears of permanent vision loss
  2. Teaching the patient to restrict activity and head movement before surgery to prevent further tearing or detachment and to promote drainage of any fluid under the retina
  3. Applying an eye patch over the affected eye to reduce eye movement
  4. Applying prescribed topical drugs to inhibit pupil constriction and accommodation
- Postoperative care
  1. Applying an eye patch and shield
  2. Monitoring the patient's vital signs and checking the eye patch and shield for any drainage
  3. Positioning the patient as prescribed to allow the agent being used to promote reattachment to press the retina against the interior surface of the eye
  4. Administering analgesics and antiemetics as prescribed
  5. Instructing the patient to report any sudden increase in pain or pain occurring with nausea, which may indicate development of complications

6. Reminding the patient to avoid activities that increase intraocular pressure (IOP)
   a. Bending from the waist
   b. Lifting objects weighing more than 10 pounds
   c. Sneezing, coughing
   d. Blowing the nose
   e. Straining to have a bowel movement
   f. Vomiting
   g. Having sexual intercourse
   h. Keeping the head in a dependent position
   i. Wearing tight shirt collars
7. Teaching the patient to avoid reading, writing, and close work, such as sewing, during the first week after surgery, because these activities cause rapid eye movements and promote detachment
8. Teaching the patient the manifestations of infection and detachment (sudden reduced visual acuity, eye pain, pupil that does not respond to light by constricting)
9. Instructing the patient to notify the surgeon immediately if these manifestations occur

ROTATOR CUFF INJURIES

- The function of the rotator cuff is to stabilize the head of the humerus in the glenoid cavity during shoulder abduction.
- It may be injured by substantial trauma and also undergoes degenerative changes with aging.
- Older adults tend to have small tears related to aging, repetitive motions, or falls.
- Younger adults sustain tears by trauma, including falling, throwing a ball, or lifting heavy objects.
- Manifestations include shoulder pain and the inability to achieve or maintain abduction of the arm at the shoulder.
- Conservative management involves use of NSAIDs, physical therapy, sling or immobilizer support, and ice or heat applications while the tear heals.
- Surgical cuff repair may be needed for patients who do not respond to conservative treatment or for those who have a complete tear.

SCABIES

- *Scabies* is a contagious skin disease that is caused by mite infestations and transmitted by close and prolonged contact with an infested companion or infested bedding.

- It is manifested by curved or linear ridges in the skin, especially between the fingers and on the palms and inner aspects of the wrists, and intense itching.
- Hypersensitivity reactions result in excoriated erythematous papules, pustules, and crusted lesions on the elbows, nipples, lower abdomen, buttocks, thighs, and penis and in the axillary folds.
- Infestation is confirmed by the presence of mites and eggs on microscopic examination of lesion scrapings.
- Treatment involves the use of scabicides, such as permethrin (Acticin), lindane (Kwell, Kildane, Scabene, Thionex), malathion (Ovide), or benzyl benzoate (Ascabiol).
- Clothing and personal items must be cleaned with hot water and detergent.
- Social contacts should also be treated.

SCLERODERMA

OVERVIEW

- Scleroderma, also called systemic sclerosis (SSc), is a chronic, inflammatory, autoimmune connective tissue disease that usually first manifests with hardening of the skin.
- The disease is often confused with systemic lupus erythematosus (SLE) but is less common and has a higher mortality rate.
- The manifestations vary widely from person to person.
- It is classified as:
  1. *Diffuse scleroderma*, with skin thickening on the trunk, face, and proximal and distal extremities
  2. *Limited scleroderma*, with thick skin limited to sites distal to the elbow and knee but also involving the face and neck. Patients have the *CREST syndrome*:
     a. *C*alcinosis (calcium deposits)
     b. *R*aynaud's phenomenon
     c. *E*sophageal dysmotility
     d. *S*clerodactyly (scleroderma of the digits)
     e. *T*elangiectasia (spider-like hemangiomas)
- Women are affected more frequently than men and usually are between 25 and 65 years old.

PATIENT-CENTERED COLLABORATIVE CARE

Assessment

- SSc manifests with joint pain and stiffness; painless, symmetric, pitting edema of the hands and fingers that may progress to include the entire upper and lower extremities and face; and taut, shiny skin that is free of wrinkles.

- When scleroderma progresses, swelling is replaced by tightening, hardening, and thickening of skin tissue with loss of elasticity and greatly decreased ROM.
- Ulcerations and joint contractures may develop, and the patient may be unable to perform ADLs.
- Major organ involvement is manifested by:
  1. GI tract changes, especially in the esophagus, with dysphagia and esophageal reflux. A small, sliding hiatal hernia may be present. Intestinal peristalsis is diminished, leading to partial bowel obstruction and malabsorption.
  2. Cardiovascular system changes, especially Raynaud's phenomenon with digit necrosis, excruciating pain, and autoamputation of the distal digits. Myocardial fibrosis may be present with cardiac dysrhythmias and chest pain.
  3. Lung changes include fibrosis of the alveoli and interstitial tissues, and pulmonary hypertension may develop.
  4. Renal involvement can lead to kidney failure and may cause malignant hypertension and death.

Interventions

- The focus of medical management is to induce disease remission and slow disease progression.
- Systemic steroids and immunosuppressants are used in large doses and often in combination.
- Nursing management includes:
  1. Local skin protective measures
     a. Teaching the patient to use mild soap and lotions and gentle cleaning techniques
     b. Inspecting the skin for further changes or open lesions
     c. Caring for skin ulcers according to their type and location
     d. Using bed cradles and foot boards.
     e. Adjusting room temperature to prevent chilling
  2. Implementing and teaching about drug therapy
  3. Teaching patients to avoid or minimize cigarette smoking
  4. Promoting nutrition
     a. Providing small, frequent meals
     b. Instructing the patient to avoid intake of foods and liquids that stimulate gastric secretion (e.g., spicy foods, caffeine, alcohol)
     c. Teaching the patient to keep the head elevated for 1 to 2 hours after a meal
  5. Reducing pain and maintaining joint mobility using interventions similar to those for rheumatoid arthritis

6. Referring patients and families to community resources such as the Arthritis Foundation (*www.arthritis.org*) and Scleroderma Foundation (*www.scleroderma.org*)

SCLEROSIS, MULTIPLE

OVERVIEW

- Multiple sclerosis (MS) is a chronic autoimmune disease that affects the myelin sheath and conduction pathway of the central nervous system (CNS).
- Women are affected twice as often as men.
- MS often mimics other neurologic diseases, which makes the diagnosis difficult and prolonged.
- The major types of MS are:
  1. Relapsing-remitting MS, which is characterized as mild or moderate, depending on the degree of disability. Symptoms develop and resolve in a few weeks to months, after which the patient may return to baseline.
  2. Primary progressive MS, which is characterized by a steady and gradual neurologic deterioration without remission of symptoms. The patient has progressive disability with no acute attacks. Patients with this type of MS tend to be between 40 and 60 years old at onset of the disease.
  3. Secondary progressive MS begins with a relapsing-remitting course that later becomes steadily progressive. Functioning continues to decline with no clear times of remission.
  4. Progressive-relapsing MS is characterized by frequent relapses with some partial recovery but not a return to baseline. Progressive, cumulative symptoms and deterioration occur over several years.

PATIENT-CENTERED COLLABORATIVE CARE

Assessment

- Assess for and document:
  1. Progression of symptoms (the patient often reports that symptoms were noticed several years earlier but disappeared, and medical attention was not sought)
  2. Factors that aggravate symptoms
     a. Stress
     b. Fatigue
     c. Overexertion
     d. Temperature extremes
     e. Hot shower or bath
  3. Motor function
     a. Fatigue

    b. Stiffness of legs
    c. Flexor spasms
    d. Increased deep tendon reflexes
    e. Clonus
    f. Positive Babinski's reflex
    g. Absent abdominal reflexes
  4. Cerebellar function
    a. Ataxic gait
    b. Intention tremor (tremor when performing activity)
    c. Dysmetria (inability to direct or limit movement)
    d. Clumsy motor movements
  5. Cranial nerve function
    a. Hearing loss
    b. Facial weakness
    c. Swallowing difficulties (dysphagia)
    d. Tinnitus
    e. Vertigo
  6. Vision
    a. Decreased visual acuity
    b. Blurred vision
    c. Diplopia
    d. Scotoma (changes in peripheral vision)
    e. Nystagmus
  7. Sensation
    a. Hypalgesia
    b. Paresthesia
    c. Facial pain
    d. Change in bowel and bladder function
    e. Impotence, difficulty sustaining an erection
    f. Decreased vaginal secretion
  8. Cognitive changes seen late in the course of the disease
    a. Memory loss
    b. Decreased ability to perform calculations
    c. Inattention
    d. Impaired judgment
  9. Psychosocial function
    a. Apathy, emotional lability, and depression
    b. Disturbed body image
- Diagnostic testing may include:
  1. MRI to determine the presence of plaques in the central nervous system (CNS)
  2. Lumbar puncture for analysis of cerebral spinal fluid (CSF)

Interventions
- Provide sufficient time to complete ADLs; as a result of weakness and fatigue, the patient requires more time or assistance.

- Collaborate with physical and occupational therapists and vocational rehabilitation specialists to assist the patient with:
  1. Implementing an exercise program to strengthen and stretch muscles
  2. Using assistive devices for ambulation, such as a cane, walker, or electric (Amigo) cart
  3. Using assistive-adaptive devices to remain independent in ADLs
  4. Valuing the importance of avoiding rigorous activities that lead to an increase in body temperature, which may lead to fatigue, decreased motor ability, and decreased visual acuity
- Drug therapy includes:
  1. Immunomodulation therapy
     a. Interferon beta, which has antiviral properties, for relapsing-remitting MS
     b. Natalizumab (Tysabri), the first monoclonal antibody approved for MS, which binds to WBCs to prevent further damage to the myelin
     c. Glatiramer acetate (Copaxone), a synthetic protein that simulates myelin-based protein
     d. Mitoxantrone (Novantrone), an antineoplastic agent, which has also been shown to be effective in reducing neurologic disability and the frequency of clinical relapses in patients with secondary-progressive, progressive-relapsing, or worsening relapsing-remitting MS
     e. Immunosuppressive therapy with a combination of cyclophosphamide (Cytoxan) and steroid therapy to stabilize the disease progression. Methotrexate (MTX) may also have a modest benefit.
  2. Steroid therapy (glucocorticoid)
  3. Adjunctive therapy to treat muscle spasticity and paresthesia
  4. Adjunctive therapy for bladder and bowel dysfunction
  5. Antispasmodics, antiepileptic drugs (AEDs), analgesics, NSAIDs, tranquilizers, or antidepressants to treat pain, paresthesia, and mood disorder
- Other interventions include:
  1. Managing cognitive problems in the areas of attention, memory, problem solving, visual perception, and use of speech
  2. Applying an eye patch to relieve diplopia and switching the eye patch every few hours
  3. Teaching scanning techniques to compensate for peripheral vision deficits

4. Teaching the patient to test the temperature of the bath water at home before placing his or her hands in hot water

5. Referring the patient to a therapist or nurse educated in issues surrounding sexuality

- Patients using complementary therapies, such as nutritional supplements, acupressure, and bee stings, report improvement in their condition, but these modalities have not been scientifically tested.

Community-Based Care

- Home care management includes:
  1. Explaining the development of MS and the factors that may exacerbate the symptoms
  2. Stressing the importance of avoiding overexertion, extremes of temperatures (fever, hot baths, overheating, excessive chilling), humidity, and exposure to infection
  3. Providing drug information, as needed
  4. Encouraging the patient to follow the exercise program developed by the physical therapist and to remain independent in all activities for as long as possible
  5. Encouraging the patient to engage in regular social activities, obtain adequate rest, and manage stress
  6. Teaching the family strategies to cope with personality changes
  7. Reviewing the established bowel and bladder, skin care, and nutrition programs
  8. Referring the patient to local and national support groups, as needed

SEIZURE DISORDERS

OVERVIEW

- A seizure is an abnormal, sudden, excessive, uncontrolled electrical discharge of neurons within the brain that may result in alteration in consciousness, motor or sensory ability, or behavior.
- Epilepsy is a chronic disorder characterized by recurrent seizure activity (two or more episodes).
- Three major categories:
  1. Generalized seizures
     a. Tonic-clonic seizure (formerly called a grand mal seizure) is characterized by stiffening or rigidity of the muscles, followed by rhythmic jerking of the extremities. Immediate unconsciousness occurs, and the patient may be incontinent of urine or feces and may bite his or her tongue.

b. Tonic seizures are characterized by an abrupt increase in muscle tone, loss of consciousness, and loss of autonomic signs lasting from 30 seconds to several minutes.

c. Clonic seizures last several minutes and are characterized by muscle contraction and relaxation.

d. Absence seizure (formerly called petit mal seizure) consists of a brief (often seconds) period of loss of consciousness and blank staring, as if the patient were daydreaming.

e. Myoclonic seizure is a brief, generalized jerking or stiffening of the extremities and may occur singly or in groups.

f. Atonic seizures (formerly called "drop attacks") are characterized by sudden loss of muscle tone, which in most cases causes the patient to fall.

2. Partial (focal) seizures

a. Complex seizure (often called a psychomotor seizure or a temporal lobe seizure) causes the patient to lose consciousness or black out for 1 to 3 minutes. Characteristic behavior, known as automatism, may occur (e.g., lip smacking, patting, picking at clothes).

b. Simple seizure consists of an aura or unusual sensation (déjà vu phenomenon, perception of an offensive smell, or sudden onset of pain) before the seizure takes place. It may be followed by unilateral movement of an extremity or autonomic or psychic symptoms. Simple seizures do not fit well into the generalized or partial classification.

3. Unclassified or idiopathic seizures, which occur for no known reason

- Status epilepticus is a seizure that lasts longer than 10 minutes or repeated seizures over the course of 30 minutes. It is a neurologic emergency and must be treated promptly or brain damage and possibly death from anoxia, cardiac dysrhythmias, or lactic acidosis may occur. Status epilepticus is usually caused by:

1. Sudden withdrawal from anticonvulsant drugs
2. Acute alcohol withdrawal
3. Head trauma
4. Cerebral edema
5. Metabolic disturbances

- Primary seizures are not associated with any identifiable brain lesions, are usually inherited, and are often age related.

- Secondary seizures often result from underlying brain pathology, such as a head injury, vascular disease, brain tumor, aneurysm, opportunistic infection from acquired immunodeficiency syndrome (AIDS), or meningitis. They may also occur in the presence of metabolic or electrolyte disorders, drug withdrawal, acute alcohol intoxication, water intoxication, or kidney or liver failure. Seizures resulting from these disorders are not considered epilepsy.

Considerations for Older Adults

Complex partial seizures are most common among older adults and account for almost 40% of all diagnosed seizures in this group. These seizures are difficult to diagnose because symptoms appear similar to dementia, psychosis, or Alzheimer's disease (AD), especially in the post-ictal stage (after the seizure). New-onset seizures in older adults are typically associated with conditions such as hypertension, cardiac disease, diabetes mellitus, stroke, or AD.

PATIENT-CENTERED COLLABORATIVE CARE

Assessment

- Obtain patient information about:
  1. Frequency, duration, and pattern of occurrence for seizure activity
  2. Description of seizure activity (aura, motor activity, sequence of progression, eye signs, consciousness, respiratory patterns) and events surrounding the seizure
  3. Current drugs, including dosage, frequency of administration, and the time at which the drug was last taken
  4. Compliance with the drug schedule and reasons for noncompliance, if appropriate
- Note whether an observed seizure is new (first occurrence) or acute. Seizures occurring in greater intensity, number, or length than the patient's usual seizures are considered *acute*. They may also appear in clusters that are different from the patient's typical seizure pattern.

Interventions

Nonsurgical Management

- Care of the patient during a tonic-clonic or complete partial seizure
  1. Protect from injury.
  2. Do not force anything into the patient's mouth.
  3. Turn the patient to the side.
  4. Loosen any restrictive clothing.
  5. Maintain the airway, and suction as needed.
  6. Do not restrain the patient; rather, guide the patient's movements.
  7. At the completion of the seizure:
     a. Take vital signs.
     b. Perform neurologic assessment.

    c. Allow the patient to rest.

    d. Document the seizure.

- Nursing observations and documentation of a seizure include:
  1. Onset and cessation of seizure activity: date, time, and duration
  2. Type of movement or activity and whether more than one type occurs
  3. Sequence of progression
     a. Where the seizure began
     b. Body parts first involved
  4. Observations during the seizure
     a. Changes in pupil size and any eye deviation
     b. Level of consciousness (LOC)
     c. Presence of apnea, cyanosis, salivation
     d. Incontinence of bowel or bladder
     e. Eye fluttering
     f. Movement and progression of motor activity
     g. Lip smacking or other automatism
     h. Tongue or lip biting
  5. How long the seizure lasted
  6. Presence and description of aura or precipitating events
  7. Post-ictal status
  8. Length of time before the patient returns to preseizure status
- Drug therapy is the major component of management; the health care provider introduces one anticonvulsant at a time to achieve seizure control.
- Serum drug levels are monitored for the first 3 days after the start of anticonvulsants and thereafter as needed.
- Follow agency policy for the implementation of Seizure Precautions.
  1. Keep oxygen, suctioning equipment, and an airway available at the bedside.
  2. Maintain IV access (a saline lock) for patients at risk for tonic-clonic seizures.
  3. Padded tongue blades do not belong at the bedside; nothing should be inserted into the patient's mouth after a seizure begins.
  4. Keep the bed in the low position and siderails up at all times. Use of padded siderails is controversial; siderails are rarely the source of significant injury, and the use of padded siderails may embarrass the patient and family.
- Convulsive status epilepticus is a neurologic emergency and must be treated promptly and aggressively. Notify the health

care provider immediately. Immediate treatment of status epilepticus includes:

1. Establishing an airway (intubation may be necessary)
2. Monitoring the patient's respiratory status carefully
3. Administering oxygen
4. Establishing an IV line and starting 0.9% saline infusion
5. Drawing blood for arterial blood gas analysis and identifying metabolic, toxic, and other causes of uncontrolled seizures
6. Administering drugs such as IV lorazepam (Ativan, Apo-Lorazepam) or possibly diazepam (Valium) to stop motor movement, followed by phenytoin (Dilantin) or fosphenytoin (Cerebyx) to prevent recurrence. General anesthesia may be used as a last resort to stop the seizure activity.
7. Monitoring vital signs every 15 minutes or more frequently until the patient's condition stabilizes

> **Critical Rescue** ◆ Ensure that oxygen and suction are available at the bedside of any patient who is at risk for seizure activity. Maintaining the airway and supporting ventilation can prevent brain injury during a seizure.

Surgical Management

- Several procedures may be performed when traditional methods fail to maintain seizure control.
  1. Vagal nerve stimulation involves surgically implanting a vagal nerve–stimulating device below the left clavicle to control partial seizures.
  2. Corpuscallostomy involves severing the corpus callosum to prevent neuronal discharges from passing through the two hemispheres of the brain. It is used to treat tonic-clonic or atonic seizures.
  3. Other procedures, including anterior temporal lobe resection for complex partial seizures of temporal origin, cortical resection, and removal of part or all of a cerebral hemisphere
- Perioperative care is as outlined in Part One, with the addition of assessing neurologic status with vital signs postoperatively.

Community Health

- Health teaching includes:
  1. The importance of taking all drugs consistently as prescribed and monitoring for effects and side effects. Dosage or effectiveness may change over time or with the occurrence of comorbid conditions.
  2. The importance of not taking any herbal remedies or OTC drugs without notifying the health care provider; anti-seizure

    medications have multiple and serious drug-drug and drug-herb interactions.

3. Components of a balanced diet and the effects of alcohol (alcohol should be avoided)
4. The role of rest, time management, and stress management in health promotion
5. The utility of keeping a seizure diary to determine whether there are factors that tend to be associated with seizure activity
6. Restrictions (if any), such as driving or operating dangerous equipment and participating in certain physical activities or sports
7. The importance of follow-up visits with the health care provider
8. The value of wearing a medical alert bracelet or necklace

- Inform the patient that state laws prohibit discrimination against people who have epilepsy.
- Refer the patient to the state Vocational Rehabilitative Services, Epilepsy Foundation of America, National Epilepsy League, or National Association to Control Epilepsy and to local support groups.

SEVERE ACUTE RESPIRATORY SYNDROME

OVERVIEW

- Severe acute respiratory syndrome (SARS) is an atypical pneumonia with a high mortality rate caused by a new coronavirus known as SARS Co-V, which is highly contagious.
- The virus infects cells of the respiratory tract, triggering an inflammatory response.
- It is easily spread by airborne droplets from infected people through sneezing, coughing, and talking and from contaminated surfaces and objects.
- People at greatest risk for SARS are those in close direct contact with an infected person. The portals of entry for infection with the virus are the mucous membranes of the eyes, nose, and mouth.

PATIENT-CENTERED COLLABORATIVE CARE

Assessment

- The manifestations of SARS are the same as those of any respiratory infection.
  1. Fever higher than 100.4° F (38.0° C)
  2. Headache and general body aches

   3. Cold symptoms of a runny nose, sore throat, and watery eyes

   4. A dry cough and dyspnea developing within 2 to 7 days

   5. Late symptoms: hypoxia with cyanosis, low oxygen saturation

- Diagnosis is made by the manifestations and the use of a rapid SARS test, the reverse transcriptase–polymerase chain reaction (RT-PCR) that detects SARS-CoV RNA in the blood within 2 days after symptoms begin.

Interventions for Patient Care

- There is no completely effective treatment at this time.
- Interventions are supportive to allow the patient's own immune system to fight the infection.

   1. Oxygen therapy

   2. Bronchodilators

   3. Intubation and mechanical ventilation

   4. Antibiotics if bacterial pneumonia occurs with SARS

Interventions for Prevention of Infection Spread

- Isolating the person with SARS and adhering to strict Isolation Precautions are effective measures for containing the infection and preventing an epidemic.

   1. Performing frequent handwashing

   2. Using Airborne and Contact Precautions if SARS is suspected

   3. Using gowns and eye protection when coming into direct contact with the patient

   4. Ensuring that the patient wears a mask and protective clothing when he or she is out of the isolation environment (the patient can contaminate surfaces with the virus)

   5. Wearing a disposable particulate mask respirator (e.g., N-95, N-99, N-100) and protective eyewear when performing procedures that normally induce coughing or promote aerosolization of particles (e.g., suctioning, using a positive-pressure face mask, obtaining a sputum culture, giving aerosolized treatments)

   6. Keeping the door to the patient's room closed

   7. Avoiding touching your face with contaminated gloves

SHOCK

OVERVIEW

- *Shock* is a widespread abnormal cellular metabolism that occurs when the human need for *oxygenation and tissue perfusion* is not met to the level needed to maintain cell function.

- It is a condition rather than a disease and represents the whole-body response that occurs when too little oxygen is delivered to the tissues.
- All body organs are affected by shock, and they work harder to adapt and compensate for reduced oxygenation or fail to function because of hypoxia.
- Shock is a "syndrome" because the cellular, tissue, and organ events that occur in response to its presence happen in a predictable sequence.
- Any problem that impairs oxygen delivery to tissues and organs can start the syndrome of shock and lead to a life-threatening emergency.
- Shock is classified as one of four types, and more than one type may be present.
    1. *Hypovolemic shock* occurs when too little circulating blood volume causes a decrease in mean arterial pressure (MAP) so that the body's total need for oxygen is not met. Common problems leading to hypovolemic shock are hemorrhage (external or internal) and dehydration.
    2. *Cardiogenic shock* occurs when the actual heart muscle is unhealthy and pumping is directly impaired. Myocardial infarction (MI) is the most common cause of direct pump failure.
    3. *Distributive shock* occurs when blood volume is not lost from the body but is distributed to the interstitial tissues, where it cannot circulate and deliver oxygen. It has several origins.
        a. Neural-induced distributive shock, in which a loss of MAP occurs because sympathetic nerve impulses controlling blood vessel smooth muscle decrease and the smooth muscles of blood vessels relax, causing widespread vasodilation.
        b. Chemical-induced distributive shock, which occurs when certain chemicals or foreign substances within the blood and blood vessels initiate widespread changes in blood vessel walls. Common conditions leading to this type of shock include:
            (1) Anaphylaxis after exposure to a specific allergen in a susceptible person, which results in widespread loss of blood vessel tone and decreased cardiac output
            (2) Sepsis due to widespread infection, which triggers a whole-body inflammatory response when pathologic microorganisms are present in the blood (also called septic shock)
            (3) Capillary leak syndrome, which is the response of capillaries to the presence of biologic chemicals

(mediators) that change blood vessel integrity and allow fluid to leak from the blood in the vascular space into the interstitial tissues. Once in the interstitial tissue, these fluids are stagnant and not able to deliver oxygen or remove tissue waste products. Problems causing fluid shifts include severe burns, liver disorders, ascites, peritonitis, paralytic ileus, severe malnutrition, large wounds, hyperglycemia, kidney disease, hypoproteinemia, and trauma.

4. *Obstructive shock* occurs when the normal heart muscle is prevented from pumping effectively. The heart itself remains normal, but conditions outside the heart prevent adequate filling of the heart or adequate contraction of the healthy heart muscle. Common causes of obstructive shock are pericarditis and cardiac tamponade.

- Although the causes and initial manifestations associated with the different types of shock vary, eventually the effects of hypotension and anaerobic cellular metabolism result in the common key features:
  1. Cardiovascular manifestations
     a. Decreased cardiac output
     b. Pulse rate increased, quality decreased
     c. Decreased systolic blood pressure
     d. Narrowed pulse pressure
     e. Postural hypotension
     f. Flat neck and hand veins in dependent positions
     g. Slow capillary refill in nail beds
     h. Diminished peripheral pulses
  2. Respiratory manifestations
     a. Increased respiratory rate
     b. Shallow depth of respirations
     c. Increased $Paco_2$; decreased Pao_2
     d. Cyanosis, especially around lips and nail beds
  3. Neuromuscular manifestations
     a. Early
        (1) Anxiety and restlessness
        (2) Increased thirst
     b. Late
        (1) Lethargy to coma
        (2) Generalized muscle weakness
        (3) Diminished or absent deep tendon reflexes
        (4) Sluggish pupillary response to light
  4. Renal manifestations
     a. Decreased urine output
     b. Increased specific gravity

S

5. Skin and mucous membrane manifestations
   a. Cool to cold
   b. Pale to mottled to cyanotic
   c. Moist, clammy
- Hypovolemic shock
  1. The basic problem of hypovolemic shock is a loss of blood volume from the vascular space, which results in a decreased mean arterial pressure (MAP) and decreased oxygen-carrying capacity from the loss of circulating RBCs.
  2. These problems decrease tissue perfusion and oxygenation, leading to anaerobic cellular metabolism.
  3. The most common problems leading to hypovolemic shock are hemorrhage (external or internal) and dehydration.
  4. Uncorrected hypovolemic shock progresses in four stages as poor cellular oxygenation continues.
     a. *Initial stage of shock (Early Shock)* occurs when the patient's baseline MAP is decreased by less than 10 mm Hg. Adaptive (compensatory) mechanisms are effective at returning MAP to normal levels, and oxygenated blood flow to all vital organs is maintained. Heart and respiratory rates are increased from the patient's baseline level, or a slight increase in diastolic blood pressure may be the only objective manifestation.
     b. *Nonprogressive stage (Compensatory Stage)* occurs when MAP decreases by 10 to 15 mm Hg from baseline. Kidney and hormonal adaptive (compensatory) mechanisms are activated because cardiovascular adjustments alone are not enough to maintain MAP and supply needed oxygen to the vital organs. Tissue hypoxia occurs in the skin, GI tract, and kidney but is not great enough to cause permanent damage. The cellular effects of this stage are reversible if the problem is recognized and appropriate interventions are started.
     c. *Progressive stage of shock (Intermediate Stage)* occurs when there is a sustained decrease in MAP of more than 20 mm Hg from baseline. Adaptive (compensatory) mechanisms are functioning but can no longer deliver sufficient oxygen, even to vital organs. As a result of poor oxygenation and a buildup of toxic metabolites, some tissues have severe cell damage and die.
     d. *Refractory stage of shock (Irreversible Stage)* occurs when too much cell death and tissue damage results from too little oxygen reaching the tissues. Vital organs have overwhelming damage, the body can no longer respond effectively to interventions, and shock continues. Widespread

release of toxic metabolites and destructive enzymes causes cell damage in vital organs to continue despite aggressive interventions, and multiple organ dysfunction syndrome (MODS) leads to death.

PATIENT-CENTERED COLLABORATIVE CARE

Assessment

- Obtain patient information about:
  1. Recent illness, trauma, procedures, or chronic health problems
     a. GI ulcers
     b. General surgery
     c. Hemophilia
     d. Liver disorders
     e. Prolonged vomiting or diarrhea
  2. Drug use, especially aspirin, diuretics, and antacids
  3. Fluid intake and output during the previous 24 hours
- Assess for and document:
  1. Bleeding of gums, wounds, and sites of dressings, drains, and vascular accesses
  2. Swelling or skin discoloration that may indicate an internal hemorrhage
  3. Cardiovascular changes
     a. Increased heart rate and decreased pulse quality
     b. Decreased peripheral pulses

> **Clinical Landmine** ◆ Changes in systolic blood pressure are not always present in the initial stage of shock and should not be used as the main indicator of shock presence or progression.

     c. Trends of decreasing systolic pressure and narrowing pulse pressure
     d. Decreasing oxygen saturation
  4. Respiratory changes
     a. Increased rate
     b. Decreased depth
  5. Renal and urinary changes
     a. Decreased urine output
     b. Increased urine specific gravity
  6. Skin changes
     a. Cool temperature
     b. Pallor or cyanosis, especially oral mucous membranes
     c. Clammy or moist skin
     d. Slow or sluggish capillary refill

7. Central nervous system (CNS) changes
   a. Thirst
   b. Decreasing alertness and level of consciousness (LOC)
8. Psychosocial changes
   a. Restlessness and sense of "impending doom"
   b. Decreasing orientation
   c. Decreased cognition
9. Laboratory changes
   a. Decreased hematocrit and hemoglobin levels if shock is caused by hemorrhage
   b. Increased hematocrit and hemoglobin levels if shock is caused by dehydration or a fluid shift

Interventions

Nonsurgical Management

- Oxygen therapy is useful whenever shock is present. It can be delivered by mask, hood, nasal cannula, nasopharyngeal tube, endotracheal tube, or tracheostomy tube.
- IV therapy (fluid resuscitation) is initiated as prescribed.
  1. Crystalloid solutions contain nonprotein substances and include normal saline and Ringer's lactate.

> **Clinical Landmine** ◆ Do not infuse Ringer's lactate with blood or blood products, because the calcium induces clotting of the infusing blood.

  2. Colloid solutions contain large molecules (usually proteins or starches) to help restore osmotic pressure and fluid volume. These fluids include whole blood, packed RBCs, plasma, plasma fractions, and synthetic plasma expanders.
  3. Drug therapy is initiated as prescribed when the volume deficit is severe and the patient does not respond sufficiently to the replacement of fluid volume and blood products.
     a. Vasoconstricting agents
        (1) Dopamine (Intropin, Revimine ❦)
        (2) Norepinephrine (Levophed)
     b. Inotropic agents
        (3) Dobutamine (Dobutrex)
        (4) Milrinone (Primacor)
     c. (5) Drugs that enhance myocardial perfusion, such as sodium nitroprusside (Nitropress, Nipride ❦)
- Additional nursing interventions include assessing the patient's response to therapy.
  1. Monitoring vital signs every 15 minutes until shock is controlled

a. Pulse
b. Blood pressure
c. Pulse pressure
d. Respiratory rate
e. Skin and mucosal color
f. Oxygen saturation
g. Urine output
2. Monitoring LOC

Surgical Management

- After a cause has been established, surgical intervention may be needed to correct the cause of shock. Such procedures include vascular repair or revision, surgical hemostasis of major wounds, closure of bleeding ulcers, and chemical scarring (chemosclerosis) of varicosities.

Infection, Sepsis, SIRS, and Septic Shock

- Sepsis and septic shock are a complex type of distributive shock that usually begins as a bacterial or fungal infection and progresses to a dangerous condition over a period of days.

Infection

- When infection is confined to a local area, it does not lead to sepsis and shock. The invasion first sets off a helpful, nonspecific series of local responses to confine and eliminate the organism and to prevent the infection from becoming worse or widespread.

- The WBCs in the area of invasion secrete cytokines to trigger a local inflammatory response and bring more phagocytic WBCs to the area to fight and kill the invading organisms. The results of this local response constrict the small veins and dilate the arterioles in the area of injury. These blood vessel changes cause redness and warmth of the locally infected tissues and increase blood flow to the area to deliver more nutrients.

- Blood flow to the area increases and edema forms at the site of injury or invasion. Capillary leak also occurs, allowing blood plasma to leak into the tissues. This response causes swelling and pain. The duration of these responses depends on the size and severity of the infection, but usually they subside within a few days, when the infection has been managed by these responses.

- An important feature of the benefit of these responses is that they are limited only to the area of infection and stop as soon as they are no longer needed. The patient does not have fever, tachycardia, decreased oxygen saturation, or reduced urine output.

Sepsis and SIRS

- Sepsis is a widespread infection coupled with a more general inflammatory response, known as *systemic inflammatory response syndrome (SIRS)*, which is triggered when an infection escapes local control.

- With the organisms and their toxins or endotoxins in the bloodstream and entering other body areas, the inflammatory responses become an enemy, leading to extensive tissue and vascular changes that further impair oxygenation and tissue perfusion.
- The WBCs are producing many pro-inflammatory cytokines, leading to widespread vasodilation and pooling of blood in some tissues.
- The patient has a low-grade fever, mild hypotension, a urine output that is lower than expected for fluid intake, and an increased respiratory rate. These actions result in a hypodynamic state with decreased cardiac output.
- Microthrombi begin to form within the capillaries of some organs, causing some cell hypoxia and reducing organ function. The microthrombi increase the number of cells that are operating under anaerobic conditions, which results in the generation of more toxic metabolites. These cause more cell damage and increase the production of pro-inflammatory cytokines, intensifying or amplifying the SIRS and leading to a vicious repeating cycle of poor oxygenation and tissue perfusion.
- These subtle manifestations indicate early sepsis and usually progress unless intervention occurs at this time.
  1. If early sepsis is identified and treated aggressively, the cycle of progression is stopped and the outcome is good.
  2. If early sepsis is not identified and treated at this stage, it almost always progresses to severe sepsis, which is much harder to control.

Severe Sepsis
- Severe sepsis is the progression of sepsis with an amplified inflammatory response. All tissues are involved, and all have some degree of hypoxia.
- Microthromi formation is widespread and consumes much of the available platelets and clotting factors, a condition is known as *disseminated intravascular coagulation (DIC)*.
- The amplified SIRS and cytokine release increase capillary leakiness, injure cells (especially endothelial cells of blood vessels), and increase cell metabolism.
- Damage to endothelial cells reduces anticlotting actions and triggers the formation of even more small clots, allowing anaerobic metabolism to continue.
- The continued stress response triggers continued release of glucose from the liver, causing hyperglycemia. The more severe the response, the higher the blood glucose level.

- At this time, cardiac function is hyperdynamic, because the pooling of blood and widespread capillary leak stimulate the heart. Heart rate is rapid, and systolic blood pressure is elevated. The patient's extremities may feel warm, and there is little or no cyanosis.
- Additional manifestations at this stage are lower oxygen saturation, rapid respiratory rate, decreased to absent urine output, and a change in the patient's cognition and affect.

Septic Shock

- Septic shock is the stage of sepsis and SIRS in which multiple organ failure is evident and uncontrolled bleeding occurs. *Even with appropriate intervention, the death rate is very high.*
- Severe hypovolemic shock is present with hypodynamic cardiac function. The clinical manifestations resemble the late stage of hypovolemic shock.

Interventions to Prevent Sepsis and Septic Shock

- Evaluate all patients for their risk for sepsis.
- Use aseptic technique during invasive procedures and when working with nonintact skin and mucous membranes in immunocompromised patients.
- Remove indwelling urinary catheters and IV access lines as soon as they are no longer needed.
- Assess vital signs often (at least twice per shift) for changes from baseline levels.
- Review laboratory data for changes in serum lactate levels, in total WBC count, and in the differential. The hallmark of sepsis is a *left shift*, an increasing serum lactate level, a normal or low total WBC count, and a decreasing segmented neutrophil level with a rising band neutrophil level.
- Assess other laboratory indicators of sepsis and septic shock, especially a low blood level of activated protein C, rising plasma D-dimer levels, rising interleukin-6 (IL-6), and normal or decreasing levels of IL-10.

Management of Sepsis and Septic Shock

- The health care team implements the Sepsis Resuscitation Bundle.
  1. Measuring serum lactate levels
  2. Obtaining blood cultures *before* administering antibiotics
  3. Administering broad-spectrum antibiotic therapy within 1 to 3 hours of establishing diagnosis
  4. If hypotension or a serum lactate level greater than 4 mmol/L (36 mg/dL) is present:
     a. Institute IV delivery of 20 mL/kg of crystalloid fluids (or the colloid equivalent).

S

    b. If hypotension does not respond to initial fluid resuscitation by increasing MAP to at least 65 mm Hg, start IV vasopressor therapy.

  5. If hypotension persists despite fluid resuscitation and vasopressor therapy and septic shock is present or the serum lactate level remains greater than 4 mmol/L (36 mg/dL), use the following parameters to monitor therapy effectiveness:

    a. Central venous pressure (CVP) of at least 8 mm Hg

    b. Central venous oxygen saturation (Scvo$_2$) of at least 70% or a mixed venous oxygen saturation (Svo$_2$) of at least 65%

- The health care team implements the Sepsis Management Bundle.

  1. When septic shock is present, administer low-dose steroids (200 to 300 mg hydrocortisone IV daily in divided doses) in accordance with ICU protocol.

  2. Administer drotrecogin alfa (activated) for patients meeting ICU and drotrecogin criteria.

  3. Administer insulin to maintain blood glucose levels at least lower than 150 mg/dL.

  4. Use mechanical ventilation to maintain inspiratory plateau pressures less than 30 cm H$_2$O.

- Blood replacement therapy is used when septic shock progresses to hemorrhage.

  1. Clotting factors (cryoprecipitate)

  2. Fresh-frozen plasma (FFP)

  3. Whole blood

  4. Packed RBCs

SJÖGREN'S SYNDROME

- Sjögren's syndrome (SS) is a group of problems that often appear with other autoimmune disorders. Inflammation and autoimmune responses obstruct certain secretory ducts and glands.
- Problems include dry eyes (sicca syndrome), dry mucous membranes of the nose and mouth (xerostomia), and vaginal dryness. Often, the patient with SS also has rheumatoid arthritis or fibromyalgia.
- Insufficient tears cause inflammation and ulceration of the cornea. Insufficient saliva decreases digestion of carbohydrates, promotes tooth decay, and increases the incidence of oral and nasal infections. Vaginal dryness increases the incidence of infection and may cause pain during sexual intercourse.
- Other manifestations include blurred vision, burning and itching of the eyes, thick mattering in the conjunctiva, difficulty

swallowing food, changes in taste sensation, nosebleeds, and frequent upper respiratory infections.

- Laboratory assessment may show increased presence of general antinuclear antibodies, anti-SS-A or anti-SS-B antibodies, and elevated levels of immunoglobulin M (IgM) rheumatoid factor.
- Most patients with SS are women between 35 and 45 years old.
- There is no cure, and management focuses on slowing the intensity and the progression of the disorder by suppressing immune and inflammatory responses.
- Drug therapy may include:
  1. Low-dose chemotherapy
     a. Methotrexate (Rheumatrex)
     b. Cyclophosphamide (Cytoxan)
  2. Corticosteroids
  3. Cyclosporine (Neoral, Sand-immune)
  4. Hydroxychloroquine (Plaquenil)
- Dry eye and dry mouth symptoms may be managed with a variety of artificial tears and artificial saliva.
- Teach patients to use humidifiers in the home to increase environmental moisture.
- Use of water-soluble vaginal lubricants and moisturizers can increase patient comfort and reduce the incidence of vaginitis.

SKIN INFECTIONS

OVERVIEW

- Skin infections can be bacterial, viral, or fungal, but most are bacterial, caused by *Staphylococcus* or *Streptococcus* microorganisms.
- *Folliculitis* is a superficial infection involving only the upper portion of the follicle. It usually manifests as a raised, red rash with small pustules.
- *Furuncles* (boils) are deeper follicle infections with a large, sore-looking, raised bump that may or may not have a pustular "head" at its point.
- *Cellulitis* is a generalized infection and involves the deeper connective tissue.
- The major cause of bacterial skin infection is minor skin trauma.
- An increasingly common skin problem is infection with methicillin-resistant *Staphylococcus aureus* (MRSA). This highly contagious specific infection is described elsewhere (see Methicillin-Resistant *Staphylococcus aureus*).

- Viral skin infections are commonly caused by the *herpes simplex virus* (HSV) and include type I infections (common cold sore), type II infections (genital herpes), and herpes zoster (shingles) (see Herpes, Genital). Viral infections differ from bacterial infections in two ways:
  1. After the first infection, the virus remains in the body in a dormant state in the nerve ganglia, and the patient has no symptoms.
  2. Reactivation stimulates the virus to travel the pathways of sensory nerves to the skin, where lesions reappear.
- Many fungal infections also affect the skin.
  1. Superficial dermatophyte infections include:
     a. Tinea pedis (athlete's foot)
     b. Tinea manus (hands)
     c. Tinea cruris (groin, "jock itch")
     d. Tinea capitis (head)
     e. Tinea corporis (ringworm)
  2. *Candida albicans*, also known as "yeast" infection, is another common superficial fungal infection of skin and mucous membranes.
     a. Risk factors include immunosuppression, long-term antibiotic therapy, diabetes mellitus, and obesity.
     b. The incidence is higher in hot, humid climates.
     c. Infected skin (most often of the mouth, perineum, vagina, axillae, and under the breasts) has a moist, red, irritated appearance, usually with itching and burning.
- Prevention of skin infections, especially bacterial and fungal infections, involves avoiding the offending organism and good personal hygiene to remove the organism before infection can occur.

> 🛟 Critical Rescue ♦ Handwashing and not sharing personal items with others are the best ways to avoid contact with some of the most easily transmitted organisms, including MRSA.

PATIENT-CENTERED COLLABORATIVE CARE
Assessment
- Obtain patient information about:
  1. Recent history of skin trauma
  2. Past or current staphylococcal or streptococcal infections
  3. Living conditions, home sanitation, personal hygiene habits, and leisure or sport activities

4. Whether fever and malaise are also present
5. Lesions locations, especially lips, mouth, or genital region
6. History of similar lesions in the same location
7. Presence of burning, tingling, or pain
8. Recent stress factors
9. Recent contact with an infected person
10. Whether the patient has had ever chickenpox or shingles
11. Whether the patient has received the shingles prevention vaccine, Zostavax
12. Social and environmental factors
    a. Direct contact with an infected person
    b. Personal hygiene practices
    c. Frequent contact with animals
    d. Type and frequency of athletic activities
- Assess for and document:
  1. Redness
  2. Warmth
  3. Edema
  4. Tenderness
  5. Pain
  6. Itching
  7. Stinging
  8. Location of areas of inflammation, rash, or infection
  9. Presence of:
     a. Blisters or vesicles
     b. Pustules
     c. Papules
     d. Scaling
     e. Single or multiple lesions

Interventions

- Most skin infections heal well with nonsurgical management, but surgery may be required if an infectious agent is present in deep tissue layers.
- Nursing interventions include:
  1. Skin care instructions
     a. Bathing daily with an antibacterial soap
     b. Not squeezing any pustules or crusts but removing them gently
     c. Applying warm compresses twice a day to furuncles or areas of cellulitis
     d. Avoiding constricting garments that might rub the lesions
     e. Keeping the skin dry between treatments
     f. Positioning for optimal air circulation to the area

2. Prevention of transmission
   a. Using proper handwashing to prevent cross-contamination
   b. Isolating the patient if infections are colonized with *Staphylococcus* that is resistant to antibiotic therapy
   c. Teaching patients to avoid sharing personal items such as hairbrushes, articles of clothing, or footwear
   d. Teaching patients to avoid sexual contact when recurrent herpes lesions are present

- Drug therapy includes:
  1. Topical agents for superficial infections and mild bacterial infections
  2. Systemic antibiotic therapy for extensive infections, especially if fever or lymphadenopathy is present
     a. Antiviral agents such as acyclovir (Zovirax), valacyclovir (Valtrex), or famciclovir (Famvir)
     b. Antifungal agents such as ketoconazole (Nizoral)

SPINAL CORD INJURY

OVERVIEW

- An injury to the vertebral column and spinal cord may be caused by motor vehicle accidents, falls, sports such as diving and football, and penetrating trauma.
- As a result of spinal cord injury (SCI), losses of or decreases in motor function, sensation, reflex activity, and bowel and bladder function may occur.
- The extent of the injury can be classified as:
  1. *Complete* if the spinal cord is severed or damaged in a way that eliminates all innervation below the level of injury, and total motor and sensory loss occurs
  2. *Incomplete* (more common) if there is preservation of a mixed pattern of motor, sensory, and reflex function
- Cervical spinal cord injuries (SCIs) may result in specific syndromes.
  1. Anterior cord injury is characterized by loss of motor function, pain, and temperature sensation below the level of the injury; sensations of touch, position, and vibration remain intact.
  2. Posterior cord injury is characterized by intact motor function and loss of vibratory sense, crude touch, and position sense.
  3. Central cord injury is characterized by loss of motor function that is more pronounced in the upper extremities than in the lower extremities.

- Complications of SCI include pressure ulcers, contractures, and deep vein thrombosis (DVT) or pulmonary emboli. Muscle spasticity and bone loss can occur over time.

PATIENT-CENTERED COLLABORATIVE CARE

Assessment

- Obtain information about:
  1. How the injury occurred and the probable mechanism of injury
  2. Position immediately after the injury
  3. Symptoms that occurred after the injury and what changes have occurred since
  4. Prehospital rescue personnel are questioned about:
     a. Problems encountered during the extrication and transport
     b. Type of immobilization devices used
     c. Medical treatment given at the scene
  5. Medical history, with particular attention to a history of arthritis of the spine, congenital deformities, osteoarthritis or osteomyelitis, cancer, previous back or spinal cord injury, and respiratory problems
- Assess for and document:
  1. Adequacy of airway, breathing, and circulation
  2. Indication of hemorrhage or bleeding around the fracture sites or in the abdomen
  3. Indications of a head injury such as a change in LOC, abnormal pupil size and reaction to light, and change in behavior or ability to respond to directions
  4. Motor strength, comparing bilateral movement; the ability to shrug the shoulders, flex and extend the arms, elevate the arms and legs off the bed, extend the wrist, wiggle the toes, and flex and extend the feet and legs; and deep tendon reflexes
  5. Spinal shock, which occurs immediately after the injury and lasts a few days to several months. It is characterized by:
     a. Flaccid paralysis
     b. Loss of reflex activity below the level of the lesion
     c. Bradycardia
     d. Paralytic ileus (occasionally)
     e. Hypotension
  6. Decreased or absent sensation, comparing bilaterally
  7. Cardiovascular dysfunction, such as bradycardia, hypotension, and cardiac dysrhythmias
  8. Change in thermoregulatory capacity, with the patient's body tending to assume the temperature of the environment (hypothermia)

9. Paralytic ileus manifested by decreased or absent bowel sounds and distended abdomen
10. Coping strategies used in the past to deal with illness, difficult situations, or disappointments

Planning and Implementation

❖**NDx:** Ineffective Tissue Perfusion (Spinal Cord)

- To preserve cord function and prevent secondary injury, implement the following management.

Nonsurgical Management

- Assess for changes in neurologic function (especially changes in movement or muscle strength) with vital signs and pain score every 4 hours.
- Observe for neurogenic shock, especially in the presence of acute cervical cord injury manifested by hypotension and bradycardia (see Shock).
- Keep the patient in optimal body alignment to prevent further cord injury or irritability.
  1. The most commonly used devices for cervical injuries are cervical tongs (Gardner-Wells, Barton, or Crutchfield tongs) and the halo fixation device to immobilize the spine.
  2. Traction is added, with the amount of weight to be used prescribed by the physician.
  3. Weights should hang free at all times; never release the traction.
  4. Monitor insertion sites for infection and clean pins per hospital policy.
- The patient with thoracic and lumbar or sacral injuries is placed on bedrest and may be immobilized with a fiberglass or plastic body cast.
- Monitor the patient for spinal shock, also called spinal shock syndrome, which occurs immediately as a concussion response to the injury. The patient has flaccid paralysis and loss of reflex activity below the level of the lesion. It usually resolves within 24 hours, and muscle spasticity begins in patients with cervical or high thoracic injuries.
- Drug therapy may include:
  1. Methylprednisolone (Solu-Medrol) may be given after the initial injury in a very high loading dose and then as a continuous drip for 24 hours.
  2. Dextran, a plasma expander, is used to increase capillary blood flow within the spinal cord and to prevent or treat hypotension.
  3. Atropine sulfate is used to treat bradycardia.
  4. Inotropic and sympathomimetic agents treat hypotension.

5. Dantrolene (Dantrium) or baclofen (Lioresal) is used to treat spasticity.

Surgical Management

- Reduce and immobilize fractured vertebrae immediately.
    1. Decompressive laminectomy is performed to relieve compression from a hematoma, to remove bone fragments, or to remove a penetrating object such as a bullet.
    2. Spinal fusion or insertion of metal or steel rods to stabilize the vertebral column may be indicated.
    3. The patient with a cervical injury may be placed in fixed skeletal traction to realign the vertebrae, facilitate bone healing, and prevent further injury, often after surgical stabilization. The most commonly used device for immobilization is the halo fixation device.
    4. Perioperative care is described in Part One with special attention to assessing neurologic status (for changes in movement or decreased strength) with vital signs.

❖**NDx:** Ineffective Airway Clearance; Ineffective Breathing Pattern; Impaired Gas Exchange

- To maintain a patent airway and adequate ventilation, implement the following management:
    1. Perform a respiratory assessment often; perform active rescue breathing, pulmonary toilet, or physician communication if the patient experiences decreased oxygenation despite repositioning, airway suctioning, or oxygen supplementation.
    2. Provide increased frequency of assessment and intervention if the patient has an injury above thoracic level 6 (T6) in the immediate 5 days after injury, when respiratory failure is most likely to occur.
    3. Provide continuous lateral rotation if the patient is mechanically ventilated. Manually reposition the patient at least every 2 hours.
    4. Teach the patient to use an incentive spirometer every 2 hours and to deep breathe at least hourly while awake.
    5. Perform tracheal suctioning based on assessment findings.
    6. Use a technique called *quad cough* or *cough assist* to help the quadriplegic patient cough: Place your hands on either side of the patient's rib cage or upper abdomen below the diaphragm. As the patient inhales, push upward to help the patient expand the lungs and cough.

❖**NDx:** Impaired Physical Mobility; Self-Care Deficit

- To prevent complications of immobility, implement the following management:
    1. Reposition the patient every 2 hours while the patient is in bed and every 30 minutes while in a chair.

S

2. Inspect the skin and teach the patient to inspect the skin every shift for signs of pressure sores or reddened areas.
3. Perform ROM exercises for all extremities at least once every 8 hours.
4. Collaborate with physical and occupational therapists to determine positioning and exercise programs; determine the need for splints and a plan to prevent foot drop.
5. Assess for signs of DVT; measure the calf and thigh if left and right are not symmetric.
6. Apply thigh-high antiembolism stockings; sequential compression devices or pneumatic compression boots may be used.
7. Observe for orthostatic hypotension when raising the head of the bed, dangling the patient on the side of the bed, and transferring the patient to a chair. Teach the patient to change positions slowly.
8. Collaborate with physical and occupational therapists to identify techniques and assistive devices to enable the patient to become as independent as possible in ADLs.

❖**NDx:** Impaired Urinary Elimination, Constipation

- To achieve control of elimination of urine and stool, implement the following management:
  1. Establish an individualized bladder program.
     a. Begin an intermittent catheterization program as soon as possible.
     b. Catheterize the patient every 4 hours or more frequently if the urinary output is more than 500 mL.
     c. Over time, intervals between catheterizations are increased and adjusted to the patient's fluid intake and sleep times.
     d. Encourage fluid intake, unless contraindicated, to 2000 to 2500 mL daily. Patients with lower motor neuron injuries may restrict fluids after 6 or 7 PM.
     e. Teach the patient with upper motor injury (spastic bladder problem) to stimulate voiding by stroking the inner thigh, pulling on pubic hair and hair of the upper thigh, pouring warm water over the perineum, or tapping the bladder area to stimulate the detrusor muscle.
     f. Teach the patient with a lower motor injury (flaccid bladder problem) to perform the Valsalva maneuver or tighten the abdominal muscles to stimulate emptying of the bladder.
     g. Catheterize for residual urine after the patient voids to determine the effectiveness of the stimulation techniques.
  2. Establish an individualized bowel program.
     a. Schedule a consistent time for evacuation.

    b. Encourage fluid intake (2000 mL daily) unless contraindicated.

    c. Provide a high-fiber diet.

    d. Assess the need for a suppository or stool softener.

    e. Place the patient on a bedside commode or bedpan at the time determined to be his or her normal time to have a bowel movement; allow for privacy.

    f. Teach the patient to use the Valsalva maneuver or to massage the abdomen from right to left to stimulate bowel evacuation.

❖**NDx:** Impaired Adjustment

- To develop an adaptive psychosocial response to significant life changes, implement the following management:

1. Refer questions about prognosis and potential for complete recovery to the health care provider, because the timing and extent of recovery vary greatly.

2. Invite the patient to ask questions; answer questions honestly and openly.

3. Explore coping strategies with the patient.

4. Redirect socially unacceptable behavior.

5. Refer the patient to clergy, a psychiatric liaison nurse, or a psychologist to help him or her adjust to unexpected life changes.

6. Refer the patient to a social worker or financial counselor for review of insurance and financial status; refer to appropriate social service agencies as needed.

❖**Collaborative Problem:** Autonomic Dysreflexia

1. Autonomic dysreflexia (hyperreflexia) is generally seen in injuries above the level of the sixth thoracic vertebra and occurs after the period of spinal shock is completed. It is usually caused by a noxious stimulus such as a distended bladder or constipation.

2. Key features of autonomic dysreflexia include:

    a. Severe, rapidly occurring hypertension

    b. Bradycardia

    c. Flushing above the level of injury

    d. Severe, throbbing headache

    e. Nasal stuffiness

    f. Sweating

    g. Nausea

    h. Blurred vision

3. Treatment of autonomic dysreflexia includes:

    a. Raising the head of the bed to a high Fowler's position

    b. Loosening tight clothing

    c. Checking the Foley catheter tubing (if present) for kinks or obstruction

    d. If a Foley catheter is not in place, checking for bladder distention and catheterizing immediately

    e. Checking the patient for fecal impaction and, if present, disimpacting immediately using anesthetic ointment

    f. Checking the room temperature to ensure that it is not too cool or drafty

    g. Monitoring blood pressure every 15 minutes; hypertension may be treated with nitrates or hydralazine

Community Health

- Discharge planning: most patients are discharged to a rehabilitation setting, where they learn more about self-care, mobility skills, and bladder and bowel retraining.
  1. Psychosocial adaptation is a crucial factor in determining the success of rehabilitation.
  2. Assist the patient to verbalize feeling and fears about body image, self-concept, role performance, and self-esteem.
  3. Talk to the patient about the expected reactions of those outside the hospital environment.
- To prepare for discharge to home or for a weekend home visit:
  1. Collaborate with the patient, family, and rehabilitation professionals to assess the home environment to ensure that it is free from hazards and can accommodate the patient's special needs.
  2. Ensure that the patient can correctly use all adaptive devices ordered for home use.
  3. Ensure that adaptive equipment is installed in the home before discharge.
- Teach the patient and family, in collaboration with other health care team members:
  1. ADL skills
  2. Bowel and bladder training program
  3. Drug regimen
  4. Skin care
  5. Sexual functioning
- Refer the patient to local, state, and national support groups.
- Provide the telephone number for the spinal cord injury hotline.

STENOSIS, AORTIC

OVERVIEW

- In aortic stenosis (AS), the aortic valve orifice narrows, obstructing left ventricular outflow during systole.
- Increased resistance to ejection or afterload results in left ventricular hypertrophy.

- As stenosis progresses, cardiac output becomes fixed and unable to meet the demands of the body during exertion and symptoms develop.
- Over time, left ventricle failure (heart failure [HF]) develops, volume backs up in the left atrium, and the pulmonary system becomes congested. Right-sided heart failure can occur late in the disease.

Considerations for Older Adults

Atherosclerosis and degenerative calcification of the aortic valve are the predominant causative factors in people older than 70 years. Aortic stenosis has become the most common valvular disorder in countries with an aging population. Of patients with aortic stenosis, 80% are men.

PATIENT-CENTERED COLLABORATIVE CARE

- Assess for and document:
  1. Dyspnea, angina, and syncope on exertion
  2. Fatigue
  3. Peripheral cyanosis
  4. Diamond-shaped systolic crescendo-decrescendo murmur
  5. Signs of heart failure
- Aortic valve surgery is the treatment of choice when the patient is symptomatic with AS.
  1. Balloon valvuloplasty may be performed to repair the valve. A balloon catheter is inserted through the femoral artery and advanced to the aortic valve, where the balloon is inflated, enlarging the orifice of the valve.
  2. In aortic valve replacement surgery, the valve is excised during cardiopulmonary bypass surgery and then replaced with a prosthetic (synthetic) or biologic (tissue) valve.
- The postoperative patient requires lifetime anticoagulation therapy to prevent thrombus formation on the valve.
- For preoperative and postoperative care, see Perioperative Care (Part One) and Surgical Management under Coronary Artery Disease.

STENOSIS, MITRAL

OVERVIEW

- Mitral stenosis causes thickening of the mitral valve by fibrosis and calcification.
- Valve leaflets fuse together, becoming stiff; the chordae tendineae contract and shorten; the valve opening narrows, preventing normal blood flow from the left atrium to the left ventricle;

and as a result, the left atrial pressure rises, the left ventricle dilates, pulmonary artery pressures increase, and the right ventricle hypertrophies.

- Pulmonary congestion and right-sided heart failure occur; later, preload is decreased and cardiac output declines.
- A history of rheumatic fever is associated with mitral stenosis.

PATIENT-CENTERED COLLABORATIVE CARE

- Assess for and document:
  1. Changes in respiratory patterns: orthopnea, dyspnea with exertion, paroxysmal nocturnal dyspnea, cough
  2. Symptoms of left ventricular failure: pulmonary edema, S_3 heart sound, crackles in lungs, frothy sputum
  3. Symptoms of right ventricular failure: hepatomegaly, neck vein distention, peripheral pitting edema
  4. Atrial fibrillation resulting from right atrial hypertrophy
  5. Rumbling, apical diastolic murmur
- Mitral valve repair or replacement surgery is the treatment of choice for symptomatic mitral valve stenosis.
  1. Balloon valvuloplasty, an invasive nonsurgical procedure, involves passing a balloon catheter from the femoral vein, through the atrial septum, to the mitral valve. The balloon is inflated to enlarge the mitral orifice.
  2. Mitral commissurotomy is performed during cardiopulmonary bypass surgery. The surgeon removes thrombi from the atria, incises the fused commissures (leaflets), and débrides calcium from the leaflets, thus widening the orifice.
  3. Mitral valve replacement is indicated if the leaflets are calcified and immobile. The valve is excised during cardiopulmonary bypass surgery, and a new valve is sutured into place.
- The postoperative patient requires lifetime anticoagulant therapy to prevent thrombus formation on the valve.
- Perioperative care
  1. For care of the patient undergoing coronary artery bypass grafting, see Coronary Artery Disease.
  2. After the procedure, observe the patient for bleeding from the catheter insertion site and institute postangiography precautions.
  3. Observe for signs of a regurgitant valve by closely monitoring heart sounds, cardiac output, and heart rhythm.
  4. Observe for signs of vascular occlusion (reduced peripheral pulses, stroke, and acute coronary syndrome) from emboli while establishing anticoagulation therapy.

Community Health
1. Provide health teaching information regarding:
   a. Drugs, especially anticoagulant therapy
   b. Plan of work, activity, and rest to conserve energy
   c. The importance of taking an antibiotic before invasive procedures (e.g., dental work, surgery)
2. Refer the patient to community resources, such as the American Heart Association.

> ⛑ **Critical Rescue** ◆ Heparin and warfarin (Coumadin) are two drugs commonly associated with significant errors in the hospital setting. Be especially vigilant in verifying the correct patient, dose, route, time of administration, and drug (including concentration!) when giving these powerful drugs.

STENOSIS, RENAL ARTERY

- Renal artery stenosis involves pathologic processes affecting the renal arteries that result in severe narrowing of the lumen and reduced blood flow to the renal parenchyma.
- Uncorrected stenosis leads to ischemia and atrophy of renal tissue.
- Renal artery stenosis is suspected when a sudden onset of hypertension occurs. Reduced renal blood flow from stenosis results in neurohormonal changes (such as activation of the renin-angiotensin-aldosterone system) that elevate blood pressure in a compensatory response to improve renal blood flow.
- Pathology may be fibrotic, atherosclerotic, or both. Fibromuscular changes of the vessel wall occur throughout the length of the renal artery from the aortic junction to the point of branching into the renal segmental arteries. Atherosclerotic changes in the renal artery are associated with similar plaque formation in other major vessels.
- The location of the defect, the overall condition of the patient, and the size of the atrophied kidney influence the decision for therapeutic intervention.
- Treatment includes:
  1. Antihypertensive drugs
  2. Percutaneous transluminal balloon angioplasty
  3. Renal artery bypass surgery

STOMATITIS

- Stomatitis is painful single or multiple ulcerations of the oral mucosa that appear as inflammation and denudation of the oral mucosa, impairing the protective lining of the mouth.

- Common causes include infection, allergy, vitamin deficiency, systemic disease, irritants, chemotherapy, and radiation therapy.
- Primary stomatitis includes aphthous stomatitis, herpes simplex infection, and traumatic insults.
- Secondary stomatitis results from infection by opportunistic viruses, fungi, or bacteria in patients who are immunocompromised.
- The patient is instructed to:
  1. Brush the teeth, gently brush the gums, and clean the oral cavity.
  2. Rinse the mouth frequently with sodium bicarbonate solution, warm saline, or hydrogen peroxide solution (do not use commercial mouthwashes because they have a high alcohol content, causing a burning sensation).
  3. Take drugs (antibiotics, antifungals, anti-inflammatory agents, immune modulators, symptomatic topical agents, and pain-relief drugs) as prescribed.

STROKE (BRAIN ATTACK)

OVERVIEW

- Stroke is caused by a change in the blood supply to the brain. The National Stroke Association now uses the term *brain attack* to describe a stroke.
- A stroke is a medical emergency that strikes suddenly, and it should be treated immediately to prevent neurologic deficit and permanent disability.
- Strokes may be classified as:
  1. Ischemic (occlusive) stroke, which is caused by the occlusion of a cerebral artery
     a. Types of ischemic strokes include:
        (1) Thrombotic stroke, which is commonly associated with the development of atherosclerosis of the blood vessel wall. Rupture of one or more atherosclerotic plaque exposes foam cells to clot-promoting elements in the blood. The end result is clot formation. The artery becomes occluded, and blood flow to the area is markedly diminished, causing transient ischemia and then complete ischemia and infarction of brain tissue. Signs and symptoms occur gradually.
        (2) A lacunar stroke is a type of thrombotic stroke that causes a soft area or cavity to develop in the white matter or deep gray matter of the brain.

(3) Embolic stroke, which is caused by an embolus or group of emboli that travel to the cerebral arteries through the carotid artery and block the artery, resulting in ischemia. Sudden and rapid development of focal neurologic deficits occurs. Cerebral hemorrhage may result if the vessel wall is damaged. Embolic strokes are associated with atrial fibrillation, coronary disease, and heart valve disease or repair.

  b. Ischemic stroke may be preceded by warning signs, including:

    (1) Transient ischemic attack (TIA), a transient focal neurologic deficit such as vertigo or blurred vision that lasts a few minutes to fewer than 24 hours

    (2) Reversible ischemic neurologic deficit (RIND), which is characterized by neurologic symptoms that last longer than 24 hours but less than 1 week

2. Hemorrhagic stroke, in which the integrity of the vessel wall is interrupted and bleeding occurs into the brain tissue or spaces surrounding the brain (ventricular, subdural, subarachnoid). Causes include hypertension, ruptured aneurysm, and arteriovenous malformation (AVM).

  a. An aneurysm is an abnormal ballooning or blister on the involved artery that may become stretched or thinned and rupture.

  b. AVM is a tangled or spaghetti-like mass of malformed, thin-walled, dilated vessels that form an abnormal communication between the arterial and venous systems.

  c. Vasospasm, a sudden and periodic constriction of a cerebral artery, often results from a cerebral hemorrhage caused by aneurysm rupture. Blood flow to distal areas of the brain supplied by the artery is markedly diminished, leading to cerebral ischemia and infarction and further neurologic dysfunction.

PATIENT-CENTERED COLLABORATIVE CARE

Assessment

- Obtain patient information about:
  1. Activity at onset of the stroke
  2. Progression and severity of symptoms, including the presence of a previous TIA or RIND
  3. LOC, orientation
  4. Motor status: gait, balance, reading and writing abilities
  5. Sensory status: speech, hearing, vision
  6. Medical history

7. Social history, with attention to identifying risk factors such as smoking, diet, and exercise
8. Current drugs and nonprescribed drugs, especially anticoagulants, aspirin, vasodilators, and illegal drugs

- Assess for and document:
  1. Neurologic function using a standard stroke screening tool such as the National Institutes of Health (NIH) Stroke Scale, including:
     a. LOC
     b. Orientation
     c. Motor ability
     d. Pupil size and reaction to light, extraocular movement, visual field deficits, ptosis (drooping eyelid)
     e. Speech and language
     f. Vital signs
     g. Blood glucose
  2. Additional neurologic assessment includes:
     a. Cognition, memory, judgment, and problem-solving and decision-making abilities
     b. Ability to concentrate and attend to tasks
     c. ROM, proprioception, head and trunk control, balance, gait, coordination, bowel and bladder control
     d. Sensory status (response to touch and painful stimuli; ability to distinguish between two tactile stimuli presented simultaneously; ability to read, write, and follow verbal directions; and ability to name objects and use them correctly)
     e. Speech pattern (rhythm, clarity, aphasia)
     f. Visual system (homonymous hemianopsia, bitemporal hemianopsia, amaurosis fugax)
     g. Cranial nerve function
     h. Cardiac system (dysrhythmias and murmurs)
     i. Coping mechanisms or personality changes
  3. Emotional lability and screen for depression
  4. Nutritional status
  5. Financial status and occupation
- Diagnostic tests
  1. CT scan of the head without contrast is performed within 30 minutes after arrival at the emergency department. This study is essential to determine patient eligibility for fibrinolytic therapy.
  2. MRI is used to identify the presence of hemorrhage or a cerebral aneurysm. Results also help differentiate stroke from other pathologic changes that mimic a stroke.
  3. CBC, serum electrolytes, and coagulation factors

4. Carotid ultrasound
5. Electrocardiogram and echocardiography to determine whether cardiac disease or dysrhythmia is a contributing factor to stroke

Planning and Implementation

❖**NDx:** Ineffective Tissue Perfusion (Cerebral)

Nonsurgical Management

- Monitor for neurologic changes or complications:
  1. Perform a neurologic assessment at least every 2 to 4 hours, checking.
     a. Verbal ability, orientation
     b. Eye opening, pupil size, and reaction to light
     c. Motor response
  2. Monitor vital signs with neurologic checks.
     a. Ask the physician for acceptable limits for blood pressure.
     b. Perform a cardiac assessment.
     c. Monitor the patient for dysrhythmias; palpate peripheral pulses to help identify new irregularities in heart rhythm in the absence of a cardiac monitor.
  3. Position the backrest to promote cerebral perfusion. In the presence of ischemic stoke, a flat backrest initially may be preferred.
  4. Avoid activities that may increase intracranial pressure.
     a. Maintain the patient's head in a midline neutral position.
     b. Position the patient to avoid extreme hip or neck flexion.
     c. Avoid clustering of nursing procedures.
     d. Provide a quiet environment; room lights should be low.
     e. Assess the need for suctioning; hyperoxygenate the patient before suctioning.
- Drug therapy
  1. Thrombolytic (fibrinolytic) therapy may be used for an acute ischemic stroke.
     a. Recombinant tissue plasminogen activator (rtPA) may be given IV within 3 hours after the onset of symptoms.
        (1) Patients who have had a stroke or serious head trauma in the past 3 months, a hemorrhagic stroke, recent myocardial infarction (MI), increased partial thromboplastin time (PTT), anticoagulant therapy, or who are pregnant are not candidates for this therapy.
     b. Catheter-directed fibrinolytic therapy may be performed as an alternative treatment for up to 6 hours after initial symptoms.

2. Anticoagulant therapy and antiplatelet therapy may be prescribed depending on the health care provider's preference.
   a. Obtain a baseline prothrombin time (for oral anticoagulation therapy) and PTT (for heparin [Hepalean] therapy) before initiating therapy, 6 to 8 hours after the start of the drug, and every morning thereafter. International normalized ratio (INR) is used to monitor warfarin therapy.
   b. Aspirin or other antiplatelet drugs may be used to prevent progression or future thrombotic and embolic strokes.
3. Other drugs used to treat symptoms associated with stroke include:
   a. Phenytoin (Dilantin) or gabapentin (Neurontin), which may be used to prevent seizures
   b. Calcium channel blockers (nimodipine [Nimotop]), which may be administered to treat vasospasm or chronic spasm of the vessel that inhibits blood flow to the area
   c. Stool softeners, analgesics for pain, and antianxiety drugs

- Monitor the patient for complications such as:
  1. Hydrocephalus—enlarged ventricles manifested by a change in the LOC, gait disturbances, and behavior changes
  2. Vasospasm, or narrowing of the cerebral arteries, which leads to cerebral ischemia and infarction and is manifested by a decreased LOC, motor and reflex changes, and increased neurologic deficits (cranial nerve deficits, aphasia)
  3. Rebleeding or rupture of an aneurysm
  4. Bleeding caused by thrombolytic, anticoagulant, or antiplatelet therapy. Observe for blood in the urine and stool, epistaxis (nosebleed), bleeding gums, and easy bruising.
- Carotid artery angioplasty is a nonsurgical intervention used to treat certain types of ischemic stroke. A distal protection device may be placed beyond the stenosis to catch any debris that breaks off during the angioplasty or stenting procedure.

Surgical Management

- Two surgical procedures that may be used for ischemic stroke are:
  1. Carotid endarterectomy to remove atherosclerotic plaque from the inner lining of the carotid artery
  2. Extracranial-intracranial bypass to bypass the occluded area and re-establish blood flow to the affected area
- Surgical procedures to treat AVM include:
  1. Injecting an embolic agent such as platinum coils, detachable silicone balloons, liquid acrylic, or polyvinyl alcohol into the

carotid artery. The agent travels to involved vessels, becomes lodged, and causes the vessels to thrombose.

2. Surgically removing involved vessels

- Surgical procedures to treat aneurysm include:
  1. Placing a clip or clamp at the base or neck of the aneurysm
  2. Wrapping the aneurysm with muscle, muslin, or plastic coating

- The nursing care for these procedures is similar to that discussed in Perioperative Care (Part One) including neurologic assessment with vital signs.

❖**NDx:** Impaired Physical Mobility; Self-Care Deficit

- Treatment includes:
  1. Performing ROM exercises and progressing to chair and ambulation
  2. Consulting with physical therapy and occupational therapy to promote mobility and evaluate for discharge placement
  3. Carefully positioning the patient in proper body alignment, using splint or brace if needed
  4. Using sequential compression devices or pneumatic compression boots to prevent deep venous thrombosis (DVT) when limited mobility is present
  5. Monitoring the patient for signs of DVT and iatrogenic pneumonia
  6. Supporting nutritional intake

❖**NDx:** Disturbed Sensory Perception

- Nursing interventions include:
  1. Providing frequent verbal and tactile cues to help the patient perform ADLs
  2. Breaking down tasks into small steps when cueing
  3. Approaching the patient from the nonaffected side
  4. Placing objects within the patient's field of vision
  5. Placing a patch over the affected eye if diplopia is present
  6. Removing clutter from the room
  7. Orienting the patient to time, place, and event with each encounter
  8. Providing a structured, repetitious, and consistent routine or schedule
  9. Presenting information in a clear, simple, concise manner
  10. Using a step-by-step approach
  11. Placing pictures and other familiar objects in the room

❖**NDx:** Unilateral Neglect

- Interventions include:
  1. Teaching the patient to use both sides of the body
  2. Teaching the patient to scan with the eyes and turn the head from side to side

❖**NDx:** Impaired Verbal Communication
- Interventions to help the patient develop communication strategies include:
  1. Giving repetitive, simple directions; breaking each task into simple steps
  2. Facing the patient and speaking slowly and distinctly
  3. Giving sufficient time for the patient to understand the direction
  4. Using pictures or a communication board if necessary
  5. Encouraging the patient to communicate and positively reinforcing this behavior
  6. Repeating the names of objects on a routine basis and teaching the family to do the same
  7. Consulting with the speech pathologist or therapist

❖**NDx:** Impaired Swallowing
- Nursing interventions include:
  1. Before feeding, assessing the patient's ability to swallow:
     a. Observe for facial drooping and a weak, hoarse voice.
     b. Assess the swallow, gag, and cough reflexes.
     c. Collaborate with the speech-language pathologist to determine the extent of the swallowing problem.
  2. Positioning the patient to facilitate swallowing
     a. Place the patient in a chair or sitting straight up in bed.
     b. Position the patient's head and neck slightly forward and flexed.
  3. Providing soft or semisoft foods and thickened fluids (e.g., mechanical soft, dental diet; custards, scrambled eggs)
  4. Maintaining a quiet room with few distractions while the patient is eating
  5. Providing supplementation if needed
  6. Encouraging family members to participate in mealtimes and feeding
  7. Weighing the patient twice a week

❖**Collaborative Problem:** Bowel and Bladder Incontinence
- Interventions to help the patient become continent include:
  1. Establishing the type (bowel or bladder) and cause of the problem
     a. Altered LOC
     b. Impaired innervation
     c. Inability to communicate the need to urinate or defecate
  2. Determining the patient's usual voiding or bowel movement pattern

3. Implementing an individualized bladder training program (see Incontinence)
   a. Place the patient on a bedpan or commode every 2 hours; encourage fluid intake to 2000 mL daily unless contraindicated.
   b. Use an intermittent catheterization program if retraining is not feasible.
4. Implementing an individualized bowel training program
   a. Determine the normal time or routine for bowel elimination.
   b. Place the patient on a bedpan or commode at the same time each day; use a suppository or stool softener, if needed.
   c. Provide a diet high in bulk or fiber (may require consultation with a nutritionist).

Community-Based Care
- Provide a detailed plan of care at the time of discharge for patients to be transferred to a rehabilitation center or long-term care facility.
- If possible, a case manager should be assigned to help coordinate plans for the patient discharged to the home setting. The case manager should collaborate with the home health agency and with physical and occupational therapists to:
  1. Identify and suggest corrections of hazards in the home before discharge.
  2. Ensure that the patient and family can correctly use all adaptive devices ordered for home use.
  3. Arrange follow-up appointments, as needed.
- Discharge teaching includes:
  1. Providing drug information as needed
  2. Reinforcing mobility skills (in collaboration with other therapists)
     a. How to safely climb stairs, transfer from bed to chair, and get into and out of a car
     b. How to use adaptive equipment
  3. Teaching the family that depression and emotional lability may occur
     a. Depression is usually self-limited; antidepressants may be needed.
     b. Advise the family to avoid being overprotective.
     c. Assist the family and patient to develop realistic and achievable goals.
- Depending on the location of the lesion, the patient may be anxious, slow, cautious, hesitant, or impulsive; may lack initiative; or may be seemingly unaware of the deficit.

- Refer the family to a social worker for further support and counseling. Family members may need a referral for respite care.
- Provide the family with a variety of publications available from the American Heart Association and National Stroke Association.

> ▨ Clinical Landmine ◆ Hand-off errors lead to patient harm. Be sure that clear, consistent communication and complete documentation are available when the patient transfers between in-hospital care units or procedural suites or to rehabilitative or home care.

SUBCLAVIAN STEAL

- Subclavian steal occurs in the upper extremities from a subclavian artery occlusion or stenosis and results in altered blood flow and ischemia in the arm.
- The disorder can occur at any age but is more common when the patient presents with risk factors for atherosclerosis.
- Assess for:
  1. Paresthesias
  2. Light-headedness
  3. Dizziness
  4. Pain and discomfort when the arms are elevated
  5. Difference in blood pressure between arms
  6. Subclavian bruit on the occluded side
  7. Subclavian pulse decreased on the occluded side
  8. Discoloration of the affected arm
- Surgical intervention involves one of three procedures:
  1. Endarterectomy of the subclavian artery
  2. Carotid-subclavian bypass
  3. Dilation of the subclavian artery
- Nursing interventions include:
  1. Frequent brachial and radial pulse checks
  2. Observation for ischemic changes of the extremity
  3. Observation for edema and redness of the extremity

SYNDROME OF INAPPROPRIATE ANTIDIURETIC HORMONE (SIADH)

OVERVIEW

- *Syndrome of inappropriate antidiuretic hormone (SIADH)* occurs when vasopressin (antidiuretic hormone [ADH]) is secreted even though plasma osmolarity is low or normal.

- Water is retained, which results in dilutional *hyponatremia* (a decreased serum sodium level) and expansion of the extracellular fluid volume.
- SIADH occurs with many pathologic conditions and specific drugs, including:
  1. Malignancies (small cell lung cancer; pancreatic, duodenal, and genitourinary carcinomas; thymoma; Hodgkin's lymphoma and non-Hodgkin's lymphoma)
  2. Pulmonary disorders (pneumonia, lung abscesses, active tuberculosis, pneumothorax, chronic lung diseases)
  3. Central nervous system (CNS) disorders (trauma, infection, tumors, strokes)
  4. Drugs
     a. Exogenous ADH
     b. Chlorpropamide
     c. Chemotherapy drugs (vincristine, cyclophosphamide)
     d. Carbamazepine
     e. Opioids
     f. Tricyclic antidepressants
     g. Selective serotonin reuptake inhibitors (SSRIs)
     h. General anesthetics

PATIENT-CENTERED COLLABORATIVE CARE

Assessment
- Obtain patient information about:
  1. Recent head trauma
  2. Cerebrovascular disease
  3. Tuberculosis or other pulmonary disease
  4. Cancer
  5. All past and current drug use
  6. Loss of appetite
  7. Nausea and vomiting
  8. Recent weight gain
- Assess for and document:
  1. Lethargy and headaches
  2. Change in LOC
  3. Decreased deep tendon reflexes
  4. Decreased responsiveness, seizures, and coma
  5. Tachycardia
  6. Hyponatremia
  7. Hypo-osmolarity of the blood
  8. Decreased urine output with high specific gravity

Interventions
- Fluid restriction
  1. Intake may be kept as low as 500 to 600 mL/24 hrs.

S

2. Dilute tube feedings with a solution other than plain water.
3. Use saline to irrigate GI tubes.
4. Mix drugs to be given by GI tube with saline.
- Assess degree of fluid retention and therapy effectiveness.
  1. Measure intake and output.
  2. Weigh the patient daily.
- Promote comfort by offering frequent oral rinsing.
- Drug therapy may include:
  1. Diuretics if heart failure results from fluid overload
  2. Hypertonic saline (i.e., 3% sodium chloride [3% NaCl]) infusions
  3. Demeclocycline (Declomycin), an antibiotic with ADH antagonist properties
     a. Check the patient's mouth daily for oral candidiasis.
     b. Teach the patient to perform meticulous mouth care at least twice daily.
- Assess for fluid overload, pulmonary edema, and heart failure.
  1. Monitor for indicators of increased fluid overload at least every 2 hours.
     a. Increased pulse quality
     b. Increasing neck vein distention
     c. Presence of crackles in lungs
     d. Increasing peripheral edema
     e. Reduced urine output

> **Critical Rescue** ◆ Pulmonary edema can occur very quickly and can lead to death. Notify the health care provider about any change that indicates the fluid overload from SIADH is not responding to therapy or is becoming worse.

- Provide a safe environment.
  1. Monitor the patient's neurologic status for:
     a. Muscle twitching
     b. Orientation to time, place, and person
  2. Reduce environmental noise and lighting to prevent overstimulation.
  3. Keep upper siderails securely in place.

SYPHILIS

OVERVIEW

- Syphilis is a complex sexually transmitted disease (STD) that can become systemic and can cause serious complications, including death.

- The causative organism is *Treponema pallidium,* a spirochete with a slender, spiral shape that resembles a corkscrew.
- In *primary syphilis,* a chancre is the first lesion. It develops at the site of entry (inoculation) of the organism, within 3 weeks on average.
  1. During this highly infectious stage, the chancre begins as a small papule that within 3 to 7 days breaks down into its typical appearance: a painless, indurated, smooth, weeping lesion.
  2. Without treatment, the chancre disappears within 6 weeks; however, the organism spreads throughout the body, and the patient is still infectious.
- *Secondary syphilis,* which develops 6 weeks to 6 months after the onset of primary syphilis, becomes a systemic disease because the spirochetes circulate throughout the bloodstream.
  1. Common manifestations include malaise, low-grade fever, headache, muscle aches and pains, and sore throat.
  2. A generalized rash on the palms and soles that tends to change from papules to squamous papules to pustules. *These lesions are highly contagious and should not be touched without gloves.*
- *Latent syphilis* is a later stage of the disease and has two phases:
  1. *Early latent* syphilis occurs during the first year after infection, and infectious lesions can recur.
  2. *Late latent* syphilis is a disease occurring more than 1 year after infection. It is not infectious except to the fetus of a pregnant woman.
- *Tertiary syphilis,* or *late syphilis,* occurs after a highly variable period, from 4 to 20 years in untreated cases. Any organ system can be affected, and manifestations vary widely. Manifestations include benign lesions (gummas) of the skin, mucous membranes, and bones; aortic valvular disease and aortic aneurysms; and neurosyphilis with central nervous system (CNS) problems (e.g., meningitis, hearing loss, generalized paresis).

PATIENT-CENTERED COLLABORATIVE CARE

Assessment

- Obtain patient information about:
  1. Sexual history
     a. Type and frequency of sexual activity
     b. Number of contacts
     c. History of STDs
     d. Possible sites of infection
     e. Sexual orientation
  2. Current health problem or manifestations

- Assess for and document:
  1. Features of the lesion or chancre (wearing gloves for this examination), including location
  2. Enlarged regional lymph nodes
  3. Presence of a rash
- Diagnosis of primary or secondary syphilis is confirmed by a finding of *T. pallidum* on microscopic examination, by a positive Venereal Disease Research Laboratory (VDRL) serum test, or by a positive rapid plasma reagin (RPR) test result. Latent and tertiary syphilis may be confirmed by the fluorescent treponemal antibody absorption *(FTA-ABS)* test or the micro-hemagglutination assay for *T. palladium* (MHA-TP).

Interventions

- Drug therapy with benzathine penicillin G, given IM as a single dose of 2.4 million units, is the treatment for primary, secondary, and early latent syphilis; the late latent stage is treated with a longer course of antibiotics.
- Nursing care includes:
  1. Testing patients who have never had penicillin for allergy
  2. Monitoring for allergic manifestations (e.g., rash, edema, shortness of breath, chest tightness, anxiety) of drug therapy
  3. Keeping all patients at the health care agency for at least 30 minutes after they have received the antibiotic
  4. Instructing patient to return for follow-up evaluations at 6, 12, and 24 months
  5. Reinforcing teaching about the cause of infection (sexual transmission); treatment, including side effects; possible complications of untreated or incompletely treated disease; and the need for follow-up care
  6. Discussing the importance of partner notification and treatment
  7. Informing patients that the disease will be reported to the local health authority and that all information will be held in strict confidence
  8. Urging the patient to practice sexual abstinence until the treatment of the patient and his or her partners is completed
  9. Encouraging the patient to discuss any feelings of fear, depression, guilt, and anxiety
  10. Referring the patient to other resources such as psychotherapy groups, self-help support groups, or STD clinics
  11. Teaching the patient about ways to avoid future episodes of syphilis by:
      a. Using a latex or polyurethane condom for genital and anal intercourse

    b. Using a condom or latex barrier (dental dam) over the genitals or anus during oral-genital or oral-anal sexual contact

    c. Using gloves for finger or hand contact with the vagina or rectum

    d. Practicing abstinence

    e. Decreasing the number of sexual partners

TETANUS

- Tetanus, also known as lockjaw, is caused by *Clostridium tetani.*
- Tetanus vaccination is initiated in childhood and re-administered every 10 years ("booster") to provide protection against this injection. Tetanus is preventable with vaccination.
- Tetanus is characterized by muscle rigidity, opisthotonos (abnormal posturing that includes arching the back), cramps, muscle spasms, stiffness, and headache.
- Treatment for infection includes prompt (within 72 hours) IM administration of antitoxin: human tetanus immune globulin or hyperimmune equine or bovine serum.
- Sedation, antianxiety agents, and muscle relaxants to decrease muscle spasms and increase comfort are provided.
- Beta blockers or another antidysrhythmic agent may be given to treat cardiac irregularities, and the patient may need aggressive respiratory support.

THORACIC OUTLET SYNDROME

- Thoracic outlet syndrome is a compression of the subclavian artery at the thoracic outlet by anatomic structures, such as a rib or muscle.
- Damage to the arterial wall can produce thrombosis or embolization in distal arteries of the arm.
- The common sites of compression of the thoracic outlet are the interscalene triangle, between the coracoid process of the scapula and the pectoralis minor tendon, and the costoclavicular space (the most common site).
- Assess for:
  1. Neck, shoulder, and arm pain
  2. Numbness of the extremity
  3. Moderate edema of the extremity
  4. Increasing pain and numbness when the arm is held over the head or out to the side

- Conservative treatment includes:
  1. Physical therapy
  2. Exercise
  3. Avoidance of aggravating positions
- Surgical treatment involves resection of the anatomic structures that are compressing the artery.

THROMBOCYTOPENIA PURPURA, AUTOIMMUNE

OVERVIEW

- In autoimmune thrombocytopenic purpura, also called idiopathic thrombocytopenic purpura (ITP), there is a greatly reduced number of circulating platelets, increasing the patient's risk for hemorrhage and death.
- In this type of thrombocytopenia, platelet production in the bone marrow is normal but an abnormal antiplatelet antibody is made, causing macrophages in the spleen to increase the rate of platelet destruction.
- When the rate of platelet destruction exceeds the rate of platelet production, the number of circulating platelets decreases and blood clotting slows.
- The problem is most common among women between the ages of 20 and 40 years and among people who have other autoimmune disorders.

PATIENT-CENTERED COLLABORATIVE CARE

- Assess for and document:
  1. Large bruises
  2. Petechial rash on the arms, legs, upper chest, and neck
  3. Mucosal bleeding
  4. Anemia
  5. Neurologic impairment as a result of an intracranial bleed–induced stroke
  6. Laboratory findings: decreased platelet count, large numbers of megakaryocytes in the bone marrow, presence of antiplatelet antibodies in the blood, low hematocrit, and low hemoglobin levels
- Interventions include:
  1. Drug therapy to suppress immune function
     a. Corticosteroids
     b. Azathioprine (Imuran)
  2. Administration of IV immunoglobulin and IV anti-Rho to prevent the destruction of antibody-coated platelets

3. Platelet transfusions (when platelet counts are less than 20,000/mm^3)
4. Maintaining safety
   a. Injury prevention
   b. Infection prevention
5. A splenectomy may be needed if there is no response to drug therapy.

TONSILLITIS

- Tonsillitis is an inflammation and infection of the tonsils and lymphatic tissues located on each side of the throat.
- It is a contagious airborne infection.
- The acute form usually lasts 7 to 10 days and often is caused by bacteria, such as *Streptococcus, Staphylococcus aureus, Haemophilus influenzae,* or *Pneumococcus,* or by viruses.
- Manifestations of acute tonsillitis include the sudden onset of:
  1. Mild to severe sore throat
  2. Fever, muscle aches, chills
  3. Dysphagia, odynophagia (painful swallowing of food)
  4. Pain in the ears
  5. Headache, anorexia, malaise
  6. "Hot potato" voice (thickened voice of poor quality)
  7. Tonsils visually swollen and red with white or yellow exudate
  8. Edematous or inflamed uvula
  9. Enlarged cervical lymph nodes
- Treatment includes:
  1. Oral antibiotics for 7 to 10 days
  2. Teaching the patient about:
     a. Supportive care (rest, increasing fluid intake, humidifying the air, analgesics for pain, gargling several times daily with warm saline, throat lozenges containing mild anesthetics)
     b. The importance of completing antibiotic therapy
- Surgical intervention may be needed for recurrent acute infections (especially group A beta-hemolytic streptococcal infections), chronic infections that have not responded to antibiotic therapy, a peritonsillar abscess, or enlarged tonsils or adenoids that obstruct the airway.
- Procedures may include:
  1. Traditional tonsillectomy and adenoidectomy
  2. Laser tonsillectomy
  3. Radiothermal ablation tonsillectomy
  4. Tonsillar "shaving"

T

TOXIC SHOCK SYNDROME

- Toxic shock syndrome (TSS) is a form of septic shock caused by *Staphylococcus aureus* or *Streptococcus* infection and is related to menstruation and tampon use.
- Other conditions associated with TSS include surgical wound infection, nonsurgical infections, and gynecologic surgeries.
- Use of a diaphragm, cervical cap, or vaginal contraceptive sponge has also been linked to this health problem.
- In menstrual-related infection, menstrual blood provides a growth medium for the bacteria, which produced endotoxins that cross the vaginal mucosa to the bloodstream. Tampon insertion or prolonged use can cause vaginal dryness and micro-abrasions that provide an entry for the microorganisms.
- Assess for:
  1. Abrupt onset of a high fever
  2. Headache and flu-like symptoms
  3. Severe hypotension
  4. Sunburn-like rash with broken capillaries in the eyes and skin
- Management includes:
  1. Removal of the infection source
  2. Restoration of fluid and electrolyte balance
  3. Drug therapy to manage hypotension
  4. IV antibiotics
  5. Other measures included in the management of sepsis and septic shock
- Patient education focuses on prevention by teaching all women about the proper use of tampons, vaginal sponges, and diaphragms.

TRACHOMA

- Trachoma is a chronic, bilateral scarring form of conjunctivitis caused by *Chlamydia trachomatis*. It is the chief cause of pre-ventable blindness in the world.
- Manifestations include tears, photophobia, edema of the eyelids and conjunctiva, and follicles on the upper eyelid conjunctiva. With disease progression, the eyelid scars and turns inward, causing the eyelashes to damage the cornea.
- Drug therapy management involves:
  1. A 4-week course of oral or topical tetracycline (Achromycin, Apo-Tetra ✤) or erythromycin (Apo-Erythro-EC ✤, E-Mycin, E.E.S.)
  2. Azithromycin (Zithromax) may be used once weekly for 1 to 3 weeks.

- Infection control management is a priority; teach patients to:
  1. Wash the hands before and after touching the eyes.
  2. Keep washcloths separate from those of unaffected people, and launder them separately.
  3. Complete the entire course of antibiotics.

TRAUMA, ABDOMINAL

OVERVIEW

- Abdominal trauma is an injury to the structures located between the diaphragm and the pelvis that occurs when the abdomen is subjected to blunt or penetrating force.
- Organs that may be injured include the large and small bowel, liver, spleen, duodenum, pancreas, kidneys, and urinary bladder.
- Two broad categories are:
  1. Blunt trauma, which commonly results from automobile accidents but is also caused by falls, assaults, and contact sports
  2. Penetrating trauma, most often caused by gunshot wounds and stab wounds

PATIENT-CENTERED COLLABORATIVE CARE

Assessment

- Assess for airway, breathing, and circulation (ABCs).
- The focus of the assessment is on the risk of hemorrhage, shock, and peritonitis. The spleen is vulnerable to blunt trauma and contributes to significant blood loss.
- The key assessment factors related to early shock detection are mental status, vital signs, and skin perfusion (see Shock for discussions of hemorrhagic and hypovolemic forms):
  1. In mild shock, the skin is pale, cool, and moist.
  2. In moderate shock, diaphoresis is marked and urine output decreased.
  3. In severe shock, changes in mental status are manifested by agitation, disorientation, and recent memory loss.
- Assess for and document:
  1. Mental status, vital signs, bowel sounds, urinary output, and changes in clinical findings every 15 to 30 minutes until stable, then hourly. Report any deterioration immediately to the physician.
  2. The patient's report about the presence, location, and quality of pain, including referred pain (e.g., right shoulder) and nausea
  3. Inspection of the abdomen, back, flanks, genitalia, and rectum for contusions, abrasions, lacerations, ecchymoses,

penetrating injuries, and symmetry. Ecchymosis around the umbilicus (Cullen's sign) and ecchymosis in either flank (Turner's sign) may indicate retroperitoneal bleeding into the abdominal wall.

4. Auscultation of the abdomen for absent or diminished bowel sounds and bruits
5. Percussion for abnormal sounds, such as resonance over the liver or dullness over the stomach or intestines (Ballance's sign)
6. Results from light palpation of the abdomen to identify areas of tenderness, guarding, rigidity, and spasm
7. Kehr's sign indicating splenic injury, which is left shoulder pain resulting from diaphragmatic irritation
8. Blood in peritoneal lavage, nasogastric tube output, or emesis

INTERVENTIONS

Nonsurgical Management

- Interventions include:
  1. Placing two large-bore IV catheters to provide rapid fluid resuscitation
  2. Infusing IV fluids at a rapid rate, as ordered, and monitoring patient responses
  3. Obtaining blood samples for analysis
  4. Inserting an indwelling Foley catheter and monitoring urine output hourly for at least 24 hours
  5. Inserting a nasogastric (NG) tube to prevent vomiting and reduce intra-abdominal pressure
  6. Some facilities may monitor intra-abdominal pressure to detect compartment syndrome, which is compression of structures in the abdominal cavity (see Compartment Syndrome).
- Diagnostic studies may include:
  1. Abdominal ultrasound in the presence of blunt trauma
  2. Peritoneal lavage
  3. Abdominal flat plate x-ray
  4. Abdominal CT scan
  5. Chest x-ray
  6. Electrocardiogram (ECG) and ongoing ECG monitoring
  7. Serum analyses: CBC, basic metabolic panel, coagulation factors, tests for liver function and blood typing with antibody screening for possible transfusion
  8. Continuous intra-abdominal pressure monitoring
- Analgesics for pain, with careful attention to maintaining airway and breathing

Surgical Management

- For patients with severe abdominal trauma, an exploratory laparotomy with repair of abdominal injuries is performed.
- Most patients with gunshot or stab wounds require an exploratory laparotomy to assess for internal damage.
- Perioperative care is performed as outlined in Part One.
- A colostomy, either temporary or permanent, may be required (see Surgical Management under Cancer, Colorectal).

National Patient Safety Goal

Before administering medications or implementing procedures, ensure that the right patient is receiving interventions by using at least two identifiers. This process is challenging to implement in the emergency department, where the fast pace of admissions and rapidly changing condition of the patient may not prioritize "routine" admission activities such a placing a nameband. Nonetheless, accurate identification is essential for risk reduction and avoidance of adverse errors.

TRAUMA, BLADDER

OVERVIEW

- Bladder trauma occurs as a result of blunt or penetrating injury to the lower abdomen.
- The most common cause is a fractured pelvis (bone fragments puncture the bladder).
- Assess for:
  1. Anuria
  2. Hematuria
  3. Bloody urinary meatus
  4. Results of cystogram and voiding cystourethrogram
- Patients with bladder trauma other than a simple contusion require surgical intervention, including closure repair of the bladder wall and peritoneal membrane.
- Patients with anterior bladder wall injury require a Penrose drain and a Foley catheter.
- Patients with posterior bladder wall injury require a Penrose drain and a Foley or suprapubic catheter.

TRAUMA, BRAIN (ACUTE BRAIN INJURY WITH OR WITHOUT SKULL FRACTURE)

OVERVIEW

- A head injury occurs as the result of blow or jolt to the head or penetration of the head by a bullet or other foreign object. As a result, the normal functioning of the brain is disrupted. Traumatic brain injury (TBI) may produce a diminished state of consciousness and changes in cognitive abilities, physical functioning, or behavioral and emotional functioning. These changes may be immediate or delayed and may resolve or persist long after the original injury.

- Direct brain injury is the result of primary forces applied to the head. The primary injury occurs at the point of injury, with potential for additional primary injury from contrecoup forces when the intracranial tissue "bounces" against the skull opposite the site of direct injury.
- Indirect brain injury results from forces applied to another body part with a rebound effect to the brain.
- Brain damage from trauma most frequently involves the frontal or temporal lobes.
- Damage to brain tissue depends on the location, degree, and mechanism of injury.
  1. Brain injury can be classified as mild, moderate, or severe, depending on the initial Glasgow Coma Scale (GCS) score, which has implications for both treatment and prognosis.
  2. It may be also described by the degree of apparent damage to the brain.
     a. A concussion is a shaking of the brain and may be associated with a brief loss of consciousness and no damage visible by CT.
     b. A contusion causes bruising of the brain tissue.
     c. A laceration causes tearing of the cortical surface ·vessels and may lead to secondary hemorrhage.
     d. Neuronal injury, ischemia, and infarct
     e. Damage to supporting structures and cells, including blood vessels, the dura, and glial and microglial cells that secrete repair and growth factors, releases substances that can extend the area of injury or interfere with normal repair.
- Brain injury can also be caused by secondary injuries that occur when delivery of oxygen and glucose to the brain is interrupted after the original trauma. Prevention of secondary injury is the focus of care during recovery. Secondary injury can result in neurologic damage and significantly increases TBI morbidity and mortality through a variety of mechanisms, including:
  1. Increased intracranial pressure (ICP)
  2. Edema: vasogenic, cytotoxic, and interstitial
  3. Hemorrhage: epidural, subdural, or intracerebral
  4. Impaired cerebral autoregulation
  5. Hydrocephalus

6. Brain herniation
7. Hypoxia
8. Systemic hypotension

- A closed head injury is caused by blunt trauma. The integrity of the skull is not violated. One severe form of closed head injury is diffuse axonal injury, in which neuronal axons are damaged due to the rotating and high-velocity force of the primary injury.
- An open head injury occurs when the skull is fractured or penetrated by an object (e.g., bullet, projectile, knife), violating the integrity of brain and dura and exposing brain tissue to extracranial contaminants.
- Brain injury may be accompanied by skull fracture, which increases the risk of central nervous system (CNS) infection and additional brain damage. Types of skull fractures include:
  1. Linear, a simple, clean break
  2. Depressed, in which bone is pressed inward into brain tissue
  3. Open, in which the scalp is lacerated along with the skull fracture
  4. Comminuted, in which the skull is fragmented and bone is depressed into the brain tissue
  5. Basilar, which occurs at the base of the skull, usually along the paranasal sinus and which may result in a cerebrospinal fluid (CSF) leak from the nose or ear and potential damage to cranial nerves I, II, VII, and VIII

PATIENT-CENTERED COLLABORATIVE CARE

Assessment

- Obtain patient information about:
  1. When, where, and how the injury occurred
  2. The patient's level of consciousness (LOC) immediately after the injury and on admission to the hospital or unit and whether there have been any changes or fluctuations
  3. Presence of seizure activity
  4. Age, gender, and race
  5. Medical and social history, especially presence of alcohol or drug use
  6. Hand dominance
  7. Allergies to drugs and foods, especially seafood (patients allergic to seafood are often allergic to the medium used in diagnostic testing)
- Assess for:
  1. Impaired airway or breathing pattern: respiratory rate, depth, and quality with peripheral oxygenation (Spo$_2$)

2. Signs and symptoms of hypovolemic shock or hemorrhage, which may indicate additional traumatic injuries, such as abdominal bleeding or bleeding into soft tissue around major fractures

3. Cardiac dysrhythmias from chest trauma, bruising of the heart, or interference with the autonomic nervous system

4. Heart rate, blood pressure, peripheral pulses, and core temperature

5. Baseline and ongoing neurologic status with a standard assessment tool such as the GCS
   a. Decreased or garbled verbal response to auditory or tactile stimulus; new aphasia
   b. Inability to follow commands; confusion
   c. Pupils that are large, pinpoint or ovoid, and nonreactive to light (indicates cranial nerve dysfunction, especially III, IV, and VII; may indicate brainstem dysfunction)
   d. Decreased or absent motor strength in the extremities; hemiparesis or hemiplegia
   e. Complaints of severe headache, nausea, or vomiting
   f. Seizure activity
   g. Drainage of CSF from the ear or nose ("halo sign")

6. Indications of post-traumatic sequelae in the patient who experienced a minor head injury (symptoms may persist for weeks or months):
   a. Persistent headache
   b. Weakness
   c. Dizziness
   d. Loss of memory
   e. Personality and behavioral changes
   f. Problems with perception, reasoning abilities, and concept formation

7. Changes in personality, behavior, and abilities, such as:
   a. Increased incidence of temper outbursts, risk-taking behavior, depression, and denial of disability
   b. Becoming more talkative and developing a very outgoing personality
   c. Decreased ability to learn new information, to concentrate, and to plan
   d. Impaired memory, especially recent or short-term memory; this should not be confused with problems of aphasia

- Assess family dynamics. Family members may be angry with the patient for being injured, especially if the patient's behavior resulted in an injury that could have been prevented, or they may feel guilty that they could not prevent the injury.

- Diagnostic studies may include:
  1. CBC, basic metabolic panel, coagulation studies, ABGs, and toxicology screen
  2. CT scan
  3. Chest x-ray and abdominal x-ray to evaluate for the presence of additional injuries

> **Critical Rescue** ♦ Level of consciousness is the most sensitive and specific indicator of neurologic deterioration. Immediately inform the physician about changes in mentation, orientation, or behavior. A decrease in GCS score of 2 points or more should be reported immediately.

Interventions
Nonsurgical Management

- Assess vital signs every 1 to 2 hours. Cardiac monitoring to detect cardiac dysrhythmias may be implemented.
- The patient may be placed in systemic or local (cranial) hypothermia devices (blanket, helmet) to slow brain metabolism during the acute phase.
- Fever may extend the area of brain damage during the acute phase; maintain normothermia.
- Position the patient to avoid extreme flexion or extension of the neck, which interferes with CSF outflow. Maintain the head in a midline, central position; log roll the patient and elevate the backrest 30 degrees unless contraindicated; use reverse Trendelenburg position if spinal cord injury is still being evaluated.
- The patient on a ventilator may receive settings to maintain the $Paco_2$ at 35 to 38 mm Hg during the first 2 to 24 hours.
- Maintain the Pao_2 at 85 to 100 mm Hg and Spo_2 at greater than 92%.
- Monitor ABGs at least twice daily if the patient receives mechanical ventilation.
- Monitor ICP with a specialized device in the ICU if the patient presents with coma; manage ICP and cerebral perfusion pressure to maintain adequate blood flow to brain tissue.
- Monitor brain tissue oxygenation with jugular venous oxygen apparatus (Sjo_2).
- Drug therapy
  1. Osmotic diuretics (mannitol) given through, or drawn up through, a needle with a filter to eliminate microscopic crystals. This is most effective when given as a bolus rather than a continuous infusion.

2. Opioids may be used if the patient is mechanically ventilated to control restlessness and agitation if activity is causing increased ICP.
3. Neuromuscular blocking agents for severe agitation or if agitation is causing elevation in ICP. These agents must be given with sedatives and an opioid.
4. Antiepileptic drugs to treat actual or risk for seizure activity

- Pulmonary management includes:
  1. Encouraging the conscious patient to breathe deeply every hour while awake; encouraging the patient to avoid coughing as it can increase ICP
  2. Turning and repositioning the patient at least once every 2 hours; consider the use of continuous lateral rotational therapy if the patient is comatose and mechanically ventilated.

- Fluid and electrolyte management includes:
  1. Monitoring electrolytes and serum and urine osmolarity
  2. Measuring intake and output every hour
  3. Measuring urine osmolality, sodium, and specific gravity when there is a significant increase in urine output (greater than 300 mL/hr for 2 hours) to evaluate for syndrome of inappropriate antidiuretic hormone (SIADH)
  4. Using a Foley catheter to monitor hourly output if acute moderate or severe brain injury is diagnosed
  5. Monitoring daily weight

- Sensory, cognitive, and behavioral management includes:
  1. Monitoring the patient for nutritional deficits that may occur secondary to loss of smell and loss of ability to taste, swallow, or feel food in the oral cavity
     a. Ensure that mealtime is a pleasant experience.
     b. Check the temperature of food and beverages on the tray before serving.
     c. Position the patient to maximize swallowing ability.
     d. Collaborate with the speech-language pathologist to develop and implement a swallowing program for the patient, as needed.
  2. Keeping the siderails up while the patient is in bed and the seat belt on while the patient is in a chair if he or she is restless or unable to provide safe self-management
  3. Initiating a sensory stimulation program, such as audiotapes used for no longer than 10 to 15 minutes for patients in coma; awake or alert patients may enjoy longer tapes
  4. Orienting the patient to environment, time, place, and the reason for hospitalization with each encounter if short-term memory loss or coma is present

5. Reassuring the patient realistically about concerns, visitation and plan for care at least once per shift
6. Providing simple, short explanations of procedures and activities immediately before any interventions
7. Collaborating with physical and occupational therapists to plan exercise and ADL programs
8. Maintaining the patient on a normal sleep-wake cycle for mild brain injury, and providing periods of rest for patients with moderate or severe injury
9. Asking the family to bring in familiar objects, such as pictures or music
10. Monitoring the patient's reaction to television or radio (the brain-injured patient is often unable to differentiate programs from what is happening within his or her own environment)
11. Keeping the bed in the low position if the patient is awake
12. Observing and documenting behavior; providing constant supervision if the patient is unable to consistently follow directions or is unsafe due to short-term memory failure

- Nutrition management includes:
  1. Beginning nutritional support as soon as possible with hyperalimentation, tube feedings (nasal or gastrostomy), or oral feedings
  2. Monitoring the patient's weight and serum albumin, prealbumin, and transferrin levels to ensure adequate protein intake

Surgical Management

- A craniotomy may be indicated to:
  1. Evacuate a subdural or epidural hematoma
  2. Treat uncontrolled increased ICP; remove ischemic tissue or tips of temporal lobe
  3. Treat hydrocephalus
- Bedside surgical insertion of an ICP-monitoring device is often performed. Types of devices include:
  1. Intraventricular catheter
  2. Epidural catheter or sensor
  3. Subarachnoid bolt or screw
  4. Fiberoptic transducer-tipped sensor

Community-Based Care

- Respite care may be needed to help the family cope with feelings of isolation, increased responsibility, financial or emotional stress, or role reversal; refer them to support groups.
- The patient may experience a sense of isolation and loneliness because personality and behavior changes make it difficult to resume or maintain pre-injury social contacts.

- Discharge planning often involves a case manager and includes:
  1. Providing a detailed plan of care at the time of transfer to a rehabilitation or long-term care facility
     a. Drugs, including dosage and possible side effects
     b. Current patient activity
     c. Techniques used to motivate or calm the patient
     d. Successful coping strategies identified by the patient or family
  2. Referring the patient to follow-up and home care to promote adjustment
  3. Informing the patient and family about resources such as the National Head Injury Foundation or a local head injury support group
- Health teaching includes:
  1. Reviewing seizure precautions
  2. Strategies to adapt to sensory dysfunction and to cope with the personality or behavior problems that may arise
  3. Explaining the purpose, dosage, schedule, and route of administration of drugs
  4. Encouraging the patient to participate in activities as tolerated
  5. Teaching the patient and family measures to treat sensory dysfunctions
     a. The home should have functioning smoke detectors (the patient may have loss of the sense of smell).
     b. Objects and furniture should be kept in consistent locations.
     c. The measures described for sensory and perceptual management also are relevant here.
     d. Help the family and patient develop a home routine that is structured, repetitious, and consistent.
  6. For minor head injury, discuss symptoms of post-traumatic syndrome. Inform the patient that these symptoms are common and refer the patient and family to a specialist in brain injury or cognitive therapy and a support group if symptoms persist. Symptoms include:
     a. Personality changes
     b. Irritability
     c. Headaches
     d. Dizziness
     e. Restlessness
     f. Nervousness
     g. Insomnia
     h. Memory loss
     i. Depression

TRAUMA, ESOPHAGEAL

OVERVIEW

- Trauma to the esophagus can result from blunt injuries, chemical burns, surgery or endoscopy, or the stress of protracted severe vomiting.
- Trauma may affect the esophagus directly, impairing swallowing and nutrition, or it may create problems and complications in related structures such as the lungs or mediastinum.
- Assess for and document:
  1. Airway patency
  2. Pain
  3. Dysphagia
  4. Vomiting
  5. Bleeding
  6. Results of x-ray examination, CT, and endoscopy
- Treatment includes:
  1. Maintaining the patient on NPO status to prevent further leakage of esophageal secretions
  2. Maintaining nasogastric (NG) or gastrostomy tube drainage to rest the patient's esophagus
  3. Administering total parenteral nutrition (TPN) during esophageal rest (usually for at least 10 days)
  4. Administering broad-spectrum antibiotics, corticosteroids, and analgesics
- Surgery may be needed to remove the tissue. A resection or replacement of the damaged esophageal segment with small bowel tissue may be required.

TRAUMA, FACIAL

OVERVIEW

- Facial trauma is defined by the specific bones (mandibular, maxillary, orbital, or nasal fractures) and the side of the face involved.
- Mandibular (lower jaw) fractures can occur at any point on the mandible and are the most common facial fractures.
- The rich blood supply of the face leads to extensive bleeding and bruising with facial trauma.

PATIENT-CENTERED COLLABORATIVE CARE

Assessment

- The first action to take for a patient with facial trauma is airway assessment.

- Assess for:
  1. Manifestations of airway obstruction
     a. Stridor
     b. Shortness of breath
     c. Anxiety and restlessness
     d. Hypoxia and hypercarbia
  2. Soft tissue trauma
     a. Edema
     b. Facial asymmetry
     c. Pain
     d. Leakage of spinal fluid through the ears or nose
     e. Vision and eye movement
     f. Bruising behind the ears in the mastoid area ("battle sign")

Interventions

- The priority action is to establish and maintain a patent airway.
- Other interventions include:
  1. Anticipating the need for emergency intubation, tracheotomy, or cricothyroidotomy
  2. Controlling hemorrhage
  3. Assessing for the extent of injury
  4. Establishing IV access and initiating fluid resuscitation
  5. Assisting in the stabilization of fractures
  6. Administering prescribed antibiotics
  7. For mandibular fixation with plates, teaching the patient about:
     a. Oral care with an irrigating device
     b. Soft diet or dental liquid diet restrictions
     c. How to cut the wires if emesis occurs

> 🔲 **Critical Rescue** ♦ Instruct the patient to keep wire cutters with him or her at all times in case this emergency arises.

TRAUMA, KIDNEY

- Renal trauma is injury to one or both kidneys. Injury can be blunt or penetrating.
- Injuries
  1. Minor injuries (contusion, small lacerations, tearing of the parenchyma and the calyx) are likely to follow falls, contact sports, and blows to the back or torso.
  2. Major injuries (lacerations to the cortex, medulla, or one of the branches of the renal artery or vein) are likely to follow penetrating abdominal, flank, or back wounds.

3. Pedicle injuries (laceration or disruption of the renal artery or vein) result in rapid and extensive hemorrhage and death unless diagnosis and intervention are prompt.

- Obtain patient information about:
  1. History of events surrounding the trauma
  2. History of renal or urologic disease, including previous surgical intervention
  3. History of diabetes or hypertension
- Assess for and document:
  1. Vital signs
  2. Abdominal or flank pain
  3. Penetrating injuries of the lower thorax, back, or abdomen
  4. Abdominal or flank bruising
  5. Abdominal distention or flank asymmetry
  6. Urine output hourly and hemoglobin or RBCs in the urine
  7. Decreased serum hemoglobin and hematocrit values
- Treatment includes drugs for vascular support, fluids to restore volume, and surgery when indicated.
  1. Administer fluids, such as crystalloids and RBCs, to restore circulatory blood volume; plasma volume expanders may also be given.
  2. Assess the need for clotting factors such as vitamin K and platelets.
- Depending on the extent of the injury, nephrectomy (surgical removal of the kidney) may be required.
- For major vascular tearing, the kidney may be surgically removed, repaired through revascularization techniques, and then surgically reimplanted.

TRAUMA, KNEE

- There are two semilunar cartilaginous structures (menisci) in the knee joint, the medial meniscus and the lateral meniscus, which act as shock absorbers.
- *Meniscus injuries* are usually tears and occur more often in the medial meniscus, usually causing the knee to lock.
- Manifestations include pain, swelling, tenderness in the knee, and a clicking or snapping sound when the knee is moved.
- A common diagnostic technique is the *McMurray test*. The examiner flexes and rotates the knee and then presses on the medial aspect while slowly extending the leg. The test result is positive if clicking is palpated or heard, but a negative finding does not rule out a tear.

- Management of a locked knee is manipulation followed by splinting or casting for 3 to 6 weeks.
- A partial or total meniscectomy may be required and is performed either as an open procedure (rare) or as a closed procedure by arthroscopy.
- Postoperative care includes:
  1. Monitoring the surgical dressing for bleeding and drainage
  2. Monitoring vital signs
  3. Performing neurovascular checks
     a. Skin temperature and color
     b. Movement and sensation
     c. Distal pulses
     d. Capillary refill
     e. Pain
  4. Teaching the patient to perform exercises (e.g., quadriceps setting, straight-leg raises)
  5. Teaching the patient to use a knee immobilizer
  6. Elevating the knee and applying ice
- Ligament injuries result in sprains and tears.
- Manifestations of an *anterior cruciate ligament (ACL)* tear include feeling a snap and the knee giving way, swelling and stiffness, and pain.
- Management may be nonsurgical (exercises, bracing, activity limitation) or surgical, depending on the severity of the injury and the anticipated activity of the patient.
- For a rupture of the patellar tendon, management includes surgical repair and casting for 6 to 8 weeks, or tendon transplantation. See Fracture for care of the patient in a cast.

TRAUMA, LARYNGEAL

- Laryngeal trauma is the result of a crushing or direct blow, fracture, or an injury such as that induced by prolonged endotracheal intubation.
- Manifestations include dyspnea, aphonia, hoarseness, subcutaneous emphysema, and hemoptysis.
- Respiratory assessment includes:
  1. Assessing the airway every 15 to 30 minutes
  2. Monitoring vital signs and pulse oximetry every 15 to 30 minutes
  3. Applying oxygen and humidification as prescribed
  4. Assessing for increased respiratory difficulty
     a. Increasing tachypnea
     b. Nasal flaring
     c. Anxiety

d. Sternal retraction
e. Dyspnea
f. Restlessness
g. Decreased oxygen saturation
h. Decreased level of consciousness
i. Stridor

> 🔲 **Critical Rescue** ◆ If the patient has respiratory difficulty, stay with him or her, and instruct other trauma team members or the Rapid Response Team to prepare for an emergency intubation or tracheostomy.

- Surgical intervention is necessary for lacerations of the mucous membranes, cartilage exposure, or paralysis of the cords.
- An artificial airway may be needed.

TRAUMA, LIVER

- The liver is one of the organs most commonly injured in patients with abdominal trauma. Damage or injury should be suspected whenever any upper abdominal or lower chest trauma is sustained.
- Common injuries to the liver include simple lacerations, multiple lacerations, avulsions (tears), and crush injuries.
- Because the liver is a vascular organ, blood loss is massive when trauma occurs (see Shock for discussion of hemorrhagic and hypovolemic types).
- Clinical manifestations of liver trauma include right upper quadrant pain with abdominal tenderness, distention, guarding, rigidity, and abdominal pain that is aggravated by deep breathing and is referred to the right shoulder.
- Exploratory laparotomy is done to determine the source and type of bleeding. Operative procedures may include suture placement, wound packing, and decompression; liver lobe resection may be necessary.
- The patient requires infusion of multiple blood products, packed RBCs, fresh-frozen plasma, and massive volume replacement to maintain hydration. Anticipate perioperative bleeding and prolonged coagulopathy with severe liver injury.

TRAUMA, PERIPHERAL NERVE

- The peripheral nerves are subject to injuries associated with mechanical or vehicular accidents, sports, the injection of particular drugs, military conflicts or wars, and acts of violence (e.g., knife or gunshot wounds).

- Specific mechanisms of injury include:
  1. Partial or complete severance of a nerve or nerves
  2. Contusion, stretching, constriction, or compression of a nerve or nerves
  3. Ischemia
  4. Electrical, thermal, or radiation injury
- Most commonly affected are the median, ulnar, and radial nerves of the arms and the peroneal, femoral, and sciatic nerves of the legs.
- Nerve damage is characterized by pain, burning, or other abnormal sensations distal to the trauma; weakness or flaccid paralysis; and change in skin color and temperature (a warm phase and a cold phase).
- Treatment consists of immobilization of the area with a splint, cast, or traction followed by physical and occupational therapy.
- Surgery may include resection and suturing to reapproximate the severed nerve ends, nerve grafting, and nerve and tendon transplantation.
- Regeneration of the damaged nerve and return of sensation may occur several years after the injury; motor movement is less likely to recover long after the event.
- Postoperative nursing care is directed toward frequent skin care and assessment, management of pain, and instructing the patient to protect the involved area from trauma.

TRAUMA, TRACHEOBRONCHIAL

- Most tears of the tracheobronchial tree result from severe blunt trauma or rapid deceleration and primarily involve the mainstem bronchi.
- Injuries to the trachea usually occur at the junction of the trachea and cricoid cartilage.
- Patients with lacerations of the trachea develop massive air leaks, causing air to enter the mediastinum and leading to extensive subcutaneous emphysema.
- Upper airway obstruction may occur, causing severe respiratory distress and inspiratory stridor.
- Large tracheal tears are managed by cricothyroidotomy or tracheotomy below the level of injury.
- Management includes:
  1. Assessing for hypoxemia by ABG assays
  2. Administering oxygen as needed

3. Maintaining mechanical ventilation
4. Assessing for subcutaneous emphysema
5. Checking lung sounds for decreased breath sounds or wheezing
6. Providing tracheostomy care if surgical repair was needed

TUBERCULOSIS, PULMONARY

OVERVIEW

- Pulmonary tuberculosis (TB) is a highly communicable disease caused by *Mycobacterium tuberculosis* infection.
- The organism is transmitted by aerosolization (airborne route) from an infected person during coughing, laughing, sneezing, whistling, or singing.
- Far more people are infected with the bacillus than actually develop active TB.
- When the bacillus is inhaled into a susceptible site, it multiplies freely, causing an exudative response and pneumonitis. Only a few people develop active TB from this initial infection.
- Initial infection is seen more often in the middle or lower lobes of the lung, and reactivation occurs more in the upper lobes.
- Progression of infection leads to an inflammatory lump that surrounds the bacilli and is filled with collagen, fibroblasts, and lymphocytes. The lump necroses, causing calcification or liquefaction and leading to destruction of lung tissue with cavity formation.
- *Miliary* or *hematogenous TB* is the spread of TB throughout the body when a large number of organisms enter the blood and can then infect the brain, meninges, liver, kidney, or bone marrow.
- An infected individual is not infectious to others until manifestations of disease occur.
- People at greatest risk for developing TB are those who have repeated close contact with an infectious person who has not yet been diagnosed with TB. People at risk include:
  1. Those in constant, frequent contact with an untreated individual
  2. Those who have immune dysfunction or HIV
  3. Those who live in crowded areas such as long-term care facilities, prisons, and mental health facilities
  4. Older people
  5. Homeless people
  6. Abusers of injection drugs or alcohol
  7. Members of lower socioeconomic groups

T

8. Foreign immigrants (especially from Mexico, the Philippines, and Vietnam)

PATIENT-CENTERED COLLABORATIVE CARE

Assessment

- Obtain patient information about:
  1. Persistent cough
  2. Weight loss
  3. Anorexia
  4. Night sweats
  5. Fever or chills
  6. Dyspnea or hemoptysis
  7. Past exposure to TB
  8. Country of origin and travel to foreign countries
  9. History of bacillus Calmette-Guérin (BCG) vaccination
- Assess for and document:
  1. Dullness with percussion over involved the lung fields
  2. Bronchial breath sounds
  3. Crackles, wheezes
  4. Enlarged lymph nodes
- TB is diagnosed on the basis of manifestations, a positive sputum smear for acid-fast bacillus, a positive purified protein derivative (PPD) two-step test, or a positive QuantiFERON-TB GOLD test. Sputum culture confirms the diagnosis.

> Clinical Landmine ◆ Do not assume that a positive PPD reaction means that active disease is present. It only indicates exposure to TB or the presence of inactive (dormant) disease.

> Clinical Landmine ◆ A reduced PPD skin reaction or a negative PPD skin test result does not rule out TB disease or infection in the very old or in anyone who is severely immunocompromised.

Interventions

- Combination drug therapy is the most effective method of treating TB and preventing transmission. Current first-line therapy uses:
  1. Isoniazid (INH) for 6 months
  2. Rifampin for 6 months
  3. Pyrazinamide for the first 2 months
  4. Ethambutol for 6 months

- Variations of the first-line drugs along with other drug types are used if the patient does not tolerate the standard first-line therapy.
- Nursing interventions include:
  1. Caring for the hospitalized patient using strict Airborne Precautions
  2. Patient teaching about drug therapy
     a. Explaining the actions, side effects, dosing, and scheduling of the drugs
     b. Stressing the importance of taking each drug regularly, exactly as prescribed
     c. Presenting drug information in multiple formats, such as pamphlets, videos, and drug-schedule worksheets
     d. Asking the patient to describe the treatment regimen, major side effects, and when to call the health care agency and physician
     e. Explaining that nausea can be prevented by taking the drugs at bedtime
  3. Patient teaching about multidrug-resistant strains of TB: higher doses of some drugs for longer periods and absolute adherence to therapy are required for survival and cure of the disease.
  4. Patient teaching about infection control
     a. Reminding patients that Airborne Precautions are not necessary in the home because family members have already been exposed
     b. Teaching family members in the household about the need to undergo TB testing
     c. Teaching the patient to cover the mouth and nose with a tissue when coughing or sneezing and to place used tissues in plastic bags
     d. Teaching the patient to wear a mask when in contact with crowds until the drugs suppress infection
  5. Patient teaching about health and general care issues
     a. Fatigue will diminish as the treatment progresses.
     b. Avoid exposure to any inhalation irritants, because they can cause further lung damage.
     c. Eat a well-balanced diet containing adequate amounts of protein and vitamins.
     d. Get adequate rest and sleep.

Community-Based Care

- Consult with the social service worker in the hospital or the community health nursing agency to ensure that the patient is discharged to the appropriate environment with continued supervision.

- Teach the patient to follow the drug regimen exactly as prescribed and always to have a supply on hand.
- Teach about side effects and ways of reducing them to ensure adherence.
- Remind the patient that the disease is usually no longer contagious after drugs have been taken for 2 to 3 consecutive weeks and clinical improvement is seen; however, *he or she must continue with the drugs for 6 months or longer as prescribed.*
- Determine the need for directly observed therapy (DOT), in which the nurse or other health care provider watches the patient swallow the drugs.
- Remind the patient to receive follow-up care by a health care provider for at least 1 year during active treatment.
- Refer the patient to community resources such as the American Lung Association (ALA).
- Urge smokers to quit, and assist them in finding an appropriate smoking-cessation program.

TUMORS, BRAIN

OVERVIEW

- Brain tumors can arise anywhere within the brain structures and are named according to the cell or tissue where they are located.
- *Primary* tumors originate within the central nervous system (CNS).
- *Secondary* brain tumors (metastatic tumors) spread to the brain from cancers in other body areas, such as the lungs, breast, kidney, and GI tract.
- Regardless of brain tumor type or location, the tumor expands and invades, infiltrates, compresses, and displaces normal brain tissue, leading to one or more problems, including:
  1. Cerebral edema/brain tissue inflammation
  2. ICP
  3. Neurologic deficits
  4. Hydrocephalus
  5. Pituitary dysfunction
  6. Seizure activity
- *Supratentorial* tumors are located within the cerebral hemispheres, and *infratentorial* tumors are located in the brainstem structures and cerebellum.
- Some brain tumors are benign and others cancerous. Regardless of type, most brain tumors must be treated or death will occur.

- Classification by cell type or tissue type includes tumors arising from:
  1. Neurons, which are responsible for nerve impulse conduction
  2. Neuroglial cells (glial cells), which provide support, nourishment, and protection
     a. Astrocytes (astrocytomas)
     b. Oligodendroglia
     c. Ependymal cells
     d. Microglia (gliomas, which are malignant)
  3. Meninges, which are the coverings of the brain (meningiomas)
  4. Pituitary (pituitary adenomas)
  5. The sheath of Schwann cells in cranial nerve VII (acoustic neuromas)
- Metastatic, or secondary, tumors from other body areas make up about 30% of brain tumors.
- The exact cause of brain tumors is unknown but may be related to genetic changes, heredity, errors in fetal development, ionizing radiation, electromagnetic fields, environmental hazards, diet, viruses, or injury.

PATIENT-CENTERED COLLABORATIVE CARE

Assessment

- Obtain patient information about general symptoms of a brain tumor, including:
  1. Headaches that are usually more severe on awakening in the morning
  2. Nausea and vomiting
  3. Vision changes (blurred or double vision)
  4. Seizures
  5. Changes in mentation or personality
  6. Papilledema (swelling of the optic disc)
  7. Specific neurologic deficits
     a. Supratentorial (cerebral) tumors usually result in paralysis, seizures, memory loss, cognitive impairment, language impairment, or vision problems.
     b. Infratentorial tumors produce ataxia, autonomic nervous system dysfunction, vomiting, drooling, hearing loss, and vision impairment.
- Diagnosis is based on the history, neurologic assessment, clinical examination, results of neurodiagnostic testing, CT, MRI, and skull x-rays. Cerebral angiography, electroencephalography (EEG), lumbar puncture (LP), brain scan, and positron emis-

T

sion tomography (PET) may be also be used to further define the tumor.

Interventions

Nonsurgical Management

- Management depends on tumor size and location, patient symptoms and general condition, and whether the tumor is primary or has recurred.
- *Drug therapy for symptom management* may include:
  1. Analgesics for headache
     a. Codeine
     b. Acetaminophen
  2. Agents to control cerebral edema
     a. Dexamethasone (Decadron)
     b. Glucocorticoids
  3. Phenytoin (Dilantin) or other antiepileptic drug for seizure activity
  4. Agents to prevent stress ulcers
     a. Histamine blockers (ranitidine hydrochloride [Zantac, Apo-Ranitidine ✦])
     b. Proton pump inhibitors (pantoprazole [Protonix])
- *Chemotherapy* may be given alone, in combination with radiation therapy and surgery, and with tumor progression. More than one agent may be given orally, IV, intra-arterially, or intrathecally through an Ommaya reservoir placed in a cranial ventricle.
  1. Commonly used agents include:
     a. CCNU (lomustine)
     b. Temozolomide (Temodar)
     c. Procarbazine (Matulane)
     d. Methotrexate (MTX)
     e. Vincristine (Oncovin)
  2. Direct drug delivery to the tumor, using a disk-shaped drug wafer (Gliadel) placed directly into the cavity created during surgical tumor removal (interstitial chemotherapy), is an emerging practice.
  3. General management issues for care of patients undergoing chemotherapy are presented in Part One, under Cancer Therapy.
- *Radiation therapy* may be used alone, after surgery, or in combination with chemotherapy and surgery.
  1. Traditional external beam radiation may be used.
  2. A radioactive monoclonal antibody may be directly injected into the cavity from which the tumor was removed.
  3. General management issues for care of patients undergoing radiation therapy are presented in Part One under Cancer Therapy.

- *Targeted therapy* is also an emerging technique for brain tumor management. Agents include:
  1. Erlotinib (Tarceva)
  2. Gefitinib (Iressa)
  3. Bevacizumab (Avastin)
- *Stereotactic radiosurgery (SRS)* is an alternative to traditional surgery. Techniques used may include:
  1. Modified linear accelerator using accelerated x-rays (LINAC)
  2. Particle accelerator using beams of protons (cyclotron)
  3. Isotope seeds implanted in the tumor (brachytherapy)
  4. Gamma knife using a single high dose of ionized radiation to focus 201 beams of gamma radiation produced by the radioisotope cobalt 60
  5. CyberKnife

Surgical Management
- Brain biopsy is done to determine the specific pathology. Then, a craniotomy (incision into the cranium) may be performed to improve symptoms related to the lesion or to decrease pressure effect from the tumor. Complete removal is possible with some tumors, which results in a "surgical cure."
  1. Minimally invasive surgery (MIS) may involve:
     a. The transnasal approach with endoscopy for pituitary tumors
     b. Stereotactic surgery using burr holes and local anesthesia
     c. Laser surgery
  2. In traditional open craniotomy, the patient's head is placed in a skull fixation device, and a piece of bone (bone flap) is removed to expose the tumor area. The tumor is removed, the bone flap is replaced, and a drain or monitoring device may be inserted.
- Provide preoperative care, including:
  1. Implementing routine preoperative care as described in Part One
  2. Allowing the patient to express anxiety and concerns about:
     a. Surgery into the brain
     b. Possibility of neurologic deficits
     c. Changes in appearance and self-image
  3. Teaching the patient and family about what to expect immediately after surgery and throughout the recovery period
  4. Ensuring that the patient had refrained from alcohol, tobacco, anticoagulants, or NSAIDs for at least 5 days before surgery

T

5. Ensuring that the patient has been NPO for at least 8 hours before surgery
- After surgery, the patient is admitted to the critical care unit.

> 🔲 **Critical Rescue** ◆ The focus of postoperative care is to monitor the patient to detect changes in status and to prevent or minimize complications, especially increased ICP.

- Provide postoperative care, including:
  1. Implementing routine postoperative care as described in Part One
  2. Assessing neurologic and vital signs every 15 to 30 minutes for the first 4 to 6 hours after surgery and then every hour
  3. Assessing for:
     a. Decreased level of consciousness (LOC)
     b. Motor weakness or paralysis
     c. Aphasia
     d. Visual changes
     e. Personality changes
  4. Ensuring appropriate positioning
     a. After supratentorial surgery
        (1) Elevating the head of the bed 30 degrees
        (2) Avoiding extreme hip or neck flexion
        (3) Maintaining the head in a midline, neutral position
        (4) Placing the patient on the nonoperative side
     b. After infratentorial (brainstem) craniotomy
        (1) Keeping the patient flat
        (2) Positioning the patient on either side for 24 to 48 hours
  5. Maintaining NPO status for at least the first 24 hours after surgery
  6. Administering prescribed drug therapy
     a. Antiepileptic drugs
     b. Histamine blockers or proton pump inhibitors
     c. Corticosteroids
     d. Analgesics
  7. Monitoring the dressing every 1 to 2 hours for:
     a. Amount, type, and color of drainage
     b. Suction of drains maintained as prescribed

> 🔲 **Critical Rescue** ◆ Immediately report a saturated head dressing or drainage greater than 50 mL in 8 hours to the surgeon.

8. Applying cold compresses for periorbital edema and ecchymosis of one or both eyes
9. Irrigating the affected eye with warm saline solution or artificial tears
10. Assessing the airway and managing mechanical ventilation
    a. Keeping $Paco_2$ at about 35 mm Hg
    b. Keeping the arterial oxygen levels higher than 95 mm Hg
    c. Preventing the patient from fighting the ventilator by administering prescribed drugs such as fentanyl citrate or midazolam (Versed)
    d. Hyperoxygenating the patient carefully before suctioning
11. Assessing the cardiac monitor for dysrhythmias
12. Precisely measuring intake and output
13. Implementing any prescribed fluid restriction
14. Ensuring that ROM exercises are performed to all extremities at least every 2 to 3 hours
15. Ensuring that the patient turns, coughs, and breathes deeply every 2 hours (if permitted)
16. Maintaining sequential compression stockings or pneumatic compression boots until the patient ambulates
17. Monitoring laboratory values for changes and abnormalities
    a. CBC
    b. Serum electrolyte levels and osmolarity
    c. Coagulation studies
    d. ABGs
18. Assessing for fluid volume overload or syndrome of inappropriate antidiuretic hormone (SIADH)
    a. Irritability
    b. Rapid weight gain
    c. Low serum sodium and potassium values
    d. Low urine output in relation to fluid intake
19. Assessing for diabetes insipidus (DI)
    a. High serum sodium and osmolarity
    b. Muscle weakness and restlessness
    c. Extreme thirst and dry mouth
    d. High output of dilute urine
20. Assessing for cerebral salt wasting (CSW)
    a. Low serum sodium and decreased osmolarity
    b. No dilution of other electrolytes or of hematocrit and hemoglobin

T

21. Preventing and assessing for other postoperative complications, including:
    a. Increased ICP
       (1) Severe headache
       (2) Deteriorating LOC
       (3) Restlessness and irritability
       (4) Dilated or pinpoint pupils that are slow to react or nonreactive to light
    b. Subdural and epidural hematomas and intracranial hemorrhage
       (1) Severe headache
       (2) Rapid change in LOC
       (3) Progressive neurologic deficits
       (4) Sudden cardiovascular and respiratory arrest
    c. Hydrocephalus (increased CSF in the brain)
    d. Respiratory complications
       (1) Atelectasis
       (2) Pneumonia
       (3) Neurogenic pulmonary edema
    e. Wound infections
       (1) Reddened and puffy wound appearance
       (2) Area is sensitive to touch
       (3) Area is warm
    f. Meningitis

Community-Based Care

- Assist the family to make the environment safe for prevention of falls (e.g., remove scatter rugs, install grab bars in the bathroom).
- When needed, work with the case manager or discharge planner to help the family select a facility with experience in providing care for neurologically impaired patients.
- Teach patients and families about:
  1. Seizure precautions and what to do if a seizure occurs
  2. Drug therapy and person to call if adverse drug events occur
  3. Avoiding any OTC drugs unless approved by the health care provider
  4. The importance of recommended follow-up health care appointments
  5. The need for adequate caloric intake during radiation therapy or chemotherapy
- Refer the patient and family to support groups and community resources such as the American Brain Tumor Association, the National Brain Tumor Foundation, the American Cancer Society, home care agencies, and hospice services or palliative care services (for those who are terminally ill).

ULCERS, PEPTIC

OVERVIEW

- A peptic ulcer is a mucosal lesion of the stomach or duodenum. The term is used to describe both gastric and duodenal ulcers.
- Peptic ulcer disease (PUD) results when mucosal defenses become impaired and no longer protect the epithelium from the effects of acid and pepsin.
- Peptic ulcer development is primarily associated with NSAID use and bacterial infection with *Helicobacter pylori*. Caffeine, smoking, alcohol, and radiation contribute to PUD.
- Recurrent ulcer can be caused by incomplete vagotomy or persistent *H. pylori* infection.
- Types of peptic ulcers include:
  1. Gastric ulcer, which occurs when there is a break in the mucosal barrier and hydrochloric acid injures the epithelium. Gastric emptying is delayed, causing regurgitation of duodenal contents. Gastric ulcers are deep and penetrating, and they usually occur on the lesser curvature of the stomach near the pylorus.
  2. Duodenal ulcer, a chronic break in the duodenal mucosa that extends through the muscularis mucosa and leaves a scar after healing. It is characterized by high gastric acid secretion and is the most common type of peptic ulcer.
  3. Stress ulcer, which occurs with acute and chronic diseases or major trauma. Bleeding resulting from gastric erosion is the principal manifestation, and multiple lesions occur in the proximal portion of the stomach, beginning with the area of ischemia and evolving into erosions.
- Complications of PUD include:
  1. Hemorrhage
  2. Perforation, with the gastroduodenal contents emptying through the anterior wall of the stomach or duodenum into the peritoneal cavity
  3. Pyloric obstruction
  4. Intractable disease, which is characterized by lack of response to conservative management and with symptoms that interfere with ADLs

PATIENT-CENTERED COLLABORATIVE CARE

Assessment

- Obtain patient information about:
  1. Tobacco use
  2. Dietary intake, including alcohol, caffeine, other irritants, and patterns of eating

3. Medical history focusing on GI problems
4. Prescribed and OTC drugs, such as corticosteroids and anti-inflammatory agents
5. Lifestyle, including actual and perceived stress
6. Symptoms, including epigastric discomfort, abdominal tenderness, cramps, indigestion, nausea, or vomiting and their onset, duration, location, and frequency, as well as aggravating and alleviating factors
7. Presence of chronic disease and recent changes in flares or medications

- Assess for and document:
  1. Epigastric pain and tenderness; rigid, boardlike abdomen accompanied by rebound tenderness (if perforation occurred)
  2. Effect of eating on GI symptoms, because gastric ulcer pain may be relieved by food, and duodenal ulcer pain occurs 90 minutes to 3 hours after eating and often awakens the patient at night
  3. Dyspepsia and effects of certain foods that may exacerbate GI symptoms
  4. Melena, especially in older adults
  5. Vomiting
  6. Orthostatic vital signs
  7. Deficient fluid volume, including orthostatic hypotension and dizziness
  8. Low hemoglobin and hematocrit levels
  9. Results of esophagogastroduodenoscopy (EGD), which visualizes the ulcer and *H. pylori* testing
  10. Family and individual stressors and the patient's usual patterns of coping and problem solving
  11. Impact of chronic disease on the patient

- Diagnostic studies may include:
  1. Hemoglobin and hematocrit
  2. Testing for *H. pylori*
  3. If perforation is suspected, the health care provider usually requests a chest and abdomen x-ray series or abdominal CT scan.
  4. The major diagnostic test for PUD is EGD, which is the most accurate means of establishing a diagnosis. Direct visualization of the ulcer crater by EGD allows the health care provider to take specimens for *H. pylori* testing and for biopsy and cytologic studies for ruling out gastric cancer.

Considerations for Older Adults

- The older adult may use OTC remedies to treat symptoms, often delaying appropriate treatment for PUD.

- Ulcer-producing drugs for chronic illnesses are often consumed by older adults.
- The older adult may be at increased risk for bleeding, complications, and death with hemorrhagic PUD.

PLANNING AND IMPLEMENTATION

❖**NDx:** Acute or Chronic Pain

- Perform a comprehensive pain assessment. Carefully assess changes in the characteristic of location or peptic ulcer pain because this may indicate the development of complications.
- Drug therapy includes:
  1. Proton pump inhibitors (PPI) or H_2 histamine receptor antagonists to inhibit gastric acid secretion
  2. An alternative to PPI or H_2 blockers, prostaglandin analogues to inhibit acid secretion and contribute to the mucosal barrier
  3. Antacids as buffering agents to decrease pain (given 2 hours after meals)
  4. Mucosal barrier fortifiers to provide a protective coat, preventing digestive action
  5. *H. pylori* infection treatment with 1-2 antibiotics and a drug to reduce gastric acidity, most often a PPI or H_2 blocker. Antibiotics may include metronidazole, amoxicillin, ciprofloxacin, or tetracycline.
- There is no evidence that dietary restrictions reduce gastric acid secretion or promote tissue healing. When diet therapy is used, teach the patient to:
  1. Avoid caffeine-containing coffee, tea, and cola and other foods that cause discomfort.
  2. Avoid alcohol and tobacco.

❖**Collaborative Problem:** Risk for GI Hemorrhage

Nonsurgical Management

- The patient is at risk for fluid volume deficit (hypovolemia), hemorrhage, and perforation.
  1. Management of hypovolemia includes:
     a. Monitoring vital signs
     b. Monitoring for fluid loss from bleeding or vomiting
     c. Maintaining strict intake and output
     d. Monitoring serum electrolytes and hematocrit and hemoglobin
     e. Inserting two large-bore peripheral IV catheters in the patient with shock symptoms (see Shock)
     f. Replacing fluids with IV fluids such as normal saline or lactated Ringer's solution

U

g. Ordering blood products in the presence of symptomatic anemia or hypoxemia from low hemoglobin

2. Management of hemorrhage includes:
   a. Monitoring for signs and symptoms indicating GI bleeding and documenting findings
      (1) Observe secretions (emesis, sputum, stool, urine, and nasogastric drainage) for frank or occult blood.
      (2) Document color, amount, and character of stools.
      (3) Monitor hematocrit, hemoglobin, and coagulation studies for changes from baseline.
   b. Inserting a nasogastric (NG) tube to ascertain the presence of blood in the stomach, assess the rate of bleeding, prevent gastric dilation, and provide lavage; irrigating the NG tube to maintain patency and prevent obstruction with blood
   c. Administering acid-decreasing drugs such as a proton pump inhibitor or H_2 histamine blocker
   d. Treatment measures include:
      (1) Esophagogastroduodenoscopy (EGD) to identify bleeding sites
      (2) Injection of the bleeding site with diluted epinephrine
      (3) Laser photocoagulation
      (4) Heater probe therapy
      (5) Electrocoagulation through an endoscope
      (6) Possible room temperature, sterile water, or saline lavage through the NG tube to remove gastric blood

3. Management of perforation includes the immediate replacement of fluid, blood, and electrolytes.
   a. Maintain nasogastric (NG) suction to drain gastric secretions.
   b. Keep the patient on NPO status, and monitor intake and output carefully.
   c. Check the patient's vital signs at least once hourly.
   d. Monitor the patient for septic shock.
   e. Anticipate emergency surgery (see Perioperative Care in Part One).

❖**Collaborative Management:** Pyloric Obstruction

- Pyloric obstruction is caused by edema, spasm, or scar tissue, and it manifests with feelings of fullness, distention, or nausea after eating, as well as vomiting copious amounts of undigested food; vomiting may be projectile.
- Treatment of pyloric obstruction is directed toward restoring fluid and electrolyte balance, decompressing the dilated stomach, and if necessary, surgical interventions.

Surgical Management

- Simple gastroenterostomy permits neutralization of gastric acid by regurgitation of alkaline duodenal contents into the stomach. A passageway is created between the body of the stomach and the small bowel, often the jejunum.
- A vagotomy eliminates the acid-secreting neural stimulus to gastric cells and decreases the responsiveness of parietal cells. This procedure occurs rarely.
- A vagotomy with pyloroplasty involves cutting the right and left branches of the vagus nerve and widening the pyloric sphincter to prevent stasis and to enhance emptying of the stomach.
- In patients with perforation, surgery entails closure of the perforation after the escaped gastric contents have been evacuated.
- Provide perioperative care as outlined in Part One with special attention postoperatively to the following interventions:
  1. Monitoring the patency of the NG tube and the type of drainage
  2. Not repositioning or irrigating the NG tube
  3. Assessing for fluid and electrolyte imbalances
  4. Assessing for the development of acute gastric dilation in the immediate postoperative period, which is manifested by:
     a. Epigastric pain
     b. Tachycardia
     c. Hypotension
     d. Feelings of fullness or hiccups
  5. Assessing for the development of the dumping syndrome, which occurs after gastric resection in which the pylorus is bypassed. This postprandial problem is associated with the rapid entry of food into the bowel, which is manifested by:
     a. Vertigo
     b. Tachycardia
     c. Syncope
     d. Sweating
     e. Pallor
     f. Palpitations
     g. Light-headedness
     h. Epigastric fullness
  6. Assisting in the management of the dumping syndrome by:
     a. Decreasing the amount of food taken by the patient at one time
     b. Providing a high-protein, high-fat, low-carbohydrate diet
     c. Administering pectin in a dry powder form

U

    d. Placing the patient in a recumbent or semirecumbent position during eating

    e. Positioning the patient in a flat position after meals

    f. Administering sedatives and antispasmodics, as ordered, to delay gastric emptying

7. Assessing for the occurrence of alkaline reflux gastritis, which is the reflux of duodenal contents with bile acids, resulting in injury to the gastric mucosal barrier and manifested by:

    a. Abdominal discomfort

    b. Early satiety

    c. Vomiting

8. Assessing for delayed gastric emptying, often present after gastric surgery, usually resolving within 1 week, and usually resulting from:

    a. Mechanical causes, such as edema at the anastomosis or adhesions obstructing the distal loop

    b. Metabolic causes, such as hypokalemia, hypoproteinemia, or hyponatremia

9. Assessing for development of afferent loop syndrome, which occurs when the duodenal loop is partially obstructed after a Billroth II resection, by monitoring for:

    a. Painful contractions

    b. Vomiting

    c. Abdominal bloating

10. Administering vitamin B_{12}, folic acid, and iron preparations to prevent problems of nutrition that develop from removal of the stomach, including deficiencies of vitamin B_{12}, folic acid, and iron; impaired calcium metabolism; and reduced absorption of calcium and vitamin D

Community-Based Care

- Collaborate with the patient and family to identify gastric irritants and lifestyle stressors and to develop strategies to make lifestyle changes.

- Instruct the patient about symptoms that should be brought to the attention of the health care provider:

    1. Abdominal pain

    2. Nausea and vomiting

    3. Black, tarry stools

    4. Weakness and dizziness

- Identify and reinforce stress management and successful coping skills to decrease ulcer recurrence.

- Instruct the patient to avoid NSAIDs unless under the care of a health care provider who may prescribe concurrent acid-reducing medication.

- Teach dietary management to the postoperative patient, especially the patient who had a partial stomach removal.
  a. Eat small, frequent meals.
  b. Avoid drinking liquids with meals.
  c. Abstain from foods that contribute to discomfort.
  d. Eliminate caffeine and alcohol consumption.
  e. Begin a smoking cessation program.
  f. Receive vitamin B_{12} injections as appropriate.

URETHRITIS

- Urethritis is inflammation of the urethra.
- Symptoms of urethritis in the male patient are:
  1. Burning on urination
  2. Urgency, frequency, and weak stream of urine
  3. Discharge from the urethral meatus
- Symptoms of urethritis in the female patient are:
  1. Bacterial cystitis (mimics)
  2. Painful urination
  3. Urgency, frequency, and incontinence
  4. Lower abdomen discomfort
  5. Pyuria (cloudy urine)
- The most common cause of urethritis in males is sexually transmitted disease (STD).
- In postmenopausal women, urethritis is probably caused by tissue changes related to low estrogen levels, and it is treated with estrogen vaginal cream.
- Nonspecific urethritis may be caused by increased serum urea levels or an STD, such as *Chlamydia* or *Trichomonas vaginalis*.
- STDs and infectious processes are treated with appropriate antibiotic therapy.

U

UROLITHIASIS

OVERVIEW

- Urolithiasis is the presence of calculi (stones) in the urinary tract. Stones often do not cause symptoms until they pass into the lower urinary tract, where they can cause excruciating pain. Nephrolithiasis is the formation of stones in the kidney. Formation of stones in the ureter is ureterolithiasis.
- The exact mechanism of formation is not known, but three factors contribute to stone formation through slow urine flow, resulting in supersaturation of the urine with the particular

element (e.g., calcium) that first becomes crystallized and later becomes the stone.

1. Damage to the lining of the urinary tract (from crystals)
2. Decreased inhibitor substances in the urine that would otherwise prevent supersaturation and crystal aggregation
3. High urine acidity (as with uric acid and cystine stones), high alkalinity (as with calcium phosphate and struvite stones), and drugs (triamterene, indinavir, and acetazolamide)

- Calculi may be formed from calcium, phosphate, oxalate, uric acid, struvite, and cystine crystals, but most stones contain calcium as one component.

Cultural Considerations

- There is an increased incidence of urolithiasis in the southeastern United States and a rising incidence in Japan and Western Europe.
- Urolithiasis is more common in men than in women and tends to occur in young adulthood or early middle adulthood.

PATIENT-CENTERED COLLABORATIVE CARE

Assessment

- Obtain patient information about:
  1. History of renal stones
  2. Family history of renal stones
  3. Diet history
  4. Previous interventions to eliminate stones
- Assess for and document:
  1. Renal colic (severe, unbearable pain); location and duration of pain
  2. Nausea and vomiting
  3. Hematuria, oliguria, or anuria
  4. Flank pain
  5. Ureteral spasm or colic
  6. Increased turbidity and odor of urine
  7. Bladder distention
  8. Diaphoresis
  9. Pale, ashen skin
  10. Presence of RBCs, WBCs, and bacteria in the urine

Planning and Implementation

❖**NDx:** Acute Pain

Nonsurgical Management

- Drug therapy includes:
  1. Opioid agents, such as morphine sulfate
  2. NSAIDs, such as ketorolac (Toradol)

3. Spasmolytic agents, such as oxybutynin chloride (Ditropan) and propantheline bromide (Pro-Banthine, Propanthel)
- Assess the patient's response to drug interventions.
- Encourage ambulation and an upright position to drain the renal calyx and pass renal calculi.
- Assist the patient to find a comfortable position and to use relaxation techniques.
- Distraction or relaxation techniques such as hypnosis, imagery, or acupuncture can be used to relieve pain.
- Lithotripsy, or extracorporeal shock wave lithotripsy (ESWL), is the application of ultrasound or dry shock wave energies to fragment the calculus. The patient receives conscious sedation as the lithotriptor and fluoroscope locate and break up the calculus. After lithotripsy, implement routine postoperative care with additional monitoring for urine output (quantity, quality, and presence of sediment or stones).

Surgical Management
- Stone removal procedures include:
  1. Ureteroscopy: The use of an endoscope through the urethra to visualize stones and to extract stones with a basket, or the use of a laser to fragment stones. Stents may be used to dilate the ureter and create a passageway for the stone.
  2. Percutaneous ureterolithotomy and nephrolithotomy: The use of an endoscope to visualize the stone with a special attachment to extract the calculus through a small flank incision
  3. Laparoscopic ureterolithotomy: The use of a laparoscope through the ureter to remove the calculus
  4. Pyelolithotomy: Direct visualization of the renal pelvis through a large flank incision and removal of the stone
  5. Nephrolithotomy: Direct visualization of the kidney through a large flank incision and removal of the stone
  6. Ureterolithotomy: Direct visualization of the ureter through a large flank or lower abdominal incision and removal of the stone
- Preoperative care includes routine care described in Part One and:
  1. Providing individualized instructions, depending on the procedure to be performed
  2. Preparing bowel according to the physician's preference
- Postoperative care includes routine care described in Part One and:
  1. Monitoring the amount and character (color, presence of sediment or clots) of urine output every 1 to 2 hours for 24 hours

2. Straining the patient's urine
3. Adherence to infection prevention guidelines, including:
   a. Monitoring for signs of infection (fever, chills, altered mental status)
   b. Obtaining a urine culture and sensitivity profile, as ordered
   c. Administering antibiotics to eliminate existing infections or prevent new ones
   d. Ensuring adequate nutrition and fluid intake
4. Administering drug therapy and assessing for adverse effects, including:
   a. Broad-spectrum antibiotics, such as aminoglycosides and cephalosporins, and monitoring blood levels of the antibiotic prescribed
   b. Acetohydroxamic acid (Lithostat) and hydroxyurea (Hydrea) for patients with struvite stones; monitoring serum creatinine levels (contraindicated for levels above 2 mg/dL)
   c. Thiazide diuretics to treat hypercalciuria (high levels of calcium in the urine)
   d. Allopurinol (Zyloprim) to treat hyperoxaluria (high levels of oxalic acid in the urine) or gout
   e. Alpha-mercaptopropionylglycine (AMPG) and captopril (Capoten) to treat cystinuria (high levels of cystine in the urine)

Community-Based Care

1. Inform the patient that:
   a. Extensive bruising may occur after lithotripsy and may take several weeks to resolve.
   b. Urine may be bloody for several days after surgical intervention.
2. Instructing the patient about:
   a. The importance of finishing all drugs
   b. The importance of balancing regular exercise with rest
   c. Diet, depending on stone type
   d. The rationale for preventing dehydration and promoting urine flow, stressing the importance of continued adequate fluid intake
   e. The importance of reporting symptoms of recurrent infection or formation of another stone, such as pain, fever, chills, and difficulty with urination
   f. The importance of keeping follow-up appointments to check on resolution of infection
3. Providing postoperative instructions, including:
   a. Keeping the incision dry

   b. Showering instead of bathing

   c. Monitoring the incision for redness, swelling, and drainage

UVEITIS

OVERVIEW

- Uveitis is a general term for inflammation of the eye's uveal tract. It may occur in the anterior or posterior portion of the eye.
- Anterior uveitis
  1. May be inflammation of the iris, inflammation of the ciliary body, or both
  2. The cause of anterior uveitis is unknown but often follows exposure to allergens, infectious agents, trauma, or systemic disease (rheumatoid arthritis, herpes simplex, herpes zoster). It can follow any local or systemic bacterial infection.
  3. Manifestations include aching around the eye; tearing; blurred vision; photophobia; a small, irregular, nonreactive pupil; and a "bloodshot" appearance of the sclera.
- Posterior uveitis
  1. Involves inflammation of the retina (retinitis) or inflammation of both the choroid and the retina (chorioretinitis)
  2. Common causes include tuberculosis, syphilis, and toxoplasmosis.
  3. Manifestations include visual impairment in the affected eye; a small, nonreactive, and irregularly shaped pupil; black dots on the optic fundus; and grayish yellow patches on the retinal surface.

PATIENT-CENTERED COLLABORATIVE CARE

- Drug therapies
  1. Resting the ciliary body with a cycloplegic agent
  2. Steroid drops given hourly to reduce the inflammation and to prevent adhesion of the iris to the cornea and lens
  3. Nonaspirin– and non–opioid-containing analgesics for pain
  4. Systemic antibiotic therapy, which may be started for posterior uveitis or when infection is present with anterior uveitis
- Symptom management
  1. Applying cool or warm compresses
  2. Darkening the room
  3. Having the patient wear dark glasses
- Safety management
  1. Instructing the patient not to drive or operate machinery

U

2. Reviewing the manifestations of bacterial and fungal ulcers and those of increased intraocular pressure (IOP)

VANCOMYCIN-RESISTANT *ENTEROCOCCUS*

OVERVIEW

- Enterococci are bacteria that live in the intestinal tract and are important for digestion. These organisms are tougher than other bacteria because they must survive pH changes, enzymes, and other environmental dangers. As long as they remain only in the intestinal tract, they pose no health problem.
- When they move to another area of the body, such as during surgery, they can cause an infection, which usually is treatable with the antibiotic vancomycin. However, in recent years, more than one fourth of these bacterial strains have become resistant to the drug, and infection with vancomycin-resistant entero-cocci (VRE) results.
- Unfortunately, VRE can live on almost any surface (e.g., toilet seats, door handles, other objects) for days or weeks and still be able to cause an infection.
- The most common infections caused by VRE include wound infections, urinary tract infections (UTIs), and bloodstream infections.
- Risk factors for this infection apply to patients who:
  1. Are hospitalized, especially in the ICU, and have received prolonged antibiotic therapy
  2. Have been previously treated with the antibiotic vancomycin or other antibiotics for long periods
  3. Are immunosuppressed (patients receiving cancer chemo-therapy, have HIV disease, have received solid organ or bone marrow transplants) or are taking immunosuppressive drugs
  4. Have extensive open wounds or have undergone surgical procedures such as abdominal or chest surgery
  5. Have a long-term internal medical device that opens to the outside, such as urinary catheters, central venous catheters, and peripherally inserted central catheters (PICCs)
- Most VRE infections occur in hospitals.

PATIENT-CENTERED COLLABORATIVE CARE

- Management
  1. People who have intestinal or mucous membrane VRE do not usually need treatment.
  2. For patients with indwelling urinary catheters and a UTI VRE, catheter removal usually halts the infection.

   3. VRE infections can be treated with antibiotics other than vancomycin after culture and sensitivity testing to determine which antibiotics are most likely to be effective.
- Prevention
  1. Performing meticulous hand-washing with soap and water is the best method of preventing VRE spread
  2. Frequently cleaning of rooms and items in contact with patients who have VRE
  3. Use Contact Precautions when coming into contact with body fluids that may contain VRE, such as stool or bandages from infected wounds.

VASCULAR DISEASE, PERIPHERAL

- Peripheral vascular disease (PVD) includes disorders that alter the natural flow of blood through the arteries and veins of the peripheral circulation.
- It affects the lower extremities much more frequently than the upper extremities.
- A diagnosis of PVD usually implies arterial disease (peripheral arterial disease [PAD]) rather than venous involvement. Some patients have arterial and venous disease.
- Atherosclerosis is the most common cause of PAD (see Atherosclerosis).

VEINS, VARICOSE

- Varicose veins are distended, protruding veins that appear darkened or tortuous.
- The vein walls weaken and dilate. Venous pressure increases, and the valves become incompetent.
- Incompetent valves enhance vessel dilation, and veins become tortuous and distended.
- Varicose veins occur primarily in patients subjected to prolonged standing. They also occur in pregnant women and in patients with systemic problems, such as heart disease or obesity, and a family history of varicose veins.
- Conservative treatment measures include:
  1. Wearing elastic stockings
  2. Elevating the extremities as often as possible
- Outpatient surgery includes routine perioperative care and restrictions to weight-bearing for several days. Procedures include:
  1. Sclerotherapy, in which the physician injects a chemical to sclerose the vein, performed on small or a limited number of varicosities

V

2. Laser treatment uses a laser fiber to heat and close the main vessel that is contributing to the varicosity.

3. Radiofrequency (RF) ablation involves heating the vein from the inside by the RF energy and shrinking the vein. Surgical intervention entails ligation (tying) and stripping (removal) the affected veins with the patient under general anesthesia.

- Collateral veins take over supplying blood to tissues after laser, RF, or surgical interventions.

VENOUS DISEASE, PERIPHERAL

OVERVIEW

- Peripheral venous disease (PVD) is a group of diseases that alter the natural flow of blood through the veins of the peripheral circulation.
- Venous blood flow may be altered by thrombus formation and defective valves.
- Thrombus formation is associated with stasis of blood flow, endothelial injury, and hypercoagulability.
- Thrombophlebitis occurs when a thrombus is associated with inflammation in superficial veins.
- Deep venous thrombophlebitis, commonly referred to as deep vein thrombosis (DVT), usually occurs in the deep veins of the lower extremities and is a major risk for pulmonary embolism. Risk factors include hip or open prostate surgeries. Other conditions that seem to promote thrombus formation are heart failure, immobility, pregnancy, and ulcerative colitis.
- Thrombus formation can lead to embolism or to breaking off of a portion of the clot, which can then travel to distal sites, impairing blood flow. This is called venothromboembolism (VTE).
- Venous insufficiency results from prolonged venous hypertension and phlebitis, which stretch the veins and damage valves, resulting in venous stasis ulcers with swelling and cellulitis.

PATIENT-CENTERED COLLABORATIVE CARE

- For the patient with DVT, assess for:
  1. Calf or groin tenderness and pain
  2. Unilateral swelling of the leg
  3. Warmth and edema of the extremity
  4. Induration along the blood vessel
  5. Size comparison with the contralateral limb
  6. Localized pitting edema

- For the patient with venous insufficiency (chronic hypertension or post-phlebitis), assess for:
  1. Discoloration along the ankles, extending up to the calf
  2. Ulcer formation
     a. Arterial ulcers develop on the toes, between the toes, or on the upper aspect of the foot; they are painful.
     b. Diabetic ulcers develop on the plantar surface of the foot, over metatarsal heads, or on the heel and pressure areas; they may not be painful.
     c. Venous stasis ulcers occur at the ankles; minimal pain is present.
- Diagnostic studies may include:
  1. Contrast venography
  2. Duplex ultrasonography
  3. Doppler flow studies
  4. Impedance plethysmography
  5. Serum for inflammatory factors and coagulation studies
- Any patient with PVD should elevate the legs if sitting or lying in bed to prevent edema and use lower extremity ROM activity to prevent venous stasis.
- To prevent DVT, the following actions may be taken:
  1. Low-molecular-weight heparin (enoxaparin), dextran, dihydroergotamine (DHE), or aspirin may be prescribed.
  2. The patient may be ambulated and mobilized early, and a thigh-high graduated compression elastic stocking and external intermittent or sequential compression devices may be used.
- For patients diagnosed with DVT, interventions include:
  1. Monitoring for pulmonary emboli and an increase in the size of the thrombus
  2. Elevating the extremity while in bed; bedrest is no longer recommended for DVT
  3. Applying warm, moist soaks to the affected area
  4. Administering anticoagulants such as warfarin (Coumadin), unfractionated heparin therapy, or low-molecular-weight heparin
     a. Teaching the patient to continue follow-up care to monitor response and therapeutic levels of anticoagulation
     b. Teaching the patient to minimize the risk for increased injury related to anticoagulation therapy, to monitor for blood in stool, and to report signs of bleeding early to health care provider
  5. Administering thrombolytic therapy to dissolve thrombus
  6. Providing surgical or interventional radiologic management of DVT, which may include a thrombectomy, inferior vena

V

caval interruption or ligation, and insertion of a filter in the inferior vena cava. Filters are recommended to be removed after six months to avoid becoming a source of clot formation.

> **⬛ Critical Rescue ◆** Instruct the patient to avoid adding new drugs (prescribed and OTC) and herbal remedies or significantly changing the diet when taking warfarin. Warfarin has multiple drug-drug, drug-herb, and drug-food interactions that can interfere with the effectiveness of the drug and contribute to increased bleeding risk.

- For venous insufficiency, interventions include:
  1. Teaching the patient to avoid standing still or sitting for long periods
  2. Having the patient wear elastic or compression stockings during the day and evening
  3. Teaching the patient to elevate his or her legs for 20 minutes four or five times a day and to avoid long periods of sitting or standing in place
  4. Teaching the patient to use a sequential gradient compression device, if ordered
  5. Treating open venous ulcers with occlusive dressings and topical agents, with or without antibiotics to chemically débride the ulcer
  6. If the patient is ambulatory, using an Unna boot

Considerations for Older Adults

- Warfarin is used with caution in older or debilitated patients to prevent bleeding.
- A reduced dose may be used to prevent spontaneous intracranial bleeding or excessive bleeding related to trauma.
- Older adults may have reduced liver or kidney function and a decreased ability to metabolize and excrete warfarin.

VISUAL IMPAIRMENT (REDUCED VISION)

OVERVIEW

- Visual impairment can range from total blindness in both eyes to various degrees and types of partial impairment.
- Patients are legally blind if their best visual acuity with corrective lenses is 20/200 or less in the better eye or if the widest diameter of the visual field in that eye is no greater than 20 degrees.

- Blindness can occur in one or both eyes. When one eye is affected, the field of vision is narrowed, and depth perception is impaired.
- Central vision can be impaired by diseases involving the macula, such as macular edema or macular degeneration.
- Peripheral vision loss affects the patient's ability to drive and awareness of hazards in the periphery.

PATIENT-CENTERED COLLABORATIVE CARE

- Nursing interventions for the patient with reduced sight focus on teaching patients techniques to make better use of existing vision, communication, safety, ambulation, self-care, and support.
  1. To make better use of existing vision, teach the patient:
     a. To move the head slightly up and down to enhance a three-dimensional effect
     b. When shaking hands or pouring water, to line up the object and move toward it
     c. To choose a position that favors the good eye; for example, people with vision in the right eye should position people and items on their right
  2. Teach the patient how to use alternative forms of communication:
     a. Auditory traffic signals
     b. Curbs that have a high-contrast paint color to let the person know when to step up or down
     c. Large-print books and books on tape
     d. "Talking" clocks, watches, and timers
     e. Playing cards, games, restaurant menus, calendars, and instruction booklets with large print sizes
     f. Computer keyboards with high-contrast, larger letters and a large screen
     g. Local resources that sell or provide adaptive items
  3. Instruct the patient about safety in the home:
     a. Teach patients to count the number of footsteps needed to move from one area to another within the home.
     b. Stress to family and friends that changes in item location should not be made without input from the person with reduced vision.
     c. Assist the patient and family in making adaptations:
        (1) Using tape and a heavy black marker, mark the 350° F temperature setting on the oven, and mark the 70° F temperature setting on the room temperature thermostat.

V

(2) Mark light switches in a deep color that contrasts with the surrounding wall.

(3) Label canned goods with large, bold, black letters on white tape.

(4) Feel for the crease in paper milk cartons that indicates the place to open the spout.

(5) Alter the shape or contours of drug bottles and containers.

4. Ensure safety in a hospital or other health care environment:

   a. Use a normal tone of voice unless the patient has a hearing problem.

   b. Orient the patient to the immediate environment, including the size of the room. Use one object in the room, such as a chair or hospital bed, as the focal point during your description. Guide the person to the focal point and describe all other objects in relation to the focal point.

   c. Go with the patient to other important areas, such as the bathroom (highlighting the location of the toilet, sink, and toilet paper holder).

> **Clinical Landmine** ◆ Never leave the patient with reduced vision in the center of an unfamiliar room.

   d. Allow the patient to establish the location of important objects, such as the call bell, water pitcher, and clock. Do not move these items after their locations have been fixed.

   e. Set up food trays using imaginary clock placement to orient the patient to the location of specific items.

5. Teach safe ambulation:

   a. Allow the patient to grasp your arm at the elbow while keeping the arm close to your body so that he or she can detect your direction of movement.

   b. Alert the patient when obstacles are in the path ahead.

   c. Teach patients the correct use of a cane to detect obstacles (the cane is held in the dominant hand several inches off the floor and sweeps the ground where the patient's foot will be placed next).

6. Promote self-care and the ability to control the environment:

   a. Knock on the door before entering the room.

   b. State your name and the reason for visiting when entering the room.

    c. Coordinate with other members of the health care team to ensure this etiquette is used consistently.

7. Provide emotional support:
   a. Allow the newly blind person a period of grieving for the "dead" (nonseeing) eye.
   b. Accept the patient's behavior.
   c. Encourage the patient and family to express feelings and concerns.
   d. Tell patients that it is normal to mourn, to cry, and to feel the loss.
   e. Encourage the mastery of one task at a time.
   f. Provide positive reinforcement for each success.

WEST NILE VIRUS

- West Nile virus infection is spread by birds, infected mosquitos, and contaminated substances such as blood products, breast milk, or organ transplantation.
- The infection is generally mild, and the patient usually is asymptomatic or has only flu-like symptoms of (e.g., fever, body aches, nausea, vomiting).
- A small percentage of patients develop severe disease with symptoms of encephalitis that include:
  1. High fever
  2. Severe headache
  3. Decreased level of consciousness
  4. Tremors
  5. Vision loss
  6. Seizures
  7. Muscle weakness or paralysis
- Diagnostic tests include enzyme-linked immunosorbent assay (ELISA) and West Nile virus–specific IgM antibody in serum or cerebrospinal fluid (CSF).
- Management is symptomatic, as for any other type of viral encephalitis.
- For the severe form of the disease, manifestations may last for several weeks, and neurologic deficits may be permanent.
- A few patients die of the disease.

W

GUIDE TO HEAD-TO-TOE PHYSICAL ASSESSMENT OF ADULTS

Guide to Head-to-Toe Physical Assessment of Adults*

Nursing Activity	Typical Finding	Changes Associated with Aging
NEUROLOGIC SYSTEM		
1. Determine level of consciousness.	1. Awake, alert	1. None
2. Test for orientation.	2. States name, place, and time	2. None
SKIN		
1. Inspect skin.	1. Intact, warm, dry, elastic skin without lesions	1a. Excessive dryness; wrinkles; "age spots" and hemangiomas; inelastic, sagging skin
		1b. Ecchymotic areas as a result of increased capillary fragility
HEAD AND FACE		
1. Inspect and palpate the scalp, hair, and skull.	1. No lesions, shiny hair	1. Thinning and dullness of hair
2. Inspect face for symmetry of expression.	2. Symmetric expression	2. None
EYE		
1. Inspect the external eye structures.	1. No structural abnormalities	1. Entropion (inverted eyelid) or ectropion (everted eyelid)
2. Inspect the conjunctivae, sclerae, corneas, and irides.	2. No abnormalities; round irides	2. None
3. Use a penlight to test pupillary response (direct and consensual).	3. Pupils are equal and round and react to light and accommodation.	3. None

4. Test vision by asking the client to read (if able). **NOTE**: Be sure that glasses or contact lenses are in place, if used.	4. No vision impairment	4. Presbyopia (farsightedness)
EAR		
1. Inspect the external structure.	1. No structural abnormalities	1. No major change
2. Inspect the auditory meatus for drainage.	2. No drainage; small amount of cerumen may be present	2. None
3. Test hearing by whispering to the client while turning head away. Note: Be sure that hearing aid, if used, is in place.	3. No difficulty in hearing	3. Hearing loss, especially high-frequency sounds
MOUTH		
1. Use a penlight to inspect mouth, teeth, and gums.	1. No lesions, extensive dental caries, or gum disease	1. None
NECK		
1. Inspect for symmetry, lesions, pulsations, and JVD.	1. Symmetric, without lesions or JVD	1. None
2. Palpate the carotid pulse, one side at a time; check for bruits.	2. No bruits; pulses equal	2. None

*Additional assessments may be needed, depending on the patient's concerns and the medical diagnoses. For more information on physical assessment, see Ignatavicius, D.D., & Workman, M.L. (2009). *Medical-surgical nursing: Critical thinking for collaborative care* (6th ed.). Philadelphia: W.B. Saunders. *ICS*, intercostal space; *JVD*, jugular venous distention; *MCL*, midclavicular line; *PMI*, point of maximal impulse; *ROM*, range of motion; *TMJ*, temporoman-dibular joint.

Continued

APPENDIX 1

Guide to Head-to-Toe Physical Assessment of Adults

Guide to Head-to-Toe Physical Assessment of Adults—cont'd

Nursing Activity	Typical Finding	Changes Associated with Aging
3. Palpate the cervical lymph nodes.	3. Unable to palpate	3. None
4. Test ROM.	4. No limitations	4. Slight decreased; possible crepitus
CHEST (POSTERIOR, ANTERIOR, AND LATERAL)		
1. Inspect the chest for deformity, symmetry, expansion, and lesions; note pulsations or heaves (lifts).	1. Symmetric; without lesions; anteroposterior-lateral ratio of 1:2; no heaves	1. Slight change in anteroposterior-lateral ratio (1:1.5)
2. Palpate any chest lesions.	2. No lesions	2. None
3. Locate the PMI.	3. PMI at the left MCL, fifth ICS	3. None
4. Palpate each vertebra of the spine.	4. No tenderness or bony spurs	4. Thoracic kyphosis
5. Auscultate breath sounds throughout all lung fields.	5. Unlabored excursion of air; no adventitious sounds	5. Shallow respirations
6. Auscultate apical rate and rhythm; auscultate heart sounds.	6. S_1 and S_2 heart sounds	6. Possible S_4 heart sound
UPPER EXTREMITIES		
1. Inspect and palpate joints for swelling, tenderness, and deformity.	1. No swelling, tenderness, or deformity	1. Tenderness of one or more joints
2. Palpate brachial and radial arteries; assess for pulse deficit.	2. Pulses equal and within normal limits	2. None
3. Test ROM in all joints and sensation.	3. No restriction	3. Slight decrease in ROM; possible crepitus
4. Test muscle strength of arms, hands, and shoulders.	4. 5/5: Movement against both gravity and resistance	4. None or slight decrease (4+/5)
5. Palpate axillary nodes.	5. Nodes not palpable	5. None

ABDOMEN

1. Inspect for contour, symmetry, lesions, and pulsations.
   1. Symmetric; without lesions or pulsations
2. Auscultate bowel sounds in all four quadrants.
   2. 5-15 sounds/min in each quadrant
3. Auscultate over abdominal aorta for bruit.
   3. No bruit
4. Palpate for liver enlargement.
   4. Liver not below costal margin

LOWER EXTREMITIES

1. Inspect and palpate for swelling, tenderness, and deformity.
   1. No swelling, tenderness, or deformity
2. Test ROM and sensation.
   2. No limitation
3. Test muscle strength.
   3. 5/5: Movement against gravity and resistance
4. Palpate femoral, popliteal, and pedal pulses.
   4. Pulses equal and within normal range
5. Palpate inguinal nodes.
   5. Nodes not palpable

GENITALIA

1. Inspect external genitalia for lesions or drainage.
   1. No lesions or drainage

1. None
2. May be slightly decreased (hypoactive)
3. None
4. None

1. Tenderness of one or more joints
2. Slight decrease in ROM; possible crepitus
3. None or slight decrease (4+/5)
4. Pedal pulses may be weak or not palpable.
5. None

1. None

ICS, intercostal space; JVD, jugular venous distention; MCL, midclavicular line; PMI, point of maxima impulse; ROM, range of motion; TMJ, temporomandibular joint.

TERMINOLOGY ASSOCIATED WITH FLUID AND ELECTROLYTE BALANCE

active transport Assisted movement of a substance through a permeable membrane between two fluid compartments; occurs against a concentration, electrical, or pressure gradient; requires the expenditure of chemical energy

adenosine triphosphate (ATP) A substance that is generated by the metabolism of glucose or fat within cells and releases chemical energy for physiologic function when a high-energy phosphate bond (~P) is broken

aldosterone A hormone secreted by the adrenal cortex that stimulates the renal reabsorption of sodium and water and the renal excretion of potassium

anion A molecule (electrolyte) that carries an overall negative charge when dissolved in water

antidiuretic hormone (ADH) A hormone secreted from the posterior pituitary gland that increases the renal reabsorption of pure water and decreases urine output

atrial natriuretic peptide (ANP) A hormone secreted by cardiac atrial cells that increases the renal excretion of sodium and water

brownian motion Inherent molecular motion

capillary (plasma) hydrostatic pressure The force generated by fluid within a capillary that tends to move fluid out from the capillary and into the interstitial space

capillary (plasma) osmotic pressure The force generated by the concentration of plasma solutes (osmotic and oncotic pressures) that tends to retain fluid within the capillary or move fluid from the interstitial space into the capillary

cation A molecule (electrolyte) that carries an overall positive charge when dissolved in water

cofactor A substance required to enhance the activity of an enzyme or a physiologic reaction

colloidal oncotic pressure The osmotic pressure exerted by the concentration of colloids (proteins) within a solution

diffusion Unimpeded movement of a substance through a permeable membrane between two fluid compartments; occurs down a concentration gradient; does not require the expenditure of chemical energy

disequilibrium A state in which two fluid compartments are unequal in at least one characteristic

electrolytes Substances that carry an electrical charge when dissolved in water

electroneutrality A state in which a body fluid has an equal number of cations and anions so that the fluid does not express an electrical charge

equilibrium A state in which two fluid compartments are equal in one or more characteristics

extracellular fluid (ECF) Body fluid present outside of cells, which includes plasma, interstitial fluid, and transcellular fluid

facilitated diffusion Assisted movement of a substance through a permeable membrane between two fluid compartments; occurs down a concentration gradient; does not require the expenditure of chemical energy

filtration The movement of fluid through a biologic membrane as a result of hydrostatic pressure differences on the two sides of the membrane

gradient A graded difference in some characteristic between two fluid compartments

hydrostatic pressure The force of pressure exerted by static water in a confined space—"water-pushing" pressure

hypertonic (hyperosmotic) Any solution with a solute concentration (osmolarity) greater than that of normal body fluids (>310 mOsm/L)

hypotonic (hyposmotic) Any solution with a solute concentration (osmolarity) less than that of normal body fluids (<270 mOsm/L)

impermeable membrane A membrane separating two fluid compartments that does not permit the movement of one or more substances through the membrane (by diffusion) from one compartment to the other

insensible fluid loss Unregulated fluid losses from the skin, gastrointestinal tract, wounds, and pulmonary epithelium

interstitial fluid Fluid in the spaces between cells

intracellular fluid (ICF) Fluid found inside cells

isotonic (isosmotic) Any solution with a solute concentration equal to the osmolarity of normal body fluids or normal saline (0.9% NaCl), or about 300 mOsm/L

obligatory urine output The minimal amount of urine output necessary to ensure the excretion of metabolic wastes (~400 mL/day)

osmolality The concentration of solute within a solution as measured by the amount of solute osmoles per kilogram of solvent

osmolarity The concentration of solute within a solution as measured by the amount of solute osmoles per liter of solution

osmoreceptor Specialized sensory nerve cells in the thalamus or hypothalamus that are sensitive to changes in the osmolarity of extracellular fluid

osmosis Diffusion of water (no other substance) through a selectively permeable membrane from an area of lower osmotic pressure to an area of greater osmotic pressure

osmotic pressure The pressure exerted by a solution that contains a relatively high concentration of solute; this pressure draws water from areas or compartments with lower concentrations of solute into the areas or compartments with higher concentrations of solute—"water-pulling" pressure

permeable membrane A membrane separating two fluid compartments that permits the movement of one or more substances through the membrane (by diffusion) from one compartment to the other

solubility The degree to which any given solute completely dissolves (dissociates) in water

solute The solid particles dissolved in a solution

solvent The fluid (water) portion of a solution

tissue hydrostatic pressure (THP) The force generated by fluid within the interstitial spaces that tends to move fluid into the capillary from the interstitial space

tissue osmotic pressure (TOP) The force generated by the concentration of interstitial fluid solutes that tend to retain fluid in the interstitial space or move fluid from the capillary into the interstitial space

transcellular fluid Extracellular fluid confined to a specific area or region of the body (cerebrospinal fluid, pericardial fluid, visceral fluid, aqueous humor, peritoneal fluid, and pleural fluid)

viscosity Gumminess or thickness of the molecules in a solution, causing friction within that solution

LABORATORY VALUES

Major Serum Electrolyte Concentrations and Functions

Electrolyte	Reference Range	International Recommended Units	Functions
Sodium (Na^+)	136-145 mEq/L	136-145 mmol/L	Maintenance of plasma and interstitial osmolarity Generation and transmission of action potentials Maintenance of acid-base balance Maintenance of electroneutrality
Potassium (K^+)	3.5-5.0 mEq/L	3.5-5.0 mmol/L	Regulation of intracellular osmolarity Maintenance of electrical membrane excitability Maintenance of plasma acid-base balance
Calcium (Ca^{2+})	9.0-10.5 mg/dL	2.25-2.75 mmol/L	Cofactor in blood-clotting cascade Excitable membrane stabilizer Adds strength and density to bones and teeth Essential element in cardiac, skeletal, and smooth muscle contraction
Chloride (Cl^-)	98-106 mEq/L	98-106 mmol/L	Maintenance of plasma acid-base balance Maintenance of plasma electroneutrality Formation of hydrochloric acid
Magnesium (Mg^{2+})	1.3-2.1 mEq/L	0.65-1.05 mmol/L	Excitable membrane stabilizer Essential element in cardiac, skeletal, and smooth muscle contraction Cofactor in blood-clotting cascade Cofactor in DNA and protein synthesis
Phosphorus (P_i)	3.0-4.5 mg/dL	0.97-1.45 mmol/L	Activation of B-complex vitamins Formation of adenosine triphosphate and other high-energy substances Cofactor in carbohydrate, protein, and lipid metabolism

Data from Pagana, K. & Pagana, T. (2007). *Mosby's manual of diagnostic and laboratory tests* (8th ed.). St. Louis: Mosby.

Major Urine Electrolytes

Electrolytes and Characteristics	Normal Value*	Significance of Abnormal Value†
Calcium	2.5-7.5 mmol/day	Increased: malignancy, thyrotoxicosis, hyperparathyroidism, osteoporosis, vitamin D intoxication
Chloride	110-250 mEq/day 110-250 mmol/day	Increased: increased salt intake, drug-induced diuresis, adrenocortical insufficiency Decreased: reduced salt intake, water retention, vomiting, cerebral edema, adrenocortical hyperfunction
Magnesium	3.0-5.0 mmol/day	Increased: alcohol intake, diuretics, corticosteroid therapy, cisplatin therapy Decreased: dietary insufficiency
Phosphorus	12.9-42.0 mmol/cay	Increased: hyperparathyroidism, renal tubular damage, immobility, nonrenal acidosis Decreased: hypoparathyroidism
Potassium	25-100 mmol/day (varies with diet)	Increased: early starvation, hyperaldosteronism, metabolic acidosis Decreased: Addison's disease, renal disease
Sodium	40-220 mEq/day 40-220 mmol/day	Increased: increased dietary intake, adrenal failure, diuretic therapy Decreased: low sodium intake, sodium and water retention, adrenocortical hyperfunction, excessive diaphoresis, diarrhea
Osmolarity (osmolality), random	50-1200 mOsm/kg water	Increased: dehydration, SIADH Decreased: diabetes insipidus, primary polydipsia
Specific gravity	1.015-1.025	Increased: dehydration, SIADH, diabetes mellitus, toxemia of pregnancy Decreased: chronic renal insufficiency, diabetes insipidus, lithium toxicity, early renal disease

*Based on a 24-hour total volume urine sample.
†Common conditions associated with abnormal values.
SIADH, syndrome of inappropriate antidiuretic hormcne.
Data from Pagana, K., & Pagana, T. (2007). *Mosby's manual of diagnostic and laboratory tests* (8th ed.). St. Louis: Mosby.

INTERVENTIONS FOR COMMON ENVIRONMENTAL EMERGENCIES

Interventions for Common Environmental Emergencies

	Clinical Manifestations	Collaborative Management
HEAT-RELATED ILLNESS Heat exhaustion	Patient complains of flu-like symptoms Headache Fatigue Anorexia Nausea Vomiting Hypotension Tachycardia May have normal temperature	Home care Move to cool environment. Remove constrictive clothing. Provide an oral rehydrating solution such as a sports drink or intravenous fluids (9% saline solution). Place cool or cold packs on neck, chest, abdomen, and groin. Place in cool water. Fan while spraying water on the skin. Hospital care (if necessary) Monitor vital signs. Rehydrate with oral or IV fluids.

Heat stroke: elevated temperature (>105° F or 40.5° C)	Hot, dry skin	Prehospital care
	Mental status changes	Call for emergency help.
	Anxiety	Rapid cooling
	Confusion	Remove clothes.
	Bizarre behavior	Place ice packs on neck, axillae, chest, and groin.
	Loss of coordination	Immerse in cold water.
	Hallucinations	Wet the body with tepid water and fan rapidly to aid
	Agitation	in cooling by evaporation.
	Seizures	Hospital care
	Coma	ABCs of airway, breathing, and circulation are a
	Hypotension	priority.
	Tachycardia	Oxygen
	Tachypnea	Intravenous fluids with 9% saline solution
		Aggressive methods to decrease temperature
		(continuously monitor temperature)
		Cooling blanket
		Iced lavage
		Peritoneal lavage
		Monitor neurologic status.
		Seizure Precautions

Continued

Interventions for Common Environmental Emergencies—cont'd

	Clinical Manifestations	Collaborative Management
COLD-RELATED INJURIES Hypothermia: core body temperature below 95° F (35° C) Mild: 32-35° C Moderate: 28-32° C Severe: <28° C	**Mild** Shivering Dysarthria Muscular incoordination, impaired cognitive abilities, and diuresis Tachycardia Increased respiratory rate **Moderate** Obvious motor impairment such as stumbling, falling Weakness Confusion, apathy Irrational, incoherent Stupor and coma Shivering stops Patient may perceive warmth and undress. Bradycardia and hypotension Decreased respiratory rate and cardiac output Dysrhythmias Coagulopathy Thrombocytopenia	**Mild** Shelter from cold environment Remove wet clothes and apply warm clothes or blankets; warm room. Provide warm, high-carbonate liquids that do not contain alcohol or caffeine. **Moderate and severe** Hospital care required Do not use external rewarming methods, which promote "after drop," a continued decrease in core body temperature after the victim is removed from the cold environment. Applying external heat may produce peripheral vasodilation, which stimulates return of cold blood from periphery to warmer core. Standard resuscitation measures, if needed Handle gently to prevent ventricular defibrillation. Place patient in horizontal position. Core rewarming methods include administration of warm IV fluids, heated oxygen, and inspired gas.

Continued

Severe	Absent neurologic reflexes; no response to pain Hypotension Acid-base abnormalities Ventricular fibrillation, asystole Coagulopathy Thrombocytopenia	Extracorporeal rewarming methods used for severe hypothermia such as cardiopulmonary bypass, hemodialysis, or continuous arteriovenous rewarming Administer medications cautiously: Metabolism is unpredictable, and a drug can accumulate without obvious therapeutic effect while the patient is cold, but it will become active and may lead to drug toxicity as effective rewarming is under way.

Frostbite	Frostnip
	  Pain, numbness, pallor of affected area (white or waxy appearance)
	First-degree frostbite
	  Hyperemia and edema
	Second-degree frostbite
	  Large, fluid-filled blisters with partial thickness skin necrosis
	Third-degree frostbite
	  Small blisters that contain dark fluid
	  Affected area cool, numb, blue, or red that does not blanch
	  Full thickness and subcutaneous necrosis
	Fourth-degree frostbite
	  No blisters or edema
	  Affected area is numb, cold, and bloodless.
	  Full-thickness necrosis extends into muscle and bone.
		Frostnip
		  Use body heat to warm affected area. For example, place warm hands over cold ears or cold hands under axillary region.
		Frostbite
		  Hospital care required
		  Rapid rewarming in a water bath at temperature of 38° C (41° C)
		  Premedicate for pain before rewarming.
		  Do not apply dry heat or rub affected area.
		  After rewarming, elevate an involved extremity above the heart to decrease tissue edema.
		  Administer tetanus prophylaxis, if needed.
		  Surgical management for deep wounds
		  Amputation may be necessary.

Interventions for Common Environmental Emergencies—cont'd

	Clinical Manifestations	Collaborative Management
SNAKE BITES North American pit viper Rattlesnake Copperhead Water moccasin (cottonmouth)	One or more puncture wounds Severe pain Swelling Redness or ecchymosis Later: vesicles or hemorrhagic bullae Minty, rubbery, or metallic taste in mouth Tingling or paresthesias of scalp, face, and lips Muscle fasciculations and weakness Nausea, vomiting Hypotension Seizures Coagulopathy Disseminated intravascular coagulation	**Prehospital care** Move patient to safe location. Encourage patient to rest to decrease venom circulation. Remove constrictive clothing and jewelry. If extremity is affected, immobilize and keep below level of heart. Keep patient warm. Provide reassurance. If hospital care and definitive treatment will be delayed, a constricting band may be applied proximal to an extremity wound to impede venom circulation through lymphatic flow but not tight enough to impair venous drainage or arterial flow. Loosen band if it becomes too tight due to edema.

Continued

Hospital care

ABCs of airway, breathing, and circulation

Assess distal circulation frequently.

Insert two large-bore IV catheters and begin fluids.

Continuous cardiac and blood pressure monitoring

Pain management

Tetanus prophylaxis

Broad-spectrum antibiotic to reduce risk of infection

Laboratory studies

CBC, electrolytes

Coagulation studies

Creatinine kinase

Type and crossmatch

Urinalysis

Electrocardiogram

Measure and record circumference of bite site every
15-30 minutes, if possible.

Monitor for bleeding due to potential of coagulopathy.

Contact the poison control center.

Administer antivenom if ordered and monitor for
adverse reactions and anaphylaxis.

Interventions for Common Environmental Emergencies—cont'd

	Clinical Manifestations	Collaborative Management

Coral snake	Pain may be only mild and transient.
	Fang marks difficult to visualize
	Coagulopathy does not occur.
	Toxic effect may be delayed 12-13 hours.
	Nausea, vomiting
	Headache
	Pallor
	Abdominal pain
	Neurologic manifestations
	  Paresthesias
	  Numbness
	  Mental status changes
	  Cranial and peripheral nerve
	    involvement
	Later may see total flaccid paralysis
	Difficulty speaking, swallowing, and
	  breathing
	Cardiovascular collapse
		Continuous cardiac, blood pressure, and pulse oximetry
		  monitoring.
		Aggressive airway management
		Monitor and initiate interventions to prevent aspiration.
		Contact the poison control center.
		Administer antivenom, if ordered, and monitor for side
		  effects.

ARTHROPOD (SPIDER) BITES

Brown recluse spider	Bite is painless, stinging, sharp, or painful.	Home care
	Intense local aching and pruritus	Cold compresses—never use heat.
	Central bite site appears as a bleb or vesicle surrounded by edema and erythema, which may expand.	Rest, elevate an extremity if affected.
		Hospital care
	Over 1-3 days, central lesion becomes dark and necrotic; eschar forms.	Wound care includes antibiotics antiseptic cream, and a sterile dressing to cover the bite area.
	When the eschar sloughs, an open would or ulcer can remain for weeks to months.	Surgical evaluation to determine the need for débridement and skin grafting
	Surgical intervention may be needed.	
	Systemic toxicity manifested by:	
	Fever, chills	
	Nausea and vomiting	
	Malaise, joint pain	
	Petechiae	
	Hemolytic reactions, renal failure, and death may occur.	

Continued

Interventions for Common Environmental Emergencies—cont'd

	Clinical Manifestations	Collaborative Management

Black widow spider	Little to severe pain
	Tiny papule or small red punctuate mark
	Systemic signs and symptoms
	Severe abdominal pain
	Muscle rigidity/spasm
	Hypertension
	Nausea and vomiting
	Facial edema
	Ptosis
	Diaphoresis
	Weakness
	Increased salivation
	Priapism
	Respiratory difficulty
	Increased respiratory secretions
	Fasciculations
	Paresthesias
		Home care
		Apply ice pack.
		Hospital care
		ABCs of airway, breathing, and circulation
		Pain medication
		Muscle relaxants
		Calcium gluconate may be used for muscle spasms, rigidity, and pain.
		Institute Seizure Precautions.
		Medications include:
		  Tetanus prophylaxis
		  Antihypertensive agents
		Monitor for pulmonary edema and shock.
		Hospital admission is recommended for pregnant women and patients with hypertension.

Tarantula	Pain at bite site Swelling Redness Numbness Lymphangitis	Supportive management Analgesics Elevate and immobilize an extremity if affected.
Scorpions	Pain and inflammation Mild systemic symptoms	Analgesics, supportive management Basic wound care

Bark scorpion	Severe pain	Vital signs
	Systemic manifestations	Continuous cardiac monitoring
	Respiratory failure	Monitor for respiratory failure.
	Pancreatitis	IV fluids
	Musculoskeletal dysfunction	Analgesics
	Cranial nerve dysfunction	Tetanus prophylaxis
		Atropine is used if hypersalivation occurs.
		Antivenom if ordered
LIGHTNING INJURIES	**Cardiovascular**	ABCs of airway, breathing, and circulation
	Asystole or ventricular fibrillation	Follow advanced life support guidelines.
	Mottled skin	Cardiac monitoring
	Absent peripheral pulses	Immobilize for spinal cord injury.
	Respiratory	Vital signs
	Arrest, hypoxia	Burn care if needed
	Central nervous system	Laboratory studies such as creatinine kinase
	Temporary paralysis lasting from	Tetanus prophylaxis if needed
	minutes to hours	Monitor for rhabdomyolysis and kidney failure.
	Loss of consciousness	
	Amnesia	
	Confusion, disorientation	
	Photophobia	
	Seizures	
	Hemorrhage	
	Cerebellar dysfunction	
	Spinal cord injury	
	Integumentary	
	Burns (superficial to full thickness)	

Continued

Interventions for Common Environmental Emergencies—cont'd

	Clinical Manifestations	Collaborative Management
ALTITUDE–RELATED ILLNESSES		
High altitude is an elevation above 5000 feet.		

Acute mountain sickness (AMS)	Throbbing headache
	Anorexia
	Nausea and vomiting
	Irritability, apathy
	Variable vital signs
	Dyspnea on exertion, at rest
		Rest and allow time to acclimate to altitude.
		Remove to lower altitude.
		Administer oxygen if available.
		Medications
		  Acetazolamide (Diamox) to prevent and treat AMS
		  Dexamethasone (Decadron) may be given while patient moves to lower altitude.

High altitude cerebral edema (HACE)	Unable to perform activities of daily living
	Extreme apathy
	Confusion, lack of judgment
	Cranial nerve dysfunction
	Seizures
	Stupor, coma, death
		Rapid descent to lower altitude
		Supplemental oxygen
		Keep patient warm.
		Medications, if available, during descent
		  Dexamethasone
		  Loop diuretics
		Hospital care required
		ABCs of airway, breathing, and circulation
		Symptom management

High altitude pulmonary edema (HAPE)	Poor exercise tolerance Dyspnea on exertion Dry cough Cyanosis of nails and lips Tachycardia, tachypnea Rales, pink frothy sputum	As above

CHEMICAL AND BIOLOGICAL AGENTS OF TERRORISM

The Centers for Disease Control and Prevention list the following indications of intentional release of a biological agent:

1. An unusual clustering of illness (e.g., persons who attended the same public event or gathering) or patients presenting with clinical signs and symptoms that suggest an infectious disease outbreak

2. An unusual age distribution for common diseases (e.g., increase in what appears to be a chickenpox-like illness among adult patients but that may be smallpox)

3. A large number of cases of acute flaccid paralysis with prominent bulbar palsies, suggesting a release of botulinum toxin

Information for this Appendix is taken from the Centers for Disease Control and Prevention website (*www.bt.cdc.gov*).

Chemical and Biological Agents of Terrorism

Agent	Clinical Manifestations	Mode of Transmission	Collaborative Management
Anthrax, cutaneous A bacterial infection caused by the gram-positive, rod-shaped organism, *Bacillus anthracis*, which lives as a spore in contaminated soil	Raised vesicle may itch and resemble an insect bite. Center of the vesicle becomes hemorrhagic and sinks inward. An area of necrosis and ulceration begins; the tissue around the wound swells and becomes edematous. It is distinguished from insect bites or other skin lesions in that it is painless and that eschar forms regardless of treatment.	Incubation period of 3-5 days after exposure Direct contact	Treatment includes Ciprofloxacin (Cipro) or doxycycline (Doryx, Vibramycin). Vaccine is not available to the general public.

Anthrax, inhalation	Prodromal stage (early) Fever Fatigue Mild chest pain Dry cough No manifestations of upper respiratory infection of rhinitis, headache, watery eyes, or sore throat Fulminant stage (late) Sudden onset of breathlessness, progressing to severe respiratory distress Diaphoresis Stridor on inhalation and exhalation Hypoxia High fever Mediastinitis and pleural effusion Hypotension Septic shock, meningitis	Incubation period of 1 day to 6 weeks Spread through direct contact Not spread by person-to-person contact	Combination therapy with ciprofloxacin, doxycycline, and amoxicillin These drugs are used individually in oral form for prophylaxis when people have been exposed to inhalation anthrax. Death within 24-36 hours after the onset of breathlessness, even if antibiotic is started at this stage

Continued

Chemical and Biological Agents of Terrorism—cont'd

Agent	Clinical Manifestations	Mode of Transmission	Collaborative Management
Botulism A muscle-paralyzing disease caused by a toxin made by the bacterium *Clostridium botulinum*	Foodborne botulism Abdominal cramps Nausea, vomiting, diarrhea Drooping eyelids Blurred or double vision Dysphagia Dry mouth Slurred speech Descending muscle weakness Inhalation botulism includes all of the above except the GI symptoms plus: Dyspnea Decreasing respirations that may lead to apnea and respiratory arrest	Incubation period is 12-72 hours. Airborne or foodborne illness	Antitoxin Intravenous fluids

Continued

Smallpox An acute, contagious, and sometimes fatal disease caused by the variola virus	Initial symptoms Fever (usually high), malaise, vomiting Head and body aches Small, red spots on the tongue and in the mouth Rash that starts on the face and legs, hands, and feet After 3 days, rash becomes raised bumps, which fill with a thick, opaque fluid and often have a depression in the center that looks like a bellybutton (a major distinguishing characteristic of smallpox). Bumps become pustules. Pustules begin to form a crust and then scab. By the end of the second week after the rash appears, most of the sores have scabbed over.	Incubation period of 7-17 days Prolonged face-to-face contact with someone who has smallpox (usually someone who already has a smallpox rash) Direct contact with infected bodily fluids or an object such as bedding or clothing that has a virus on it Exposure to an aerosol release of smallpox Infected person is contagious to others until all of the scabs have fallen off.	No proven treatment Intravenous fluids Medication to control fever or pain and antibiotics for any secondary bacterial infections that may occur Smallpox vaccination is not available to the general public.
Plague Disease caused by *Yersinia pestis* (*Y. pestis*), a bacterium found in rodents and their fleas	Fever, weakness Rapidly developing pneumonia Dyspnea chest pain Cough, bloody or watery sputum Nausea, vomiting, and abdominal pain May lead to respiratory failure, shock, and rapid death	Incubation period of 2-4 days Respiratory droplets Intentional aerosol release	Tetracycline (e.g., doxycycline) and/or Fluoroquinolone (e.g., ciprofloxacin). Possibly streptomycin or gentamicin

Chemical and Biological Agents of Terrorism—cont'd

Agent	Clinical Manifestations	Mode of Transmission	Collaborative Management
Tularemia Inhalational *Francisella tularensis*	Resembles the flu Fever, fatigue Swollen glands Sore throat Pneumonia	Incubation period of 3-7 days	
Hemorrhagic fever Caused by Ebola, Marburg, Lassa, and Crimean-Congo hemorrhagic fever viruses and resulting in multisystem organ failure syndrome	Specific signs and symptoms vary by the type of viral hemorrhagic fever (VHF). Marked fever, fatigue Dizziness Muscle aches Loss of strength Bleeding under the skin, in internal organs, or from body orifices such as the mouth, eyes, and ears Signs of shock Nervous system malfunction, coma, delirium, and seizures Renal failure	Carried by rodents, mosquitoes, and tics Incubation period of 5-10 days May spread from one person to another after an initial person has become infected Secondary transmission of the virus can occur directly through close contact with infected people or their body fluids. It can also occur indirectly through contact with objects contaminated with infected body fluids.	Supportive therapy; no other treatment or established cure for VHFs Ribavirin, an antiviral drug, has been effective in treating some individuals with Lassa fever. Treatment with convalescent-phase plasma has been used with success in some patients with Argentine hemorrhagic fever.

Ricin			
A toxic protein made from castor beans. The poison can be extracted from the beans, purified, and treated to form a powder that can be inhaled.	**Inhalation:** Respiratory distress (difficulty breathing), tightness in the chest Fever, cough, nausea Heavy sweating Pulmonary edema Hypotension and respiratory failure, leading to death **Ingestion:** Vomiting and diarrhea that may be bloody and result in severe dehydration Hypotension Hallucinations Seizures Blood in the urine **Skin and eye exposure:** Redness and pain of the skin and the eyes	Symptoms within 8 hours of inhalation	No antidote exists Supportive care Death may take place within 36-72 hours of exposure, depending on the route of exposure and the dose received. If death has not occurred in 3-5 days, the victim usually recovers.

Continued

Chemical and Biological Agents of Terrorism—cont'd

Agent	Clinical Manifestations	Mode of Transmission	Collaborative Management
Sarin (GB) and soman (GD) Both are human-made chemical warfare agents classified as nerve agents, which can evaporate into a vapor (gas) and spread into the environment.	Runny nose Watery eyes Small, pinpoint pupils Eye pain Blurred vision Drooling and excessive sweating Cough Chest tightness Rapid breathing Diarrhea Increased urination Confusion Drowsiness Weakness Headache Nausea, vomiting, abdominal pain Slow or fast heart rate Low or high blood pressure Loss of consciousness Convulsions Paralysis Respiratory failure possibly leading to death	Incubation is a few minutes to several hours. Clothing can give off vapors for up to 30 minutes after exposure. The patient can be exposed through skin or eye contact; breathing air that contains the agents; touching or drinking contaminated water, eating contaminated food, or touching contaminated clothes	Full protective gear for emergency responders and emergency department personnel Remove patient's clothing. Rapidly wash the patient's entire body with soap and water. Give antidote, as ordered. Provide airway, breathing, and circulatory support. Supportive care based on patient's signs and symptoms

Continued

Tabun
The manmade chemical warfare agent is classified as a nerve agent.

Same as sarin and soman

Tabun is an immediate but short-lived threat and does not last a long time in the environment.
Tabun is more volatile than VX, and it remains on exposed surfaces for a shorter period than VX.
Tabun is less volatile than sarin, and it remains on exposed surfaces for a longer period than sarin.

Chemical and Biological Agents of Terrorism—cont'd

Agent	Clinical Manifestations	Mode of Transmission	Collaborative Management
VX The human-made chemical warfare agent is classified as a nerve agent. It is the most potent of all nerve agents and affects breathing function.	Same as sarin and soman	Symptoms appear within a few seconds after exposure to the vapor form of VX and within a few minutes to up to 18 hours after exposure to the liquid form. Under average weather conditions, VX can last for days on objects that it has come in contact with. Under very cold conditions, VX can last for months. It evaporates slowly and can be a long-term threat as well as a short-term threat. Surfaces contaminated with VX should be considered a long-term hazard.	Recovery from VX exposure is possible with treatment, but the antidotes available must be used quickly to be effective.

DISCHARGE PLANNING

- Discharge planning begins on admission.
- Information to ask the patient to assist with discharge planning:
  1. Where do you live?
  2. How will you get home?
  3. Can you describe your home?
  4. How many stairs must you climb to get into your house?
  5. Is your bedroom, bathroom, and kitchen on the same floor, or will you need to use steps?
  6. Do you live alone, or does someone live with you?
     a. Who lives with you?
     b. Will the person be able to help you after your discharge?
     c. Is there a neighbor or church member who can help you after you are discharged?
     d. Is anyone available to help you with grocery shopping or driving to doctors' appointments?
- Collaborate with social worker, case manager, or discharge planner to identify the patient's needs related to care after hospitalization, including meal preparation, dressing changes, activities of daily living, and personal hygiene.
- If equipment or supplies are needed for use at home, make sure they are ordered and delivered before the patient is discharged.
- Ensure that the patient and family know how to use the specific type of supplies and equipment that are to be used at home.
- Refer to social services, rehabilitation (physical, occupational, or speech therapy), and community and health care agencies, as appropriate.
- The patient may need referrals for or help with planning housing, finances, insurance, legal services, funeral arrangements, and spiritual counseling.
- Support the patient and family as they make discharge arrangements.
- Provide patient and family education:
  1. Provide information about the disease process, how to recognize complications (if appropriate), and how to manage the disease at home.

2. Teach the patient about drugs:
    a. Name of drugs
    b. Purpose
    c. Dosage
    d. Side effects
    e. Interactions, if any, with foods or other drugs
    f. Importance of taking drugs as prescribed
- Teach the patient and family members how to perform any dressing changes, suctioning, tube feeding, or other special care that may be required at home.
- Signs and symptoms should be reported to the health care provider. Focus on information that must be reported immediately.
- Collaborate with the registered dietitian to provide dietary information.
- Stress the importance of follow-up care with the health care provider.

ELECTROCARDIOGRAPHIC COMPLEXES, SEGMENTS, AND INTERVALS

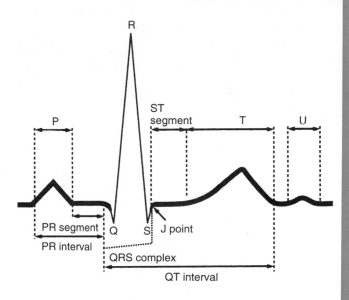

The electrocardiogram (ECG) is the graphic record of electrical activity of the heart. The spread of electrical current in the heart is detected by surface electrodes, and the amplified electrical signals are recorded on calibrated paper.

The first step in reading an electrocardiogram is to analyze the rhythm. Determine whether the rhythm is regular or irregular, then calculate the heart rate by counting the number of PP or RR intervals that occur in 6 seconds, and multiply that number by 10. A normal rate is 60-100 beats per minute (bpm).

The second step is to systematically examine the waveforms, intervals, and segments:

P wave represents atrial depolarization.

PR segment represents the time required for the impulse to travel through the atrioventricular (AV) node (where it is delayed) and through the bundle of His, bundle branches, and Purkinje fiber network, just before ventricular depolarization.

PR interval represents the time required for atrial depolarization and impulse travel through the conduction system and Purkinje fiber network, inclusive of the P wave and PR segment. It is measured from the beginning of the P wave to the end of the PR segment, and a normal time is 0.12 to 0.2 second.

QRS complex represents depolarization of both ventricles and is measured from the point at which the complex first leaves the baseline to the end of the last appearing wave (from the end of the PR interval to the J point). This is normally 0.04 to 0.1 second. A widened QRS complex indicates a delay in the conduction time in the ventricles and is typically the result of myocardial ischemia, injury, or infarct; it may also result from ventricular hypertrophy or electrolytes imbalances.

J point represents the junction where the QRS complex ends and the ST segment begin.

ST segment represents early ventricular repolarization. It is measured from the J point to the beginning of the T wave.

T wave represents ventricular repolarization.

U wave represents late ventricular repolarization. It is not normally seen in all leads.

QT interval represents the total time required for ventricular depolarization and repolarization. It is measured from the beginning of the QRS complex to the end of the T wave. It varies with age, gender, and heart rate. It must be corrected to a heart rate of 60 after measurement (QTc). The upper limit of normal QTc is less than 0.43 second in men and less than 0.45 second in women with a normal rate of 60-100 bpm.

The third and final step is to interpret the recoding.

NORMAL SINUS RHYTHM

In the figure on p. 721, notice that the atrial and ventricular rhythms are essentially regular (a slight variation in rhythm is normal). Both atrial and ventricular rates are 92 beats/min. One P wave occurs before each QRS complex, and all P waves are of a consistent morphology (shape). The PR interval measures 0.14 second and is constant; the QRS complex measures 0.08 second and is constant. The T waves vary in amplitude because of respirations; they are flat with inspiration and positive with expiration.

Shortest R-R interval (0.72 s)

Longest R-R interval (1.0 s)

Sinus Arrhythmia ■ All P waves have the same morphology, indicating that they are from the sinus node. The rhythm is slightly irregular, indicating a normal respiratory variation. The shortest RR interval (0.72 second) varies about 20% (or less than 0.14 second) from the longest RR interval (1 second). The actual variation is 0.12 second; actual variation is 0.12 second.

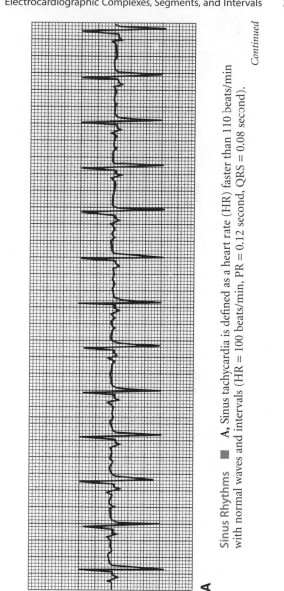

Sinus Rhythms ■ *A,* Sinus tachycardia is defined as a heart rate (HR) faster than 110 beats/min with normal waves and intervals (HR = 100 beats/min, PR = 0.12 second, QRS = 0.08 second).

Continued

B

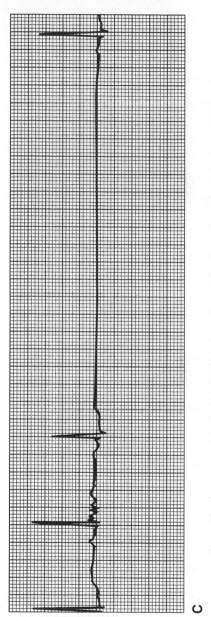

Sinus Rhythms—cont'd   ■ **B,** Sinus bradycardia is defined as a heart rate less than 60/min with all other waves and segments within normal values (HR = 35 beats/min, PR = 0.16 second, QRS = 0.10 second). **C,** Sinus pause (underlying HR = 60 beats/min, PR = 0.20 second, QRS 5 0.08 second, with just under a 5-second pause).

C

A

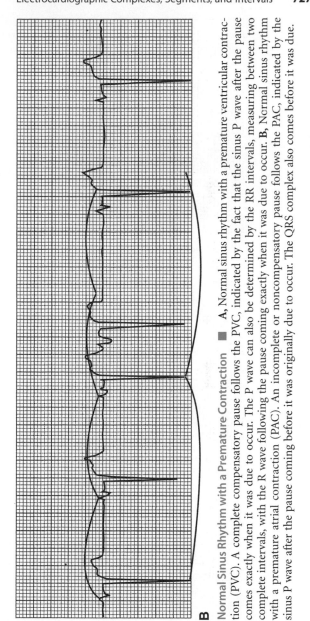

B

Normal Sinus Rhythm with a Premature Contraction ■ **A,** Normal sinus rhythm with a premature ventricular contraction (PVC). A complete compensatory pause follows the PVC, indicated by the fact that the sinus P wave after the pause comes exactly when it was due to occur. The P wave can also be determined by the RR intervals, measuring between two complete intervals, with the R wave following the pause coming exactly when it was due to occur. **B,** Normal sinus rhythm with a premature atrial contraction (PAC). An incomplete or noncompensatory pause follows the PAC, indicated by the sinus P wave after the pause coming before it was originally due to occur. The QRS complex also comes before it was due.

A

Atrial Dysrhythmias ■ **A**, Normal sinus rhythm with an 11-beat run of paroxysmal atrial tachycardia (PAT) with 1:1 conduction. **B**, In patients with atrial fibrillation (AF), multiple rapid impulses from many atrial foci depolarize the atria in a totally disorganized manner at a rate of 350 to 600 times per minute. The result is a chaotic rhythm with no clear P waves, no atrial contractions, loss of atrial kick, and an irregular ventricular response. Notice the wavy baseline with atrial electrical activity and irregular ventricular rhythm.

B

A

Continued

Ventricular Dysrhythmias ■ *A,* Normal sinus rhythm with unifocal premature ventricular complexes (PVCs). Notice the pair of PVCs. *B,* Normal sinus rhythm with a three-beat run of ventricular tachycardia (three consecutive PVCs) and another unifocal PVC.

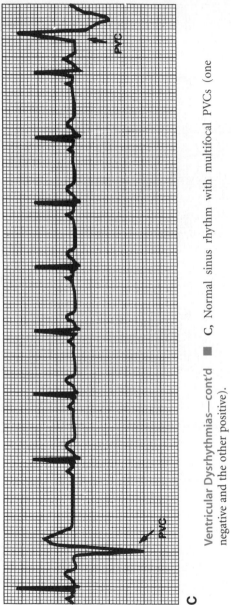

Ventricular Dysrhythmias—cont'd ■ C, Normal sinus rhythm with multifocal PVCs (one negative and the other positive).

Continued

Ventricular Dysrhythmias ■ **A,** Coarse ventricular fibrillation.

A

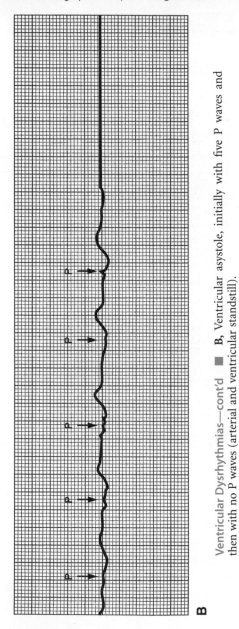

Ventricular Dysrhythmias—cont'd ■ **B,** Ventricular asystole, initially with five P waves and then with no P waves (arterial and ventricular standstill).

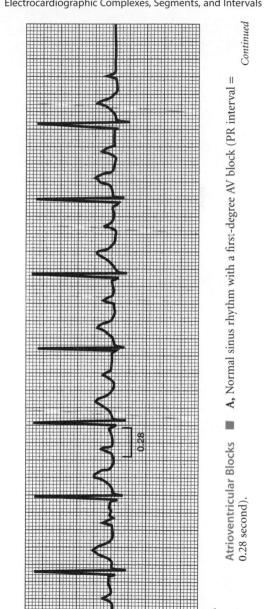

0.28

Atrioventricular Blocks ■ **A,** Normal sinus rhythm with a first-degree AV block (PR interval = 0.28 second). *Continued*

A

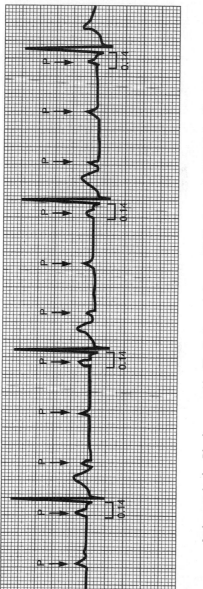

Atrioventricular Blocks—cont'd ■ **B,** Second-degree AV block type I (Wenckebach) with an irregular rhythm, grouped beating, and progressive prolongation of the PR interval until a P wave is completely blocked and not followed by a QRS complex. **C,** Second-degree AV block type II (Mobitz II) with 3:1 conduction and a constant PR interval.

C

A

Atrioventricular Blocks ■ **A,** Third-degree AV block (complete heart block) with regular atrial and ventricular rhythms. This dysrhythmia indicates no communication between the atria and ventricles at the AV node and is typically treated with a pacemaker. Note the inconsistent PR intervals (AV dissociation), and a junctional escape focus (normal QRS complexes) pacing the ventricles at a rate of 38/min. **B,** Third-degree AV block with regular atrial and ventricular rhythms, inconsistent PR intervals (AV dissociation), and ventricular escape focus pacing the ventricles at a rate of 35/min, with wide QRS complexes.

Continued

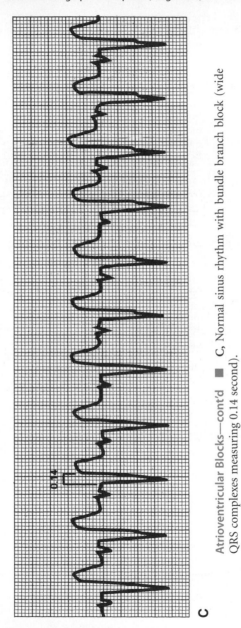

Atrioventricular Blocks—cont'd ■ C, Normal sinus rhythm with bundle branch block (wide QRS complexes measuring 0.14 second).

THE PATIENT REQUIRING INTUBATION AND VENTILATION

OVERVIEW

- Mechanical ventilation is usually a temporary life-support technique, although it may be lifelong for those with severe, restrictive lung disease and those with chronic, progressive neuromuscular diseases that reduce effective ventilation.
- It is most often used for patients with hypoxemia and progressive alveolar hypoventilation with respiratory acidosis.
- Mechanical ventilation requires intubation to establish an artificial airway.
- The purposes of intubation are to maintain a patent airway, provide a means to remove secretions, and provide ventilation and oxygen.
- The most common type of airway for a short-term basis is the endotracheal (ET) tube.

PATIENT-CENTERED COLLABORATIVE CARE

- Endotracheal intubation
  1. Most often, the long polyvinyl chloride ET tube is passed through the mouth into the trachea, usually by an anesthesiologist, nurse anesthetist, or pulmonologist. The nasal route is reserved for facial or oral traumas and surgeries and when oral intubation is not possible.
  2. When properly positioned, the tip of the ET tube rests about 2 cm above the carina.
  3. The main parts of the ET are:
     a. The shaft, with a radiopaque line running its length
     b. The cuff at the distal end, which is inflated after placement to create a seal between the trachea and the cuff
     c. The pilot balloon, which is a one-way valve, allows air to be inserted into the cuff, and prevents air from escaping
     d. The adaptor, which connects the ET tube to ventilator tubing or to other types of oxygen delivery systems
  4. Prepare for emergency intubation by:
     a. Summoning intubation personnel in the facility to the bedside in an emergency situation
     b. Explaining the procedure to the patient as clearly as possible

    c. Ensuring that the code ("crash") cart, airway equipment box, and suction equipment (often already on the code cart) are at the bedside

    d. Maintaining a patent airway through positioning and inserting an oral or nasopharyngeal airway until the patient is intubated

    e. During the intubation, continuously monitoring for changes in vital signs, signs of hypoxia or hypoxemia, dysrhythmias, and aspiration

    f. Ensuring that each intubation attempt lasts no longer than 30 seconds, preferably less than 15 seconds and after 30 seconds, providing oxygen by means of a mask and manual resuscitation bag to prevent hypoxia and cardiac arrest

    g. Suctioning, as necessary

    h. Verifying tube placement by assessing for:
       (1) End-tidal carbon dioxide levels
       (2) Bilateral breath sounds
       (3) Symmetrical chest movement
       (4) Air emerging from the ET tube

    i. Stabilizing ET tube at the mouth or nose and marking the tube where it touches the lip, incisor tooth or naris

    j. Inserting an oral airway to keep the patient from biting the ET tube

5. Providing nursing care, including:

    a. Regularly assessing tube placement, minimal cuff leak, breath sounds, and chest wall movement

    b. Preventing pulling or tugging on the tube by the patient to prevent dislodgment or "slipping" of the tube
       (1) Ensuring proper positioning
       (2) Ensuring adequate sedation
       (3) Providing constant supervision, often with the help of family members
       (4) Applying soft wrist restraints as a last resort

    c. Checking the pilot balloon to ensure that the cuff is inflated

    d. Assessing and changing the device or tape that secures the ET tube
       (1) If using adhesive tape, always taping the tube to the upper lip, never the lower
       (2) Inspecting the device or tape at least every shift for signs of loosening or skin irritation or breakdown
       (3) Checking anchoring each shift if swelling in the face and neck occurs or if there is an increase in fluid retention

(4) Applying skin protectants to the areas under the tape or device
(5) Keeping the ET tube from touching the corners of the mouth

- Mechanical ventilation
  1. The purposes of mechanical ventilation are to improve gas exchange and to decrease the work needed for an effective breathing pattern.
  2. Mechanical ventilation does not cure diseased lungs; it provides ventilation until the patient is able to resume the process of breathing.
  3. Positive-pressure ventilators generate pressure that pushes air into the lungs and expands the chest. There are four types:
     a. *Pressure-cycled ventilators* (bi-level positive airway pressure [BiPAP], positive end-expiratory pressure [PEEP]) push air into the lungs until a preset airway pressure is reached.
     b. *Time-cycled ventilators* push air into the lungs until a preset time has elapsed.
     c. *Volume-cycled ventilators* push air into the lungs until a preset volume is delivered.
     d. *Microprocessor ventilators* are computer-managed, positive-pressure ventilators that often have the components of volume-, time-, and pressure-cycled ventilators.
  4. Modes of ventilation are the way in which the patient receives breaths from the ventilator:
     a. *Assist-control ventilation* (ACV) in which the ventilator takes over the work of breathing for the patient. The tidal volume and ventilatory rate are preset to establish a minimal ventilatory pattern if the patient does not trigger spontaneous breaths.
     b. *Synchronized intermittent mandatory ventilation* (SIMV), in which the tidal volume and ventilatory rate are preset to establish a minimal ventilatory pattern when the patient does not trigger breaths, but it also allows spontaneous breathing at the patient's own rate and tidal volume between the ventilator breaths.
     c. *Bi-level positive airway pressure* (BiPAP) provides noninvasive pressure support ventilation by nasal mask or facemask.
     d. Additional, less commonly used modes include:
        (1) Pressure support
        (2) Continuous flow (flow-by)
        (3) Maximum mandatory ventilation (MMV)

(4) Inverse inspiration-expiration (I/E) ratio

(5) Permissive hypercarbia

(6) Airway pressure–release ventilation

(7) Proportional assist ventilation

(8) High-frequency ventilation

(9) High-frequency oscillation

5. Common ventilator controls and settings include:

   a. *Tidal volume* (V_T): The volume of air the patient receives with each breath ranges between 7 and 10 mL/kg of body weight. In the presence of acute lung injury (ALI) or acute respiratory distress syndrome (ARDS), a reduced tidal volume of 5 to 6 mL/kg is used to prevent additional lung injury.

   b. *Rate*: The number of ventilator breaths delivered per minute is usually between 10 and 14 breaths/min.

   c. *Fraction of inspired oxygen* (F_{IO_2}): The oxygen level delivered to the patient can range between 21% and 100% oxygen.

   d. *Peak airway (inspiratory) pressure* (PIP): This is the pressure needed by the ventilator to deliver a set tidal volume at a given lung compliance.

   e. *Continuous positive airway pressure* (CPAP): Positive airway pressure is applied throughout the entire respiratory cycle for spontaneously breathing patients. It keeps the alveoli open during inspiration and prevents alveolar collapse during expiration. Normal levels of CPAP are 5 to 15 cm H_2O.

   f. *Positive end-expiratory pressure* (PEEP): Positive pressure is exerted during the expiratory phase of ventilation to improve oxygenation by enhancing gas exchange and preventing atelectasis. The amount of PEEP is usually 5 to 15 cm H_2O.

   g. *Flow:* This rate is how fast each breath is delivered, and it is usually set at 40 L/min.

> ⚙ **Critical Rescue** ♦ If a patient is agitated or restless, has a widely fluctuating pressure reading on inspiration, or has other signs of air hunger, the flow may be set too low. Increasing the flow and investigating oxygenation status (SpO_2, PaO_2) should be tried before using chemical restraints.

6. Three nursing priorities in caring for the patient during mechanical ventilation are monitoring and evaluating patient responses, managing the ventilator system safely, and preventing complications.

7. Provide nursing care, including:
   a. Explaining all procedures and treatments, providing access to a call bell, and visiting the patient frequently
   b. Providing a letter board or pencil and paper for communication
   c. Assessing the patient's respiratory status at least every 4 hours and then as needed
      (1) Taking vital signs at least every 4 hours
      (2) Observing the patient's color (especially lips and nail beds)
      (3) Observing the patient's chest for bilateral expansion
      (4) Assessing the placement of the nasotracheal or endotracheal tube
      (5) Measuring oxygen saturation
      (6) Evaluating arterial blood gases (ABGs), as indicated
      (7) Maintaining head of the bed higher than 30 degrees to prevent microaspiration and ventilator-associated pneumonia
      (8) Noting the peak and plateau inspiratory pressures from the ventilator, because increasing pressure may indicate a need for suctioning or worsening lung disease
   d. Documenting pertinent observations in the patient's medical record (chart)
   e. Checking at least every 4-8 hours to be sure the ventilator settings are set as prescribed
   f. Checking to be sure alarms are set (especially low-pressure and low-exhaled volume)

> **Critical Rescue** ♦ Alarm systems must be activated and functional at all times. If the cause of the alarm cannot be determined, ventilate the patient manually with a resuscitation bag until the problem is corrected by another health care professional.

   g. If the patient is on PEEP, observing the peak airway pressure dial to determine the proper level of PEEP
   h. Observing the exhaled volume digital display to be sure the patient is receiving the prescribed tidal volume
   i. Emptying ventilator tubing when moisture collects

> **Clinical Landmine** ♦ Never empty fluid in the tubing back into the cascade.

   j. Ensuring humidity by keeping delivered air temperature maintained at body temperature

k. Ensuring the tracheostomy cuff (or endotracheal cuff) is adequately inflated to provide adequate tidal volume

l. Auscultating the lungs for crackles, wheezes, equal breath sounds, and decreased or absent breath sounds

m. Observing the patient's need for tracheal, oral, or nasal suctioning every 2 hours

n. Performing suctioning, as needed

o. Inspecting the patient's mouth around the endotracheal tube for pressure ulcers

p. Performing mouth care every 2 hours and brushing teeth every 8 hours

q. Changing the tracheostomy or endotracheal tube tape or holding device, as needed
   (1) Carefully move the oral endotracheal tube to the opposite side of the mouth once daily to prevent ulcers.
   (2) Provide tracheostomy care every 8 hours.

r. Assessing patients for GI distress (diarrhea, constipation, tarry stools)

s. Maintaining accurate intake and output records to monitor fluid balance

t. Turning the patient at least every 2 hours to promote lung expansion. Consider continuous lateral rotation therapy if the patient is comatose or at high risk for or experiences ALI or ARDS.

u. Scheduling treatments and nursing care at intervals for rest

v. Monitoring for the effectiveness of mechanical ventilation in terms the patient's physiologic and psychological status

w. Monitoring for adverse effects of mechanical ventilation: infection, barotrauma, and reduced cardiac output

x. Positioning the patient to facilitate ventilation-perfusion matching ("good lung down"), as appropriate

y. Administering prescribed muscle-paralyzing agents, sedatives, and narcotic analgesics

8. Preventing these complications (most are caused by the positive pressure from the ventilator)

   a. Cardiac problems include hypotension and fluid retention.
      (1) Teach the patient to avoid a Valsalva maneuver (bearing down while holding the breath).
      (2) Prevent constipation.
      (3) Monitor the patient's fluid intake and output, weight, hydration, and signs of hypovolemia.

b. Lung problems include barotrauma (damage to the lungs by positive pressure), volutrauma (damage to the lung by excess volume delivered to one lung over the other), and acid-base imbalance.

c. GI and nutritional problems result from the stress of mechanical ventilation.

   (1) Administer prescribed drug therapy (antacids, sucralfate [Carafate, Sulcrate ✤], histamine blockers such as ranitidine [Zantac], or proton-pump inhibitors such as esomeprazole [Nexium]).

   (2) Consult with a nutritionist to provide balanced nutrition through the diet, enteral feedings, or parenteral feedings.

   (3) Closely monitor potassium, calcium, magnesium, and phosphate levels, and replenish deficits as prescribed.

d. Monitor for infection, especially ventilator-associated pneumonia (VAP), and implement these practices for the *ventilator bundle*:

   (1) If possible, perform oral care with a disinfecting oral rinse *immediately before* the intubation.

   (2) Do not wear hand jewelry, especially rings, when providing care to ventilator patients.

   (3) Wash hands before and after contact with the patient.

   (4) Provide oral care every 2-4 hours with toothbrushing every 8 hours.

   (5) Remove subglottic secretions frequently (at least every 2 hours) or continuously (when the endotracheal tube has a separate lumen that opens directly above the tube cuff).

   (6) Keep the head of the bed elevated to at least 30 degrees unless another health problem is a contraindication for this position.

   (7) Verify that an initial x-ray has been obtained to confirm the placement of any nasogastric tube before instilling drugs, fluids, or feedings into the tube.

   (8) Work with the patient and health care team to assist in the weaning process as soon as possible.

e. Muscle deconditioning and weakness are caused by immobility.

   (1) Get the patient out of bed as soon as possible.

   (2) Ambulate the patient with assistance.

   (3) Encourage the patient to perform active ROM exercises.

9. Perform extubation (ET tube removal).
   a. Explain the procedure to the patient.
   b. Set up the prescribed oxygen delivery system.
   c. Have the equipment for emergency reintubation at the bedside.
   d. Hyperoxygenate the patient.
   e. Thoroughly suction the ET tube and the oral cavity.
   f. Rapidly deflate the cuff of the ET tube, and remove the tube at peak inspiration.
   g. Immediately instruct the patient to cough.
   h. Give oxygen by facemask or nasal cannula.
   i. Assess the patient's responses, ability to maintain adequate gas exchange, and the possible need for reintubation.

> 🔲 **Critical Rescue** ◆ Monitor the vital signs every 5 minutes at first, and assess the ventilatory pattern for manifestations of respiratory distress (dyspnea, coughing, and the inability to expectorate secretions). Notify the physician or Rapid Response Team at the onset of these problems.

> 🔲 **Critical Rescue** ◆ If stridor (high-pitched, crowing noise during inspiration) develops at any time, immediately call the Rapid Response Team.

THE PATIENT REQUIRING CHEST TUBES

OVERVIEW

- A chest tube is a drain placed in the pleural space to restore intrapleural pressure and allow re-expansion of the lung through the use of gravity and pressure.
- The drainage system consists of one or more chest tubes or drains, a collection container placed below the chest level, and a water seal to keep air from entering the chest.
- The tip of the tube used to drain air is placed near the front lung apex. The tube that drains liquid is placed on the side near the base of the lung. The sites are covered with airtight dressings.
- The chest tube is connected to about 6 feet of tubing that leads to a collection device placed several feet below the chest.
- Standard stationary chest tube drainage systems usually have three chambers connected to each other:
  1. Chamber 1 is the drainage collection container with the tube(s) from the patient is (are) connected to it, penetrating shallowly and never having the tip touch the fluid collection.
  2. Chamber 2 is the water seal that prevents air from entering the patient's pleural space. Air from the pleural space also enters chamber 1 but moves immediately to chamber 2 through the connecting tube. This tube must always be under the water level in chamber 2 to prevent air from returning to the patient. The tube acts as a one-way valve, allowing air to move into the water and preventing air in this chamber from re-entering the tube. As long as the tip of the tube from the first chamber is under water in the water seal chamber, air that has escaped from the patient's chest tube cannot re-enter the patient.
     a. Bubbling of the water here indicates air drainage from the patient and is usually seen when the patient exhales, coughs, or sneezes.
     b. When the air in the pleural space has been removed, bubbling stops. A blocked or kinked chest tube also can cause bubbling to stop.
     c. Excessive bubbling in this chamber may indicate an air leak.

3. Chamber 3 is the suction control of the system. The health care provider prescribes the amount of water to be placed and maintained in this chamber. While suction is applied, gentle bubbling is seen in this chamber. It has three connections:
   a. One from the second chamber
   b. A long open tube dipped into the water to serve as an air vent
   c. A short tube connecting to the suction unit

PATIENT-CENTERED COLLABORATIVE CARE

- Initial care includes:
  1. Checking hourly to ensure the sterility and patency of any chest drainage system
  2. Taping tubing junctions to prevent accidental disconnections
  3. Keeping an occlusive dressing at the chest tube insertion site
  4. Keeping sterile gauze at the bedside to cover the insertion site immediately if the chest tube becomes dislodged
  5. Keeping padded clamps at the bedside for use if the drainage system is interrupted
  6. Positioning the drainage tubing to prevent kinks and large loops of tubing, which can block drainage and prevent lung re-expansion
- Specific nursing care includes:
  1. Ensuring that the dressing on the chest around the tube is tight and intact
  2. Reinforcing or changing loose dressings according to agency policy and surgeon preference
  3. Assessing for difficulty breathing
  4. Assessing breathing effectiveness by pulse oximetry
  5. Listening to breath sounds in each lung
  6. Checking alignment of the trachea
  7. Checking the tube insertion site for condition of the skin and palpating the area for puffiness or crackling that may indicate subcutaneous emphysema
  8. Inspecting the site for signs of infection (redness, purulent drainage) or excessive bleeding
  9. Checking to see if the tube "eyelets" are visible
  10. Assessing for pain and its location and intensity, and administering prescribed drugs for pain as prescribed
  11. Assisting the patient to deep breathe, cough, perform maximal sustained inhalations, and use incentive spirometry

12. Repositioning the patient who reports a "burning" pain in the chest
- Manage the drainage system by:
  1. Not "stripping" the chest tube
  2. Keeping drainage system lower than the level of the patient's chest
  3. Keeping the chest tube as straight as possible, avoiding kinks and dependent loops
  4. Ensuring the chest tube is securely taped to the connector and that the connector is taped to the tubing going into the collection chamber
  5. Assessing bubbling in the water seal chamber, which should be gentle bubbling during the patient's exhalation, forceful cough, or position changes. If the system is "dry", then assess fluctuation of the sealed chamber.
  6. Assessing for normal "tidaling" (water in the long tube of the second chamber rises and falls 2 to 4 inches during inhalation and exhalation)
  7. Checking water level in the water seal chamber and keeping the level at that recommended by the manufacturer
  8. Checking the water level in the suction control chamber and keeping it at the level prescribed by the surgeon
  9. Clamping the chest tube only for brief periods to change the drainage system or when checking for air leaks
  10. Checking and documenting the amount, color, and characteristics of fluid in the collection chamber as often as needed according to the patient's condition and agency policy
  11. Emptying the collection chamber or changing the system before the drainage makes contact with the bottom of the tube
  12. Obtaining drainage samples (when indicated for culture and sensitivity) from the chest tube by cleansing using a 20-gauge (or smaller) needle and drawing it up into a syringe
  13. Immediately notifying the physician or Rapid Response Team about:
      a. Tracheal deviation
      b. Sudden onset or increased intensity of dyspnea
      c. Oxygen saturation less than 90%
      d. Drainage greater than 70 mL/hr
      e. Visible eyelets on the chest tube
      f. Chest tube falling out of the patient's chest (first, cover the area with dry, sterile gauze)

g. Chest tube disconnecting from the drainage system (first put end of tube in a container of sterile water, and keep below the level of the patient's chest)

h. Drainage in the tube stopping in the first 24 hours

HEALTH CARE ORGANIZATIONS AND RESOURCES

NURSING ORGANIZATIONS

Academy of Medical-Surgical Nurses
(866) 877-2676
www.medsurgnurse.org

American Academy of Ambulatory Care Nursing
(800) 262-6877
www.aaacn.org

American Academy of Nurse Practitioners
(512) 442-4262
www.aanp.org

American Association of Critical-Care Nurses
(800) 899-2226
www.aacn.org

American Association of Diabetes Educators
(800) 338-3633
www.aadenet.org

American Association of Legal Nurse Consultants
(877) 402-2562
www.aalnc.org

American Association of Managed Care Nurses, Inc.
(804) 747-9698
www.aamcn.org

American Association of Neuroscience Nurses
(888) 557-2266
www.aann.org

American Association of Nurse Anesthetists
(847) 692-7050
www.aana.com

The American Association of Nurse Attorneys
(877) 538-2262
www.taana.org

American Association of Occupational Health Nurses, Inc.
(770) 455-7757
www.aaohn.org

American Association of Spinal Cord Injury Nurses
(718) 803-3782
www.aascin.org

American College of Nurse-Midwives
(240) 485-1800
www.acnm.org, www.midwife.org

American College of Nurse Practitioners
(703) 740-2529
www.acnpweb.org

American Forensic Nurses
(760) 322-9925
www.amrn.com

American Holistic Nurses Association
(800) 278-2462
www.ahna.org

American Nephrology Nurses Association
(888) 600-2662
www.annanurse.org

American Nurses Association
(800) 274-4262
www.ana.org

American Radiological Nurses Association
(850) 474-7292
www.arna.net

American Society of Ophthalmic Registered Nurses
(415) 561-8513
http://webeye.ophth.uiowa.edu/asorn

American Society for Pain Management Nursing
(913) 895-4606
www.aspmn.org

American Society of PeriAnesthesia Nurses
(877) 737-9696
www.aspan.org

American Society of Plastic and Reconstructive Surgical Nurses
(856) 256-2340
http://asprsn.inurse.com

Association of Nurses in AIDS Care
(800) 260-6780
www.anacnet.org

Association of Occupational Health Professionals
(800) 362-4347
www.aohp.org

Association of Perioperative Registered Nurses (AORN)
(800) 755-2676
www.aorn.org

Association for Professionals in Infection Control and Epidemiology, Inc.
(202) 789-1890
www.apic.org

Association of Women's Health, Obstetric and Neonatal Nurses
(800) 673-8499
www.awhonn.org

Canadian Association of Critical Care Nurses
(866) 477-9077
www.caccn.ca

Case Management Society of America
(501) 225-2229
www.cmsa.org

Dermatology Nurses' Association
(800) 454-4362
www.dnanurse.org

Emergency Nurses Association
(800) 243-8362
www.ena.org

Home Healthcare Nurses Association
www.nahc.org

Hospice and Palliative Nurses Association
(412) 787-9301
www.hpna.org

Infusion Nurses Society
(781) 440-9408
www.ins1.org

International Society of Nurses in Genetics
(412) 344-1414
www.isong.org

International Transplant Nurses Society
(412) 343-4867
www.itns.org

National Association of Clinical Nurse Specialists
(717) 234-6799
www.nacns.org

National Association of Orthopaedic Nurses
(800) 289-6266
www.orthonurse.org

National Association of School Nurses
(240) 821-1130
www.nasn.org

National Black Nurses Association
(301) 589-3200
www.nbna.org

National Gerontological Nursing Association
(800) 723-0560
www.ngna.org

National League for Nursing
(800) 669-1656
www.nln.org

National Nursing Staff Development Organization
(800) 489-1995
www.nnsdo.org

National Student Nurses' Association
(718) 210-0705
www.nsna.org

Oncology Nursing Society
(412) 859-6100
www.ons.org

Sigma Theta Tau International
(888) 634-7575
www.nursingsociety.org

Society of Gastroenterology Nurses and Associates, Inc.
(800) 245-7462
www.sgna.org

Society of Otorhinolaryngology and Head-Neck Nurses, Inc.
(386) 428-1695
www.sohnnurse.com

Society of Urologic Nurses and Associates
(888) 827-7862
http://suna.inurse.com

Society for Vascular Nursing
(888) 536-4786
www.svnnet.org

Wound, Ostomy and Continence Nurses Society
(888) 224-9626
www.wocn.org

COMMUNITY ORGANIZATIONS AND OTHER RESOURCES

ALTERNATIVE AND COMPLEMENTARY THERAPIES

American Holistic Nurses' Association
(800) 278-2462
www.ahna.org

American Massage Therapy Association
(847) 864-0123
www.amtamassage.org

Healing Touch International, Inc.
(303) 989-7982
www.healingtouchinternational.org

HealthAtoZ
(609) 301-2169
www.healthatoz.com

Integrative Imagery Training for Health Care Professionals
(650) 570-6157
www.integrativeimagery.com

Whole Nurse
www.wholenurse.com

CANCER/DEATH AND DYING

American Brain Tumor Association
(847) 827-9910
www.abta.org

American Cancer Society
(404) 320-3333
www.cancer.org

Breast Cancer Helpline of Susan G. Komen for the Cure
(800) 462-9273
www.komen.org

Canadian Cancer Society, National Office
(416) 961-7223
www.cancer.ca

Cancer Information Services Hotline
(800) 4-CANCER
www.cancer.gov

Cancer411.org
(877) CANCR411
www.cancer411.org

CDC: Smoking and Tobacco Use
(800) 232-4636
www.cdc.gov/tobacco

Funeral Consumers Alliance
(800) 765-0107
www.funerals.org

Hospice Association of America
(202) 546-4759
www.nahc.org/HAA/

Leukemia & Lymphoma Society
(914) 949-5213
www.leukemia.org

National Cancer Institute
www.nci.nih.gov

National Hospice and Palliative Care Organization
(703) 837-1500
www.nhpco.org

National Ovarian Cancer Coalition
(469) 587-3826
www.ovarian.org

Partnership for Caring, National Office
(202) 296-8071
www.partnershipforcaring.org

QuitNet (smoking cessation)
(615) 665-1122
www.quitnet.com

Susan G. Komen Breast Cancer Foundation
(972) 855-1600
www.komen.org

Y-ME National Breast Cancer Organization
(312) 986-8338
www.y-me.org

CARDIOVASCULAR AND HEMATOLOGIC PROBLEMS

American Association of Blood Banks
(301) 907-6977
www.aabb.org

American Heart Association, National Center
(800) AHA-USA1
www.americanheart.org

American Heart Association—Take Wellness to Heart
(888) MY HEART
www.women.americanheart.org

Heart Information Network
www.heartinfo.org

Mended Hearts, Inc.
(214) 360-6149
www.mendedhearts.org

National Hemophilia Foundation
(212) 328-3700
www.hemophilia.org

Sickle Cell Disease Association of America, Inc.
(800) 421-8453
www.sicklecelldisease.org

DIABETES MELLITUS

American Diabetes Association
(800) 342-2383
www.diabetes.org

American Dietetic Association
(800) 877-1600
www.eatright.org

CDC: Diabetes
(800) 232-4636
www.cdc.gov/diabetes/

National Institute of Diabetes & Digestive & Kidney
Diseases (NIDDK)
(301) 496-3583
www.niddk.nih.gov

EYE AND EAR PROBLEMS

American Foundation for the Blind
(212) 502-7600
www.afb.org

American Speech-Language-Hearing Association
(800) 638-8255
www.asha.org

Deafness Research Foundation
(866) 454-3924
www.drf.org

The Ear Foundation
(800) 545-4327
www.earfoundation.org

Eye Bank Association of America
(202) 775-4999
www.restoresight.org

GASTROINTESTINAL PROBLEMS

American Anorexia Bulimia Association, Inc.
(212) 734-1114
www.aabainc.org

Crohn's and Colitis Foundation of America
(800) 932-2423
www.ccfa.org

IMMUNOLOGIC PROBLEMS/INFECTION CONTROL AND PREVENTION

American Academy of Allergy, Asthma & Immunology
(414) 272-6071
www.aaaai.org

Centers for Disease Control and Prevention (CDC)
(404) 498-1515
www.cdc.gov

HIV/AIDS Surveillance Report of the CDC
(404) 498-1515
www.cdc.gov/hiv/stats/hasrlink.htm

Immune Deficiency Foundation
(800) 296-4433
www.primaryimmune.org

National AIDS Treatment Advocacy Project
(212) 219-0106
www.natap.org

The Safer Sex Page
www.safersex.org

MUSCULOSKELETAL PROBLEMS

Arthritis Foundation
(404) 872-7100
www.arthritis.org

Back Pain Hotline: Texas Back Institute
(800) 247-2225
www.texasback.com

National Institute of Arthritis and Musculoskeletal and Skin Diseases
(877) 226-4267
www.niams.nih.gov

Osteoporosis and Related Bone Diseases—National Resource Center
(800) 624-BONE
www.osteo.org

Spondylitis Association of America
(800) 777-8189
www.spondylitis.org

NEUROLOGIC PROBLEMS AND REHABILITATION

The ALS Association
(818) 880-9007
www.alsa.org

Christopher Reeve Paralysis Foundation
(800) 225-0292
www.christopherreeve.org

The Epilepsy Foundation
(800) 332-1000
www.efa.org

Epilepsy Ontario
(416) 229-2291
www.epilepsyontario.org

Huntington's Disease Society of America
(212) 242-1968
www.hdsa.org

Michael J. Fox Foundation for Parkinson's Research
(800) 708-7644
www.michaeljfox.org

National Headache Foundation
(888) 643-5552
www.headaches.org

National Multiple Sclerosis Society
(212) 463-7787
www.nmss.org

National Parkinson's Foundation, Inc.
(800) 327-4545
www.parkinson.org

National Stroke Association
(800) 787-6537
www.stroke.org

Neurosciences on the Internet
www.neuroguide.com

Parkinson's Society of Canada
www.parkinson.ca

OLDER ADULTS/GERONTOLOGY

Alzheimer's Association
(312) 335-8700
www.alz.org

American Association of Retired Persons
(888) 687-2277
www.aarp.org

American Federation for Aging Research
(212) 703-9977
www.afar.org

National Institute on Aging
(301) 496-1752
www.nih.gov/nia/

REPRODUCTIVE HEALTH PROBLEMS

Bair PMS Home Page
www.bairpms.com

Center for Human Reproduction
(630) 916-8630 (Chicago), (212) 994-4400 (New York)
www.centerforhumanreprod.com

Endometriosis Association, International Headquarters
(414) 355-2200
www.endometriosisassn.org

Georgia Reproductive Specialists
www.ivf.com/endohtml.html

North American Menopause Society
(440) 442-7550
www.menopause.org

Planned Parenthood Federation of America, Inc.
(212) 541-7800
www.ppfa.org

Sexual Health InfoCenter
www.sexhealth.org

RESPIRATORY PROBLEMS

American Lung Association
(212) 315-8700
www.lungusa.org

Cystic Fibrosis Foundation
(800) 344-4823
www.cff.org

URINARY AND RENAL PROBLEMS

American Urogynecologic Society
(202) 367-1167
www.augs.org

National Association for Continence
(843) 377-0900
www.nafc.org

National Kidney Foundation
(800) 622-9010
www.kidney.org

The Simon Foundation for Continence
(800) 23-SIMON
www.simonfoundation.org

WOMEN'S HEALTH CONSIDERATIONS

Breast Cancer Helpline of Susan G. Komen for the Cure
(800) 462-9273
www.komen.org

Endometriosis Association
(414) 355-2200
www.endometriosisassn.org

Estronaut: A Forum for Women's Health
(312) 335-0095
www.womenshealth.org

Healthy Weight
www.healthyweight.com

National Ovarian Cancer Coalition, Inc.
(469) 587-3826
www.ovarian.org

Osteoporosis and Related Bone Diseases—National Resource Center
(800) 624-BONE
www.osteo.org

MISCELLANEOUS RESOURCES

Agency for Health Care Research and Quality (AHRQ)
(301) 427-1364
www.ahcpr.gov

American Academy of Dermatology
(847) 240-1280
www.aad.org

American Academy of Pain Management
(209) 533-9744
www.aapainmanage.org

American Council on Alcoholism
(800) 527-5344
www.aca-usa.org

American Hospital Association
(312) 422-3000
www.aha.org

American Red Cross National Headquarters
(703) 206-6000
www.redcross.org

American Thyroid Association, Inc.
(703) 998-8890
www.thyroid.org

Lupus Foundation of America, Inc.
(800) 558-0121
www.lupus.org

MedicAlert Foundation
(888) 633-4298
www.medicalert.org

Medicare
(800) 633-4227
www.medicare.gov

National Graves' Disease Foundation
(828) 877-5251
www.ngdf.org

National Institutes of Health (NIH)
(301) 496-4000
www.nih.gov

National Institute of Nursing Research (NINR)
(301) 496-0207
www.nih.gov/ninr

National Psoriasis Foundation
(800) 723-9166
www.psoriasis.org

Transplant Recipients International Organization (TRIO)
www.trioweb.org

United Network for Organ Sharing
(804) 782-4800
www.unos.org

US Department of Health and Human Services (DHHS)
(877) 696-6775
www.hhs.gov

U.S. Food and Drug Administration (FDA)
(888) 463-6332
www.fda.gov

COMMUNICATION QUICK REFERENCE FOR SPANISH-SPEAKING PATIENTS

The Body • El Cuerpo (ehl KOO-ehr-poh)

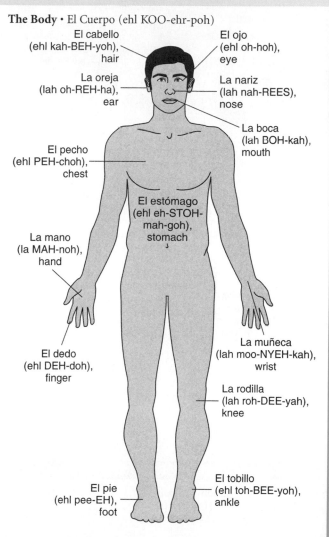

El cabello (ehl kah-BEH-yoh), hair

El ojo (ehl oh-hoh), eye

La oreja (lah oh-REH-ha), ear

La nariz (lah nah-REES), nose

La boca (lah BOH-kah), mouth

El pecho (ehl PEH-choh), chest

El estómago (ehl eh-STOH-mah-goh), stomach

La mano (la MAH-noh), hand

El dedo (ehl DEH-doh), finger

La muñeca (lah moo-NYEH-kah), wrist

La rodilla (lah roh-DEE-yah), knee

El pie (ehl pee-EH), foot

El tobillo (ehl toh-BEE-yoh), ankle

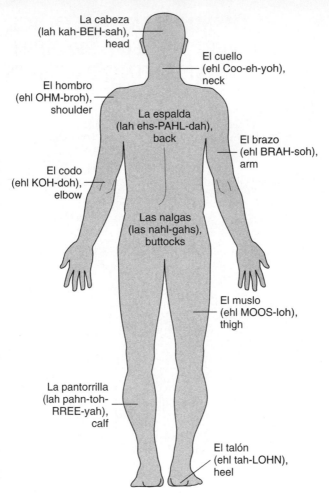

La cabeza
(lah kah-BEH-sah),
head

El cuello
(ehl Coo-eh-yoh),
neck

El hombro
(ehl OHM-broh),
shoulder

La espalda
(lah ehs-PAHL-dah),
back

El brazo
(ehl BRAH-soh),
arm

El codo
(ehl KOH-doh),
elbow

Las nalgas
(las nahl-gahs),
buttocks

El muslo
(ehl MOOS-loh),
thigh

La pantorrilla
(lah pahn-toh-
RREE-yah),
calf

El talón
(ehl tah-LOHN),
heel

COMMON TERMS FOR BODY PARTS

Move the, Mueva (mooh-EH-bah)
Touch the, Toque (TOH-keh)
Point to the, Señale (seh-NYAH-leh)

MORE PARTS OF THE BODY

Armpit, la axila (lah ahk-SEE-lah)
Breasts, los senos (lohs SEH-nohs)
Collarbone, la clavícula (lah klah-BEE-koo-lah)
Diaphragm, el diafragma (ehl dee-ah-FRAHG-mah)
Forearm, el antebrazo (ehl ahn-teh-BRAH-soh)
Groin, la ingle (lah EEN-gleh)
Hip, la cadera (lah kah-DEH-rah)
Kneecap, la rótula (lah ROH-too-lah)
Nail, la uña (lah OON-yah)
Pelvis, la pelvis (lah PEHL-bees)
Rectum, el recto (ehl REHK-toh)
Rib, la costilla (lah kohs-TEE-yah)
Spine, la espina dorsal (lah ehs-pee-NAH dohr-sahl)
Throat, la garganta (lah gahr-GAHN-tah)
Tongue, le lengua (lah LEHN-goo-ah)

ORGANS

Appendix, el apéndice (ehl ah-PEHN-dee-seh)
Bladder, la vejiga (lah beh-HEE-gah)
Brain, el cerebro (ehl seh-REH-broh)
Colon, el colon (ehl KOH-lohn)
Esophagus, el esófago (ehl eh-SOH-fah-goh)
Gallbladder, la vesícula biliar (lah beh-SEE-koo-lah bee-lee-AHR)
Genitals, los genitales (lohs heh-nee-TAH-lehs)
Heart, el corazón (ehl koh-rah-SOHN)
Kidney, el riñón (ehl ree-NYOHN)
Large intestine, el intestino grueso (ehl een-tehs-TEE-noh groo-EH-soh)
Liver, el hígado (ehl EE-gah-doh)
Lungs, los pulmones (lohs pool-MOH-nehs)
Pancreas, el páncreas (ehl PAHN-kreh-ahs)
Small intestine, el intestino delgado (ehl een-tehs-TEE-noh dehl-GAH-doh)
Spleen, el bazo (ehl BAH-soh)
Thyroid gland, la tiroides (lah tee-ROH-ee-dehs)
Tonsils, las amígdalas (lahs ah-MEEG-dah-lahs)
Uterus, el útero (ehl OO-teh-roh)

ESSENTIAL PHRASES

Good morning.	Buenos días.	Boo-eh-nohs dee-ahs.
Good afternoon.	Buenas tardes.	Boo-eh-nahs TAHR-dehs.
Good night.	Buenas noches.	Boo-eh-nahs NOH-chehs.
Hello.	Hola.	OH-lah.
How are you?	¿Cómo está?	¿Koh-moh ehs-TAH?
Good (fine).	Bien.	Bee-ehn.
Bad, Better, worse	Mal, Mejor, Peor	Mahl, Meh-HOHR, peh-ohr
The same	Igual	Ee-GOO-ahl
Do you speak English?	¿Habla Inglés?	¿Ah-blah een-glehs?
I don't understand.	No comprendo.	Noh kom-PREHN-doh.
Excuse me.	Discúlpeme.	Dees-KOOL-peh-meh.
Please speak slowly.	Por favor, hable más lento	Pohr fah-VOHR, AH-bleh MAHS LEHN-toh
Are you in pain?	¿Está adolorido(a)?	¿Ehs-TAH ah-doh-loh-REE-doh(dah)?
Yes, no	Sí, No	SEE, noh
Tell me where it hurts.	Digame donde le duele.	DEE-gah-meh DOHN-deh leh doo-eh-leh.
Here, there	Aquí, ahi	Ah-KEE, ah-EE

DESCRIPTION OF PAIN

Is your pain ... burning?	Tiene un dolor ... ¿que arde?	Tee-EH-neh oon doh-LOHR ... ¿keh ahr-deh?
... constant?	¿constante?	¿kohns-TAHN-teh?
... dull?	¿amortiguado?	¿ah-mohr-tee-goo-ah-doh?
... intermittent?	¿intermitente?	¿een-tehr-mee-TEHN-teh?
... mild?	¿moderado?	¿moh-deh-RAH-doh?
... severe?	¿muy fuerte?	¿MOO-ee Foo-ehr-teh?
... sharp?	¿agudo?	¿ah-GOO-doh?
... throbbing?	¿pulsante?	¿pool-SAHN-teh?
... worse?	¿peor?	¿peh-OHR?
Are you allergic to any medication?	¿Es usted alérgico(a) a algun medicamento?	¿Ehs oos-TEHD ah-LEHR-hee-koh(kah) ah ahl-GOON meh-dee-kah-mehn-toh?

I'm here to help you.	Estoy aquí para ayudarle.	Ehs-TOH-ee ah-KEE pah-rah ah-yoo-DAHR-leh.
Calm down.	Cálmese.	KAHL-meh-she.
Please.	Por favor.	Pohr fah-VOHR.
Thank you.	Gracias.	GRAH-see-ahs.
You're welcome.	De nada.	Deh NAH-dah
May I?	¿Puedo?	¿poo-eh-doh?
Who, what, when, where?	¿Quién, qué, cuándo, dónde?	¿Kee-ehn, keh, koo-AHN-doh, DOHN-deh?
Zero, one, two, three, four	Cero, uno, dos, tres, cuatro	SEH-roh, oo-noh, dohs, trehs, Koo-ah-troh
Five, six, seven, eight, nine, ten	Cinco, seis, siete, ocho, nueve, diez	SEEN-koh, seh-ees, See-eh-teh, OH-choh, Noo-eh-beh, dee-EHS

PRELIMINARY EXAMINATION

My name is _____, and I am your nurse.	Me llamo _____, y soy su enfermera(o).	Meh YAH-moh ___, ee Soh-ee soo ehn-fehr-MEH-rah(roh).
I'm going to … take your vital signs.	Le voy a … tomar los signos vitales.	Leh voh-ee ah … toh-MAHR lohs SEEG-nohs vee-TAH-lehs.
… weigh you.	pesar.	Leh voy ah … peh-sahr.
… take your blood pressure.	tomar la presión.	toh-MAHR lah preh-See-ohn.
Extend your arm and relax.	Extienda su brazo y descánselo.	Ehks-tee-ehn-dah soo BRAH-soh ee dehs-KAHN-seh-loh.
I'm going to take your … pulse	Le voy a tomar … el pulso	Leh voy ah toh-MAHR…ehl POOL-soh.
… temperature	su temperatura	soo tehm-peh-rah-TOO-rah
I'm going to count your respirations.	Voy a contar sus respiraciones.	Voy ah kohn-TAHR soos rehs-pee rah-See-oh-nehs.

OBTAINING A BLOOD SAMPLE

| I need to draw a blood sample. | Necesito tomar una muestra de la sangre. | Neh-seh-SEE-toh toh-MAHR oo-nah Moo-ehs-trah deh lah SAHN-greh. |
| Please give me your arm. | Por favor, déme el brazo. | Pohr fah-VOHR, DEH-meh ehl BRAH-soh. |

It may cause a little discomfort.	Le puede causar alguna molestia.	Leh Poo-eh-deh kah-oo-sahr ahl-GOO-nah moh-LEHS-tee-ah.
I am going to put a tourniquet around your arm.	Le voy a poner una liga alrededor del brazo.	Leh voh-ee ah poh-NEHR OO-nah LEE-gah ahl-reh-deh-dohr dehl BRAH-soh.
I am going to draw blood from this vein.	Voy a sacar la sangre de esta vena.	Voy ah sah KAHR lah SAHN-greh deh EHS-tah VEH-nah.

OBTAINING BLOOD FROM A FINGER STICK

| I need to take a few drops of blood from your finger. | Necesito sacar unas gotas de sangre de uno de sus dedos. | Neh-seh-SEE-toh sah-KAHR oo-nahs goh-tahs deh sahn-greh deh oo-noh dehsoos DEH-dohs. |

OBTAINING A URINE SAMPLE

We also need a urine sample.	También necesitamos una muestra de la orina.	Tahm-Bee-ehn neh-seh-see-TAH-mohs oo-nah Moo-ehs-trah deh lah oh-REE-nah.
It has to be from the middle of the stream.	Tiene que ser de la mitad del chorro.	Tee-eh-neh keh sehr deh lah mee-TAHD dehl CHOH-rroh.
Put the urine in this cup.	Ponga la orina en esta tasa.	POHN-gah lah oh-REE-nah ehn EHS-tah tah-sah.

OBTAINING A STOOL SPECIMEN

| I need a sample of your stool. | Necesito una muestra de su excremento. | Neh-seh-SEE-tohOO-nah Moo-ehs-trah deh soo ehx-kreh-MEHN-toh. |
| Please put a small amount in this cup. | Por favor ponga un poco en esta tasa. | Pohr fah-VOHR POHN-gah oon POH-koh ehn EHS-tah tah-sah. |

OBTAINING A SPUTUM SPECIMEN

| I need a sample of your sputum. | Necesito una muestra de su esputo. | Neh-seh-SEE-toh OO-nah Moo-ehs-trah deh soo ehs-POO-toh. |

Please spit in this cup.	Por favor, escupa en esta tasa.	Pohr fah-VOHR, ehs-KOO-pah ehn EHS-tah tah-sah.
ORDERS		
You need … a bandage.	Necesita … un vendaje.	Neh-seh-see-TAH … oon behn-DAH-heh.
… blood transfusion.	transfusión de sangre.	oo-nah trahns-foo-see-ohn deh SAHN-greh.
… a cast.	un molde de yeso.	oon mohl-deh deh yeh-soh.
… gauze.	la gasa.	lah GAH-sah.
… intensive care.	cuidado intensivo.	koo-ee-dah-doh een-tehn-SEE-boh.
… intravenous fluids.	líquidos intravenosos.	LEE-kee-dohs een-trah-beh-noh-sohs.
… an operation.	una operación	oo-nah oh-peh-rah-see-OHN.
… physical therapy.	terapia física	teh-RAH-pee-ah FEE-see-kah.
… a shot.	una inyección	Oo-nah een-yehk-see-OHN.
… x-rays.	rayos equis.	RAH-yohs EH-kees.
We're going to … change the bandage.	Vamos a … cambiarle el vendaje.	VAH-mohs ah … kahm-bee-AHR leh ehl behn-DAH-heh.
… give you a bath.	darle un baño.	DAHR-leh oon BAH-nyoh.
… take out the IV.	sacarle el tubo intravenoso.	sah-KAHR-leh ehl TOO-boh een-trah-beh-NOH-soh.
DESCRIPTION OF TUBES		
The tube in your … arm is for IV fluids.	El tubo en su … brazo es para líquidos intravenosos.	Ehl TOO-boh ehn soo … BRAH-soh ehs PAH-rah LEE-kee-dohs een-trah-beh-NOH-sohs.
… bladder is for urinating.	vejiga es para orinar.	beh-HEE-gah ehs PAH-rah oh-ree-NAHR.
… stomach is for the food.	estómago es para los alimentos.	ehs-TOH-mah-goh ehs PAH-rah lohs ah-lee-mehn-tohs.
… throat is for breathing.	garganta es para respirar.	gahr-GAHN-tah ehs PAH-rah rehs-pee-RAHR.

Trauma *(Continued)*
  head, 637–644
    ARDS from, 95–96
    respiratory acidosis from, 93
    seizure disorders and, 590
  kidney, 646–647
  laryngeal, 648–649
  penetrating
    to abdomen, 635
    to head, 639
  peripheral nerve, 649–650
  tracheobronchial, 650–651
Traumatic amputation, 102
Travatan. *See* Travoprost
Travoprost (Travatan), 336
Trazodone (Desyrel), 52
  for fibromyalgia syndrome, 306
Trelstar. *See* Triptorelin
Treponema palladium, 628
Treprostinil (Remodulin), 559
Triamterene (Dyrenium), 431
Trichomonas vaginalis, 667
Tricyclic antidepressants, 52
  for AD, 266
  for DM, 282
  for IBS, 450
  for migraine headache, 350
  SIADH and, 627
  for UI, 445, 447
Trigeminy, 290
Trimethoprim (Proloprim, Trimpex), 259
Trimethoprim/sulfamethoxazole (Bactrim, Septra)
  for diverticular disease, 287
  for gastroenteritis, 332
  for HIV, 387
  for PKD, 451
Trimox. *See* Amoxicillin
Trimpex. *See* Trimethoprim
Triptans
  for cluster headache, 349
  for migraine headache, 351
Triptorelin (Trelstar), 198
Trivalent botulism antitoxin (ABE), 311
Trousseau's sign, 411
Truphylline. *See* Aminophylline
TRUS. *See* Transrectal ultrasound
Trusopt. *See* Dorzolamide
Truss, 375

T_S cells, 44
TSH. *See* Thyroid stimulating hormone
TSIs. *See* Thyroid-stimulating immunoglobulins
TSS. *See* Toxic shock syndrome
Tubal abscess
  PID and, 536
Tuberculosis (TB), 651–654
  anal fistula and, 307
  respiratory acidosis from, 93
  SIADH and, 627
  uveitis from, 671
TULIP. *See* Transurethral ultrasound-guided laser incision of the prostate
Tumor lysis syndrome (TLS), 18, 21
Tumor ploidy, 3
Tumors. *See also Specific sites and types*
  ARDS from, 95–96
  chromosomes and, 3
  grading of, 3
TUMT. *See* Transurethral microwave therapy
TUNA. *See* Transurethral needle ablation
TURBT. *See* Transurethral resection of the bladder tumor
Turner's sign, 528, 635–636
TURP. *See* Transurethral resection of the prostate
Tylenol. *See* Acetaminophen
Tympanoplasty reconstruction, 354
Type 1 diabetes, 272
Type 1 multiple endocrine neoplasia (MEN1), 411
Type 2 diabetes, 272
  age and, 274
  insulin for, 275–277
  obesity and, 274
Tysabri. *See* Natalizumab
TZDs. *See* Thiazolidinediones

U

UAP. *See* Unlicensed assistive personnel
UE. *See* Upper extremity
UFE. *See* Uterine fibroid embolization
UI. *See* Urinary incontinence
Ulcerative colitis, 232–237.
  See also Crohn's disease
  pain with, 235–236